Neonatal Care

A Compendium of AAP Clinical Practice Guidelines and Policies

American Academy of Pediatrics
DEDICATED TO THE HEALTH OF ALL CHILDREN®

AMERICAN ACADEMY OF PEDIATRICS
PUBLISHING STAFF

Mary Lou White
Chief Product and Services Officer/SVP, Membership, Marketing, and Publishing

Mark Grimes
Vice President, Publishing

Jennifer McDonald
Senior Editor, Digital Publishing

Sean Rogers
Digital Content Specialist

Leesa Levin-Doroba
Production Manager, Practice Management

Linda Smessaert, MSIMC
Senior Marketing Manager, Professional Resources

Mary Louise Carr
Marketing Manager, Clinical Publications

Published by the American Academy of Pediatrics
345 Park Blvd
Itasca, IL 60143
Telephone: 630/626-6000
Facsimile: 847/434-8000
www.aap.org

The American Academy of Pediatrics is an organization of 67,000 primary care pediatricians, pediatric medical subspecialists, and pediatric surgical specialists dedicated to the health, safety, and well-being of infants, children, adolescents, and young adults.

The recommendations in this publication do not indicate an exclusive course of treatment or serve as a standard of medical care. Variations, taking into account individual circumstances, may be appropriate.

Products are mentioned for informational purposes only. Inclusion in this publication does not imply endorsement by the American Academy of Pediatrics.

Every effort has been made to ensure that the drug selection and dosage set forth in this publication are in accordance with the current recommendations and practice at the time of publication. It is the responsibility of the health care professional to check the package insert of each drug for any change in indications and dosage and for added warnings and precautions.

This publication has been developed by the American Academy of Pediatrics. The authors, editors, and contributors are expert authorities in the field of pediatrics. No commercial involvement of any kind has been solicited or accepted in the development of the content of this publication.

Special discounts are available for bulk purchases of this publication. E-mail Special Sales at aapsales@aap.org for more information.

Printed in the United States of America
9-423/REPO222   3 4 5 6 7 8 9 10
MA0913

ISBN: 978-1-61002-303-0
eBook ISBN: 978-1-61002-304-7
Library of Congress Control Number: 2018907928

INTRODUCTION

Clinical practice guidelines have long provided physicians with evidence-based decision-making tools for managing common pediatric conditions. Policy statements issued by the American Academy of Pediatrics (AAP) are developed to provide physicians with a quick reference guide to the AAP position on child health care issues. We have combined these 2 authoritative resources into 1 comprehensive manual to provide easy access to important clinical and policy information.

This manual contains an AAP clinical practice guideline, as well as AAP policy statements, clinical reports, and technical reports related to neonatal care.

Additional information about AAP policy can be found in a variety of professional publications such as *Guidelines for Perinatal Care,* 8th Edition; *Red Book®*, 31st Edition; and *Red Book® Online* (http://redbook.solutions.aap.org).

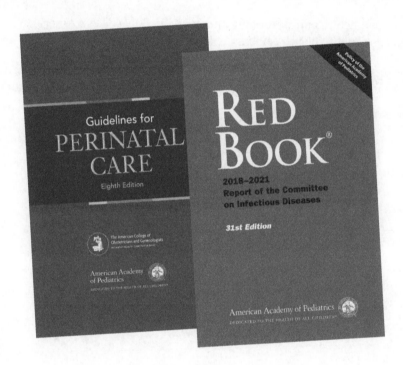

AMERICAN ACADEMY OF PEDIATRICS

The American Academy of Pediatrics (AAP) and its member pediatricians dedicate their efforts and resources to the health, safety, and well-being of infants, children, adolescents, and young adults. The AAP has approximately 67,000 members in the United States, Canada, and Latin America. Members include pediatricians, pediatric medical subspecialists, and pediatric surgical specialists.

Core Values. *We believe*
- In the inherent worth of all children; they are our most enduring and vulnerable legacy.
- Children deserve optimal health and the highest quality health care.
- Pediatricians, pediatric medical subspecialists, and pediatric surgical specialists are the best qualified to provide child health care.
- Multidisciplinary teams, including patients and families, are integral to delivering the highest quality health care.
- The AAP is the organization to advance child health and well-being and the profession of pediatrics.

Vision. Children have optimal health and well-being and are valued by society. American Academy of Pediatrics members practice the highest quality health care and experience professional satisfaction and personal well-being.

Mission. The mission of the AAP is to attain optimal, physical, mental, and social health and well-being for all infants, children, adolescents, and young adults. To accomplish this mission, the AAP shall support the professional needs of its members.

TABLE OF CONTENTS

SECTION 9
OTHER RELATED POLICIES

FOREWORD

The core mission of the American Academy of Pediatrics (AAP) is "to attain optimal physical, mental, and social health and well-being for all infants, children, adolescents, and young adults." In order to reach these goals, the AAP advocates for the needs of children and supports the professional needs of its members who provide care to those children. With a commitment to evidence-based medicine, the AAP has established leadership entities—committee, councils, and sections—that are charged with providing policy, educational programming, and resources for AAP members.

The AAP Committee on Fetus and Newborn (COFN) is one of 26 AAP committees. Its members include academic newborn specialists from throughout the United States, as well as liaisons from the AAP Section on Neonatal-Perinatal Medicine, Centers for Disease Control and Prevention, National Association of Neonatal Nurses, Eunice Kennedy Shriver National Institutes of Child Health and Development, AAP Neonatal Resuscitation Program, Canadian Paediatric Society Fetus and Newborn Committee, and AAP Section on Surgery. COFN also works closely with the American College of Obstetricians and Gynecologists (ACOG) and includes a representative from the ACOG Committee on Obstetric Practice. Most recently, COFN has added a representative from the Neonatal-Perinatal Medicine Section Training and Early Career Neonatologists Council, as an educational and training opportunity for early career academic neonatologists. COFN is supported by AAP staff, including the Director of Hospital and Surgical Services and staff from the AAP Advocacy and External Affairs office.

The primary charge to COFN is the creation and revision of AAP policy statements, clinical reports, and technical reports. In many instances, this is done in collaboration with other AAP committees, councils, sections, or task forces. Oftentimes, COFN will reach out to external consultants for their expertise and review. Although COFN statements differ in content and purpose, they must all be evidence-based and formally developed. These statements and reports are intended to serve as clinical practice guidelines, to provide the pediatric provider with an organized, analytic framework for evaluating and treating common neonatal conditions. As noted in each COFN statement and report, they are not intended as an exclusive course of action or a standard of care. Rather, they represent expert review of all available data, evidence-based recommendations, and consensus where data may be lacking. AAP policy statements, clinical reports, and technical reports provide guidance, while allowing for flexibility in individual situations and encouraging sound clinical judgment.

Within this compendium, you will find the collected results of COFN efforts for the past several years, in addition to select policies from other AAP groups. A wide range of perinatal topics, from antenatal counseling for periviable gestations, to hospital discharge of the high-risk infant, to post-discharge follow-up of infants with congenital diaphragmatic hernia, is captured in these pages. More than 40 different topics, organized into 9 sections for easy reference, are included. Each statement or report contains an abstract overview, a concise presentation and critique of the available data, and a summary of the findings and/or recommendations, along with a current and comprehensive bibliography. It is important to note that COFN is continually working on new statements and reports, and each published statement or report is revised as new information becomes available.

As chairperson of COFN, I can attest to the hard work, dedication, and meticulous preparation that goes into each of the statements and reports presented in this compendium. As a practicing neonatologist, I guarantee that you will find this resource indispensable.

James J. Cummings, MD, MS, FAAP
Chairperson, AAP Committee on Fetus and Newborn

SECTION 1

Delivery/ Discharge

American Academy
of Pediatrics

DEDICATED TO THE HEALTH OF ALL CHILDREN™

POLICY STATEMENT

Hospital Discharge of the High-Risk Neonate

Organizational Principles to Guide and
Define the Child Health Care System and/or
Improve the Health of All Children

Committee on Fetus and Newborn

ABSTRACT

This policy statement updates the guidelines on discharge of the high-risk neonate first published by the American Academy of Pediatrics in 1998. As with the earlier document, this statement is based, insofar as possible, on published, scientifically derived information. This updated statement incorporates new knowledge about risks and medical care of the high-risk neonate, the timing of discharge, and planning for care after discharge. It also refers to other American Academy of Pediatrics publications that are relevant to these issues. This statement draws on the previous classification of high-risk infants into 4 categories: (1) the preterm infant; (2) the infant with special health care needs or dependence on technology; (3) the infant at risk because of family issues; and (4) the infant with anticipated early death. The issues of deciding when discharge is appropriate, defining the specific needs for follow-up care, and the process of detailed discharge planning are addressed as they apply in general to all 4 categories; in addition, special attention is directed to the particular issues presented by the 4 individual categories. Recommendations are given to aid in deciding when discharge is appropriate and to ensure that all necessary care will be available and well coordinated after discharge. The need for individualized planning and physician judgment is emphasized. *Pediatrics* 2008;122:1119–1126

INTRODUCTION

The decision of when to discharge an infant from the hospital after a stay in the NICU is complex.[1] This decision is made primarily on the basis of the infant's medical status but is complicated by several factors. These factors include the readiness of families for discharge, differing opinions about what forms of care can be provided at home, and pressures to contain hospital costs by shortening the length of stay. Insofar as possible, determination of the readiness for discharge should be based on peer-reviewed scientific evidence. Shortening the length of a hospital stay may benefit the infant and family by decreasing the period of separation of infant and parents; moreover, the infant may benefit from shortening its exposure to the risks of hospital-acquired morbidity. However, the overriding concern is that infants may be placed at risk of increased mortality and morbidity by discharge before physiologic stability is established. Infants born preterm with low birth weight who require neonatal intensive care experience a much higher rate of hospital readmission and death during the first year after birth compared with healthy term infants.[2–5] Careful preparation for discharge and good follow-up after discharge may reduce these risks. It takes time for the family of a high-risk infant to prepare to care for their infant in a home setting and to obtain the necessary support services and mobilize community resources. With increased survival of very preterm and very ill infants, many infants are discharged with unresolved medical issues that complicate their subsequent care. Infants are often discharged requiring more care and closer follow-up than was typical in the past. In addition, societal and economic forces have come to bear on the timing and process of discharge and follow-up care. As a result, health care professionals need guidance in assessing readiness for discharge and planning for subsequent care. This policy statement, therefore, addresses 4 broad categories of high-risk infants: (1) the preterm infant; (2) the infant with special health care needs or dependence on technology; (3) the infant at risk because of family issues; and (4) the infant with anticipated early death. This policy statement updates a previous guideline published by the American Academy of Pediatrics in 1998.[1]

CATEGORIES OF HIGH-RISK INFANTS

The Preterm Infant

Historically, preterm infants were discharged only when they achieved a certain weight, typically 2000 g (5 lb). However, randomized clinical trials[6–8] have shown that earlier discharge is possible without adverse health effects

www.pediatrics.org/cgi/doi/10.1542/
peds.2008-2174

doi:10.1542/peds.2008-2174

All policy statements from the American
Academy of Pediatrics automatically expire
5 years after publication unless reaffirmed,
revised, or retired at or before that time.

Key Words
discharge, high risk, premature, neonate,
infant

Abbreviation
SIDS—sudden infant death syndrome

PEDIATRICS (ISSN Numbers: Print, 0031-4005;
Online, 1098-4275). Copyright © 2008 by the
American Academy of Pediatrics

when preterm infants are discharged on the basis of physiologic criteria rather than body weight. Although the population characteristics, the nature and results of the outcome measures, and the content of the early discharge programs in these studies varied, the common elements included:

- physiologic stability;
- an active program of parental involvement and preparation for care of the infant at home;
- arrangements for health care after discharge by a physician or other health care professional who is experienced in the care of high-risk infants; and
- an organized program of tracking and surveillance to monitor growth and development.

The 3 physiologic competencies that are generally recognized as essential before hospital discharge of the preterm infant are oral feeding sufficient to support appropriate growth, the ability to maintain normal body temperature in a home environment, and sufficiently mature respiratory control. These competencies are achieved by most preterm infants between 36 and 37 weeks' postmenstrual age,[7,9] but maturation of respiratory control to a point that allows safe discharge may take longer, occasionally up to 44 weeks' postmenstrual age.[10,11] Although interrelated, not all competencies are achieved by the same postnatal age in a given infant. The pace of maturation is influenced by the birth weight, the gestational age at birth, and the degree and chronicity of neonatal illnesses. Infants born earlier in gestation and with more complicated medical courses tend to take longer to achieve these physiologic competencies.

Home monitors are rarely indicated for detection of apnea solely because of immature respiratory control, in part because infants with immature respiratory control, in general, are still hospitalized until they are no longer at risk of apnea of prematurity. Use of a home monitor does not preclude the need for demonstrated maturity of respiratory control before discharge and should not be used to justify discharge of infants who are still at risk of apnea. Home monitors are not indicated for prevention of sudden infant death syndrome (SIDS) in preterm infants,[12] although preterm infants are at increased risk of SIDS.[13] Formal laboratory analyses of breathing patterns (ie, "pneumograms") are of no value in predicting SIDS[12] and are not helpful in identifying patients who should be discharged with home monitors.

Preterm infants should be placed supine for sleeping,[14–17] just as term infants should, and the parents of preterm infants should be counseled about the importance of supine sleeping in preventing SIDS. Hospitalized preterm infants should be kept predominantly in the supine position, at least from the postmenstrual age of 32 weeks onward, so that they become acclimated to supine sleeping before discharge. Supine positioning for sleep has led to an increase in positional skull deformity, especially in preterm infants but also in term infants[16,18,19]; although only cosmetic, these deformities can be quite disturbing to parents. Ways of safely preventing and treating deformation of the skull have been identified and are the subject of further investigation.[15,18,20]

Late-preterm infants, those born between 34 and 37 weeks' gestation, are at increased risk of having feeding problems and hyperbilirubinemia after discharge. These problems can be minimized but not wholly prevented by careful discharge planning and close follow-up after discharge.[21]

The Infant With Special Health Care Needs or Dependence on Technology

In recent years, increasing numbers of children with unresolved medical problems or special health care needs have been discharged requiring some form of supportive technology.[22] For newborn infants, the main types of technological support needed are nutritional support and respiratory support, including supplemental oxygen. This discussion will focus on nutritional and respiratory support, although other forms of home technological support are sometimes needed, including intravenous medications, bladder catheterization, and renal replacement therapy.

For most preterm infants and those with complex medical problems, oral feeding is best learned in the hospital under the care of expert physicians, nurses, and feeding therapists. Gavage feeding has been used safely in the home setting for infants who are not able to feed well enough by breast or bottle.[23–25] This practice has a limited role and should be considered only when feeding is the last issue requiring continued hospitalization. Not all parents are capable of safely managing home gavage feedings. When little or no progress is being made with oral feeding skills and long-term tube feeding seems inevitable, placement of a feeding gastrostomy tube provides another alternative method of feeding.[26] Unless precluded by neurologic deficits that threaten airway defense, oral feeding should be continued along with tube feeding so that oral feeding skills can continue to develop. Ordinarily, gavage or gastrostomy tube feedings are used to complement what is eaten orally to ensure adequate total intake. Home intravenous nutritional support is sometimes needed when enteral feeding is not possible or is limited by short-bowel syndrome or poor gastrointestinal function. Parenteral nutrition in the home requires careful assessment of the caregivers and home environment, thorough education of caregivers, and the support of a well-qualified home-care company.[27]

Home oxygen therapy for infants with bronchopulmonary dysplasia has been used as a means of achieving earlier hospital discharge while avoiding the risks of growth failure and cor pulmonale resulting from marginal oxygenation.[28–33] Sufficient oxygen should be delivered to maintain oxygen saturation at an acceptable level during a range of activities.[34–36] Infants who are discharged on supplemental oxygen are often also discharged on a cardiorespiratory monitor or pulse oximeter in case the oxygen should become dislodged or the supply depleted. Reducing or stopping supplemental oxygen should be supervised by the physician or other health care professional and attempted only when the infant demonstrates normal oxygen saturation, good growth velocity, and sufficient stamina for a full range of activity.[36] Tracheostomy is sometimes required for neonates with upper airway abnormalities or occasionally for infants who cannot be weaned from assisted ventilation.[37–40] Good parental teaching and coordinated multidisciplinary follow-up care are essential for these infants. Infants who require home ventilation should also be on a cardiorespiratory monitor in case the airway should become obstructed, but the home ventilator should also have a disconnect alarm to alert caregivers to ventilator disconnection. Home ventilation requires qualified personnel to provide bedside care; in most cases, home-nursing support will be needed for at least part of the day.

The Infant at Risk Because of Family Issues

Preterm birth and prolonged hospitalization are known family stressors and risk factors for subsequent family dysfunction and child abuse.[41–43] In addition to preterm birth and prolonged hospital stay, birth defects and disabling conditions are also risk factors.[44] Maternal factors include lower educational level, lack of social support, marital instability, and fewer prenatal care visits.[41,42] In 1 study, significantly fewer family visits during the stay in the NICU had occurred for infants in whom subsequent maltreatment was documented.[41] Parental substance abuse is another factor that places the infant at risk, both because of adverse effects on the developing fetus in utero and because of possible postnatal exposure to drugs through breastfeeding or by inhalation. Moreover, the drug-seeking behaviors of parents may compromise the safety of the child's environment. Sequelae such as attachment disturbances, behavioral and developmental disorders, and child maltreatment have been observed frequently among children born to substance abusers.

Identifying effective strategies to help protect the infant who is at increased risk because of family reasons has been elusive. Most interventions have focused on multidisciplinary teams that provide follow-up monitoring, including home visits.[45] However, the efficacy of these interventions has been difficult to demonstrate. At the very least, it is hoped that an organized approach to planning for discharge can identify infants who require extra support or whose home environments present unacceptable risks.

The Infant With Anticipated Early Death

For many infants with incurable, terminal disorders, the best place to spend the last days or weeks of life is at home.[46] In these situations, the family provides most of the care, often with support by staff from a community hospice organization. In rare instances, withdrawal of assisted ventilation can occur in the home.[47] In preparing to discharge an infant for home hospice care, several aspects must be considered in addition to the usual factors.[48] These preparations include arrangements for medical follow-up and home-nursing visits; management of pain and other distressing symptoms; arrange-

ments for home oxygen or other equipment and supplies; providing the family with information on bereavement support for the parents, siblings, and others; discussion of possible resources for respite of caregivers; and assistance in addressing financial issues. If appropriate, a letter should be provided for the family to show to other caregivers or emergency medical workers indicating that the child should not be resuscitated. The focus of planning efforts should be to enhance the quality of the infant's remaining life for the benefit of both the infant and his or her family.

TIMING OF DISCHARGE

The appropriate time for discharge is when the infant demonstrates the necessary physiologic maturity (in the case of the preterm infant), discharge planning and arrangements for follow-up and any home care have been completed, and the parents have received the necessary teaching and have demonstrated their mastery of the essential knowledge and skills. In selected cases, an infant may be discharged before one of the infant's physiologic competencies has been met, provided the health care team and the parents agree that this is appropriate and suitable plans have been made to provide additional support needed to ensure safe care at home, such as tube feeding, cardiorespiratory monitoring, or home oxygen. The standard, default criterion remains that the infant should be sufficiently mature to need no such assistance at home. The decision to facilitate earlier discharge by providing such additional support should be made only as a mutual decision by the health care team and the parents.

Before discharge, the eyes of qualifying infants should be examined at specified times by an ophthalmologist with expertise in the diagnosis of retinopathy of prematurity.[49] The infant's hearing should be evaluated[50,51]; the results of the newborn metabolic screen should be reviewed[52]; appropriate immunizations should be given, if not given previously; and palivizumab should be given to qualifying infants during respiratory syncytial virus season.[53,54]

Sometimes infants are transferred to a hospital closer to home so that the family may visit more easily. This is appropriate provided appropriate medical care is available in the receiving hospital, including capabilities for ophthalmologic examinations to screen for retinopathy of prematurity and the experience and resources for planning discharge and follow-up care.

DISCHARGE PLANNING

High-risk infants should receive primary medical care from a physician with expertise in the care of patients who have spent time in the NICU, often in partnership with 1 or more specialized clinics in the discharging medical center. To ensure continuity of care after discharge, infants with unresolved medical issues that persist after their hospital stay, such as bronchopulmonary dysplasia or feeding dysfunction, should be comanaged by a neonatologist or other medical subspecialist from the hospital at which most of the care was provided. The subspecialist provides consultation to the primary physician about issues such as the weaning and discontinuation of supplemental oxygen. Most high-risk infants should also be enrolled in a follow-up clinic that specializes in the neurodevelopmental assessment of high-risk infants. This neurodevelopmental follow-up is sometimes integrated with the child's visits to the neonatologist. Standardized assessments should be performed in the follow-up clinic at specific ages through early childhood.[55-57]

The care of each high-risk neonate after discharge must be coordinated carefully to provide ongoing multidisciplinary support of the family. The discharge-planning team should include parents, the neonatologist, neonatal nurses and nurse practitioners, and the social worker. Other professionals, such as surgical specialists and pediatric medical subspecialists, respiratory, physical, occupational, and speech therapists, infant educators, nutritionists, home-health care company staff, and others may be included as needed.

Discharge planning should begin early in the hospital course. The goal of the discharge plan is to ensure successful transition to home care. Essential discharge criteria are a physiologically stable infant, a family who can provide the necessary care with appropriate support services in the community, and a primary care physician who is prepared to assume the responsibility with appropriate backup from specialist physicians and other professionals as needed.[55,56] Six critical components must be included in discharge planning.

1. Parental Education

Parental contact and involvement in the care of the infant should be encouraged from the time of admission. The participation of the parents in whatever way possible from the beginning has a positive effect on their confidence in handling the infant and readiness to assume full responsibility for the infant's care at home.

The development of an individualized teaching plan helps parents to acquire the skills and judgment needed to care for their infant. A written checklist or outline of the specific areas and tasks to be mastered increases the likelihood that parents and other caregivers will receive complete instructions and experience. Caregivers and parents must understand that the infant's immaturity and medical status will require increased care and vigilance at home beyond that of the usual parental role. Thus, ample time for teaching the parents and caregivers the techniques and the rationale for each item in the care plan is essential. Requesting return demonstrations by the parents of their new knowledge, parent rooming-in, and telephone follow-up by hospital staff all facilitate parental education and adaptation to their infant's care. Although it is important for the parents to understand that their child may need extra care and surveillance, the infant's fragility should not be overstated. If this occurs, the parents may become excessively protective, which can restrict the child's social development and lead to behavior problems.[58] Parents should be coached in communicating about the infant with any older siblings, who may not fully understand the infant's condition and may

even imagine themselves to be responsible for the vulnerable state of their younger brother or sister.

Insofar as possible, at least 2 responsible caregivers should be identified and learn the necessary care for each infant. The demands of home care can be physically and emotionally draining, especially at first, for infants who require frequent feeding. Young mothers who do not live with a parent or the father of the infant have been shown to be especially vulnerable to the strains of home care. Even in a 2-parent family, the primary caregiver may become ill and need relief.

2. Completion of Appropriate Elements of Primary Care in the Hospital

Preparing the infant for transition to primary care begins early in the hospitalization with administration of immunizations at the recommended postnatal ages, regardless of prematurity or medical condition,[59] completion of metabolic screening,[52] assessment of hearing by an acceptable electronic measurement,[50,51] and baseline neurodevelopmental and neurobehavioral assessment. For infants at risk, appropriate funduscopic examination for retinopathy of prematurity should be performed by an ophthalmologist who is skilled in the evaluation of the retina of the preterm infant.[49] Assessment of hematologic status is recommended for all infants because of the high prevalence of anemia after neonatal intensive care. Very preterm infants and those who have received parenteral nutrition for prolonged periods may be at risk of hypoproteinemia, vitamin deficiencies, and bone mineralization abnormalities; therefore, evaluation for nutritional or metabolic deficiencies may be indicated. When discharge is near, the high-risk infant should be evaluated to ensure physiologic stability in an appropriate car seat or car bed.[60-62]

3. Development of Management Plan for Unresolved Medical Problems

Review of the hospital course and the active problem list of each infant and careful physical assessment will reveal any unresolved medical issues and areas of physiologic function that have not reached full maturation. From such a review, the diagnostic studies required to document the current clinical status of the infant can be identified and management can be continued or adjusted as appropriate. The intent should be to ensure implementation of appropriate home-care and follow-up plans.

4. Development of the Comprehensive Home-Care Plan

Although the content of the home-care plan may vary with the infant's diagnoses and medical status, the common elements include (1) identification and preparation of the in-home caregivers, (2) formulation of a plan for nutritional care and administration of any required medications, (3) development of a list of required equipment and supplies and accessible sources, (4) identification and mobilization of the primary care physician, the necessary and qualified home-care personnel and community support services, (5) assessment of the adequacy of the physical facilities within the home, (6) development of an emergency care and transport plan, and (7) assessment of available financial resources to ensure the capability to finance home-care costs. The input of the primary care physician in formulating the home-care plan of the technology-dependent infant is essential. Many infants, particularly extremely preterm and technology-dependent infants, require continued care by multiple specialists and subspecialists, who should be included in the predischarge assessment and discharge planning.

5. Identification and Involvement of Support Services

The infant's optimal outcome ultimately depends on the capacity and effort of the family. The psychological, social, economic, and educational condition and needs of the family should be addressed from the beginning of the infant's hospitalization, noting strengths that can support the infant's continued adaptation, growth, and development and any risk factors that may contribute to an adverse infant outcome. The availability of social support is essential for the success of every parent's adaptation to the home care of a high-risk infant. Before discharge and periodically thereafter, a review of the family's needs, coping skills, use of available resources, financial problems, and progress toward goals in the home care of their infant should be evaluated. After the social support needs of the family have been identified, an appropriate, individualized intervention plan using available community programs, surveillance, or alternative care placement of the child may be implemented.

6. Determination and Designation of Follow-Up Care

In general, the attending neonatologist or other discharging physician has the responsibility for coordination of follow-up care, although in some institutions this responsibility may be delegated to another professional. A primary care physician (or "medical home") should be identified well before discharge to facilitate the coordination of follow-up care planning between the staff responsible for planning the discharge and the primary health care professionals. Pertinent information about the nursery course, including a discharge summary, and the home-care plan should be given to the primary care physician before the infant's discharge. In specialty center units, the primary care attending physician should work with the neonatologist in coordinating the discharge planning.

Arrangements for an initial appointment with the primary care physician should be made before discharge. Specific follow-up appointments with each involved surgical specialist and pediatric medical subspecialist should be made, giving attention to grouping the appointments as much as possible for the convenience of the family. A plan should be developed and discussed for emergency care and transportation to a hospital, should it be necessary.

Periodic evaluation of the developmental progress of every infant is essential for identifying deviations in neurodevelopmental progress at the earliest possible point, thereby facilitating entry into early intervention programs. The primary care physician with appropriate skills, the pediatric medical subspecialist, or clinic personnel may provide longitudinal developmental follow-up. When need for input from multiple disciplines is identified before discharge, a clinic that provides multidisciplinary care, usually in an academic or tertiary center, may be the least cumbersome option for the family.

SPECIAL CONSIDERATIONS

Many infants are transported to hospitals nearer to their family homes for convalescent care. In these hospitals, the discharge-planning process should follow the same principles as those outlined previously in this statement for an infant being discharged from a subspecialty center. It is especially important that periodic examination by a qualified ophthalmologist be available for infants who still require evaluation for retinopathy of prematurity.

In caring for the discharged high-risk infant, use of community resources, both public and private, should be encouraged. The goal should be to provide coordinated care and family support. Efficient teamwork by health care professionals is imperative. Home-nursing visits are often indicated. When this is so, it is important to use experienced nurses who are qualified to perform the required assessments. When choosing a home-care company or agency for technology-dependent infants, it is essential that previous performance and existing quality-control programs be considered.

RECOMMENDATIONS

The following recommendations are offered as a framework for guiding decisions about the timing of discharge. It is prudent for each institution to establish guidelines that ensure a consistent approach yet allow some flexibility on the basis of physician and family judgment. It is of foremost importance that the infant, family, and community be prepared for the infant to be safely cared for outside the hospital.

Infant Readiness for Hospital Discharge

The infant is considered ready for discharge if, in the judgment of the responsible physician, the following have been accomplished:

- A sustained pattern of weight gain of sufficient duration has been demonstrated.
- The infant has demonstrated adequate maintenance of normal body temperature fully clothed in an open bed with normal ambient temperature (20–25°C).
- The infant has established competent feeding by breast or bottle without cardiorespiratory compromise.
- Physiologically mature and stable cardiorespiratory function has been documented for a sufficient duration.
- Appropriate immunizations have been administered.
- Appropriate metabolic screening has been performed.

- Hematologic status has been assessed and appropriate therapy has been instituted, if indicated.

- Nutritional risks have been assessed and therapy and dietary modification has been instituted, if indicated.

- Hearing evaluation has been completed.

- Funduscopic examinations have been completed, as indicated.

- Neurodevelopmental and neurobehavioral status has been assessed and demonstrated to the parents.

- Car seat evaluation has been completed.

- Review of the hospital course has been completed, unresolved medical problems have been identified, and plans for follow-up monitoring and treatment have been instituted.

- An individualized home-care plan has been developed with input from all appropriate disciplines.

Family and Home Environmental Readiness

Assessment of the family's caregiving capabilities, resource availability, and home physical facilities has been completed as follows:

- identification of at least 2 family caregivers and assessment of their ability, availability, and commitment;

- psychosocial assessment for parenting strengths and risks;

- a home environmental assessment that may include on-site evaluation; and

- review of available financial resources and identification of adequate financial support.

In preparation for home care of the technology-dependent infant, it is essential to complete an assessment documenting availability of 24-hour telephone access, electricity, safe in-house water supply, and adequate heating. Detailed financial assessment and planning are also essential. Parents and caregivers should have demonstrated the necessary capabilities to provide all components of care, including:

- feeding, whether by breast, bottle, or an alternative technique, including formula preparation, if required;

- basic infant care, including bathing; skin, cord, and genital care; temperature measurement; dressing; and comforting;

- infant cardiopulmonary resuscitation and emergency intervention;

- assessment of clinical status, including understanding and detection of the general early signs and symptoms of illness as well as the signs and symptoms specific to the infant's condition;

- infant safety precautions, including proper infant positioning during sleep and proper use of car seats or car bed;

- specific safety precautions for the artificial airway, if any; feeding tube; intestinal stoma; infusion pump;

and other mechanical and prosthetic devices, as indicated;

- administration of medications, specifically proper storage, dosage, timing, and administration and recognition of potential signs of toxicity;

- equipment operation, maintenance, and problem solving for each mechanical support device required; and

- the appropriate technique for each special care procedure required, including special dressings for infusion entry site, intestinal stoma, or healing wounds; maintenance of an artificial airway; oropharyngeal and tracheal suctioning; and physical therapy, as indicated.

Specific modification of home facilities must have been completed if needed to accommodate home-care systems. Plans must be in place for responding to loss of electrical power, heat, or water and for emergency relocation mandated by natural disaster.

Community and Health Care System Readiness

An emergency intervention and transportation plan have been developed and emergency medical services providers have been identified and notified, if indicated.

Follow-up care needs have been determined, appropriate providers have been identified, and appropriate information has been exchanged, including the following:

- A primary care physician has been identified and has accepted responsibility for care of the infant.

- Surgical specialty and pediatric medical subspecialty follow-up care requirements have been identified and appropriate arrangements have been made.

- Neurodevelopmental follow-up requirements have been identified and appropriate referrals have been made.

- Home-nursing visits for assessment and parent support have been arranged, as indicated by the complexity of the infant's clinical status and family capability, and the home-care plan has been transmitted to the home health agency.

- For breastfeeding mothers, information on breastfeeding support and availability of lactation counselors has been provided.

The determination of readiness for care at home of an infant after neonatal intensive care is complex. Careful balancing of infant safety and well-being with family needs and capabilities is required while giving consideration to the availability and adequacy of community resources and support services. The final decision for discharge, which is the responsibility of the attending physician, must be tailored to the unique constellation of issues posed by each infant's situation.

REFERENCES

1. American Academy of Pediatrics, Committee on Fetus and Newborn. Hospital discharge of the high-risk neonate: proposed guidelines. *Pediatrics.* 1998;102(2 pt 1):411–417
2. Hulsey TC, Hudson MB, Pittard WB III. Predictors of hospital postdischarge infant mortality: implications for high-risk infant follow-up efforts. *J Perinatol.* 1994;14(3):219–225
3. Lamarche-Vadel A, Blondel B, Truffert P, et al. Re-hospitalization in infants younger than 29 weeks' gestation in the EPIPAGE study. *Acta Paediatr.* 2004;93(10):1340–1345
4. Smith VC, Zupanic JA, McCormick MC, et al. Rehospitalization in the first year of life among infants with bronchopulmonary dysplasia. *J Pediatr.* 2004;144(6):799–803
5. Resch B, Pasnocht A, Gusenleitner W, Muller W. Rehospitalisations for respiratory disease and respiratory syncytial virus infection in preterm infants of 29–36 weeks gestational age. *J Infect.* 2005;50(5):397–403
6. Davies DP, Herbert S, Haxby V, McNeish AS. When should pre-term babies be sent home from neonatal units? *Lancet.* 1979;1(8122):914–915
7. Brooten D, Kumar S, Brown L, et al. A randomized clinical trial of early hospital discharge and home follow-up of very-low-birth-weight infants. *N Engl J Med.* 1986;315(15):934–939
8. Casiro OG, McKenzie ME, McFadyen L, et al. Earlier discharge with community-based intervention for low birth weight infants: a randomized trial. *Pediatrics.* 1993;92(1):128–134
9. Powell PJ, Powell CVE, Holli S, Robinson JM. When will my baby go home? *Arch Dis Child.* 1992;67(10 Spec No.):1214–1216
10. Eichenwald EC, Aina A, Stark AR. Apnea frequently persists beyond term gestation in infants delivered at 24 to 28 weeks. *Pediatrics.* 1997;100(3 pt 1):354–359
11. Darnall RA, Kattwinkel J, Nattie C, Robinson M. Margin of safety for discharge after apnea in preterm infants. *Pediatrics.* 1997;100(5):795–801

12. American Academy of Pediatrics, Committee on Fetus and Newborn. Apnea, sudden infant death syndrome, and home monitoring. *Pediatrics.* 2003;111(4 pt 1):914–917
13. Thompson JMD, Mitchell EA; New Zealand Cot Death Study Group. Are the risk factors for SIDS different for preterm and term infants? *Arch Dis Child.* 2006;91(2):107–111
14. Øyen N, Markestad T, Skjærven R, et al. Combined effects of sleeping position and prenatal risk factors in sudden infant death syndrome: the Nordic Epidemiological SIDS Study. *Pediatrics.* 1997;100(4):613–621
15. American Academy of Pediatrics, Task Force on Infant Sleep Position and Sudden Infant Death Syndrome. Changing concepts of sudden infant death syndrome: implications for infant sleeping environment and sleep position. *Pediatrics.* 2000;105(3 pt 1):650–656
16. American Academy of Pediatrics, Task Force on Sudden Infant Death Syndrome. The changing concept of sudden infant death syndrome: diagnostic coding shifts, controversies regarding the sleeping environment, and new variables to consider in reducing risk. *Pediatrics.* 2005;116(5):1245–1255
17. Blair PS, Platt MW, Smith IJ, Fleming PJ; CESDI SUDI Research Group. Sudden infant death syndrome and sleeping position in pre-term and low birth weight infants: an opportunity for targeted intervention. *Arch Dis Child.* 2006;91(2):101–106
18. Persing J; American Academy of Pediatrics, Committee on Practice and Ambulatory Medicine, Section on Plastic Surgery, and Section on Neurological Surgery. Prevention and management of positional skull deformities in infants. *Pediatrics.* 2003;112(1 pt 1):199–202
19. Graham JM Jr, Kreutzman J, Earl D, Halberg A, Samayoa C, Guo X. Deformational brachycephaly in supine-sleeping infants. *J Pediatr.* 2005;146(2):253–257
20. Graham JM Jr, Gomez M, Halberg A, et al. Management of deformational plagiocephaly: repositioning versus orthotic therapy. *J Pediatr.* 2005;146(2):258–262
21. Engle WA, Tomashek KM, Wallman C; American Academy of Pediatrics, Committee on Fetus and Newborn. "Late-preterm" infants: a population at risk. *Pediatrics.* 2007;120(6):1390–1401
22. American Academy of Pediatrics, Section on Home Health Care. *Guidelines for Pediatric Home Health Care.* McConnell MS, Imaizumi SO, eds. Elk Grove Village, IL: American Academy of Pediatrics; 2002
23. Collins CT, Makrides M, McPhee AJ. Early discharge with home support of gavage feeding for stable preterm infants who have not established full oral feeds. *Cochrane Database Syst Rev.* 2003;(4):CD003743
24. Örtenstrand A, Waldenström U, Winbladh B. Early discharge of preterm infants needing limited special care, followed by domiciliary nursing care. *Acta Paediatr.* 1999;88(9):1024–1030
25. Örtenstrand A, Winbladh B, Nordström G, Waldenström U. Early discharge of preterm infants followed by domiciliary nursing care: parents' anxiety, assessment of infant health and breastfeeding. *Acta Paediatr.* 2001;90(10):1190–1195
26. Åvitsland TL, Kristensen C, Emblem R, Veenstra M, Mala T, Bjørnland K. Percutaneous endoscopic gastrostomy in children: a safe technique with major symptom relief and high parental satisfaction. *J Pediatr Gastroenterol Nutr.* 2006;43(5):624–628
27. George DE; American Academy of Pediatrics, Section on Home Health Care. Home parenteral and enteral nutrition. In: McConnell MS, Imaizumi SO, eds. *Guidelines for Pediatric Home Health Care.* Elk Grove Village, IL: American Academy of Pediatrics; 2002:113–123
28. Pinney MA, Cotton EK. Home management of bronchopulmonary dysplasia. *Pediatrics.* 1976;58(6):856–859
29. Halliday HL, Dumpit FM, Brady JP. Effects of inspired oxygen

on echocardiographic assessment of pulmonary vascular resistance and myocardial contractility in bronchopulmonary dysplasia. *Pediatrics*. 1980;65(3):536–540

30. Groothuis JR, Rosenberg AA. Home oxygen promotes weight gain in infants with bronchopulmonary dysplasia. *Am J Dis Child*. 1987;141(9):992–995

31. Sekar KC, Duke JC. Sleep apnea and hypoxemia in recently weaned premature infants with and without bronchopulmonary dysplasia. *Pediatr Pulmonol*. 1991;10(2):112–116

32. Garg M, Kurzner SI, Bautista DB, Keens TG. Clinically unsuspected hypoxia during sleep and feeding in infants with bronchopulmonary dysplasia. *Pediatrics*. 1988;81(5):635–642

33. Moyer-Mileur LJ, Nielson DW, Pfeffer KD, Witte MK, Chapman DL. Eliminating sleep-associated hypoxemia improves growth in infants with bronchopulmonary dysplasia. *Pediatrics*. 1996;98(4 pt 1):779–783

34. Kotecha S, Allen J. Oxygen therapy for infants with chronic lung disease. *Arch Dis Child Fetal Neonatal Ed*. 2002;87(1): F11–F14

35. Allen J, Zwerdling R, Ehrenkranz R, et al. Statement on the care of the child with chronic lung disease of infancy and childhood. *Am J Respir Crit Care Med*. 2003;168(3):356–396

36. Pannitch H; American Academy of Pediatrics, Section on Home Health Care. Bronchopulmonary dysplasia. In: McConnell MS, Imaizumi SO, eds. *Guidelines for Pediatric Home Health Care*. Elk Grove Village, IL: American Academy of Pediatrics; 2002: 323–342

37. Quint RD, Chesterman E, Crain LS, Winkleby M, Boyce WT. Home care for ventilator-dependent children. *Am J Dis Child*. 1990;144(11):1238–1241

38. Storgion S; American Academy of Pediatrics, Section on Home Health Care. Care of children requiring home mechanical ventilation. In: McConnell MS, Imaizumi SO, eds. *Guidelines for Pediatric Home Health Care*. Elk Grove Village, IL: American Academy of Pediatrics; 2002:307–321

39. Edwards EA, O'Toole M, Wallis C. Sending children home on tracheostomy dependent ventilation: pitfalls and outcomes. *Arch Dis Child*. 2004;89(3):251–255

40. Edwards EA, Hsiao K, Nixon GM. Paediatric home ventilatory support: the Auckland experience. *J Paediatr Child Health*. 2005; 41(12):652–658

41. Hunter RS, Kilstrom N, Kraybill EN, Loda F. Antecedents of child abuse and neglect in premature infants: a prospective study in a newborn intensive care unit. *Pediatrics*. 1978;61(4): 629–635

42. Murphy JF, Jenkins J, Newcombe RG, Sibert JR. Objective birth data and the prediction of child abuse. *Arch Dis Child*. 1981;56(4):295–297

43. Spencer N, Wallace A, Sundrum R, Bacchus C, Logan S. Child abuse registration, fetal growth, and preterm birth: a population based study. *J Epidemiol Community Health*. 2006;60(4): 337–340

44. Spencer N, Devereux E, Wallace A, et al. Disabling conditions and registration for child abuse and neglect: a population-based study. *Pediatrics*. 2005;116(3):609–613

45. Rosen TS, Rosen J; American Academy of Pediatrics, Section on Home Health Care. Comprehensive home care program for the socially high-risk infant. In: McConnell MS, Imaizumi SO, eds. *Guidelines for Pediatric Home Health Care*. Elk Grove Village, IL: American Academy of Pediatrics; 2002:297–305

46. Leuthner SR, Boldt AM, Kirby RS. Where infants die: examination of place of death and hospice/home health care options in the state of Wisconsin. *J Palliat Med*. 2004;7(2):269–277

47. Zwerdling T, Hamann KC, Kon AA. Home pediatric compassionate extubation: bridging intensive and palliative care. *Am J Hosp Palliat Care*. 2006;23(3):224–228

48. Leuthner SR, Pierucci R. Experience with neonatal palliative care consultation at the Medical College of Wisconsin-Children's Hospital of Wisconsin. *J Palliat Med*. 2001;4(1): 39–47

49. American Academy of Pediatrics, Section on Ophthalmology; American Academy of Ophthalmology; American Association of Pediatric Ophthalmology and Strabismus. Screening examination of premature infants for retinopathy of prematurity [published correction appears in *Pediatrics*. 2006;118(3):1324]. *Pediatrics*. 2006;117(2):572–576

50. American Academy of Pediatrics, Task Force on Newborn and Infant Hearing Loss. Newborn and infant hearing loss: detection and intervention. *Pediatrics*. 1999;103(2):527–530

51. Joint Committee on Infant Hearing. Year 2000 position statement: principles and guidelines for early hearing detection and intervention programs. *Pediatrics*. 2000;106(4):798–817

52. Kaye CI; American Academy of Pediatrics, Committee on Genetics. Newborn screening facts sheet. *Pediatrics*. 2006;118(3): 934–963

53. American Academy of Pediatrics, Committee on Infectious Diseases and Committee on Fetus and Newborn. Policy statement: revised indications for the use of palivizumab and respiratory syncytial virus immune globulin intravenous for the prevention of respiratory syncytial virus infections. *Pediatrics*. 2003; 112(6 pt 1):1442–1446

54. Meissner HC, Long SS; American Academy of Pediatrics, Committee on Infectious Diseases and Committee on Fetus and Newborn. Technical report: revised indications for the use of palivizumab and respiratory syncytial virus immune globulin intravenous for the prevention of respiratory syncytial virus infections. *Pediatrics*. 2003;112(6 pt 1):1447–1452

55. Vohr BR, O'Shea M, Wright LL. Longitudinal multicenter follow-up of high-risk infants: why, who, when, and what to assess. *Semin Perinatol*. 2003;27(4):333–342

56. Vohr B, Wright LL, Hack M, Aylward G, Hirtz D. Follow-up care of high-risk infants. *Pediatrics*. 2004;114(5 suppl): 1377–1397

57. Hummel P, Cronin J. Home care of the high-risk infant. *Adv Neonatal Care*. 2004;4(6):354–364

58. Pearson SR, Boyce WT. The vulnerable child syndrome. *Pediatr Rev*. 2004;25(10):345–348

59. Saari TN; American Academy of Pediatrics, Committee on Infectious Diseases. Immunization of preterm and low birth weight infants. *Pediatrics*. 2003;112(1 pt 1):193–198

60. American Academy of Pediatrics, Committee on Injury and Poison Prevention and Committee on Fetus and Newborn. Safe transportation of premature and low birth weight infants. *Pediatrics*. 1996;97(5):758–760

61. American Academy of Pediatrics, Committee on Injury and Poison Prevention. Transporting children with special health care needs. *Pediatrics*. 1999;104(4 pt 1):988–992

62. Bull MJ, Sheese J. Update for the pediatrician on child passenger safety: five principles for safer travel. *Pediatrics*. 2000; 106(5):1113–1116

POLICY STATEMENT · Organizational Principles to Guide and Define the Child Health Care System and/or Improve the Health of all Children

American Academy
of Pediatrics

DEDICATED TO THE HEALTH OF ALL CHILDREN™

Hospital Stay for Healthy Term Newborn Infants

William E. Benitz, MD, FAAP, COMMITTEE ON FETUS AND NEWBORN

abstract

The hospital stay of the mother and her healthy term newborn infant should be long enough to allow identification of problems and to ensure that the mother is sufficiently recovered and prepared to care for herself and her newborn at home. The length of stay should be based on the unique characteristics of each mother-infant dyad, including the health of the mother, the health and stability of the newborn, the ability and confidence of the mother to care for herself and her newborn, the adequacy of support systems at home, and access to appropriate follow-up care in a medical home. Input from the mother and her obstetrical care provider should be considered before a decision to discharge a newborn is made, and all efforts should be made to keep a mother and her newborn together to ensure simultaneous discharge.

www.pediatrics.org/cgi/doi/10.1542/peds.2015-0699

DOI: 10.1542/peds.2015-0699

PEDIATRICS (ISSN Numbers: Print, 0031-4005; Online, 1098-4275).

PURPOSE

The purpose of this policy statement is to review issues related to length of stay and readmission of healthy term newborns and to identify specific criteria that should be met to ensure that discharge and subsequent follow-up are appropriate.

BACKGROUND

The hospital stay of the mother and her healthy term newborn infant (mother-infant dyad) should be long enough to allow identification of problems and to ensure that the mother is sufficiently recovered and prepared to care for herself and her newborn at home. Many neonatal cardiopulmonary problems related to the transition from the intrauterine to the extrauterine environment usually become apparent during the first 12 hours after birth.[1] Other neonatal problems, such as jaundice,[2,3] ductal-dependent cardiac lesions,[4,5] and gastrointestinal obstruction,[6] may require a longer period of observation by skilled health care professionals.[7] Likewise, significant maternal complications, such as endometritis, may not become apparent during the first day after delivery.

The average length of stay of the mother-infant dyad after delivery declined steadily from 1970 until the mid-1990s.[8] Early newborn discharge was implemented in the 1990s, but in response to the ensuing debate on the care and safety of mothers and their infants, most states and the US Congress enacted legislation that ensured hospital stay for up to 48 hours for a vaginal delivery and up to 96 hours after birth by cesarean delivery. Several subsequent studies have reported that the postpartum length-of-stay legislation has led to an increase in postpartum length of stay, but the impact of this increase in length of stay on the rate of neonatal readmissions has been inconsistent.[8–11]

Risk of Readmission

Criteria for newborn discharge include physiologic stability, family preparedness and competence to provide newborn care at home, availability of social support, and access to the health care system and resources. An inadequate assessment by health care providers in any of these areas before discharge can place an infant at risk and may result in readmission. In several large epidemiologic studies, readmission rates were used to assess the adequacy of the newborn hospital length of stay. In these reports, readmissions after an early discharge varied from no increase to a significant increase.[8,12–15] However, the differences in the definition of early discharge, postdischarge follow-up and support, and the timing of readmissions make it difficult to compare the results. In some of these studies, the risk factors for readmission to identify infants who may benefit from either a longer hospital stay or close postdischarge follow-up also were evaluated. These studies identified jaundice, dehydration, and feeding difficulties as the most common reasons for readmission.[16,17] Other frequently reported risk factors for readmission were Asian race, primiparity, associated maternal morbidities, shorter gestation or lower birth weight, instrumented vaginal

delivery, and small size for gestational age.[13,15–18] Close follow-up and better coordination of postdischarge care were important factors in decreasing the readmission rates.[13,17]

Readiness for Discharge

Readiness for discharge of a healthy term infant is traditionally determined by pediatric care providers after a review of the mother's and family members' ability to provide care to a newborn infant at home. However, perceptions about the degree of readiness at the time of discharge often differ among pediatric care providers, obstetrical care providers, and mothers.[18] Factors associated with perceived unreadiness for maternal or neonatal discharge, primarily as reported by mothers themselves, include first live birth, maternal history of chronic disease or illness after birth, in-hospital neonatal illness, intent to breastfeed, mothers with inadequate prenatal care and poor social support, and black non-Hispanic maternal race.[13,18] Although no specific clinical tool is currently available to evaluate mothers' or families' perception of readiness for discharge after delivery, the American Academy of Pediatrics Safe and Healthy Beginnings toolkit contains a discharge-readiness checklist that can aid clinicians with preparation of a newborn for discharge. This tool was tested by 22 clinical practice teams during the Safe and Healthy Beginnings improvement project and focuses on risk for severe hyperbilirubinemia, availability of breastfeeding support, and coordination of newborn care.[19] All efforts should be made to keep mothers and infants together to promote simultaneous discharge. To accomplish this, a pediatric care provider's decision to discharge a newborn should be made jointly with input from the mother, her obstetrical care provider, and other health care providers, such as nursing staff and social workers, who are involved in the care of the mother and her infant.

RECOMMENDATIONS

The length of stay of a healthy term newborn should be based on the unique characteristics of each mother-infant dyad, including the health of the mother, the health and stability of the infant, the ability and confidence of the mother to care for her infant, the adequacy of support systems at home, and access to appropriate follow-up care. Input from the mother and her obstetrical care provider and nursing staff should be considered before a decision to discharge a newborn is made, and all efforts should be made to keep a mother and her newborn together to encourage on-demand breastfeeding and to ensure simultaneous discharge. It is recommended that the following minimum criteria be met before discharge of a term newborn, defined as an infant born between 37-0/7 and 41-6/7 weeks of gestation[20] after an uncomplicated pregnancy, labor, and delivery.

1. Clinical course and physical examination reveal no abnormalities that require continued hospitalization.

2. The infant's vital signs are documented as being within normal ranges, with appropriate variations based on physiologic state, and stable for the 12 hours preceding discharge. These ranges include an axillary temperature of 36.5°C to 37.4°C (97.7–99.3°F, measured properly in an open crib with appropriate clothing),[21] a respiratory rate below 60 per minute[22] and no other signs of respiratory distress, and an awake heart rate of 100 to 190 beats per minute.[23] Heart rates as low as 70 beats per minute while sleeping quietly, without signs of circulatory compromise and responding appropriately to activity, also are acceptable. Sustained heart rates near or above the upper end of this range may require further evaluation.

3. The infant has urinated regularly and passed at least 1 stool spontaneously.

4. The infant has completed at least 2 successful feedings. If the infant is breastfeeding, a caregiver knowledgeable in breastfeeding, latch, swallowing, and infant satiety should observe an actual feeding and document successful performance of these tasks in the medical record.[24] If the infant is bottle-feeding, it is documented that the newborn is able to coordinate sucking, swallowing, and breathing while feeding.

5. There is no evidence of excessive bleeding at the circumcision site for at least 2 hours.

6. The clinical significance of jaundice, if present before discharge, has been determined, and appropriate management and/or follow-up plans have been instituted as recommended in American Academy of Pediatrics clinical practice guidelines for management of hyperbilirubinemia.[2]

7. The infant has been adequately evaluated and monitored for sepsis on the basis of maternal risk factors and in accordance with current guidelines for management of neonates with suspected or proven early-onset sepsis.[25]

8. Maternal and infant laboratory tests are available and have been reviewed, including the following:
   - maternal syphilis, hepatitis B surface antigen, and HIV status; and
   - umbilical cord or newborn blood type and direct Coombs test result, if clinically indicated.[2]

9. Initial hepatitis B vaccine has been administered as indicated by the infant's risk status and according to the current immunization schedule.[26]

10. If the mother has not previously been vaccinated, she should receive tetanus toxoid, reduced diphtheria toxoid, and acellular pertussis, adsorbed (Tdap) vaccine immediately after the infant is born. Other adolescents and adults who will have or anticipate having close contact with the infant should be encouraged to receive a single dose of Tdap if they have not previously received Tdap.[27] If a mother who delivers during the flu season has not been previously immunized, she also should receive an influenza vaccination.[28]

11. Newborn metabolic,[29] hearing,[30,31] and pulse oximetry[32–34] screenings have been completed per hospital protocol and state regulations. If screening metabolic tests were performed before 24 hours of milk feeding, a system for repeating the test during the follow-up visit must be in place in accordance with local or state policy.

12. The mother's knowledge, ability, and confidence to provide adequate care for her infant are documented by the fact that training and information has been received in the following areas:
   - the importance and benefits of breastfeeding for both mother and infant;
   - appropriate urination and stooling frequency for the infant;
   - umbilical cord, skin, and newborn genital care, as well as temperature assessment and measurement with a thermometer;
   - signs of illness and common infant problems, particularly jaundice;
   - infant safety, such as use of an appropriate car safety seat, supine positioning for sleeping, maintaining a smoke-free environment, and sleeping in proximity but not bed-sharing[35,36]; and
   - hand hygiene, especially as a way to reduce infection.

13. A car safety seat appropriate for the infant's maturity and medical condition that meets Federal Motor Vehicle Safety Standard 213 has been obtained and is available before hospital discharge, and the mother has demonstrated to trained hospital personnel appropriate infant positioning and use.

14. Family members or other support persons, including health care providers who are familiar with newborn care and are knowledgeable about lactation and the recognition of jaundice and dehydration, are available to the mother and infant after discharge.

15. A physician-directed source of continuing health care (medical home) for the mother and infant has been identified. Instructions to follow in the event of a complication or emergency have been provided. The mother should know how to reach the medical home and should have scheduled the infant's first visit, if possible, or know how to do so.

16. Family, environmental, and social risk factors have been assessed, and the mother and her other family members have been educated about safe home environment. When the following or other risk factors are present, discharge should be delayed until they are resolved or a plan to safeguard the newborn is in place. This plan may involve discussions with social services and/or state agencies, such as child protective services. These risk factors may include, but are not limited to the following:
   - untreated parental use of illicit substances or positive urine

toxicology results in the mother or newborn consistent with maternal abuse or misuse of drugs;

- history of child abuse or neglect by any anticipated care provider;
- mental illness in a parent or another person in the home;
- lack of social support, particularly for single, first-time mothers;
- no fixed home;
- history of domestic violence, particularly during this pregnancy;
- adolescent mother, particularly if other previously listed conditions apply; or
- barriers to adequate follow-up care for the newborn, such as lack of transportation to medical care services, lack of easy access to telephone communication, and non–English-speaking parents.

17. For newborns discharged before 48 hours after delivery, an appointment should be made for the infant to be examined by a health care practitioner within 48 hours of discharge.[10,12,16,37,38] If this cannot be ensured, discharge should be deferred until a mechanism for follow-up is identified. The follow-up visit can take place in a home, clinic, or hospital outpatient setting as long as the health care professional who examines the infant is competent in newborn assessment and the results of the follow-up visit are reported to the infant's primary care provider or his or her designee on the day of the visit. The purpose of the follow-up visit is to
   - promote establishment of a relationship with the medical home by verifying the plan for health care maintenance, including a method for obtaining emergency services, preventive care and immunizations, periodic evaluations and physical examinations, and necessary screenings;
   - weigh the infant and assess the infant's general health, hydration, and degree of jaundice, and identify any new problems;
   - review feeding patterns and technique, and encourage and support breastfeeding by observation of the adequacy of position, latch, and swallowing;
   - obtain historical evidence of adequate stool and urine patterns;
   - provide or make a referral for lactation support if the foregoing evaluations are not reassuring;
   - assess quality of mother-infant attachment and details of infant behavior;
   - reinforce maternal or family education in infant care, particularly regarding feeding and sleep position, avoidance of co-sleeping, and appropriate use of car safety seats, which should be used only for travel and not for positioning in the home;
   - review results of outstanding laboratory tests, such as newborn metabolic screens, performed before discharge;
   - perform screenings in accordance with state regulations and other tests that are clinically indicated, such as serum bilirubin; and
   - assess for parental well-being with focus on screening for maternal postpartum depression.

CONCLUSIONS

The timing of discharge from the hospital should be the decision of the health care provider caring for the mother and her newborn. This decision should be made in consultation with the family and should not be based on arbitrary policies established by third-party payers. A shortened hospital stay (less than 48 hours after delivery) for healthy, term newborns can be accommodated but is not appropriate for every mother and newborn. If possible, institutions are encouraged to develop processes to prevent the necessity for early discharge of uninsured or underinsured newborn infants for purely financial reasons, however. Institutions should develop guidelines through their professional staff in collaboration with appropriate community agencies, including third-party payers, to establish hospital-stay programs for mothers and their healthy newborns. State and local public health agencies also should be involved in the oversight of existing hospital-stay programs for quality assurance and monitoring. Obstetrical care, newborn nursery care, and follow-up care should be considered independent services to be paid as separate packages and not as part of a global fee for maternity-newborn labor and delivery services. Adoption of standardized processes, such as predischarge checklists, may facilitate more uniform implementation of these recommendations across the full spectrum of health care settings where care for newborn infants is provided.

LEAD AUTHOR

William E. Benitz, MD, FAAP

COMMITTEE ON FETUS AND NEWBORN, 2014–2015

Kristi L. Watterberg, MD, FAAP, Chairperson
Susan Aucott, MD FAAP
William E. Benitz, MD, FAAP
James J. Cummings, MD, FAAP
Eric C. Eichenwald, MD, FAAP
Jay Goldsmith, MD, FAAP
Brenda B. Poindexter, MD, FAAP
Karen Puopolo, MD, FAAP
Dan L. Stewart, MD, FAAP
Kasper S. Wang, MD, FAAP

LIAISONS

CAPT Wanda D. Barfield, MD, MPH, FAAP – *Centers for Disease Control and Prevention*

James Goldberg, MD – *American College of Obstetricians and Gynecologists*
Thierry Lacaze, MD – *Canadian Pediatric Society*
Erin L. Keels, APRN, MS, NNP-BC – *National Association of Neonatal Nurses*
Tonse N. K. Raju, MD, DCH, FAAP – *National Institutes of Health*

STAFF

Jim Couto, MA

REFERENCES

1. Desmond MM, Rudolph AJ, Phitaksphraiwan P. The transitional care nursery. A mechanism for preventive medicine in the newborn. *Pediatr Clin North Am*. 1966;13(3):651–668

2. American Academy of Pediatrics Subcommittee on Hyperbilirubinemia. Management of hyperbilirubinemia in the newborn infant 35 or more weeks of gestation. *Pediatrics*. 2004;114(1): 297–316

3. Maisels MJ, Bhutani VK, Bogen D, Newman TB, Stark AR, Watchko JF. Hyperbilirubinemia in the newborn infant > or =35 weeks' gestation: an update with clarifications. *Pediatrics*. 2009;124(4):1193–1198

4. Gentile R, Stevenson G, Dooley T, Franklin D, Kawabori I, Pearlman A. Pulsed Doppler echocardiographic determination of time of ductal closure in normal newborn infants. *J Pediatr*. 1981;98(3):443–448

5. Lambert EC, Canent RV, Hohn AR. Congenital cardiac anomalies in the newborn. A review of conditions causing death or severe distress in the first month of life. *Pediatrics*. 1966;37(2): 343–351

6. Juang D, Snyder CL. Neonatal bowel obstruction. *Surg Clin North Am*. 2012; 92(3):685–711, ix–x

7. Jackson GL, Kennedy KA, Sendelbach DM, et al. Problem identification in apparently well neonates: implications for early discharge. *Clin Pediatr (Phila)*. 2000;39(10):581–590

8. Datar A, Sood N. Impact of postpartum hospital-stay legislation on newborn length of stay, readmission, and mortality in California. *Pediatrics*. 2006; 118(1):63–72

9. Madden JM, Soumerai SB, Lieu TA, Mandl KD, Zhang F, Ross-Degnan D; Health maintenance organization. Effects of a law against early postpartum discharge on newborn follow-up, adverse events, and HMO expenditures. *N Engl J Med*. 2002;347(25):2031–2038

10. Meara E, Kotagal UR, Atherton HD, Lieu TA. Impact of early newborn discharge legislation and early follow-up visits on infant outcomes in a state Medicaid population. *Pediatrics*. 2004;113(6): 1619–1627

11. Madden JM, Soumerai SB, Lieu TA, Mandl KD, Zhang F, Ross-Degnan D. Length-of-stay policies and ascertainment of postdischarge problems in newborns. *Pediatrics*. 2004;113(1 pt 1):42–49

12. Kotagal UR, Atherton HD, Eshett R, Schoettker PJ, Perlstein PH. Safety of early discharge for Medicaid newborns. *JAMA*. 1999;282(12):1150–1156

13. Watt S, Sword W, Krueger P. Longer postpartum hospitalization options— who stays, who leaves, what changes? *BMC Pregnancy Childbirth*. 2005;5:13

14. Grupp-Phelan J, Taylor JA, Liu LL, Davis RL. Early newborn hospital discharge and readmission for mild and severe jaundice. *Arch Pediatr Adolesc Med*. 1999;153(12):1283–1288

15. Paul IM, Lehman EB, Hollenbeak CS, Maisels MJ. Preventable newborn readmissions since passage of the Newborns' and Mothers' Health Protection Act. *Pediatrics*. 2006;118(6): 2349–2358

16. Escobar GJ, Greene JD, Hulac P, et al. Rehospitalisation after birth hospitalisation: patterns among infants of all gestations. *Arch Dis Child*. 2005; 90(2):125–131

17. Danielsen B, Castles AG, Damberg CL, Gould JB. Newborn discharge timing and readmissions: California, 1992-1995. *Pediatrics*. 2000;106(1 pt 1):31–39

18. Bernstein HH, Spino C, Finch S, et al. Decision-making for postpartum discharge of 4300 mothers and their healthy infants: the Life Around Newborn Discharge study. *Pediatrics*. 2007;120(2). Available at: www.pediatrics.org/cgi/content/full/120/2/e391

19. Safe and Healthy Beginnings. A resource toolkit for hospitals and physicians' offices. 2009. Available at: https://www.aap.org/en-us/professional-resources/practice-support/quality-improvement/ Quality-Improvement-Innovation-Networks/Pages/Safe-and-Healthy-Beginnings-A-Resource-Toolkit-for-Hospitals-and-Physicians-Offices.aspx?aid=2577. Accessed March 3, 2014

20. American College of Obstetricians and Gynecologists. ACOG Committee Opinion No 579: definition of term pregnancy. *Obstet Gynecol*. 2013;122(5):1139–1140

21. Mayfield SR, Bhatia J, Nakamura KT, Rios GR, Bell EF. Temperature measurement in term and preterm neonates. *J Pediatr*. 1984;104(2):271–275

22. Taylor WC, Watkins GM. Respiratory rate patterns in the newborn infant. *Can Med Assoc J*. 1960;83:1292–1295

23. Semizel E, Öztürk B, Bostan OM, Cil E, Ediz B. The effect of age and gender on the electrocardiogram in children. *Cardiol Young*. 2008;18(1):26–40

24. Hagan JF, Shaw JS, Duncan PM, eds. Bright Futures: Guidelines for Health Supervision of Infants, Children, and Adolescents. 3rd ed. Elk Grove Village, IL: American Academy of Pediatrics; 2008

25. Polin RA, Papile LA, Baley JE, et al; Committee on Fetus and Newborn. Management of neonates with suspected or proven early-onset bacterial sepsis. *Pediatrics*. 2012;129(5):1006–1015

26. Centers for Disease Control and Prevention. Recommended immunization schedule for persons aged 0 through 18 years: United States—2014. Available at: www.cdc.gov/vaccines/schedules/downloads/child/0-18yrs-schedule.pdf. Accessed March 10, 2014

27. Centers for Disease Control and Prevention (CDC). Updated recommendations for use of tetanus toxoid, reduced diphtheria toxoid, and acellular pertussis vaccine (Tdap) in pregnant women—Advisory Committee on Immunization Practices (ACIP), 2012. *MMWR Morb Mortal Wkly Rep*. 2013; 62(7):131–135

28. Centers for Disease Control and Prevention. Prevention and control of seasonal influenza with vaccines. Recommendations of the Advisory Committee on Immunization Practices—United States, 2013-2014. *MMWR Recomm Rep*. 2013;62(RR-07): 1–43

29. American Academy of Pediatrics Newborn Screening Authoring

Committee. Newborn screening expands: recommendations for pediatricians and medical homes—implications for the system. *Pediatrics*. 2008;121(1):192–217

30. American Academy of Pediatrics, Joint Committee on Infant Hearing. Year 2007 position statement: principles and guidelines for early hearing detection and intervention programs. *Pediatrics*. 2007;120(4):898–921

31. Harlor AD Jr, Bower C; Committee on Practice and Ambulatory Medicine; Section on Otolaryngology-Head and Neck Surgery. Hearing assessment in infants and children: recommendations beyond neonatal screening. *Pediatrics*. 2009;124(4):1252–1263

32. Kemper AR, Mahle WT, Martin GR, et al. Strategies for implementing screening for critical congenital heart disease. *Pediatrics*. 2011;128(5). Available at:

www.pediatrics.org/cgi/content/full/128/5/e1259

33. Mahle WT, Martin GR, Beekman RH III, Morrow WR; Section on Cardiology and Cardiac Surgery Executive Committee. Endorsement of Health and Human Services recommendation for pulse oximetry screening for critical congenital heart disease. *Pediatrics*. 2012;129(1):190–192

34. US Department of Health and Human Services. HHS Secretary adopts recommendation to add critical congenital heart disease to the Recommended Uniform Screening Panel. 2012. Available at: www.hrsa. gov/advisorycommittees/mchbadvisory/heritabledisorders/recommendations/correspondence/cyanoticheartsecre09212011.pdf. Accessed November 3, 2013

35. Durbin DR; Committee on Injury, Violence, and Poison Prevention. Child passenger safety. *Pediatrics*. 2011; 127(4):788–793

36. Moon RY; Task Force on Sudden Infant Death Syndrome. SIDS and other sleep-related infant deaths: expansion of recommendations for a safe infant sleeping environment. *Pediatrics*. 2011; 128(5):1030–1039

37. Escobar GJ, Braveman PA, Ackerson L, et al. A randomized comparison of home visits and hospital-based group follow-up visits after early postpartum discharge. *Pediatrics*. 2001;108(3): 719–727

38. Nelson VR. The effect of newborn early discharge follow-up program on pediatric urgent care utilization. *J Pediatr Health Care*. 1999;13(2): 58–61

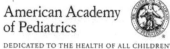

DEDICATED TO THE HEALTH OF ALL CHILDREN™

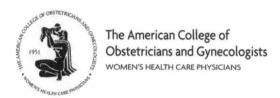

The American College of
Obstetricians and Gynecologists
WOMEN'S HEALTH CARE PHYSICIANS

CLINICAL REPORT

Immersion in Water During Labor and Delivery

abstract

Immersion in water has been suggested as a beneficial alternative for labor, delivery, or both and over the past decades has gained popularity in many parts of the world. Immersion in water during the first stage of labor may be associated with decreased pain or use of anesthesia and decreased duration of labor. However, there is no evidence that immersion in water during the first stage of labor otherwise improves perinatal outcomes, and it should not prevent or inhibit other elements of care. The safety and efficacy of immersion in water during the second stage of labor have not been established, and immersion in water during the second stage of labor has not been associated with maternal or fetal benefit. Given these facts and case reports of rare but serious adverse effects in the newborn, the practice of immersion in the second stage of labor (underwater delivery) should be considered an experimental procedure that only should be performed within the context of an appropriately designed clinical trial with informed consent. Facilities that plan to offer immersion in the first stage of labor need to establish rigorous protocols for candidate selection, maintenance and cleaning of tubs and immersion pools, infection control procedures, monitoring of mothers and fetuses at appropriate intervals while immersed, and immediately and safely moving women out of the tubs if maternal or fetal concerns develop. *Pediatrics* 2014;133:758–761

AMERICAN ACADEMY OF PEDIATRICS Committee on Fetus and Newborn and AMERICAN COLLEGE OF OBSTETRICIANS AND GYNECOLOGISTS Committee on Obstetric Practice

KEY WORDS
labor, delivery, water birth, immersion, perinatal care

ABBREVIATIONS
CI—confidence interval
RCT—randomized controlled trial
RR—risk ratio

www.pediatrics.org/cgi/doi/10.1542/peds.2013-3794

doi:10.1542/peds.2013-3794

All clinical reports from the American Academy of Pediatrics automatically expire 5 years after publication unless reaffirmed, revised, or retired at or before that time.

PEDIATRICS (ISSN Numbers: Print, 0031-4005; Online, 1098-4275).

INTRODUCTION

Immersion in water has been suggested as a beneficial alternative for labor, delivery, or both and over the past decades has gained popularity in many parts of world.[1–4] Approximately 1% of births in the United Kingdom include at least a period of immersion,[5] and a 2006 joint statement from the Royal College of Obstetricians and Gynaecologists and Royal College of Midwives supported immersion in water during labor for healthy women with uncomplicated pregnancies and stated that to achieve best practice with water birth, it is necessary for organizations to provide systems and structure to support this service.[6] The prevalence of this practice in the United States is unknown, because such data are not collected as part of vital statistics. A 2001 survey found that at least 143 US birthing centers offered immersion in water during labor, delivery, or both.[7] A 2005 commentary by the Committee on Fetus and Newborn of the American Academy of Pediatrics did not endorse underwater birth.[8] This clinical report reviews the literature concerning the reported risks and benefits of immersion in water during labor and delivery.

EVIDENCE REGARDING IMMERSION IN WATER DURING LABOR AND DELIVERY

Before examining available evidence concerning immersion during childbirth, it is important to recognize the limitations of studies and evidence in this area. Most published articles that recommend underwater births are retrospective reviews of a single center experience, observational studies using historical controls, or personal opinions and testimonials, often in publications that are not peer reviewed.[1–3,9–11] Also of importance, there are no basic science studies in animals or humans to confirm the physiologic mechanisms proposed to underlie the reported benefits of underwater births.

Other issues, in addition to the nature and design of studies, complicate the interpretation of the published findings, including the absence of a uniform definition of the exposure itself. Often, immersion is referred to as "underwater birth," but effects and outcomes may be different for immersion during the first stage and second stage of labor. This clinical report, accordingly, avoids the term underwater birth and makes an effort to distinguish data and outcomes related separately to immersion in the first stage and second stage of labor. Not all studies, however, distinguish when in the course of labor and delivery immersion was undertaken.

Outcomes indicating safety or risk in association with immersion at 1 stage may not translate into equivalent outcomes at a different stage of labor; specifically, safety during labor may not translate into safety during delivery. In addition to this important limitation, immersion therapies have varied between studies in the duration of immersion, the depth of the bath or pool, the temperature of the water, and whether or not agitation (jets or whirlpool) was used. In considering the evaluation of outcomes, it is important to note that health care providers involved in providing or studying immersion therapy are not masked to either the treatment or outcomes, and especially in nonrandomized studies, outcomes may be influenced by differences in the environment attending a particular choice of delivery. Finally, most trials of immersion therapy are small, which limits their power to detect rare outcomes.

Randomized controlled trials (RCTs) would be ideal to address many of the aforementioned concerns. A 2009 Cochrane review identified 12 relevant and appropriately designed RCTs of immersion during labor, which involved 3243 women. Nine of these trials involved immersion during the first stage of labor alone (1 of 9 trials compared early versus later immersion during the first stage), 2 trials involved first stage and second stage of labor, and 1 trial involved comparing only the second stage of labor with the controls. Even among these RCTs, however, some of the aforementioned limitations remain, including concerns about power and how the absence of blinding might affect definition of outcomes. The systematic review also noted that most trials have small sample sizes and, thus, a high risk of bias. These factors limit comparison across trials and the reliability and validity of the trial findings.[5]

PROPOSED BENEFITS FROM IMMERSION DURING LABOR AND DELIVERY

There have been claims concerning the positive effects of immersion during labor.[12–14] Immersion is known to affect maternal cardiovascular physiology as hydrostatic pressure promotes increased venous return and mobilization of extravascular fluid and edema.[15,16] In part as a result of these effects, proponents of underwater immersion during labor and delivery argue that there are a variety of benefits to such treatment, including a decrease in perinatal pain, a greater sense of well-being and control, and a decreased rate of perineal trauma. Some advocates argue that immersion during labor and delivery decreases maternal stress and stress-associated hormone levels. It could also potentially benefit the newborn infant with a gentler transition from the in utero to ex utero environment.[1–7]

Individual retrospective analyses and case series argue in support of 1 or more of the benefits listed previously, but among RCTs studying immersion in the first stage of labor that were included in the 2009 Cochrane systematic review,[5] results were inconsistent. Although many individual RCTs reported no benefit, the combined data indicated that immersion during the first stage of labor was associated with decreased use of epidural, spinal, or paracervical analgesia among those allocated to water immersion compared with controls (478/1254 vs 529/1245; risk ratio [RR] 0.90; 95% confidence interval [CI], 0.82 to 0.99; 6 trials). There was a reduction in duration of the first stage of labor (mean difference −32.4 minutes; 95% CI, −58.7 to −6.13). However, considering each of these effects (particularly the latter), it is difficult to know how factors other than immersion, such as the structure of care (including health care providers and timing and frequency of examinations) affected outcome. Furthermore, there were no differences in perineal trauma or tears (RR, 1.16; 95% CI, 0.99 to 1.35; 5 trials) or need for either assisted vaginal deliveries (RR, 0.86; 95% CI, 0.71 to 1.05; 7 trials) or cesarean delivery (RR, 1.21; 95% CI, 0.87 to 1.65; 8 trials) between those allocated to the immersion and control arms in the meta-analysis results.

Among the 2 trials that reported outcomes from immersion in the second stage of labor included in this systematic review,[5] the only difference in maternal outcomes from immersion during the second stage was an improvement in satisfaction among those allocated to immersion in 1 trial. None of the individual trials or the Cochrane systematic review[5] has reported any benefit to the newborn infant from maternal immersion during labor or delivery.

REPORTED COMPLICATIONS FROM IMMERSION DURING LABOR AND DELIVERY

Individual case reports and case series have noted complications for the mother and the neonate[17–25] that highlight potential risks from immersion during labor and delivery. Because the denominators are not uniformly reported, the exact incidence of complications is difficult to assess. Some of the reported concerns include higher risk of maternal and neonatal infections, particularly with ruptured membranes; difficulties in neonatal thermoregulation; umbilical cord avulsion and umbilical cord rupture while the newborn infant is lifted or maneuvered through and from the underwater pool at delivery, which leads to serious hemorrhage and shock; respiratory distress and hyponatremia that results from tub-water aspiration (drowning or near drowning); and seizures and perinatal asphyxia.[23]

Among this list of complications, given its potential seriousness, the possibility of a neonate aspirating water during birth while immersed has been the focus of understandable concern. Alerdice et al[26] summarized case reports of adverse neonatal outcomes, including drownings and near drownings. The case reports included immersion births in hospitals and at home. Subsequently, a study by Byard and Zuccollo reported 4 cases of severe respiratory distress in neonates after water birth, 1 of whom died of overwhelming sepsis from *Pseudomonas aeruginosa*.[19] Although it has been claimed that neonates delivered into the water do not breathe, gasp, or swallow water because of the protective "diving reflex," studies in experimental animals and a vast body of literature from meconium aspiration syndrome demonstrate that, in compromised fetuses and neonates, the diving reflex is overridden,[27,28] which leads potentially to gasping and aspiration of the surrounding fluid.

Morbidity and mortality, including respiratory complications, suggested in case series were not seen in the 2009 Cochrane synthesis of RCTs, which concluded that "there is no evidence of increased adverse effects to the fetus/neonate or woman from laboring in water or water birth."[5] This conclusion, however, should be tempered by several concerns, including the issue of the power of the sample size to identify rare but potentially serious outcomes. In this regard, in an RCT[29] excluded from the Cochrane analysis (because included labors all involved dystocia), 12% of neonates who were delivered in the immersion arm required admission to the NICU, as compared with none in the group delivered without immersion.

SUMMARY

Immersion in water during the first stage of labor may be appealing to some and may be associated with decreased pain or use of anesthesia and decreased duration of labor; however, there is no evidence that immersion during the first stage of labor otherwise improves perinatal outcomes. Immersion therapy during the first stage of labor should not prevent or inhibit other elements of care, including appropriate maternal and fetal monitoring.

In contrast, the safety and efficacy of immersion in water during the second stage of labor have not been established, and immersion in water during the second stage of labor has not been associated with maternal or fetal benefit. Given these facts and case reports of rare but serious adverse effects in the newborn, the practice of immersion in the second stage of labor (underwater delivery) should be considered an experimental procedure that only should be performed within the context of an appropriately designed clinical trial with informed consent.

Although not the focus of specific trials, facilities that plan to offer immersion in the first stage of labor need to establish rigorous protocols for candidate selection, maintenance and cleaning of tubs and immersion pools, infection control procedures, monitoring of mothers and fetuses at appropriate intervals while immersed, and protocols for moving women from tubs if urgent maternal or fetal concerns develop.

AAP COMMITTEE ON FETUS AND NEWBORN, 2012–2013
Lu-Ann Papile, MD, Chairperson
Jill E. Baley, MD
William Benitz, MD
Waldemar A. Carlo, MD
James Cummings, MD
Praveen Kumar, MD
Richard A. Polin, MD
Rosemarie C. Tan, MD, PhD
Kristi L. Watterberg, MD

LIAISONS
CAPT Wanda Denise Barfield, MD, MPH – *Centers for Disease Control and Prevention*

Ann L. Jefferies, MD – *Canadian Pediatric Society*

George Macones, MD – *American College of Obstetricians and Gynecologists*

Rosalie O. Mainous, PhD, RNC, NNP – *National Association of Neonatal Nurses*

*Tonse N. K. Raju, MD, DCH – *National Institutes of Health*

Kasper S. Wang, MD – *Section on Surgery*

STAFF

Jim Couto, MA

*The views expressed in this document are not necessarily those of the Eunice Kennedy Shriver National Institute of Child Health and Human Development, the National Institutes of Health, or the Department of Health and Human Services.

REFERENCES

1. Geissbühler V, Eberhard J. Waterbirths: a comparative study. A prospective study on more than 2,000 waterbirths. *Fetal Diagn Ther.* 2000;15(5):291–300

2. Geissbuehler V, Stein S, Eberhard J. Waterbirths compared with landbirths: an observational study of nine years. *J Perinat Med.* 2004;32(4):308–314

3. Woodward J, Kelly SM. A pilot study for a randomised controlled trial of waterbirth versus land birth. *BJOG.* 2004;111(6):537–545

4. Chaichian S, Akhlaghi A, Rousta F, Safavi M. Experience of water birth delivery in Iran. *Arch Iran Med.* 2009;12(5):468–471

5. Cluett ER, Burns E. Immersion in water in labour and birth. *Cochrane Database Syst Rev.* 2009;(2):CD000111

6. Immersion in Water During Labour and Birth. RCOG/Royal College of Midwives Joint Statement No. 1. London, England: Royal College of Obstetricians and Gynaecologists, Royal College of Midwives; 2006. Available at: www.rcog.org.uk/womens-health/clinical-guidance/immersion-water-during-labour-and-birth. Accessed February 6, 2013

7. Mackey MM. Use of water in labor and birth. *Clin Obstet Gynecol.* 2001;44(4):733–749

8. Batton DG, Blackmon LR, Adamkin DH, et al; Committee on Fetus and Newborn, 2004–2005. Underwater births [commentary]. *Pediatrics.* 2005;115(5):1413–1414

9. Enning C. How to support the autonomy of motherbaby in second stage of waterbirth. *Midwifery Today Int Midwife.* 2011;(98):40–41

10. Maude RM, Foureur MJ. It's beyond water: stories of women's experience of using water for labour and birth. *Women Birth.* 2007;20(1):17–24

11. Moore M. How to make a portable waterbirth tub. *Midwifery Today Int Midwife.* 2002;(61):38–39

12. Edlich RF, Towler MA, Goitz RJ, et al. Bioengineering principles of hydrotherapy. *J Burn Care Rehabil.* 1987;8(6):580–584

13. Ginesi L, Niecierowicz R. Neuroendocrinology and birth 2: the role of oxytocin. *Br J Midwifery.* 1998;6(12):791–796

14. Garland D, Jones KC. Waterbirth: supporting practice with clinical audit. *MIDIRS Midwifery Dig.* 2000;10(3):333–336

15. Katz VL, Rozas L, Ryder R, Cefalo RC. Effect of daily immersion on the edema of pregnancy. *Am J Perinatol.* 1992;9(4):225–227

16. Katz VL, McMurray R, Berry MJ, Cefalo RC, Bowman C. Renal responses to immersion and exercise in pregnancy. *Am J Perinatol.* 1990;7(2):118–121

17. Bowden K, Kessler D, Pinette M, Wilson E. Underwater birth: missing the evidence or missing the point? [published correction appears in *Pediatrics.* 2004;113:433] *Pediatrics.* 2003;112(4):972–973

18. Pinette MG, Wax J, Wilson E. The risks of underwater birth. *Am J Obstet Gynecol.* 2004;190(5):1211–1215

19. Byard RW, Zuccollo JM. Forensic issues in cases of water birth fatalities. *Am J Forensic Med Pathol.* 2010;31(3):258–260

20. Eckert K, Turnbull D, MacLennan A. Immersion in water in the first stage of labor: a randomized controlled trial. *Birth.* 2001;28(2):84–93

21. Franzin L, Cabodi D, Scolfaro C, Gioannini P. Microbiological investigations on a nosocomial case of *Legionella pneumophila* pneumonia associated with water birth and review of neonatal cases. *Infez Med.* 2004;12(1):69–75

22. Gilbert R. Water birth—a near-drowning experience. *Pediatrics.* 2002;110(2 pt 1):409

23. Kassim Z, Sellars M, Greenough A. Underwater birth and neonatal respiratory distress. *BMJ.* 2005;330(7499):1071–1072

24. Mottola MF, Fitzgerald HM, Wilson NC, Taylor AW. Effect of water temperature on exercise-induced maternal hyperthermia on fetal development in rats. *Int J Sports Med.* 1993;14(5):248–251

25. Nguyen S, Kuschel C, Teele R, Spooner C. Water birth—a near-drowning experience. *Pediatrics.* 2002;110(2 pt 1):411–413

26. Alderdice F, Renfrew M, Marchant S, et al. Labour and birth in water in England and Wales. *BMJ.* 1995;310(6983):837

27. Johnson P. Birth under water—to breathe or not to breathe. *Br J Obstet Gynaecol.* 1996;103(3):202–208

28. Cammu H, Clasen K, Van Wettere L, Derde MP. "To bathe or not to bathe" during the first stage of labor. *Acta Obstet Gynecol Scand.* 1994;73(6):468–472

29. Cluett ER, Pickering RM, Getliffe K, St George Saunders NJ. Randomised controlled trial of labouring in water compared with standard of augmentation for management of dystocia in first stage of labour. *BMJ.* 2004;328(7435):314

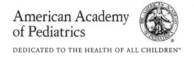

American Academy
of Pediatrics
DEDICATED TO THE HEALTH OF ALL CHILDREN®

Organizational Principles to Guide and Define the Child
Health Care System and/or Improve the Health of all Children

POLICY STATEMENT

Planned Home Birth

abstract

The American Academy of Pediatrics concurs with the recent statement of the American College of Obstetricians and Gynecologists affirming that hospitals and birthing centers are the safest settings for birth in the United States while respecting the right of women to make a medically informed decision about delivery. This statement is intended to help pediatricians provide supportive, informed counsel to women considering home birth while retaining their role as child advocates and to summarize the standards of care for newborn infants born at home, which are consistent with standards for infants born in a medical care facility. Regardless of the circumstances of his or her birth, including location, every newborn infant deserves health care that adheres to the standards highlighted in this statement, more completely described in other publications from the American Academy of Pediatrics, including *Guidelines for Perinatal Care*. The goal of providing high-quality care to all newborn infants can best be achieved through continuing efforts by all participating health care providers and institutions to develop and sustain communications and understanding on the basis of professional interaction and mutual respect throughout the health care system. *Pediatrics* 2013;131:1016–1020

COMMITTEE ON FETUS AND NEWBORN

KEY WORDS
birth, delivery, newborn infant, home birth, midwife, obstetrician, pediatrician

ABBREVIATIONS
ACOG—American College of Obstetricians and Gynecologists
AAP—American Academy of Pediatrics

INTRODUCTION

Women and their families may desire a home birth for a variety of reasons, including hopes for a more family-friendly setting, increased control of the process, decreased obstetric intervention, and lower cost. Although the incidence of home birth remains below 1% of all births in the United States, the rate of home birth has increased during the past several years for white, non-Hispanic women.[1] However, a woman's choice to plan a home birth is not well supported in the United States. Obstacles are pervasive and systemic and include wide variation in state laws and regulations, lack of appropriately trained and willing providers, and lack of supporting systems to ensure the availability of specialty consultation and timely transport to a hospital. Geography also may adversely affect the safety of planned home birth, because travel times >20 minutes have been associated with increased risk of adverse neonatal outcomes, including mortality.[2] Whether for these reasons or others, planned home birth in the United States appears to be associated with a two- to threefold increase in neonatal mortality or an absolute risk increase of approximately 1 neonatal death per 1000 nonanomalous live births.[3–5] Evidence also suggests that infants born at home in the United States

www.pediatrics.org/cgi/doi/10.1542/peds.2013-0575

doi:10.1542/peds.2013-0575

PEDIATRICS (ISSN Numbers: Print, 0031-4005; Online, 1098-4275).

have an increased incidence of low Apgar scores and neonatal seizures.[3,4] In contrast, a smaller study of all planned home births attended by midwives in British Columbia, Canada, from 2000 to 2004 revealed no increase in neonatal mortality over planned hospital births attended by either midwives or physicians.[6] Registered midwives in British Columbia are mandated to offer women the choice to deliver in a hospital or at home if they meet the eligibility criteria for home birth defined by the College of Midwifery of British Columbia (Table 1).

In a recent position statement, the Committee on Obstetric Practice of the American College of Obstetricians and Gynecologists (ACOG) stated, "although the Committee on Obstetric Practice believes that hospitals and birthing centers are the safest setting for birth, it respects the right of a woman to make a medically informed decision about delivery. Women inquiring about planned home birth should be informed of its risks and benefits based on recent evidence."[7] The statement reviewed appropriate candidates for home delivery and outlined the health care system components "critical to reducing perinatal mortality rates and achieving favorable home birth outcomes" (Table 1).

Pediatricians must be prepared to provide supportive, informed counsel to women considering home birth while retaining their role as child advocates in assessing whether the situation is appropriate to support a planned home birth (Table 1). In addition to apprising the expectant mother of the increase in neonatal mortality and other neonatal complications with planned home birth, the pediatrician should advise her that the American Academy of Pediatrics (AAP) and ACOG support provision of care only by midwives who are certified by the American Midwifery Certification Board and should make her aware that some women who plan to deliver at home will need transfer to a hospital before delivery because of unanticipated complications. This percentage varies widely among reports, from approximately 10% to 40%, with a higher transfer rate for primiparous women.[8,9] The mother should be encouraged to see successful transfer not as a failure of the home birth but rather as a success of the system.

Care of the newborn infant born at home is a particularly important topic, because infants born at home are cared for outside the safeguards of the systems-based protocols required of hospitals and birthing centers. This situation places a larger burden on individual health care providers to remember and carry out all components of assessment and care of the newborn infant. To assist providers, this policy statement addresses 2 specific areas: resuscitation and evaluation of the newborn infant immediately after birth and essential elements of care and follow-up for the healthy term newborn infant.

ASSESSMENT, RESUSCITATION, AND CARE OF THE NEWBORN INFANT IMMEDIATELY AFTER BIRTH

As recommended by the AAP and the American Heart Association, there should be at least 1 person present at every delivery whose primary responsibility is the care of the newborn infant.[10] Situations in which both the mother and the newborn infant simultaneously require urgent attention are infrequent but will nonetheless occur. Thus, each delivery should be attended by 2 individuals, at least 1 of whom has the appropriate training, skills, and equipment to perform a full resuscitation of the infant in accordance of the principles of the Neonatal Resuscitation Program.[10] To facilitate obtaining emergency assistance when needed, the operational integrity of the telephone or other communication system should be tested before the delivery (as should every other piece of medical equipment), and the weather should be monitored. In addition, a previous arrangement with a medical facility needs to be in place to ensure a safe and timely transport in the event of an emergency.

Care of the newborn infant immediately after delivery should adhere to standards of practice as described in *Guidelines for Perinatal Care*[11] and include provision of warmth, initiation of appropriate resuscitation measures,

---

TABLE 1 Recommendations When Considering Planned Home Birth

Candidate for home delivery[a]
- Absence of preexisting maternal disease
- Absence of significant disease occurring during the pregnancy
- A singleton fetus estimated to be appropriate for gestational age
- A cephalic presentation
- A gestation of 37 to <41 completed weeks of pregnancy
- Labor that is spontaneous or induced as an outpatient
- A mother who has not been referred from another hospital

Systems needed to support planned home birth
- The availability of a certified nurse-midwife, certified midwife, or physician practicing within an integrated and regulated health system
- Attendance by at least 1 appropriately trained individual (see text) whose primary responsibility is the care of the newborn infant
- Ready access to consultation
- Assurance of safe and timely transport to a nearby hospital with a preexisting arrangement for such transfers

Data are from refs 6, 7, 10, 11, and 13.
[a] ACOG considers previous cesarean delivery to be an absolute contraindication to planned home birth.[7]

and assignment of Apgar scores. Although skin-to-skin contact with mother is the most effective way to provide warmth, portable warming pads should be available in case a newborn infant requires resuscitation and cannot be placed on the mother's chest. A newborn infant who requires any resuscitation should be monitored frequently during the immediate postnatal period, and infants who receive extensive resuscitation (eg, positive-pressure ventilation for more than 30–60 seconds) should be transferred to a medical facility for close monitoring and evaluation. In addition, any infant who has respiratory distress, continued cyanosis, or other signs of illness should be immediately transferred to a medical facility.

CARE OF THE NEWBORN

Subsequent newborn care should adhere to the AAP standards as described in *Guidelines for Perinatal Care* as well as to the AAP statement regarding care of the well newborn infant.[11–13] Although a detailed review of these standards would be far too lengthy to include in this statement, a few practice points are worthy of specific mention:

- *Transitional care (first 4–8 hours)*: The infant should be kept warm and undergo a detailed physical examination that includes an assessment of gestational age and intrauterine growth status (weight, length, and head circumference), as well as a comprehensive risk assessment for neonatal conditions that require additional monitoring or intervention. Temperature, heart and respiratory rates, skin color, peripheral circulation, respiration, level of consciousness, tone, and activity should be monitored and recorded at least once every 30 minutes until the newborn's condition is considered normal and

has remained stable for 2 hours. An infant who is thought to be <37 weeks' gestational age should be transferred to a medical facility for continuing observation for conditions associated with prematurity, including respiratory distress, poor feeding, hypoglycemia, and hyperbilirubinemia, as well as for a car safety seat study.

- *Monitoring for group B streptococcal disease*: As recommended by the Centers for Disease Control and Prevention and the AAP, all pregnant women should be screened for group B streptococcal colonization at 35 to 37 weeks of gestation.[14] Women who are colonized should receive ≥4 hours of intravenous penicillin, ampicillin, or cefazolin. If the mother has received this intrapartum treatment and both she and her newborn infant remain asymptomatic, they can remain at home if the infant can be observed frequently by an experienced and knowledgeable health care provider. If the mother shows signs of chorioamnionitis or if the infant does not appear completely well, the infant should be transferred rapidly to a medical facility for additional evaluation and treatment.[14]

- *Glucose screening*: Infants who have abnormal fetal growth (estimated to be small or large for gestational age) or whose mothers have diabetes should be delivered in a hospital or birthing center because of the increased risk of hypoglycemia and other neonatal complications. If, after delivery, an infant is discovered to be small or large for gestational age or has required resuscitation, he or she should be screened for hypoglycemia as outlined in the AAP statement.[15] If hypoglycemia is identified and persists after feeding (glucose <45 mg/dL), the infant should be

transferred promptly to a medical facility for continuing evaluation and treatment.

- *Eye prophylaxis*: Every newborn infant should receive prophylaxis against gonococcal ophthalmia neonatorum.

- *Vitamin K*: Every newborn infant should receive a single parenteral dose of natural vitamin K_1 oxide (phytonadione [0.5–1 mg]) to prevent vitamin K–dependent hemorrhagic disease of the newborn. Oral administration of vitamin K has not been shown to be as efficacious as parenteral administration for the prevention of late hemorrhagic disease. This dose should be administered shortly after birth but may be delayed until after the first breastfeeding.

- *Hepatitis B vaccination*: Early hepatitis B immunization is recommended for all medically stable infants with a birth weight >2 kg.

- *Assessment of feeding*: Breastfeeding, including observation of position, latch, and milk transfer, should be evaluated by a trained caregiver. The mother should be encouraged to record the time and duration of each feeding, as well as urine and stool output, during the early days of breastfeeding.

- *Screening for hyperbilirubinemia*: Infants whose mothers are Rh negative should have cord blood sent for a Coombs direct antibody test; if the mother's blood type is O, the cord blood may be tested for the infant's blood type and direct antibody test, but it is not required provided that there is appropriate surveillance, risk assessment, and follow-up.[16] All newborn infants should be assessed for risk of hyperbilirubinemia and undergo bilirubin screening between 24 and 48 hours. The bilirubin value should be plotted on the hour-specific nomogram to determine the risk of severe hyperbilirubinemia and the need for repeat determinations.[13]

- *Universal newborn screening*: Every newborn infant should undergo universal newborn screening in accordance with individual state mandates, with the first blood specimen ideally collected between 24 and 48 hours of age. (A list of conditions for which screening is performed in each state is maintained online by the National Newborn Screening and Genetic Resource Center, available at http://genes-r-us.uthscsa.edu/resources/consumer/statemap.htm.)

- *Hearing screening*: The newborn infant's initial caregiver should ensure that the hearing of any infant born outside the hospital setting is screened by 1 month of age, in accordance with AAP recommendations.

- *Provision of follow-up care*: Comprehensive documentation and communication with the follow-up provider are essential. Written records should describe prenatal care, delivery, and immediate postnatal course, clearly documenting which screenings and medications have been provided by the birth attendant, and which remain to be performed. All newborn infants should be evaluated by a health care professional who is knowledgeable and experienced in pediatrics within 24 hours of birth and subsequently within 48 hours of

that first evaluation. The initial follow-up visit should include infant weight and physical examination, especially for jaundice and hydration. If the mother is breastfeeding, the visit should include evaluation of any maternal history of breast problems (eg, pain or engorgement), infant elimination patterns, and a formal observed evaluation of breastfeeding, including position, latch, and milk transfer. The results of maternal and neonatal laboratory tests should be reviewed; clinically indicated tests, such as serum bilirubin, should be performed; and screening tests should be completed in accordance with state regulations. Screening for congenital heart disease should be performed by using oxygen saturation testing as recommended by the AAP.[17]

CONCLUSIONS

The AAP concurs with the recent position statement of the ACOG, affirming that hospitals and birthing centers are the safest settings for birth in the United States, while respecting the right of women to make a medically informed decision about delivery.[7] In addition, the AAP in concert with the ACOG does not support the provision of care by lay midwives or other midwives who are not certified by the American Midwifery Certification Board.[7]

Regardless of the circumstances of his or her birth, including location, every newborn infant deserves health care

that adheres to the standards highlighted in this statement and more completely described in other AAP publications.[11–16] The goal of providing high-quality care to all newborn infants can best be achieved through continuing efforts by all participating providers and institutions to develop and sustain communications and understanding on the basis of professional interaction and mutual respect throughout the health care system.

LEAD AUTHOR

Kristi L. Watterberg, MD

COMMITTEE ON FETUS AND NEWBORN, 2012–2013

Lu-Ann Papile, MD, Chairperson
Jill E. Baley, MD
William Benitz, MD
James Cummings, MD
Waldemar A. Carlo, MD
Eric Eichenwald, MD
Praveen Kumar, MD
Richard A. Polin, MD
Rosemarie C. Tan, MD, PhD

PAST COMMITTEE MEMBER

Kristi L. Watterberg, MD

LIAISONS

Capt. Wanda Denise Barfield, MD, MPH – *Centers for Disease Control and Prevention*
George Macones, MD – *American College of Obstetricians and Gynecologists*
Ann L. Jefferies, MD – *Canadian Pediatric Society*
Erin L. Keels, APRN, MS, NNP-BC – *National Association of Neonatal Nurses*
Tonse N. K. Raju, MD, DCH – *National Institutes of Health*
Kasper S. Wang, MD – *Section on Surgery*

STAFF

Jim Couto, MA

REFERENCES

1. MacDorman MF, Mathews TJ, Declercq E. Home births in the United States, 1990–2009. *NCHS Data Brief.* 2012;Jan(84):1–8
2. Ravelli AC, Jager KJ, de Groot MH, et al. Travel time from home to hospital and adverse perinatal outcomes in women at term in the Netherlands. *BJOG.* 2011;118(4):457–465
3. Malloy MH. Infant outcomes of certified nurse midwife attended home births: United States 2000 to 2004. *J Perinatol.* 2010;30(9):622–627
4. Chang JJ, Macones GA. Birth outcomes of planned home births in Missouri: a population-based study. *Am J Perinatol.* 2011;28(7):529–536
5. Wax JR, Lucas FL, Lamont M, Pinette MG, Cartin A, Blackstone J. Maternal and newborn

outcomes in planned home birth vs planned hospital births: a meta-analysis [published correction appears in *Am J Obstet Gynecol.* 2011;204(4):e7–e13]. *Am J Obstet Gynecol.* 2010;203(3):243.e1–243.e8

6. Janssen PA, Saxell L, Page LA, Klein MC, Liston RM, Lee SK. Outcomes of planned home birth with registered midwife versus planned hospital birth with midwife or physician [published correction appears in *CMAJ.* 2009;181(9):617]. *CMAJ.* 2009;181(6–7):377–383

7. ACOG Committee on Obstetric Practice. ACOG Committee opinion no. 476: planned home birth [published correction appears in *Obstet Gynecol.* 2011;117(5):1232]. *Obstet Gynecol.* 2011;117(2 pt 1):425–428

8. Lindgren HE, Rådestad IJ, Hildingsson IM. Transfer in planned home births in Sweden—effects on the experience of birth: a nationwide population-based study. *Sex Reprod Healthc.* 2011;2(3):101–105

9. Symon A, Winter C, Inkster M, Donnan PT. Outcomes for births booked under an independent midwife and births in NHS maternity units: matched comparison study. *BMJ.* 2009;Jun 11(338):b2060

10. Kattwinkel J, Perlman JM, Aziz K, et al; American Heart Association. Neonatal resuscitation: 2010 American Heart Association guidelines for cardiopulmonary resuscitation and emergency cardiovascular care. *Pediatrics.* 2010;126(5). Available at: www.pediatrics.org/cgi/content/full/126/5/e1400

11. American Academy of Pediatrics; American College of Obstetricians and Gynecologists. Care of the newborn. In: Riley LE, Stark AR, Kilpatrick SJ, Papile L-A, eds. *Guidelines for Perinatal Care.* 7th ed. Elk Grove Village, IL: American Academy of Pediatrics; 2012:265–320

12. American Academy of Pediatrics Committee on Fetus and Newborn. Hospital stay for healthy term newborns. *Pediatrics.* 2010;125(2):405–409

13. American Academy of Pediatrics; American College of Obstetricians and Gynecologists. Neonatal complications and management of high-risk infants. In: Riley LE, Stark AR, Kilpatrick SJ, Papile L-A, eds. *Guidelines for Perinatal Care.* 7th ed. Elk Grove Village, IL: American Academy of Pediatrics; 2012:321–382

14. Baker CJ, Byington CL, Polin RA; Committee on Infectious Diseases; Committee on Fetus and Newborn. Policy statement—recommendations for the prevention of perinatal group B streptococcal (GBS) disease. *Pediatrics.* 2011;128(3):611–616

15. Adamkin DH; Committee on Fetus and Newborn. Postnatal glucose homeostasis in late-preterm and term infants. *Pediatrics.* 2011;127(3):575–579

16. American Academy of Pediatrics Subcommittee on Hyperbilirubinemia. Management of hyperbilirubinemia in the newborn infant 35 or more weeks of gestation [published correction appears in *Pediatrics.* 2004;114(4):1138]. *Pediatrics.* 2004;114(1):297–316

17. Kemper AR, Mahle WT, Martin GR, et al. Strategies for implementing screening for critical congenital heart disease. *Pediatrics.* 2011;128(5). Available at: www.pediatrics.org/cgi/content/full/128/5/e1259

American Academy
of Pediatrics

DEDICATED TO THE HEALTH OF ALL CHILDREN™

CLINICAL REPORT

Safe Transportation of Preterm and Low Birth Weight Infants at Hospital Discharge

Guidance for the Clinician in Rendering Pediatric Care

Marilyn J. Bull, MD, William A. Engle, MD, the Committee on Injury, Violence, and Poison Prevention and the Committee on Fetus and Newborn

ABSTRACT

Safe transportation of preterm and low birth weight infants requires special considerations. Both physiologic immaturity and low birth weight must be taken into account to properly position such infants. This clinical report provides guidelines for pediatricians and other caregivers who counsel parents of preterm and low birth weight infants about car safety seats. *Pediatrics* 2009;123:1424–1429

www.pediatrics.org/cgi/doi/10.1542/peds.2009-0559

doi:10.1542/peds.2009-0559

All clinical reports from the American Academy of Pediatrics automatically expire 5 years after publication unless reaffirmed, revised, or retired at or before that time.

The guidance in this report does not indicate an exclusive course of treatment or serve as a standard of medical care. Variations, taking into account individual circumstances, may be appropriate. This document is copyrighted and is property of the American Academy of Pediatrics and its Board of Directors. All authors have filed conflict-of-interest statements with the American Academy of Pediatrics. Any conflicts have been resolved through a process approved by the Board of Directors. The American Academy of Pediatrics has neither solicited nor accepted any commercial involvement in the development of the content of this publication.

Key Words
safe transportation, preterm, premature, low birth weight, car safety seats, car beds

Abbreviation
FMVSS—Federal Motor Vehicle Safety Standard

PEDIATRICS (ISSN Numbers: Print, 0031-4005; Online, 1098-4275). Copyright © 2009 by the American Academy of Pediatrics

INTRODUCTION

Improved survival rates and earlier discharge of preterm (<37 weeks' gestation at birth) and low birth weight (<2500 g at birth) infants have increased the number of small infants who are being transported in private vehicles. Car safety seats that are used correctly are 71% effective in preventing fatalities attributable to passenger car crashes in infants.[1] To ensure that preterm and low birth weight infants are transported safely, the proper selection and use of car safety seats or car beds are necessary.

Federal Motor Vehicle Safety Standard (FMVSS) 213, which establishes design and dynamic performance requirements for child-restraint systems, applies to children weighing up to 65 lb. However, the standard has no minimum weight limit and does not address the relative hypotonia and risk of airway obstruction in preterm or low birth weight infants. Most rear-facing car safety seats are designated by the manufacturer for use by infants weighing more than 4 or 5 lb, with some designated for use from birth regardless of weight.

Infant dummies as small as 3.3 lb have been shown to be satisfactorily restrained in standard rear-facing car safety seats during crash tests.[2,3] Test dummies, however, cannot replicate the airway and tone variables that occur in preterm infants, and there is no information on restraint of infants who weigh less than 3.3 lb (1.5 kg).

Rear-facing car safety seats provide the best protection in a frontal crash, because the forces are transferred from the back of the restraint to the infant's back, the strongest part of an infant's body. The restraint also supports the infant's head. Severe tensile forces on the neck in flexion are also prevented by use of rear-facing car safety seats.[4]

The long-term experience and documented protective value of car safety seats make them the preferred choice for travel for all infants who can maintain cardiorespiratory stability in the semireclined position.[4] A car bed that meets FMVSS 213 may be indicated for infants who manifest apnea, bradycardia, or low oxygen saturation when positioned semireclined in a car safety seat.[2,5] Of note, some preterm and term infants positioned in car beds and car safety seats seem to have similar rates of apnea, bradycardia, and oxygen desaturation.[6,7]

A car bed is designed to accommodate an infant in a fully reclined position and is oriented in the vehicle seat perpendicular to the direction of travel. An infant is secured in the car bed with an internal harness, and the car bed is secured to the vehicle with the vehicle's seat belt. Car beds, like car safety seats, have specific weight requirements designated by the manufacturer and, like car safety seats, should be used according to manufacturer recommendations.

The size of the infant, especially for those born preterm, is an important consideration when selecting a car safety seat or car bed.[2,8] Weight, length, neurologic maturation, and associated medical conditions (especially bronchopulmonary dysplasia) all influence the potential risk of respiratory compromise for infants in seating devices.[6,9]

Preterm infants are subject to an increased risk of oxygen desaturation, apnea, and/or bradycardia,[10] especially when placed in a semireclined position in car safety seats.[5,11–13] Furthermore, frequent cardiorespiratory events and intermittent hypoxia may adversely affect later neurodevelopment, psychosocial behavior, and academic achievement.[14,15] In 1 study, mental development in preterm infants with 5 or more cardiorespiratory events during 210 hours or more of cardiorespiratory monitoring was associated with a lower mental development index on the Bayley Scales of Infant Development (95.8 vs 100.4; $P = .04$)[14]; physical developmental indices were not different (94.4 vs 91.7; $P = .37$). It is unclear whether the association of cardiorespiratory events and lower mental development reflects an underlying abnormality or a negative consequence of the events. It is rational, if practical, to attempt to reduce the frequency and severity of cardiorespiratory events experienced by preterm infants seated in car safety seats to minimize potential neurodevelopmental sequelae. Therefore, car safety seat monitoring in the infant's own car safety seat before discharge from the hospital should be considered for all infants less than 37 weeks' gestation at birth to determine if physiologic maturity and stable cardiorespiratory function are present, as recommended in the American Academy of Pediatrics publication *Guidelines for Perinatal Care*.[16] Because information is limited about the severity and frequency of adverse outcomes in preterm infants who experience cardiorespiratory events, including those events that occur while in car safety seats, additional research is needed.[17]

Many infants are discharged from the hospital with cardiac/apnea monitors, supplemental oxygen, and, occasionally, portable ventilators, suction machines, batteries, and other equipment. These objects are heavy and could cause injury if they were to hit the child or another vehicle occupant in the event of a sudden stop or crash. Although there is no commercially available securement system for portable medical equipment, restraint is recommended.[18]

No data are available to establish a specific age or neurodevelopmental status at which an infant with respiratory compromise who was discharged from the hospital in a car bed can safely transition to a semireclined car safety seat. Before discontinuing use of a car bed, the physician can consider arranging for a follow-up study to determine when the infant can travel semireclined without apnea, bradycardia, or oxygen desaturation. The time to perform the test may vary depending on the rate of growth and neurologic maturation of the infant and the infant's respiratory status and should be determined by the treating physician.

Car safety seats are used frequently for positioning infants for purposes other than travel. Potential detrimental effects of excessive use of infant seating devices, including exacerbation of gastroesophageal reflux and potentiation of plagiocephaly, have been documented.[19,20] Use of car safety seats for purposes other than travel also may increase the risk of adverse cardiorespiratory and other adverse medical events.

CLINICAL IMPLICATIONS

Several important considerations for transportation of preterm and low birth weight infants at risk for recurrent oxygen desaturation, apnea, or bradycardia include the following.

1. The increased frequency of oxygen desaturation and episodes of apnea or bradycardia while sitting in car safety seats suggests that preterm infants should have a period of observation in a car safety seat, preferably their own, before hospital discharge. This period of observation should be performed with the infant carefully positioned for optimal restraint and the car safety seat placed at an angle that is approved for use in the vehicle. A period of observation for a minimum of 90 to 120 minutes or the duration of travel, whichever is longer, is suggested.[5,6,11,21]

2. Hospital staff who are trained in positioning infants properly in the car safety seat and in detecting apnea, bradycardia, and oxygen desaturation should conduct the car safety seat observation.

3. Hospitals should develop protocols to include car safety seat observation before discharge for infants born at less than 37 weeks' gestation.[22] Some hospital protocols include car safety seat observations for infants at risk of obstructive apnea, bradycardia, or oxygen desaturation other than those born at less than 37 weeks' gestation. Examples include infants with hypotonia (eg, Down syndrome or congenital neuromuscular disorders), infants with micrognathia (Pierre Robin sequence), and infants who have undergone congenital heart surgery.[9]

4. Families should be taught by trained hospital staff how to position the infant properly in the car safety seat.

5. The duration of time the infant is seated in a car safety seat should be minimized. Parents should be advised that car safety seats should be used only for travel.

6. A conventional car safety seat that allows for proper positioning of the preterm infant should be selected if a semiupright position can be maintained safely by the infant. Better observation of the infant may be possible when the child is in a rear-facing car safety seat adjacent to an adult rather than in a car bed. In addition, the protection provided by a rear-facing car safety seat is better documented than the protection provided by car beds.[4]

7. If events documented on cardiorespiratory monitoring in a car safety seat are deemed significant by the treating physician or the hospital policy, interventions to reduce the frequency of desaturation and episodes of apnea and bradycardia are recommended (eg, use of car bed; supplemental oxygen; continued hospitalization or further medical assessment). If a car bed is considered, a similar period of cardiorespiratory monitoring while the infant is in the car bed should be performed before discharge.

8. Infants with documented oxygen desaturation, apnea, or bradycardia in a semiupright position should travel in a supine or prone position in an FMVSS 213–approved car bed after an observation period

that is free of such events as described in point 1 above. This may need to be revised as new evidence becomes available from future research. Specific information regarding currently available car beds can be obtained from several resources.[23]

9. Before transitioning from a car bed, a period of observation of an infant for apnea, bradycardia, and oxygen desaturation in the infant's own semireclined car safety seat should be considered. The study can be performed as a home oxypneumocardiogram, as an outpatient polysomnogram, or as an observed outpatient clinical evaluation performed similarly to that described in point 1 above.

10. Infants at risk of respiratory compromise in car safety seats may be at similar risk with use of other upright equipment, including infant swings, infant seats, backpacks, slings, and infant carriers. Consideration should also be given to limiting the use of these devices until the child's respiratory status in a semireclined position is stable.[24]

11. Infants for whom home cardiac and apnea monitors are prescribed should use this monitoring equipment during travel and have portable, self-contained power available for at least twice the duration of the expected transport time.

12. Commercially available securement systems for portable medical equipment such as monitors are not available; therefore, this equipment should be wedged on the floor or under the vehicle seat to minimize the risk of it becoming a dangerous projectile in the event of a crash or sudden stop.[2,8]

Proper positioning of preterm and low birth weight infants in car safety seats is important for minimizing the risk of respiratory compromise. Specific national guidance for selecting car safety seats and positioning preterm and low birth weight infants includes the following.

1. Infants should ride facing the rear as long as possible and to the highest weight and length allowed by the manufacturer of the seat for greatest protection.[25-27] By the time infants weigh 20 lb or reach the top length allowed by the manufacturer of the seat, they should ride facing the rear in infant seats or convertible car safety seats approved for rear-facing use at higher weights and lengths. Most convertible car safety seats are approved for rear-facing use up to 30 to 35 lb and 36 in. Parents of infants born preterm may benefit from specific counseling about this concept.

2. Infant-only car safety seats with 3-point or 5-point harness systems or convertible car safety seats with 5-point harness systems provide optimum comfort, fit, and positioning for the preterm or low birth weight infant. A small infant should not be placed in a car safety seat with a shield, abdominal pad, or arm rest because of potential breathing difficulty behind the shield or injury to an infant's face and neck during a sudden stop or crash.[2,21]

3. Car safety seats with the shortest distances from the crotch strap to the seat back should be selected to reduce

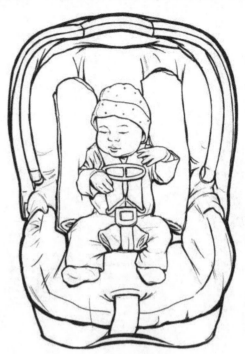

FIGURE 1
Car safety seat with a small cloth between crotch strap and infant, retainer clip positioned at the midpoint of the infant's chest, and blanket rolls on both sides of the infant.

the potential for the infant to slip forward feet-first under the harness (ie, "submarining"). Some car safety seats have crotch-to-seat back distances as short as 5.5 in, which may accommodate some preterm or low birth weight infants well. A small rolled diaper or blanket between the crotch strap and the infant may be added to reduce the risk of submarining (Fig 1) in smaller infants. A car safety seat with multiple harness-strap slots provides more choice and may be more suitable for small but rapidly growing infants. Ideally, car safety seats with harness straps that can be positioned at or below the shoulders should be selected.[21]

4. The infant should be properly positioned in the car safety seat, with buttocks and back flat against the back of the car safety seat. The harness must be snug, and the car safety seat's retainer clip should be positioned at the midpoint of the infant's chest, not on the abdomen or in front of the neck (Fig 1).

5. Some car safety seats come with head-support systems as standard equipment. Many head-support systems, however, are sold as aftermarket products and may decrease the safety provided by the seat and harness system, because they introduce slack into harness straps. Only products that come with the seat or are sold by the manufacturer for use with their specific seat should be used. Most very small infants require positioning support in addition to the head support that comes with the seat. Blanket rolls may be placed on both sides of the infant to provide lateral support for the head and trunk (Fig 1).

6. The rear-facing car safety seat should be reclined approximately 45° or as directed by the instructions

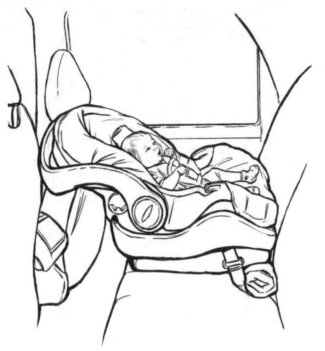

FIGURE 2
Seat with tightly rolled towel to recline seat halfway back at a 45° angle.

provided with the car safety seat. If the vehicle seat slopes and the seat is too upright, the infant's head may fall forward. A lightweight, noncompressible object, such as a tightly rolled blanket or pool "noodle," may be placed under the car safety seat to achieve the appropriate angle. Some car safety seats have built-in angle indicators and angle adjusters to assist with achieving the proper angle (Fig 2).

7. A rear-facing car safety seat should never be placed in the front passenger seat of any vehicle equipped with a passenger-side front air bag because of risk of death or serious injury from the impact of the air bag. In some vehicles without rear seating positions, the air bag can be deactivated when the front seat is used for a child passenger. The back seat is the safest place for all children to travel.[28,29]

8. Infants riding in the rear seat may be more difficult to observe, and whenever possible, parents should arrange for an adult to be seated in the rear seat adjacent to the infant. In the event of a monitor alarm, if a second caregiver is not available, the driver may need to come safely to a stop and assess the infant.

9. An infant should never be left unattended in a car safety seat inside or out of the car.

RESEARCH IMPLICATIONS

1. Studies are needed to gather more information on the severity and frequency of adverse outcomes in preterm infants who experience cardiorespiratory events, including those events that occur while in car safety seats.

2. Studies need to be conducted to determine the risk factors associated with cardiorespiratory events among preterm and low birth weight infants and criteria that indicate neurodevelopmental and physiologic maturity required for an infant to be positioned upright without respiratory compromise.

3. Studies should be designed to assess the correlation of car safety seat monitoring performed in the hospital, while stationary in the car, and while traveling.

4. Methods should be developed to better determine the relative protection provided by rear-facing car safety seats and car beds.

5. Design of car safety seats should be encouraged to specifically meet the positioning and transportation needs of preterm and low birth weight infants.

6. Methods should be developed to better secure heavy medical equipment, such as monitors and oxygen, in vehicles.

7. The efficacy of various protocols for car safety seat monitoring and car safety seats for different patient populations of at-risk infants needs to be determined.

SUMMARY

Proper selection and use of car safety seats or car beds are important for ensuring that preterm and low birth weight infants are transported as safely as possible.

The increased frequency of oxygen desaturation or episodes of apnea or bradycardia experienced by preterm and low birth weight infants positioned semireclined in car safety seats may expose them to increased risk of cardiorespiratory events and adverse neurodevelopmental outcomes.

It is suggested that preterm infants should have a period of observation of 90 to 120 minutes (or longer, if time for travel home will exceed this amount) in a car safety seat before hospital discharge. Educating parents about the proper positioning of preterm and low birth weight infants in car safety seats is important for minimizing the risk of respiratory compromise. Providing observation and avoiding extended periods in car safety seats for vulnerable infants and using car seats only for travel should also minimize risk of adverse events.

COMMITTEE ON INJURY, VIOLENCE AND POISON PREVENTION, 2006–2007
Gary A. Smith, MD, DrPH, Chairperson
Carl R. Baum, MD
M. Denise Dowd, MD, MPH
Dennis R. Durbin, MD, MSCE
Kyran P. Quinlan, MD, MPH
Robert D. Sege, MD, PhD
Michael S. Turner, MD
Jeffrey C. Weiss, MD
Joseph L. Wright, MD, MPH

LIAISONS
Julie Gilchrist, MD
　　Centers for Disease Control and Prevention

Lynne Haverkos, MD, MPH
   Eunice Kennedy Shriver National Institute of Child
   Health and Human Development
Jonathan D. Midgett, PhD
   Consumer Product Safety Commission
Lori Roche
   Health Resources and Services Administration
Alexander "Sandy" Sinclair
   National Highway Traffic Safety Administration
Lynne J. Warda, MD
   Canadian Paediatric Society

STAFF

Bonnie Kozial

COMMITTEE ON FETUS AND NEWBORN, 2006–2007

Ann R. Stark, MD, Chairperson
David H. Adamkin, MD
Daniel G. Batton, MD
Edward F. Bell, MD
Vinod K. Bhutani, MD
Susan E. Denson, MD
Gilbert I. Martin, MD
Kristi L. Watterberg, MD

LIAISONS

Keith J. Barrington, MD
   Canadian Paediatric Society
Gary D. V. Hankins, MD
   American College of Obstetrics and Gynecology
Tonse N. K. Raju, MD
   National Institutes of Health
Kay M. Tomashek, MD
   Centers for Disease Control and Prevention
Carol Wallman, MSN, RNC, NNP
   National Association of Neonatal Nurses and
   Association of Women's Health, Obstetric and
   Neonatal Nurses

STAFF

Jim Couto, MA

REFERENCES

1. National Highway Traffic Administration. *Research Note: Revised Estimates of Child Restraint Effectiveness*. Washington, DC: US Department of Transportation, National Center for Statistics and Analysis; 1996. Available at: www.nhtsa.dot.gov/portal/site/nhtsa/menuitem.e649cd1b2b018c7d8eca01046108a0c/. Accessed March 10, 2008
2. Bull M, Weber K, Stroup K. Automotive restraint systems for premature infants. *J Pediatr*. 1988;112(3):385–388
3. National Center for Safe Transportation of Children With Special Needs. Child Restraint System Test Results. Available at: www.preventinjury.org/uploads/researchinfo/ResearchInfo_11.pdf. Accessed April 9, 2009
4. Weber K. Crash protection for child passengers: a review of best practice. *UMTRI Res Rev*. 2000;31(3):1–28
5. Willett LD, Leuschen MP, Nelson LS, Nelson RM Jr. Risk of hypoventilation in premature infants in car seats. *J Pediatr*. 1986;109(2):245–248
6. Salhab WA, Khattak A, Tyson JE, et al. Car seat or car bed for very low birth weight infants at discharge home. *J Pediatr*. 2007;150(3):224–228
7. Kinane TB, Murphy J, Bass JL, Corwin MJ. Comparison of respiratory physiologic features when infants are placed in car safety seats or car beds [published correction appears in *Pediatrics*. 2006;118(5):2270]. *Pediatrics*. 2006;118(2):522–527
8. Bull MJ, Stroup KB. Premature infants in car seats. *Pediatrics*. 1985;75(2):336–339
9. Simsic JM, Masterson K, Kogon BE, Kirshbom PM, Kanter K. Pre-hospital discharge car safety seat testing in infants after congenital heart surgery. *Pediatr Cardiol*. 2008;29(1):142–145
10. Ramanathan R, Corwin MJ, Hunt CE, et al. Cardiorespiratory events recorded on home monitors: comparison of healthy infants with those at increased risk for SIDS. *JAMA*. 2001;285(17):2199–2207
11. Willett LD, Leuschen MP, Nelson LS, Nelson RM Jr. Ventilatory changes in convalescent infants positioned in car seats. *J Pediatr*. 1989;115(3):451–455
12. Merchant JR, Worwa C, Porter S, Coleman JM, deRegnier RA. Respiratory instability of term and near-term healthy newborn infants in car safety seats. *Pediatrics*. 2001;108(3):647–652
13. Bass JL, Mehta KA, Camara J. Monitoring premature infants in car seats: implementing the American Academy of Pediatrics policy in a community hospital. *Pediatrics*. 1993;91(6):1137–1141
14. Hunt CE, Corwin MJ, Baird T, et al. Cardiorespiratory events detected by home memory monitoring and one-year neurodevelopmental outcome. *J Pediatr*. 2004;145(4):465–471
15. Bass JL, Corwin M, Gozal D, et al. The effect of chronic or intermittent hypoxia on cognition in childhood: a review of the evidence. *Pediatrics*. 2004;114(3):805–816
16. American Academy of Pediatrics; American College of Obstetricians and Gynecologists. Neonatal complications. In: *Guidelines for Perinatal Care*. 6th ed. Washington DC: American College of Obstetricians and Gynecologists; 2007:251–301
17. Côté A, Bairam A, Deschenes M, Hatzakis G. Sudden infant deaths in sitting devices. *Arch Dis Child*. 2008;93(5):384–389
18. American Academy of Pediatrics, Committee on Injury and Poison Prevention. Transporting children with special health care needs. *Pediatrics*. 1999;104(4 pt 1):988–992
19. Callahan CW. Increased gastroesophageal reflux in infants: can history provide an explanation? *Acta Paediatr*. 1998;87(12):1219–1223
20. Orenstein SR, Whittington PF, Orenstein DM. The infant seat as treatment for gastroesophageal reflux. *N Engl J Med*. 1983;309(13):760–763
21. National Highway Traffic Safety Administration. National Standardized Child Passenger Safety Training Program. Available at: www.safekids.org/certification/index.html. Accessed March 12, 2008
22. American Academy of Pediatrics, Committee on Injury and Poison Prevention. Safe transportation of newborns at hospital discharge. *Pediatrics*. 1999;104(4 pt 1):986–987
23. National Center for Safe Transportation of Children With Special Needs. Special Needs Transportation: Restraints. Available at: www.preventinjury.org/SNTrestraints.asp. Accessed March 12, 2008
24. Stening W, Nitsch P, Wassmer G, Roth B. Cardiorespiratory stability of premature and term infants carried in infant slings. *Pediatrics*. 2002;110(5):879–883
25. American Academy of Pediatrics, Committee on Injury and Poison Prevention. Selecting and using the most appropriate car safety seats for growing children: guidelines for counseling parents. *Pediatrics*. 2002;109(3):550–553

26. Henary B, Sherwood C, Crandall J, et al. Car safety seats for children: rear facing for best protection. *Inj Prev.* 2007;13(6): 398–402

27. National Highway Traffic Safety Administration. Child Passenger Safety: A Parent's Primer. Available at: www.nhtsa.gov/ staticfiles/DOT/NHTSA/Traffic%20Injury%20Control/Articles/ Associated%20Files/4StepsFlyer.pdf. Accessed April 9, 2009

28. Braver ER, Whitifield R, Ferguson SA. Seating positions and children's risk of dying in motor vehicle crashes. *Inj Prev.* 1998;4(3):181–187

29. Durbin D, Chen I, Smith R, Elliott M, Winston F. Effects of seating position and appropriate restraint use on the risk of injury to children in motor vehicle crashes. *Pediatrics.* 2005;115(3). Available at: www.pediatrics.org/cgi/content/full/115/3/e305

CLINICAL REPORT   Guidance for the Clinician in Rendering Pediatric Care

American Academy
of Pediatrics

DEDICATED TO THE HEALTH OF ALL CHILDREN™

Umbilical Cord Care in the Newborn Infant

Dan Stewart, MD, FAAP, William Benitz, MD, FAAP, COMMITTEE ON FETUS AND NEWBORN

abstract

Postpartum infections remain a leading cause of neonatal morbidity and mortality worldwide. A high percentage of these infections may stem from bacterial colonization of the umbilicus, because cord care practices vary in reflection of cultural traditions within communities and disparities in health care practices globally. After birth, the devitalized umbilical cord often proves to be an ideal substrate for bacterial growth and also provides direct access to the bloodstream of the neonate. Bacterial colonization of the cord not infrequently leads to omphalitis and associated thrombophlebitis, cellulitis, or necrotizing fasciitis. Various topical substances continue to be used for cord care around the world to mitigate the risk of serious infection. More recently, particularly in high-resource countries, the treatment paradigm has shifted toward dry umbilical cord care. This clinical report reviews the evidence underlying recommendations for care of the umbilical cord in different clinical settings.

DOI: 10.1542/peds.2016-2149

PEDIATRICS (ISSN Numbers: Print, 0031-4005; Online, 1098-4275).

Copyright © 2016 by the American Academy of Pediatrics

FINANCIAL DISCLOSURE: The authors have indicated they do not have a financial relationship relevant to this article to disclose.

FUNDING: No external funding.

POTENTIAL CONFLICT OF INTEREST: The authors have indicated they have no potential conflicts of interest to disclose.

To cite: Stewart D, Benitz W, AAP COMMITTEE ON FETUS AND NEWBORN. Umbilical Cord Care in the Newborn Infant. *Pediatrics.* 2016;138(3):e20162149

INTRODUCTION

Despite significant global progress in recent decades,[1] bacterial infections (sepsis, meningitis, and pneumonia) continue to account for approximately 700 000 neonatal deaths each year, or nearly one-quarter of the 3 million neonatal deaths that occur worldwide.[1,2] Although the magnitude of its contribution to these deaths remains uncertain, the umbilical cord may be a common portal of entry for invasive pathogenic bacteria,[3] with or without clinical signs of omphalitis. Neonatal mortality associated with bacterial contamination of the umbilical stump may therefore rank among the greatest public health opportunities of the 21st century.

Common risk factors for the development of neonatal omphalitis include unplanned home birth or septic delivery, low birth weight, prolonged rupture of membranes, umbilical catheterization, and chorioamnionitis.[4,5] In countries with limited resources, the risk of omphalitis may be 6 times greater for infants delivered at home than for hospital births.[6] Multiple studies have delineated the susceptibility of the umbilical cord to bacterial colonization. The method of caring for the umbilical cord after birth affects both bacterial colonization and time to cord separation.[7-10] The devitalized umbilical cord provides an ideal medium for bacterial growth. Sources of potentially pathogenic bacteria that colonize the umbilical cord include the mother's birth canal and various local bacterial sources at the site of delivery, most prominently the nonsterile hands of any person assisting with the delivery.[11] *Staphylococcus aureus* remains the most frequently reported organism.[5-7,12] Other common pathogens include group A and group B *Streptococci* and Gram-negative bacilli including *Escherichia coli*, *Klebsiella* species, and *Pseudomonas* species. Rarely, anaerobic and polymicrobial infections also may occur. In addition to omphalitis, tetanus in neonates can result from umbilical cord colonization, particularly in countries with limited resources. This infection results from contamination of the umbilical separation site by *Clostridium tetani* acquired from a nonsterile device used to separate the umbilical cord during the peripartum period or from application of unhygienic substances to the cord stump.

Multiple complications can occur from bacterial colonization and infection of the umbilical cord because of its direct access to the bloodstream. These complications include the development of intraabdominal abscesses, periumbilical cellulitis, thrombophlebitis in the portal and/or umbilical veins, peritonitis, and bowel ischemia.[13-16] Neonatal omphalitis may present at 4 grades of severity: (1) funisitis/umbilical discharge (an unhealthy-appearing cord with purulent, malodorous discharge), (2) omphalitis with abdominal wall cellulitis (periumbilical erythema and tenderness in addition to an unhealthy-appearing cord with

discharge), (3) omphalitis with systemic signs of infection, and (4) omphalitis with necrotizing fasciitis (umbilical necrosis with periumbilical ecchymosis, crepitus, bullae, and evidence of involvement of superficial and deep fascia; frequently associated with signs and symptoms of overwhelming sepsis and shock).[6]

The incidence of omphalitis reported in different communities varies greatly, depending on prenatal and perinatal practices, cultural variations in cord care, and delivery venue (home versus hospital). Reliable current data on rates in untreated infants are surprisingly scant. In high-resource countries, neonatal omphalitis now is rare, with an estimated incidence of approximately 1 per 1000 infants managed with dry cord care (eg, a total of 3 cases among 3518 infants described in 2 reports from Canada[17,18]). In low-income communities, omphalitis occurs in up to 8% of infants born in hospitals and in as many as 22% of infants born at home, in whom omphalitis is moderate to severe in 17% and associated with sepsis in 2%.[19] Depending on how omphalitis is defined, case-fatality rates as high as 13% have been reported.[4] The development of necrotizing fasciitis, with predictable complications from septic shock, is associated with much higher case-mortality rates.[5] These disparate observations in different settings have resulted in divergent recommendations for cord care by the World Health Organization (WHO), which advocates dry cord care for infants born in a hospital or in settings of low neonatal mortality and application of chlorhexidine solution or gel for infants born at home or in settings of high neonatal mortality.[20]

EVIDENCE-BASED PRACTICE

Best practices for antisepsis of the umbilical cord continue to remain

somewhat controversial and variable, even in high-resource countries with relatively aseptic conditions at the time of delivery. In resource-limited countries, in accordance with cultural traditions, unhygienic substances continue to be applied to the umbilicus, creating a milieu ideal for the development neonatal omphalitis. To achieve the goal of preventing omphalitis worldwide, deliveries must be clean and umbilical cord care must be hygienic. The cord should be cut with a sterile blade or scissors, preferably using sterile gloves, to prevent bacterial contamination leading to omphalitis or neonatal tetanus. As discussed later, dry cord care without the application of topical substances is preferable under most circumstances in high-resource countries and for in-hospital births elsewhere; the application of topical chlorhexidine is recommended for infants born outside the hospital setting in communities with high neonatal mortality rates.[20]

Methods of umbilical cord care have been the subject of 4 recent meta-analyses,[21-24] including 2 Cochrane reviews.[23,24] Although the scope and methodologies of these reviews differed, all 4 stratified results according to the study setting, distinguishing results reported from communities with high proportions of births at home and high neonatal mortality rates from those obtained in hospitals and settings with low neonatal mortality rates. These analyses concluded that 3 studies (including >44 000 subjects) in community settings in South Asia with a high neonatal mortality rate[3,25,26] support the effectiveness of application of 4% chlorhexidine solution or gel to the umbilical cord stump within 24 hours after birth, which results in a significant reduction in both omphalitis (relative risk [RR]: 0.48; 95% confidence interval [CI]: 0.40–0.57) and neonatal mortality

(RR: 0.81; 95% CI: 0.71–0.92) compared with dry cord care.[24] No other cord-management strategies have been evaluated systematically in such settings, but the application of traditional materials (eg, ash, herbal or other vegetal poultices, and human milk) may provide a source of contamination with pathogenic bacteria, including *C tetani*.[27] In contrast, the meta-analyses found little evidence of benefit from topical treatments for infants born in hospitals.[22-24] The meta-analyses used different criteria for inclusion of trials and compared a variety of treatments versus dry cord care or versus one another. Only a single trial[28] reported mortality data, which did not differ between topical chlorhexidine and dry care (RR: 0.11; 95% CI: 0.01–2.04). However, the low mortality rate and the small contribution made by bacterial infection[29] in these settings provide only a small opportunity for a reduction in mortality rates. In 5 such trials[30-33] analyzed by Karumbi et al,[22] no treatment was found to significantly reduce omphalitis and sepsis when compared against one another, although the sample sizes were small and the evidence was deemed of low quality.[22] The Cochrane review by Imdad et al,[23] which compared a variety of pairs of topical agents, reached similar conclusions. The most recent meta-analysis, by Sinha et al,[24] considered 2 studies[28,34] comparing chlorhexidine with dry cord care. In the first of these, 140 infants admitted to the NICU at a hospital in north India were randomly assigned to receive cord treatment with chlorhexidine solution or dry cord care.[28] Enrollment criteria included gestational age >32 weeks and birth weight >1500 g, but the provided demographic data suggest that the infants were predominantly late-preterm, and they experienced high rates of complications of prematurity (including asphyxia, respiratory distress, mechanical ventilation, and necrotizing enterocolitis). No cases of umbilical sepsis were reported in either group, but culture-proven sepsis was more common in the dry cord care group than in the chlorhexidine group (15 of 70 vs 2 of 70; *P* = .002). These observations cannot be generalized to all healthy infants born in a hospital. The second enrolled 669 subjects, who were randomly assigned to receive treatment with chlorhexidine powder or dry cord care.[34] Cord-related adverse events (erosion, irritation, lesion, omphalitis, erythema, umbilical granuloma, purulence, bleeding, discharge, or weeping of the navel) were more common in the dry cord care group (29% vs 16%; *P* = .001), but there were no differences in serious adverse events (2.1% in both groups) or in the incidence of omphalitis (2.1% vs 0.6%; *P* = .1). Although the meta-analysis reported a significant difference in the pooled risk of omphalitis (RR: 0.48; 95% CI: 0.28–0.84), combining culture-proven sepsis cases[28] with omphalitis cases[34] is not appropriate. This analysis provides only very weak, or perhaps no, evidence for a benefit of chlorhexidine treatment.

Since 1998, the WHO has advocated the use of dry umbilical cord care in high-resource settings.[35] Dry cord care includes keeping the cord clean and leaving it exposed to air or loosely covered by a clean cloth. If it becomes soiled, the remnant of the cord is cleaned with soap and sterile water. In situations in which hygienic conditions are poor and/or infection rates are high, the WHO recommends chlorhexidine.[16]

There is some uncertainty as to the effect of chlorhexidine on mortality when applied to the umbilical cords of newborn infants in the hospital setting, but there is moderate evidence for its effects on infection prevention.[24] Although the application of chlorhexidine is regarded as safe,[35] trace levels of the compound have been detected in the blood of infants after umbilical cord cleaning.[36,37] In addition, contact dermatitis has been reported in up to 15% of very low birth weight infants after placement of a 0.5% chlorhexidine impregnated dressing over a central venous catheter.[38] The data on the safety of chlorhexidine application are incomplete, and the amount of exposure to chlorhexidine that can be considered safe is not known.[24] In addition to the incremental increase in the cost of using chlorhexidine, the practice of reducing bacterial colonization may have the unintended consequences of selecting more virulent bacterial strains without demonstrable benefits.[24] Because the incidence of omphalitis is very low in high-resource countries and the severity is mild, the preponderance of evidence favors dry cord care.

PROMOTING NONPATHOGENIC COLONIZATION OF THE UMBILICAL CORD

Promoting colonization of the umbilical cord by nonpathogenic bacteria may prevent the development of neonatal omphalitis. By allowing neonates to "room-in" with their mothers, one can create an environment conducive for colonization from less pathogenic bacteria acquired from the mother's flora.[39] This type of colonization helps to reduce colonization and infection from potentially pathogenic organisms that are ubiquitous in the hospital environment. Over time, attempts to decrease bacterial colonization with topical antimicrobial agents may actually select for resistant and more pathogenic organisms[35] (level of evidence: III).

IMPLICATIONS FOR CLINICAL PRACTICE

1. Application of select antimicrobial agents to the umbilical cord may be beneficial for infants born at home in resource-limited

countries where the risks of omphalitis and associated sequelae are high.

2. Application of select antimicrobial agents to the umbilical cord does not provide clear benefit in the hospital setting or in high-resource countries, where reducing bacterial colonization may have the unintended consequence of selecting more virulent bacterial strains. In high-resource countries, there has been a shift away from the use of topical antimicrobial agents in umbilical cord care for this reason.

3. For deliveries outside of birthing centers or hospital settings and in resource-limited populations (eg, Native American communities), the application of prophylactic topical antimicrobial agents to the umbilical cord remains appropriate.

4. At the time of discharge, parental education regarding the signs and symptoms of omphalitis might decrease significant morbidities and even associated mortalities.

5. Of paramount importance is the need for all primary care providers to be diligent in reporting infections associated with umbilical cord care. The development of a local reporting system regarding the occurrence of omphalitis and/or its morbidities to the health care providers at the site of delivery will create more robust data, allowing for improvement in treatment paradigms in the future.

LEAD AUTHORS

Dan L. Stewart, MD, FAAP
William E. Benitz, MD, FAAP

COMMITTEE ON FETUS AND NEWBORN, 2015–2016

Kristi L. Watterberg, MD, FAAP, Chairperson
James J. Cummings, MD, FAAP
William E. Benitz, MD, FAAP
Eric C. Eichenwald, MD, FAAP
Brenda B. Poindexter, MD, FAAP

Dan L. Stewart, MD, FAAP
Susan W. Aucott, MD, FAAP
Jay P. Goldsmith, MD, FAAP
Karen M. Puopolo, MD, PhD, FAAP
Kasper S. Wang, MD, FAAP

LIAISONS

Tonse N.K. Raju, MD, DCH, FAAP – *National Institutes of Health*
Wanda D. Barfield, MD, MPH, FAAP – *Centers for Disease Control and Prevention*
Erin L. Keels, APRN, MS, NNP-BC – *National Association of Neonatal Nurses*
Thierry Lacaze, MD – *Canadian Paediatric Society*
Maria Mascola, MD – *American College of Obstetricians and Gynecologists*

STAFF

Jim R. Couto, MA

ABBREVIATIONS

CI: confidence interval
RR: relative risk
WHO: World Health Organization

REFERENCES

1. Lawn JE, Blencowe H, Oza S, et al; Lancet Every Newborn Study Group. Every Newborn: progress, priorities, and potential beyond survival. *Lancet.* 2014;384(9938):189–205

2. Liu L, Johnson HL, Cousens S, et al; Child Health Epidemiology Reference Group of WHO and UNICEF. Global, regional, and national causes of child mortality: an updated systematic analysis for 2010 with time trends since 2000. *Lancet.* 2012;379(9832):2151–2161

3. Mullany LC, Darmstadt GL, Khatry SK, et al. Topical applications of chlorhexidine to the umbilical cord for prevention of omphalitis and neonatal mortality in southern Nepal: a community-based, cluster-randomised trial. *Lancet.* 2006;367(9514):910–918

4. Güvenç H, Aygün AD, Yaşar F, Soylu F, Güvenç M, Kocabay K. Omphalitis in term and preterm appropriate for gestational age and small for gestational age infants. *J Trop Pediatr.* 1997;43(6):368–372

5. Mason WH, Andrews R, Ross LA, Wright HT Jr. Omphalitis in the newborn infant. *Pediatr Infect Dis J.* 1989;8(8):521–525

6. Sawardekar KP. Changing spectrum of neonatal omphalitis. *Pediatr Infect Dis J.* 2004;23(1):22–26

7. Verber IG, Pagan FS. What cord care—if any? *Arch Dis Child.* 1993;68(5 spec no):594–596

8. Ronchera-Oms C, Hernández C, Jimémez NV. Antiseptic cord care reduces bacterial colonization but delays cord detachment. *Arch Dis Child Fetal Neonatal Ed.* 1994;71(1):F70

9. Novack AH, Mueller B, Ochs H. Umbilical cord separation in the normal newborn. *Am J Dis Child.* 1988;142(2):220–223

10. Arad I, Eyal F, Fainmesser P. Umbilical care and cord separation. *Arch Dis Child.* 1981;56(11):887–888

11. Mullany LC, Darmstadt GL, Katz J, et al. Risk factors for umbilical cord infection among newborns of southern Nepal. *Am J Epidemiol.* 2007;165(2):203–211

12. Airede AI. Pathogens in neonatalomphalitis. *J Trop Pediatr.* 1992;38(3):129–131

13. Forshall I. Septic umbilical arteritis. *Arch Dis Child.* 1957;32(161):25–30

14. Lally KP, Atkinson JB, Woolley MM, Mahour GH. Necrotizing fasciitis: a serious sequela of omphalitis in the newborn. *Ann Surg.* 1984;199(1):101–103

15. Monu JU, Okolo AA. Neonatal necrotizing fasciitis—a complication of poor cord hygiene: report of three cases. *Ann Trop Paediatr.* 1990;10(3):299–303

16. Samuel M, Freeman NV, Vaishnav A, Sajwany MJ, Nayar MP. Necrotizing fasciitis: a serious complication of omphalitis in neonates. *J Pediatr Surg.* 1994;29(11):1414–1416

17. Dore S, Buchan D, Coulas S, et al. Alcohol versus natural drying for newborn cord care. *J Obstet Gynecol Neonatal Nurs.* 1998;27(6):621–627

18. Janssen PA, Selwood BL, Dobson SR, Peacock D, Thiessen PN. To dye or not to dye: a randomized, clinical trial of a triple dye/alcohol regime versus dry cord care. *Pediatrics.* 2003;111(1):15–20

19. Mir F, Tikmani SS, Shakoor S, et al. Incidence and etiology of omphalitis

in Pakistan: a community-based cohort study. *J Infect Dev Ctries.* 2011;5(12):828–833

20. World Health Organization. *WHO Recommendations on Postnatal Care of the Mother and Newborn.* Geneva, Switzerland: WHO Press; 2014

21. Imdad A, Mullany LC, Baqui AH, et al. The effect of umbilical cord cleansing with chlorhexidine on omphalitis and neonatal mortality in community settings in developing countries: a meta-analysis. *BMC Public Health.* 2013;13(suppl 3):S3–S15

22. Karumbi J, Mulaku M, Aluvaala J, English M, Opiyo N. Topical umbilical cord care for prevention of infection and neonatal mortality. *Pediatr Infect Dis J.* 2013;32(1):78–83

23. Imdad A, Bautista RM, Senen KA, Uy ME, Mantaring JB III, Bhutta ZA. Umbilical cord antiseptics for preventing sepsis and death among newborns. *Cochrane Database Syst Rev.* 2013;5:CD008635

24. Sinha A, Sazawal S, Pradhan A, Ramji S, Opiyo N. Chlorhexidine skin or cord care for prevention of mortality and infections in neonates. *Cochrane Database Syst Rev.* 2015;3:CD007835

25. Arifeen SE, Mullany LC, Shah R, et al. The effect of cord cleansing with chlorhexidine on neonatal mortality in rural Bangladesh: a community-based, cluster-randomised trial. *Lancet.* 2012;379(9820):1022–1028

26. Soofi S, Cousens S, Imdad A, Bhutto N, Ali N, Bhutta ZA. Topical application of chlorhexidine to neonatal umbilical cords for prevention of omphalitis and neonatal mortality in a rural district of Pakistan: a community-based,

cluster-randomised trial. *Lancet.* 2012;379(9820):1029–1036

27. Mrisho M, Schellenberg JA, Mushi AK, et al. Understanding home-based neonatal care practice in rural southern Tanzania. *Trans R Soc Trop Med Hyg.* 2008;102(7):669–678

28. Gathwala G, Sharma D, Bhakhri B. Effect of topical application of chlorhexidine for umbilical cord care in comparison with conventional dry cord care on the risk of neonatal sepsis: a randomized controlled trial. *J Trop Pediatr.* 2013;59(3):209–213

29. Centers for Disease Control and Prevention. QuickStats: leading causes of neonatal and postneonatal deaths—United States, 2002. *MMWR.* 2005;54(38):966

30. Ahmadpour-Kacho M, Zahedpasha Y, Hajian K, Javadi G, Talebian H. The effect of topical application of human milk, ethyl alcohol 96%, and silver sulfadiazine on umbilical cord separation time in newborn infants. *Arch Iran Med.* 2006;9(1):33–38

31. Erenel AS, Vural G, Efe SY, Ozkan S, Ozgen S, Erenoğlu R. Comparison of olive oil and dry-clean keeping methods in umbilical cord care as microbiological. *Matern Child Health J.* 2010;14(6):999–1004

32. Hsu WC, Yeh LC, Chuang MY, Lo WT, Cheng SN, Huang CF. Umbilical separation time delayed by alcohol application. *Ann Trop Paediatr.* 2010;30(3):219–223

33. Pezzati M, Rossi S, Tronchin M, Dani C, Filippi L, Rubaltelli FF. Umbilical cord care in premature infants: the effect of two different cord-care

regimens (salicylic sugar powder vs chlorhexidine) on cord separation time and other outcomes. *Pediatrics.* 2003;112(4):e275

34. Kapellen TM, Gebauer CM, Brosteanu O, Labitzke B, Vogtmann C, Kiess W. Higher rate of cord-related adverse events in neonates with dry umbilical cord care compared to chlorhexidine powder: results of a randomized controlled study to compare efficacy and safety of chlorhexidine powder versus dry care in umbilical cord care of the newborn. *Neonatology.* 2009;96(1):13–18

35. World Health Organization. *Care of the Umbilical Cord: A Review of the Evidence.* Geneva, Switzerland: World Health Organization; 1998

36. Aggett PJ, Cooper LV, Ellis SH, McAinsh J. Percutaneous absorption of chlorhexidine in neonatal cord care. *Arch Dis Child.* 1981;56(11):878–880

37. Johnsson J, Seeberg S, Kjellmer I. Blood concentrations of chlorhexidine in neonates undergoing routine cord care with 4% chlorhexidine gluconate solution. *Acta Paediatr Scand.* 1987;76(4):675–676

38. Garland JS, Alex CP, Mueller CD, et al. A randomized trial comparing povidone-iodine to a chlorhexidine gluconate-impregnated dressing for prevention of central venous catheter infections in neonates. *Pediatrics.* 2001;107(6):1431–1436

39. Pezzati M, Biagioli EC, Martelli E, Gambi B, Biagiotti R, Rubaltelli FF. Umbilical cord care: the effect of eight different cord-care regimens on cord separation time and other outcomes. *Biol Neonate.* 2002;81(1):38–44

SECTION 2

Newborn Screening

American Academy
of Pediatrics
DEDICATED TO THE HEALTH OF ALL CHILDREN™

CLINICAL REPORT

Newborn Screening Expands: Recommendations for Pediatricians and Medical Homes—Implications for the System

Guidance for the Clinician in Rendering Pediatric Care

Newborn Screening Authoring Committee

ABSTRACT

Advances in newborn screening technology, coupled with recent advances in the diagnosis and treatment of rare but serious congenital conditions that affect newborn infants, provide increased opportunities for positively affecting the lives of children and their families. These advantages also pose new challenges to primary care pediatricians, both educationally and in response to the management of affected infants. Primary care pediatricians require immediate access to clinical and diagnostic information and guidance and have a proactive role to play in supporting the performance of the newborn screening system. Primary care pediatricians must develop office policies and procedures to ensure that newborn screening is conducted and that results are transmitted to them in a timely fashion; they must also develop strategies to use should these systems fail. In addition, collaboration with local, state, and national partners is essential for promoting actions and policies that will optimize the function of the newborn screening systems and ensure that families receive the full benefit of them.

INTRODUCTION

It's another busy day in pediatric practice, even before you receive the telephone call from the state newborn screening program. One of your newborn patients has an out-of-range result* on the screen for a rare but serious congenital condition. "Now what?" you wonder, as you begin to take down the notes. What additional testing is needed? What is the treatment regimen, and when does it begin? What do you tell the parents? And, what do you do about the rest of your schedule?

In the past decade, new technologies have led to a rapid expansion in the number of congenital conditions that are targeted in state newborn screening programs. As newborn screening programs expand, the likelihood increases that individual pediatricians will one day receive an out-of-range screening result for an unfamiliar congenital condition for one of their patients.

In 2005, the American Academy of Pediatrics (AAP) endorsed a report from the American College of Medical Genetics (ACMG), which recommended that all states screen newborn infants for a core panel of 29 treatable congenital conditions and an additional 25 conditions that may be detected by screening (Appendix 1).[1] The Secretary of Health and Human Services' Advisory Committee on Heritable Disorders and Genetic Diseases in Newborns and Children (ACHDGDNC)† also adopted that report. Some states are now screening for more than 50 congenital conditions, many of which are rare and unfamiliar to pediatricians and other

www.pediatrics.org/cgi/doi/10.1542/
peds.2007-3021

doi:10.1542/peds.2007-3021

All clinical reports from the American Academy of Pediatrics automatically expire 5 years after publication unless reaffirmed, revised, or retired at or before that time.

The guidance in this report does not indicate an exclusive course of treatment or serve as a standard of medical care. Variations, taking into account individual circumstances, may be appropriate.

Key Words
newborn screening, genetic disorders, children with special health care needs, medical home

Abbreviations
AAP—American Academy of Pediatrics
ACMG—American College of Medical Genetics
ACHDGDNC—Advisory Committee on Heritable Disorders and Genetic Diseases in Newborns and Children
MCHB—Maternal Child Health Bureau
HRSA—Health Resources and Services Administration
PCP—primary care pediatrician
CPT—*Current Procedural Terminology*
ACOG—American College of Obstetricians and Gynecologists
SNSAC—state newborn screening advisory committee

PEDIATRICS (ISSN Numbers: Print, 0031-4005; Online, 1098-4275). Copyright © 2008 by the American Academy of Pediatrics

---

*A note about language: although physicians often think of screening results as being "normal/abnormal" or "negative/positive," laboratories use the more specific language of "in range" and "out of range" to report results. We felt that it was appropriate to use and promote this language for the sake of clarity and consistency. For ease of reading, we use "parent" as a generic term to connote the adult who is responsible for a child's health care; we recognize that adults other than the biological parent may serve in this role. Where implications of congenital disorders are discussed, these obviously affect only those persons who are related biologically. In some circumstances, a primary care physician may suggest that the biological parent be contacted regarding congenital conditions, even if that parent is not the current primary caregiver for the child.

†A federal advisory committee to the Secretary of Health and Human Services, the ACHDGDNC advises and guides the Secretary regarding the most appropriate application of universal newborn screening tests, technologies, policies, guidelines, and programs for effectively reducing morbidity and mortality in newborns and children having or being at risk for heritable disorders.

primary health care professionals. In the foreseeable future, screening programs will likely adopt screening technologies that will further expand the number of conditions screened and tests offered.

The ACMG, with the support of the Health Resources and Services Administration (HRSA) Maternal and Child Health Bureau (MCHB), has developed and maintains Web-based resources it calls action (ACT) sheets to guide pediatricians through preliminary responses to out-of-range newborn screening results. These brief reference resources provide a focused, single-page summary of differential diagnoses, descriptions of the condition, actions to be taken by the pediatrician, diagnostic evaluation, clinical considerations, reporting requirements, and links to additional resources. ACT sheets are designed to be supplemented by state-specific information regarding referral resources. Many state-program Web sites have additional program-specific educational information; links to these program Web sites are readily accessible through an interactive map maintained by the National Newborn Screening and Genetics Resource Center (http://genes-r-us.uthscsa.edu/resources/consumer/statemap.htm).

Advances in newborn screening technologies and the availability of resources such as ACT sheets are aimed at improving health outcomes for affected children. To optimize this potential, primary care pediatricians (PCPs) must effectively engage the newborn screening program in their state. PCPs who treat patients who routinely cross state borders for care will likely engage multiple newborn screening programs.

The primary goals of this statement are to:

- delineate the responsibilities of PCPs and pediatric medical subspecialists within the newborn screening program;

- introduce 2 algorithms that, together, outline a clear and efficient pathway through the process of fulfilling those responsibilities; and

- outline resources that will support PCPs in addressing these responsibilities.

In addition to these primary goals, this statement addresses the steps that individual PCPs and practices must take to prepare for these responsibilities. We also recognize the significant roles other health care professionals and agencies have on the newborn screening system and identify ways these other entities can support PCPs and improve newborn screening and, therefore, advance improved health outcomes for newborns across the nation.

Limitations of This Statement

State newborn screening systems vary in their specific structure, procedures, and practices; this statement is focused on the core elements that are common to most state newborn screening systems. Newborn screening is increasingly being offered by commercial laboratories that market directly to parents and pediatric health care professionals. These programs introduce another layer of variation, which is beyond the scope of this statement.

Adequate funding of all aspects of newborn screening

systems is necessary to ensure optimal performance of the system. This statement includes some general recommendations to promote such funding, and the AAP supports efforts to address financing for the nation's newborn screening systems and their constituent parts. Detailed recommendations for addressing the myriad challenges of system financing lie beyond the purview of this document.‡

Limitations of Newborn Screening

It is important to emphasize that newborn screening panels do not include all possible congenital conditions, and results for conditions on the panel should not be considered diagnostic. Thus, an in-range newborn screening result does not eliminate the possibility that a clinically symptomatic child has a congenital condition. Congenital conditions must be considered whenever an infant has signs or symptoms that are suggestive of (or consistent with) one of the disorders that can be detected by newborn screening.

An important goal of newborn screening is to identify infants with treatable congenital conditions before they become symptomatic. However, clinicians who care for children must be aware that some screened conditions may present with clinical deterioration before notification of newborn screening results. Pediatricians and emergency care physicians are often among the first health care professionals to encounter symptomatic infants, so they should be knowledgeable about the newborn screening program, ACT sheets for suspected conditions, and local or regional pediatric medical subspecialists to whom infants can be referred. The state newborn screening program usually can provide information about suspected conditions and expedite the newborn's follow-up confirmatory testing and care.

THE ALGORITHMS

The PCP plays several significant roles in the newborn screening system. In addition to responding to out-of-range newborn screening results, the PCP serves as a central source of education for parents regarding multiple aspects of the newborn screening system; the PCP also has responsibility for ensuring that newborn screening has been conducted, which can include providing education and encouragement to parents who decline screening. Finally, the PCP must ensure coordinated and comprehensive care for children affected by congenital conditions that are identified through newborn screening. The medical home provides a model for such care; the algorithms presented here address the specific roles of a medical home provider within the newborn screening system (Figs 1 and 2).

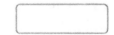

3- to 5-Day-Old Visit

The AAP[2] and *Bright Futures*[3] recommend neonatal follow-up visits in a child's medical home shortly after

---

‡For guidance on the *Current Procedural Terminology* (CPT) codes appropriate for use in the care of children who are identified as having congenital disorders, PCPs should refer to Rappo MA, Rappo PD. A special issue: coding for children with special health care needs. *AAP Pediatric Coding Newsletter*. January 2007. Available at: http://coding.aap.org/newsletterarchive.aspx.

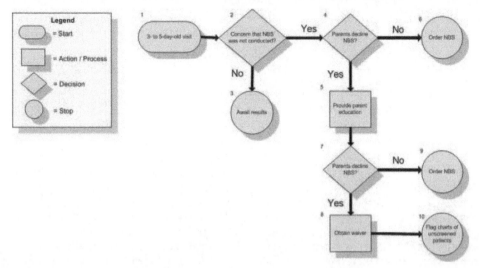

FIGURE 1
Algorithm 1. NBS indicates newborn screening program (see Appendix 2).

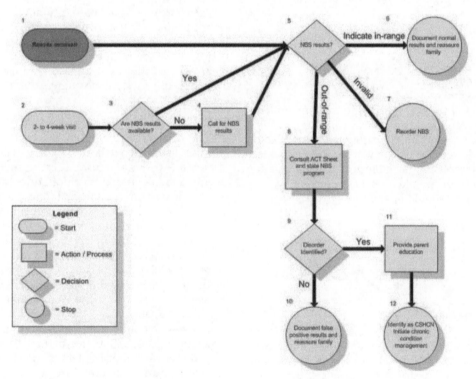

FIGURE 2
Algorithm 2. NBS indicates newborn screening program; CSHCN, child with special health care needs (see Appendix 3).

hospital discharge (3 to 5 days of life) and again by 1 month of age to ensure adequate weight gain, resolve neonatal concerns such as hyperbilirubinemia, and address parental questions. At the 3- to 5-day-old visit, the PCP should check for circumstances suggesting that newborn screening might not have been conducted.

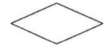

Concern That Newborn Screening Was Not Conducted?

In most cases, newborn screening will occur as a result of standing orders at a hospital or birthing facility. In these cases, the PCP can address other aspects of the visit.

There are circumstances, however, under which the PCP might have cause for concern that the newborn screening was not performed. These circumstances include, but are not limited to, home births, emergency births, hospital transfers, and international adoption. In addition, although most states mandate newborn screening, most jurisdictions provide parents with the right of refusal (see "Parents Decline Newborn Screening?").

If available discharge papers do not indicate that the newborn screening has been performed, the PCP should make arrangements for specimen acquisition.

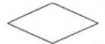

Parents Decline Newborn Screening?
If parental refusal is the reason that newborn screening has not been conducted, or if parents refuse newborn screening suggested by the PCP, the PCP should discuss the possible implications of nontesting and supply the parents with printed materials on newborn screening. Educational materials for parents and PCPs can be accessed through the AAP Web site (www.medicalhomeinfo.org/screening/newborn.html).

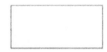

Provide Parent Education
Parent concerns and questions should be addressed fully, and a discussion of the general benefits and limited risks of newborn screening is recommended. More familiar conditions, such as congenital hearing loss, phenylketonuria, and sickle cell disease, may be used as examples.

If parental permission is obtained, arrangements for specimen acquisition should be made immediately, and newborn screening should be ordered.

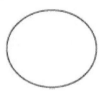

Order Newborn Screening
Newborn screening is conducted through the state newborn screening program, and protocols for ordering the screening vary by state. Contact information for each state's newborn screening program is available (see Appendix 4 and http://genes-r-us.uthscsa.edu/resources/consumer/statemap.htm).

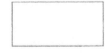

Obtain Waiver
If parental permission is not obtained, parents or guardians should be asked to sign a waiver that documents their decision to decline newborn screening. In many cases, parents already will have signed a waiver at the hospital. PCPs should document the additional conversation and the parents' decision in the patient's chart and may wish to include a waiver signed in the PCP's office. A sample waiver form is included as Appendix 5;

appropriate waiver forms should also be available through the state health department.

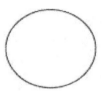

Flag the Charts of Unscreened Patients
In addition to documenting the discussion of newborn screening and the parents' refusal to consent to the screening, PCPs should flag the chart of any patients who are not screened so that the lack of screening will be taken into account should any subsequent concerns emerge regarding the child's growth or development. Vomiting, poor growth, seizures, developmental delay, lethargy, recurrent pneumonia, or poor feeding should prompt an evaluation that includes consideration of heritable conditions.

The chart note should also prompt the pediatrician to return to the question of newborn screening on subsequent visits to determine if the parents have changed their minds. The usefulness of screening after the neonatal period varies by condition, and use of state newborn screening systems for older infants varies by program.

Special Circumstances
For cases in which newborn screening is delayed because of previous parental refusal, because the infant was receiving total parenteral nutrition, or because of circumstances such as international adoption or an older infant entering care, the PCP should consult with the state newborn screening program regarding the availability and usefulness of the newborn screening protocol.

Newborn screening may not be ordered or may require an additional specimen in the case of preterm births, transfusion before screening, and other circumstances.[4] In these cases, the PCP should consult with a neonatal specialist.

In every circumstance, until and unless newborn screening is conducted, the patient's chart should be flagged to ensure that the lack of newborn screening is considered during ongoing care.

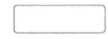

Results Received
In the case of an invalid or out-of-range screening result, the pediatrician identified on the newborn screening card should be called by the state newborn screening program in accordance with the urgency of the need for clinical intervention. In-range results are often transmitted by mail and should arrive before the 2- to 4-week visit.

2- to 4-Week Visit

The PCP cannot assume a "no news is good news" approach with regard to newborn screening. Delays or procedural failures at hospitals, state laboratories, other facilities, or within the newborn screening program may result in late or lost results. An infant's medical follow-up may not occur as planned, or newborn screening results may go directly to the child's birth facility instead of the infant's medical home.

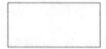

Are Newborn Screening Results Available?

Office staff should check routinely for newborn screening results before the 2- to 4-week visit and pursue missing results before the visit. Using electronic-chart prompts or paper-chart templates for newborn visits will remind office staff to seek out newborn screening results.

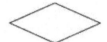

Call for Newborn Screening Results

If newborn screening results are not available before the 2- to 4-week visit, the PCP should contact the state newborn screening program or the birthing facility for the results. An increasing number of state newborn screening programs have automated interactive telephone- or Internet-based systems through which pediatric offices can check for newborn screening results at any time.

Special Circumstances

Occasionally, newborn screening results may be sent to the nonprimary physician; a physician who provides hospital or perinatal care for the infant may be noted on the newborn screening card even if he or she is not the infant's medical home physician. Clerical or other errors also may result in a physician who is unconnected to the child receiving the newborn screening results. However, the name on the card implies responsibility for the results, and physicians who receive results for patients who are no longer in their care should collaborate with the state newborn screening program and, in some instances, the hospital or birthing facility to locate the infant's family and/or current provider and to proceed with appropriate follow-up until the responsibility for subsequent care is clearly established. Physicians who receive results for patients with whom they or their colleagues have had no interaction should also notify the state newborn screening program immediately.

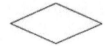

Screening Results?

The state newborn screening program will report results to the child's physician of record as being in range, invalid, or out of range. Appropriate responses to each of these results are discussed in the next sections.

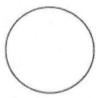

Document In-Range Screening Results and Reassure Family

In-range newborn screening results should be noted in the infant's chart and shared with the parents or guardians. In reassuring the family, the PCP should keep in mind that newborn screening does not rule out congenital conditions that are not included in the panel and does not absolutely guarantee the absence of the conditions that are screened. The PCP might note, however, that false in-range results are quite rare and the family can be reassured that their child is unlikely to be affected by conditions for which screening was performed.

Special Circumstances

Nine states (Arizona, Colorado, Delaware, Nevada, New Mexico, Oregon, Texas, Utah, and Wyoming) mandate an additional screening when the infant is 1 to 2 weeks old on the basis of the belief that a second screening is necessary to identify the maximum number of children with genetic disorders. A second screening is recommended for all infants in several other states, and approximately 25% of all US newborn infants currently receive 2 screenings. The relevance of second screenings for endocrinopathies is the subject of a study currently being designed by the MCHB. PCPs should familiarize themselves with their state's policies and procedures. If a second screening is ordered, it can be introduced and explained to parents within the context of state policies and the current limitations to newborn screening technologies discussed previously.

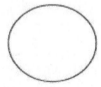

Reorder Newborn Screening

If the specimen is invalid (eg, collected too early, inadequate specimen, poor drying or application technique, inadequate or illegible patient information), the infant's newborn screening must be reordered and blood redrawn. This screen should be completed promptly to optimize the availability of results. PCPs must be familiar with local protocols for rescreening and should contact parents immediately to direct them to the site at which the second blood specimen will be obtained.

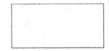

Consult ACT Sheets and State Newborn Screening Program

An out-of-range result on the newborn screening panel is not a diagnosis. However, some congenital conditions can be rapidly fatal in infants who appeared entirely healthy a few days earlier; thus, out-of-range screening results should always lead to prompt action by the PCP.

If the state newborn screening program does not provide the ACT sheet specific to the condition for which an out-of-range result was obtained, the PCP should download it (www.acmg.net/resources/policies/ACT/condition-analyte-links.htm).

The ACT sheet should be reviewed and followed in its entirety, but the most important actions are highlighted. These actions include:

- when to contact the family;
- whom to consult and whether an appointment is needed immediately;
- when the patient must be seen by the PCP;
- whether additional confirmatory testing is needed and what tests should be conducted;
- whether treatment is necessary and what treatment to initiate;
- how to educate parents about the condition; and
- when findings need to be reported back to the newborn screening program.

In addition to following ACT sheet recommendations, the PCP should consult with the state newborn screening program regarding out-of-range results. The state program should be familiar with local or regional experts for the conditions on their screening panels. In some states, the programs fund subspecialty clinics to conduct diagnostic evaluations and provide short-term and/or long-term subspecialty care to infants with out-of-range screening results.

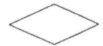

Condition Identified?

After an out-of-range screening result is obtained, confirmatory testing and/or definitive consultation with subspecialists are required before a final diagnosis can be made.

To increase the sensitivity of a population screening test for rare conditions (and hopefully minimize the number of false in-range results missed), false out-of-range results are expected to occur, and false out-of-range results are significantly more frequent than true out-of-range results for most newborn screening tests. However, given the seriousness of the congenital conditions included in the newborn screening panel, the PCP must avoid complacency in the face of out-of-range results. Until confirmatory testing and/or definitive con-

sultation with subspecialists can be accomplished, all out-of-range results must be taken very seriously.

Special Circumstances

In addition to true or false out-of-range results, confirmatory tests may identify the child as a carrier of the condition or may lead to an indeterminate result.

Carriers are individuals who are heterozygous for an autosomal-recessive condition and are usually not at risk of health problems themselves, although this may vary with the condition. Many state programs notify the PCP that the infant has been identified as a carrier, and it may be the responsibility of the PCP to disclose and discuss these results with the parents.

Knowledge of carrier status has 2 implications. First, because most of the conditions tested for on newborn screening are autosomal-recessive in inheritance, it is highly probable that at least 1 of the parents is a carrier also, and both parents might be carriers. If both parents are carriers, they have a 1-in-4 chance with each pregnancy of having an affected child. Alerting parents to the carrier status of their child serves to alert them that they may be at increased risk of having an affected infant with their next pregnancy. (When newborn screening results lead to genetic testing of the parents, pediatricians should be aware that misattributed paternity could be identified. Discussion with a geneticist or genetic counselor about how to manage these sensitive results may be helpful.)

The second implication of identifying a newborn as a carrier is that the infant will be at an increased risk of bearing an affected child when he or she achieves reproductive age if his or her future partner also is a carrier for the same condition. The risk is largely determined by the prevalence of the condition within the population, and additional genetic counseling may be warranted.

Occasionally, confirmatory diagnostic test results will not result in a definitive diagnosis. Uncertain results can be distressing to parents and PCPs, so thorough consultation with a subspecialist is essential. Unfortunately, indeterminate results may not be possible to resolve without more knowledge about some of these conditions and longer-term follow-up of these children.

At this point, it is incumbent on the PCP and the subspecialist to maintain an ongoing collaboration and continue to monitor the infant for signs and symptoms of a suspected condition. Children with uncertain results should have their chart identified for close monitoring. Good communication between the PCP and the consulting subspecialist is essential at this point to ensure that a unified message is conveyed to parents.

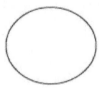

Document False Out-of-Range Results and Reassure Parents

In the event that the initial out-of-range result proves to be a false out-of-range result, the PCP can provide reassurance to parents. However, research that evaluated parents of infants with false out-of-range results has suggested that 5% to 20% of these parents will persist in their concerns about the health of their children for months or years after screening.[5–9] Therefore, PCPs should not take the event of a false out-of-range result too lightly and may wish to discuss this issue with parents on subsequent visits to provide additional reassurance and eliminate any misconceptions.

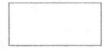

Provide Parent Education

To lay the foundation for comprehensive and collaborative care, it is critical during this time of uncertainty that the parents and family of the neonate be provided with condition-specific information and support as they await final clarification of the child's diagnosis and begin to plan for treatment and management. Parents are usually intensely anxious about the health of their child while the diagnosis is being pursued, and increasingly, parents are adept at tapping into resources on the Internet about specific conditions. Frequent, specific, and supportive communication from the PCP will help to avoid confusion and build trust. Appropriate materials for distribution to parents have been produced by the AAP (www. aap.org), the American College of Obstetricians and Gynecologists (ACOG [www.acog.org]), and MCHB/ HRSA (www.mchb.hrsa.gov/screening). State newborn screening programs may also make educational materials available to health care professionals.

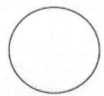

Identify the Child as a Child With Special Health Care Needs and Initiate Chronic Care Management

Any child who is given a diagnosis of a significant medical condition should be identified by the medical home physician as a child with special health care needs. Such a child should be entered into the practice's children with special health care needs registry, and chronic condition management should be initiated. Chronic care management provides proactive care for children with special health care needs, including condition-related office visits, written care plans, explicit comanagement with subspecialists, appropriate patient education, and effective information systems for monitoring and tracking the child's condition.[10]

IMPLEMENTING THE ALGORITHM

Role of the Medical Home

Regardless of diagnosis, every child needs a medical home to ensure coordinated and comprehensive care such that all of the medical, psychosocial, and educa-

tional needs of the child and family are met successfully within the local community. The PCP is responsible for providing a medical home.

Some conditions identified by newborn screening are relatively mild and or/transitory, and others have a wide spectrum of severity from asymptomatic to life-threatening crises. Plans for continuing care should be made in consultation with the family and appropriate subspecialists in light of the condition affecting the child and the severity of its manifestation. In some cases, the PCP may provide all or most of the ongoing care.

In other cases, the family may view their subspecialist as their primary care physician. Although a subspecialist may provide substantial ongoing care for a child who has been diagnosed with a severe and complex condition, the PCP retains the responsibility for providing a central source of "family centered, accessible, continuous, coordinated, comprehensive, compassionate, and culturally effective" care for the family.[11] The parents and family should be encouraged to maintain their relationship with their PCP. This relationship is critical, especially for cases in which the subspecialist is located at some distance from the family. In a crisis, the PCP may be the only available provider with knowledge of the child; he or she must have up-to-date information regarding the child's treatment.

The complex nature of many conditions identified by newborn screening may require care by a team of medical subspecialists, therapists, nutritionists, and educators.[12] The PCP and other professionals involved in the child's care must collaborate in the provision of acute care for illness or injury; surveillance of growth and development; anticipatory guidance to the family; immunizations; communications with schools, social services, and camps; transitions in care; and communication with other care professionals. In any case, clearly defined roles may help to reduce redundancies of services and prevent fragmentation of care.

The medical home should actively engage public and private resources to aid in the management of chronic conditions. Public health nursing provided through some state public health departments' maternal and child health programs often has a role in assisting PCPs, subspecialists, and families of children with conditions that are diagnosed through newborn screening. The level of public health nursing may vary from simply providing information and referrals to assisting with chronic condition management for a family.

If there is not a local health department or nursing service, PCPs may contact their state maternal and child health department (Title V) and the directors of programs for children with special health care needs through the state department of public health to obtain information on the availability of local family services; the state department of education for contacts with school nurses; and the early intervention agency (Individuals With Disabilities Education Act Part C) for contact information for the local early childhood connections program. Although the state resources for public health vary greatly from state to state, almost all communities have one or all of these resources available for families. The national organization Family Voices (www. familyvoices.org) can provide information on local organizations and agencies that can offer resources to families with children with special health care needs and can assist families in accessing community services.

For additional information regarding care coordination, see the AAP policy statement "Care Coordination in the Medical Home: Integrating Health and Related Systems of Care for Children With Special Health Care Needs."[13]

Role of the Subspecialist

For most of the conditions that may be detected through newborn screening, the subspecialist will confirm the diagnosis, develop the treatment plan, educate the family about the treatment, monitor treatment, identify complications related to the disease process that may require additional referral, and work with other consultants in coordination of care. When acute illness exacerbates the condition, the PCP should work with the subspecialist to diagnose the acute illness and manage it appropriately to reduce morbidity.

Some children with conditions identified through newborn screening will have long-term sequelae that will require ongoing subspecialty management despite appropriate early intervention. Many of these children will have mild neurodevelopmental disabilities that may present as learning difficulties, attention-deficit/hyperactivity disorder, or other behavioral problems. However, in some instances, more significant cognitive and motor deficits and/or problems that adversely affect the child's feeding skills and respiratory status may be present. It is essential that the PCP provide ongoing screening and surveillance for these developmental disabilities.

Even with appropriate treatment, patients with certain conditions identified through newborn screening can undergo metabolic decompensation during an acute febrile illness. PCPs need to be aware of the initial clinical signs and laboratory abnormalities that may be found when metabolic decompensation occurs and be able to provide immediate intervention to stabilize the child until more specific advice can be obtained from the appropriate treating subspecialist. Effective communication among subspecialists as well as between each subspecialist and the PCP is essential for optimal long-term management of these children.[14] Long-term responsibilities of the subspecialist, in collaboration with the PCP, include:

- Providing genetic counseling and evaluation: Because the majority of conditions diagnosed through newborn screening are hereditary, genetic evaluation and counseling will be necessary for the parents. Older siblings may be affected with the condition but not yet symptomatic; diagnostic studies may be indicated for the siblings, and other relatives may wish to undergo carrier testing. The PCP, the state newborn screening program, and subspecialists are jointly responsible for ensuring that referral for genetic services occurs.

- Providing ongoing parent education and links to available resources: Resources for managing the condition should be made available to the patients and their families. Subspecialists, the PCP, and the state newborn screening program should collaborate in making appropriate referrals to programs for children with special health care needs, childhood early intervention programs, community-based support services, and additional subspecialists who are needed to evaluate and manage associated disabilities. Information from disease-specific advocacy organizations, along with parent brochures and guidance for child health care professionals, may be available through the subspecialist. The Genetic Alliance, a coalition of advocacy groups, serves as another national resource for parents (www. geneticalliance.org). The National Library of Medicine also has material on every condition in the expanded ACMG-recommended panel (http://ghr.nlm.nih.gov).

- Assisting in the transition to adult care: When transition to adult care is appropriate, the subspecialist will work with the PCP to identify a new team of physicians to care for the young adult. As adolescence proceeds, additional genetic counseling and preparation for family planning are appropriate.

RECOMMENDATIONS

Preparing the Practice

Before receiving notice of an out-of-range newborn screening result from their state newborn screening system, PCPs can take several steps to enhance their ability to successfully address their roles and responsibilities within the newborn screening program.

1. PCPs should familiarize themselves with their state newborn screening program via available (online) resources or, if necessary, by contacting the state program. PCPs should develop some familiarity with the conditions being screened and basic operations of their state newborn screening program, including protocols for retesting invalid screening results and conducting second screenings. PCPs should identify the person(s) with whom they should consult in the case of an out-of-range screening result and ensure that contact information is readily available.

2. State-specific contact information for regional pediatric medical subspecialists should be collected and kept on file in the PCP's office.

3. Procedures to address several steps of the algorithm should be developed in advance. These procedures include:

   a. updating contact information for the state newborn screening program and regional pediatric medical subspecialists;

   b. identifying children who are most likely not to have had newborn screening;

   c. confirming receipt of newborn screening results on all patients;

d. obtaining newborn screening results when they are not received from the state program;

e. documenting parental refusal of newborn screening; and

f. obtaining newborn screening specimens in the case of lost, delayed, or invalid results (the CPT code for retesting is 84030, and the diagnosis code is 270.10; PCPs should check with insurers to assess reimbursement).

4. PCPs should establish registries to identify, follow, and provide chronic condition management for children with special health care needs.

5. Educational materials regarding newborn screening should be on hand to distribute to expectant parents, parents who may decline newborn screening, and parents whose child's screening returns an out-of-range or inconclusive result. These materials should be available in languages and at literacy levels appropriate to all patients served. Appropriate materials for distribution to parents have been produced by the AAP (www.medicalhomeinfo.org/screening/newborn.html), ACOG (www.acog.org), and MCHB/HRSA (www.mchb.hrsa.gov/screening). State newborn screening programs may also make educational materials available to health care professionals.

Care coordination plays an essential role in ongoing efforts to integrate health and related systems of care for children and youth with special health care needs.[15] Becoming aware of available resources, being involved in the care coordination process, and developing unique care coordination approaches within one's own practice and community and in relationship with existing tertiary care centers are essential for providing optimal care for children with special health care needs. Families, PCPs, and other professionals can collaborate meaningfully to provide effective coordinated care.[13,15]

PCPs are also encouraged to participate in state, regional, or national registries; quality assurance programs; and/or research projects designed to enhance the care of children with the rare and complex conditions included in the newborn screening panel. They are also encouraged to seek opportunities for additional training and learning about state newborn screening programs and the conditions for which infants are screened and to work with their local AAP chapter and state newborn screening advisory committee (SNSAC) to advance the quality and effectiveness of the newborn screening system at the state and federal levels.

Collaboration With Other Health Care Professionals

The goals of ensuring the successful operation of the newborn screening system and advancing optimal care for infants and their families cannot be accomplished by PCPs alone. Effective collaboration and communication among PCPs and other clinicians and among the systems of care that engage the newborn screening system will ensure the best outcomes for infants and families. In light of this necessary collaboration, recommendations have been developed for prenatal health care professionals, hospitals and other birthing facilities, pediatric medical subspecialists, states and SNSACs, and federal agencies.

Prenatal Health Care Professionals

The prenatal period provides an ideal opportunity to begin to educate a family regarding the importance of newborn screening and the risks and benefits of early identification of the conditions identified through screening. The ACOG Committee on Genetics has asserted that "[o]bstetricians need to be aware of the status of newborn screening in their states and should be prepared to address questions or refer their patients to appropriate sources for additional information."[16] The following specific steps can help bring the awareness and knowledge of the obstetrician to bear in preparing a family for newborn screening and promoting the function of the newborn screening system.

1. Prenatal health care professionals are ideally positioned to educate expectant parents about the newborn screening program in conjunction with the prenatal screening program. The obstetrician is encouraged to begin the education early enough to allow patients the opportunity to ask questions that will assist them in understanding the purpose of newborn screening, its implementation, and the importance of test results and follow-up. Concise, clear, and comprehensive educational materials and/or video presentations already in existence should be made available to expectant parents during the prenatal period. Appropriate materials are available from the AAP (www.medicalhomeinfo.org/screening/newborn.html) and the National Library of Medicine (ghr.nlm.nih.gov/nbs).

2. Prenatal health care professionals should strongly encourage prospective parents to identify a medical home for their infant early in pregnancy. When the mother presents for postpartum care, the prenatal health care professional can further support the medical home by inquiring about the infant's well-being and follow-up care.

3. If an infant is lost to follow-up to the newborn screening program, prenatal health care professionals should assist in locating the family.

Hospitals and Other Birthing Facilities

In most cases, it is the facility at which the infant is delivered that is initially responsible for processing the newborn screening specimen. It is essential that these facilities have policies and procedures in place to ensure high-quality specimen processing and prompt delivery to the designated screening laboratory.

1. Particular attention should be brought to the development of protocols for:

   a. Repeat screening of invalid specimens.

   b. Documenting parental refusal to consent to newborn screening: Parents should be asked to sign a waiver form that documents not only their refusal to consent to newborn screening but also their understanding of the program and its purpose and the risks associated with their refusal.

c. Adequate training of clinical and laboratory staff and quality assurance programs focused on high-quality specimen processing: Appropriate and complete information regarding the infant, contact information, and medical follow-up must be gathered and submitted with specimens.

d. Assisting public health authorities in locating infants who are lost to follow-up: If the infant's medical home is not clearly identified, the facility at which the child was born should assume responsibility for notifying the family of an out-of-range screening result and referring for additional diagnostic testing and subspecialty care.

2. Identification of the medical home or site of medical follow-up should be established as a condition for discharge.

3. Discharge materials should clearly indicate whether newborn screening was conducted and should identify the PCP and the in-hospital managing physician for later contact, if needed.

4. Hospitals and other birthing facilities should ensure the availability of printed and/or video educational materials, presented in concise and understandable language, to all families, including those whose primary language is not English. These materials should address the purpose of newborn screening, the risks and benefits associated with newborn screening, and the consequences of delaying or refusing newborn screening.

5. Opportunities for further discussion or questions should be made available with either the family's chosen PCP or staff members who are knowledgeable about the screening process and the conditions for which screening is conducted.

Pediatric Medical Subspecialists

Pediatric medical subspecialists play several roles in the care of children who have out-of-range results from newborn screening: they conduct confirmatory testing, care for the primary condition of infants who are affected by congenital diseases, and collaborate in the care of children with disabilities associated with some of the diseases identified through newborn screening. In fulfillment of these roles:

1. Pediatric medical subspecialists should assist the state newborn screening program in the development of educational materials for the public, families, PCPs, the state newborn screening program, and policy makers on specific conditions identified by newborn screening.

2. Pediatric medical subspecialists should serve on their SNSAC.

3. Pediatric medical subspecialists should respond promptly to requests for diagnostic and management services to infants with out-of-range screening results

and children with conditions identified by newborn screening. Findings from clinic visits, laboratory studies, imaging studies, and diet and medication changes should be communicated promptly to the PCP, state newborn screening programs, other pediatric medical subspecialists, and the family (as appropriate).

4. Pediatric medical subspecialists should underscore the importance of maintaining a medical home relationship with the PCP for the infant identified with a condition through newborn screening.

5. Pediatric medical subspecialists should assist in the identification of associated disabilities and appropriate referral to other subspecialists for management.

6. Pediatric medical subspecialists should assist in the development of condition-specific protocols for the treatment of acute illness or injury and in the development of the child's care plan for school, activity restrictions, and special feeding/diet programs. Pediatric medical subspecialists should also work with the PCP, the family, and other subspecialists to delineate each person's role in managing acute illnesses, establishing relationships with schools and therapists, providing immunizations, working with social services and camps, and maintaining contact with insurers.

7. Pediatric medical subspecialists should provide ongoing education to the family and PCP about new developments and treatments for the condition and associated disabilities.

8. Pediatric medical subspecialists should work with the PCP and other subspecialists in identifying appropriate adult health care professionals for the transition to adult care.

State Systems

The state's role in newborn screening is to design, coordinate, and manage an effective newborn screening system. It has traditionally been the state's responsibility to oversee key aspects of the newborn screening system, including initial screening, confirmation of diagnosis, and coordination of short-term follow-up for infants with out-of-range screening results as well as longer-term care for children with special health care needs. Ultimately, the state must maintain an adequate public health infrastructure to ensure that every newborn infant receives appropriate care.

The AAP Newborn Screening Task Force set forth a broad agenda for state newborn screening systems in its statement published in 2000.[17] In addition to addressing the recommendations that follow, states are urged to consult that AAP statement for guidance in developing and supporting an effective and comprehensive newborn screening system.

To ensure the appropriate and effective function of newborn screening systems, the following recommendations must be addressed immediately:

1. States must monitor specimen collection and transmission of information between screening hospitals, the testing laboratory, and individual practitioners.

2. Identification of the follow-up medical home must be required on all newborn screening specimens.[16,18]

3. Laboratory collection and handling procedures must be clearly delineated at every site at which newborn screens are obtained or processed. State newborn screening laboratories are expected to maintain up-to-date technology and procedures and be prepared to implement recommended changes in the newborn screening process.[11]

4. Practical mechanisms should be established for re-testing infants whose newborn screening results are indeterminate/invalid regardless of the cause.

5. Procedures should be adopted to ensure that the medical home is notified of out-of-range screening results by telephone on a schedule consistent with the urgency of the need for intervention. In the case of urgent out-of-range results, a designated medical subspecialist may be notified in addition to the medical home; the newborn screening program may need to contact the family if efforts to contact physicians are not successful.

6. Procedures should be adopted to ensure that in-range and invalid screening results are available to the medical home within 2 weeks of an infant's birth.

7. When out-of-range screen results are reported, the appropriate updated ACT sheet (or equivalent) and state-specific referral information should be forwarded immediately to the PCP.

8. States must have policies and procedures in place to locate children who have not established a medical home and to ensure that all newborn infants with out-of-range screening results receive appropriate diagnostic follow-up and subspecialty care.

9. States must provide clinicians with contact information for their newborn screening program coordinator and ensure that clinicians are updated promptly should any changes occur.

10. Public health agencies and maternal and child health programs should assist with care coordination for patients with special health care needs and their families.

Because states play a significant educational role in the newborn screening system, the following are recommended:

11. With direction from the SNSAC, states should develop and facilitate distribution of clear and concise educational materials for families at prenatal visits and in the hospital at the time of delivery. Condition-specific materials must be developed for families whose infants have out-of-range screening results; these materials include an explanation of test results, appropriate educational materials on the tested condition, referral for additional diagnostic testing, and referral for subspecialty care. Educational materials developed by the AAP, ACOG, and HRSA/MCHB may be used and/or supplemented with materials developed by the state. These materials can be accessed at www.medicalhomeinfo.org/screening/newborn.html or mchb.hrsa.gov/screening.

12. The state must develop educational information for medical professionals that outlines their responsibilities in the newborn screening process.

Finally, there are a number of steps that can be taken to improve the operation of the newborn screening system, including the following:

13. To prevent delays in processing when screening occurs on the weekend, the newborn screening laboratory responsible for state screening should operate at least 6 days a week, with coverage for holidays. Rapid turnaround time for results is essential for prompt diagnosis and treatment of metabolic conditions.

14. Information systems through which clinicians could directly download newborn screening results should be developed. Policies and regulations must be developed concurrently to protect privacy and confidentiality rights.

15. States should develop and implement information systems that facilitate the tracking of infants across state lines through communication and integration of data across newborn screening systems.

16. States must develop and implement policies that allow for interstate licensure and practice of medicine (including the use of telemedicine) to facilitate consultation and communication to underserved areas and ensure the free flow of information across state lines. There is a shortage of pediatric medical subspecialists across the country and a complete absence from more sparsely populated regions. This challenge must be addressed cooperatively by the states.

17. States should ensure the availability of ongoing care for infants with out-of-range screening results who lack health insurance and for those whose insurance does not provide coverage for necessary services and treatments. Medically required diets and vitamins are among the treatments often excluded from coverage provided by third-party payers.[19]

18. To promote greater understanding of the effects and benefits of the newborn screening system, states should develop information systems that are capable of tracking the multitude of performance measures for the newborn screening system and long-term outcomes of children with special health care needs identified through newborn screening. Performance measures include diagnosis for and treatment of infants with out-of-range screening results, cases missed by newborn screening, false out-of-range result rates, time to diagnosis, parental involvement and satisfaction, the social and psychological effects on families of infants with out-of-range and false out-of-range results, and family access to appropri-

ate and necessary services. Data to support the analysis of cost-effectiveness and cost benefit should also be collected.

19. To provide national data for newborn screening system quality assurance and program comparison, state programs should contribute timely case findings and laboratory data to the national newborn screening data-collection system operated by the National Newborn Screening and Genetics Resource Center (www2.uthscsa.edu/nnsis).

20. SNSACs should be authorized in each state to help implement and ensure the establishment of principles of universal access, clinician and community education, remedial surveillance for accountability, and quality of services for all infants. SNSACs should be chartered with appropriate authority and provided adequate support to effectively fulfill the roles outlined as follows.

State Newborn Screening Advisory Committees

1. SNSACs should comprise a balanced, representative, and diverse membership. Representation by diverse families and societal leaders should be balanced by members of the health care community, including clinicians in practice, representatives of hospitals and professional organizations, and public health experts, including the laboratories and the state. A diverse clinician representation would include pediatricians, obstetricians, family physicians, and nurse and midwife practitioners. In addition, the panel must have access to expert medical subspecialists, health care researchers, and biostatisticians.

2. SNSACs should cooperate with the US Department of Health and Human Services ACHDGDNC and other federal agencies to promote consistency in newborn screening throughout the nation.

3. SNSACs must work to advance state support and development of the newborn screening system, with particular attention to:

   a. efforts to use health information technology to advance clinician and family access to information about newborn screening as well as screening and follow-up services;

   b. optimization and accurate interpretation of privacy laws;

   c. implementation of a systems approach based on the Institute of Medicine principles for patient-centered safety, effectiveness, efficiency, timeliness, and equity[20];

   d. efforts to provide unfettered access, through both print and electronic media, to understandable education materials for families with diverse reading and language abilities; and

   e. development and distribution of resources for PCPs.

4. SNSACs must address identified challenges of frag-

mented service delivery as well as geographic, cultural, social, and financing barriers across county and state lines.

5. SNSACs should promote a statewide report on newborn health status for identifiable conditions and a national newborn health report that provides data on incidence, outcome, and community participation.

6. SNSACs must develop a mechanism for receiving feedback from parents, medical home practitioners, and subspecialists on the appropriateness of including particular conditions in the newborn screening program. This feedback should then be transmitted to the ACHDGDNC.

7. Each SNSAC is encouraged to develop its own charter and seek statutory establishment and state support.

National Partnerships

Although states remain responsible for newborn screening systems, federal agencies and national organizations play a significant role in the newborn screening system and in supporting families of children with genetic conditions. Strengthening national partnerships between federal agencies and professional, nonprofit, and family organizations provides the opportunity for a coordinated effort to increase the services offered to children with genetic and congenital conditions in all stages of diagnosis, treatment, and follow-up. There are 4 critical points of partnership for these groups: collaboration, funding, oversight, and follow-up.

Collaboration

1. Health care professionals, nonprofit agencies, state and federal public health programs, and families should seek to build relationships with other groups that focus on the newborn screening system. Relationships can be fostered through partnering on national initiatives, inviting other perspectives to serve on project advisory committees, and establishing a systematic method of receiving feedback from families.

2. Research should be performed on all aspects of newborn screening systems, including parent and provider education, results management, laboratory quality, residual specimen storage and use, and, most importantly, efficacy of newborn screening for each proposed condition. A national research agenda for newborn screening should be outlined. Input from federal agencies, professional associations, nonprofit organizations, and family support organizations should be coordinated. Multistate or national collaborations are often necessary to recruit a sufficient number of affected infants to understand the clinical spectrum of the disease and to compare treatment strategies. Collaboration will be key in conducting this research.

3. National partnerships should be developed and coordinated to support state newborn screening sys-

tems and encourage coordination, effective collaboration, and decrease duplication.

Funding

4. Adequate third-party reimbursement, grant applications, nonprofit fundraising efforts, and other sources of funding for newborn screening programs should be pursued by those who seek to improve the newborn screening system. Funding for the components of the newborn screening system and long-term care of children with genetic conditions comes from a variety of sources including screening fees, federal programs, state programs, nonprofit fundraising, insurance companies, and others, and such funding is critical at all levels.

5. Because ongoing research in the areas of education, results management, laboratory quality, and identifying and treating genetic diseases is important as the world of newborn screening continues to expand, funding for the implementation of these research projects should be provided.

6. Because establishing and funding a 24-hour hotline for access to online state-specific newborn screening program contact information can be useful in supporting state newborn screening programs, physicians, and families, a dedicated newborn screening hotline should be considered as part of preparing for national emergencies, natural disasters, or other circumstances.

7. Funding should be provided for demonstration projects directed toward strengthening the communication process between pediatricians and the newborn screening program. These efforts can include the development of telemedicine, effective health information exchanges, and linked information systems to facilitate the communication process.

8. Because the increased level of services required to comanage and coordinate care for patients with special needs identified through newborn screening can pose a significant financial burden for the PCP and the subspecialist, appropriate CPT coding that is aimed at enhanced reimbursement for chronic condition management should be developed.

Oversight

9. ACHDGDNC policies and activities should promote and facilitate uniformity across newborn screening programs, promote coordination between state newborn screening programs, support public health infrastructure for these programs, monitor the quality of these programs, and coordinate and promote research efforts related to newborn screening.

10. The ACHDGDNC should promote federal interagency collaboration and federal agency collaboration with state public health newborn screening programs to encourage coordination and effective collaboration between federal and state agencies.

11. Family involvement in all levels of newborn screening and follow-up care is important and should be encouraged. Families can give feedback on services provided, make suggestions on improving systems of care, advocate for needed services, and support other families that are going through similar situations.

Follow-up

12. Appropriate treatment and chronic condition management for children with congenital conditions should be ensured. Federal agencies, state newborn screening programs, and others can collaborate to create a national definition for follow-up to newborn screening systems.

13. Because enrolling children onto long-term research studies can provide the opportunity to test new treatments and better understand the natural history of chronic conditions, federal agencies and national organizations should promote opportunities for such research and create materials to educate parents about research in general and specific opportunities to participate in research.

National Medical Specialty Organizations, Including the AAP
National medical specialty organizations and their state chapters can play specific roles in the continued development of the collaboration necessary to ensure optimal performance of the newborn screening system throughout the country.

1. They should maintain communication with and participation on the ACHDGDNC to provide information to their constituencies and communicate any concerns to the ACHDGDNC.

2. They should foster education regarding newborn screening and promote pediatric medical subspecialties that focus on metabolic diseases among medical students and residents.

3. They should promote the development and implementation of a Health Plan Employer Data and Information Set (HEDIS) measure on newborn screening.

4. They should comment on the appropriateness of adding new tests to the core screening panel, ensuring that any newborn screening provides clear benefit to all children screened and to their families. These comments should be presented to the ACHDGDNC for consideration and adoption.

CONCLUSIONS
Advances in newborn screening technology, coupled with recent advances in the diagnosis and treatment of rare but serious congenital conditions that affect newborn infants, provide increased opportunities for positively affecting the lives of children and their families. These advantages, however, also pose new challenges to PCPs, both educationally and in response to the management of affected infants.

To respond appropriately, PCPs require immediate

access to clinical and diagnostic information and guidance; ACT sheets from the ACMG are a valuable source of such guidance. PCPs, however, have a proactive role to play in supporting the performance of the newborn screening system and ensuring the successful completion of their responsibilities to the program. PCPs must develop office policies and procedures to ensure that newborn screening is conducted and that results are transmitted to them in a timely fashion. PCPs must also develop strategies to use should these systems fail.

The newborn screening system extends well beyond the PCP's office, and many other stakeholders are essential for ensuring that the system functions well and supporting PCPs in their role within the system. The system is challenged by error, lack of education or information on the part of families and health care professionals, and systemic challenges such as the national shortage of pediatric medical subspecialists and barriers inherent in state licensing requirements. Lack of universal health care coverage and limited funding for newborn screening programs present additional significant challenges.

State and federal entities, hospitals, prehospital health care professionals, pediatricians, and pediatric medical subspecialists should act collaboratively to address these challenges or reduce their effects on the newborn screening system. AAP chapters and individual pediatricians should work together with the AAP and SNSACs to promote actions and policies that will optimize the function of newborn screening systems and ensure that children and families receive the full benefit of them.

NEWBORN SCREENING AUTHORING COMMITTEE

E. Stephen Edwards, MD, Chairperson
Vinod K. Bhutani, MD
    Committee on Fetus and Newborn
Jeffrey Botkin, MD
    Committee on Bioethics
Barbara Deloian, PhD, RN, CPNP
    Bright Futures Early Childhood Expert Panel
Stephen Deputy, MD
    Section on Neurology
Timothy Geleske, MD
    Medical Home Initiatives for Children With Special
    Needs Project Advisory Committee
Joseph H. Hersh, MD
    Council on Children With Disabilities
Celia Kaye, MD, PhD
    Committee on Genetics
Jennifer Lail, MD
    Quality improvement expert
Michele A. Lloyd-Puryear, MD, PhD
    Maternal and Child Health Bureau
Michael Watson, PhD
    American College of Medical Genetics

CONSULTANT

Aaron Carroll, MD, MS
    Medical Informatician

WRITING CONSULTANT

Melissa Capers

STAFF

Anne Gramiak, MPH
Jennifer Mansour

ACKNOWLEDGMENTS

This project was funded by the Health Resources and Services Administration's Maternal and Child Health Bureau, through a contract in the American College of Medical Genetics cooperative agreement (U22 MC 03957-01-00). The views expressed in this report are those of the American Academy of Pediatrics, not necessarily that of HRSA/MCHB.

REFERENCES

1. American College of Medical Genetics. Newborn screening: toward a uniform screening panel and system. *Genet Med.* 2006; 8(suppl):1S–252S
2. American Academy of Pediatrics, Committee on Practice and Ambulatory Medicine, Bright Futures Steering Committee. Recommendations for preventive pediatric health care. *Pediatrics.* 2007;120:1376–1378
3. American Academy of Pediatrics, Bright Futures Steering Committee. *Bright Futures: Guidelines for Health Supervision of Infants, Children, and Adolescents.* Hagan JF Jr, Shaw JS, Duncan P, eds. 3rd ed. Elk Grove Village, IL: American Academy of Pediatrics; 2007
4. Kaye CI; American Academy of Pediatrics, Committee on Genetics. Newborn screening fact sheets. *Pediatrics.* 2006;118(3). Available at: www.pediatrics.org/cgi/content/full/118/3/e934
5. Bodegård G, Fyro K, Larsson A. Psychological reactions in 102 families with a newborn who has a falsely positive screening test for congenital hypothyroidism. *Acta Paediatr Scand Suppl.* 1983;304:1–21
6. Dobrovoljski G, Kerbl R, Strobl C, Schwinger W, Dornbusch HJ, Lackner H. False-positive results in neuroblastoma screening: the parents' view. *J Pediatr Hematol Oncol.* 2003;25: 14–18
7. Fyrö K, Bodegard G. Four-year follow-up of psychological reactions to false positive screening tests for congenital hypothyroidism. *Acta Paediatr Scand.* 1987;76:107–114
8. Sorenson JR, Levy HL, Mangione TW, Sepe SJ. Parental response to repeat testing of infants with "false-positive" results in a newborn screening program. *Pediatrics.* 1984;73:183–187
9. Waisbren SE, Albers S, Amato S, et al. Effect of expanded newborn screening for biochemical genetic disorders on child outcomes and parental stress. *JAMA.* 2003;290:2564–2572
10. American Academy of Pediatrics, Council on Children With Disabilities, Section on Developmental and Behavioral Pediatrics; Bright Futures Steering Committee, Medical Home Initiatives for Children With Special Needs Project Advisory Committee. Identifying infants and young children with developmental disorders in the medical home: an algorithm for developmental surveillance and screening [published correction appears in *Pediatrics.* 2006;118:1808–1809]. *Pediatrics.* 2006;118:405–420
11. Sia C, Tonniges TF, Osterhus E, Taba S. History of the medical home concept. *Pediatrics.* 2004;113:1473–1478
12. Pass KA, Lane PA, Fernhoff PM, et al. US Newborn Screening System guidelines II: follow-up of children, diagnosis, management, and evaluation. Statement of the Council of Regional Networks for Genetics Services (CORN). *J Pediatr.* 2000;137(4 suppl):S1–S46

13. American Academy of Pediatrics, Council on Children With Disabilities. Care coordination in the medical home: integrating health and related systems of care for children with special health care needs. *Pediatrics.* 2005;116:1238–1244

14. Dionisi-Vici C, Deodato F, Roschinger W, Rhead W, Wilcken B. "Classical" organic acidurias, propionic aciduria, methylmalonic aciduria and isovaleric aciduria: long-term outcome effects of expanded newborn screening using tandem mass spectrometry. *J Inherit Metab Dis.* 2006;29:383–389

15. American Academy of Pediatrics, Medical Home Initiatives for Children With Special Needs Project Advisory Committee. The medical home. *Pediatrics.* 2002;110:184–186

16. American College of Obstetricians and Gynecologists. ACOG committee opinion number 287, October 2003: newborn screening. *Obstet Gynecol.* 2003;102:887–889

17. Newborn Screening Task Force. Serving the family from birth to the medical home. Newborn screening: a blueprint for the future—a call for a national agenda on state newborn screening programs. *Pediatrics.* 2000;106:389–427

18. Kim S, Lloyd-Puryear MA, Tonniges TF. Examination of the communication practices between state newborn screening programs and the medical home. *Pediatrics.* 2003;111(2). Available at: www.pediatrics.org/cgi/content/full/111/2/e120

19. American Academy of Pediatrics, Committee on Nutrition. Reimbursement for foods for special dietary use. *Pediatrics.* 2003; 111:1117–1119

20. Institute of Medicine, Committee on Quality of Health Care in America. *Crossing the Quality Chasm: A New Health System for the 21st Century.* Washington, DC: National Academies Press; 2001

APPENDIX 1   2005 ACMG Recommended Screening Panel

OA	FAO	AA	Hemoglobinopathies	Other
Core panel				
Isovaleric acidemia	Medium-chain acyl-CoA dehydrogenase deficiency	Phenylketonuria	Sickle cell anemia (Hb SS disease) Hb	Congenital hypothyroidism
Glutaric acidemia type I	Very long-chain acyl-CoA dehydrogenase deficiency	Maple syrup disease	Hb S/β-thalassemia	Biotinidase deficiency
3-Hydroxy-3-methylglutaryl-CoA lyase deficiency	Long-chain L-3-hydroxy acyl-CoA dehydrogenase deficiency	Homocystinuria (caused by cystathionine β-synthase)	Hb S/C disease	Congenital adrenal hyperplasia (21-hydroxylase deficiency)
Multiple carboxylase deficiency	Trifunctional protein deficiency	Citrullinemia		Classical galactosemia
Methylmalonic acidemia (mutase deficiency)	Carnitine-uptake defect	Argininosuccinic acidemia		Hearing loss
3-Methylcrotonyl-CoA carboxylase deficiency		Tyrosinemia type I		Cystic fibrosis
Methylmalonic acidemia (Cbl A,B)				
Propionic acidemia				
β-ketothiolase deficiency				
Secondary targets				
Methylmalonic acidemia (Cbl C,D)	Short-chain acyl-CoA dehydrogenase deficiency	Benign hyperphenylalaninemia	Variant hemoglobinopathies (including Hb E)	Galactokinase deficiency
Malonic acidemia	Glutaric acidemia type II	Tyrosinemia type II		Galactose epimerase deficiency
Isobutyryl-CoA dehydrogenase deficiency	Medium/short-chain L-3-hydroxy acyl-CoA dehydrogenase deficiency	Defects of biopterin cofactor biosynthesis		
2-Methyl 3-hydroxy butyric aciduria	Medium-chain ketoacyl-CoA thiolase deficiency	Argininemia		
2-Methylbutyryl-CoA dehydrogenase deficiency	Carnitine palmitoyltransferase II deficiency	Tyrosinemia type III		
3-Methylglutaconic aciduria	Carnitine: acylcarnitine translocase deficiency	Defects of biopterin cofactor regeneration		
	Carnitine palmitoyltransferase I deficiency (liver)	Hypermethioninemia		
	Dienoyl-CoA reductase deficiency	Citrullinemia type II		

OA indicates disorders of organic acid metabolism; FAO, disorders of fatty acid metabolism; AA, disorders of amino acid metabolism; CoA, coenzyme A.

APPENDIX 2.

Algorithm 1

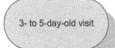

At the 3- to 5-day-old visit, the PCP should check for circumstances suggesting newborn screening might *not* have been conducted. Concerning situations include home or emergency births or international adoption.

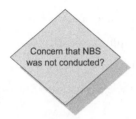

If the PCP has cause for concern that the newborn screening was not ordered and available discharge papers do not indicate the newborn screening has been ordered, the PCP should make arrangements for sample acquisition.

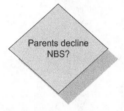

If newborn screening has not been conducted because of parental refusal or if parents refuse newborn screening suggested by the PCP, the PCP should discuss the general benefits and limited risks of newborn screening as well as possible implications of not testing.

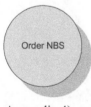

Educational materials for parents and PCPs can be accessed through the AAP Web site (www.medicalhomeinfo.org/screening/newborn.html). Parent concerns and questions should be addressed fully, and a discussion of the general benefits and limited risks of newborn screening is recommended. Very treatable conditions, such as phenylketonuria (PKU) and congenital hypothyroidism (CH), may be used as examples. If parental permission is obtained, arrangements for sample acquisition should be made immediately, and newborn screening should be ordered, as noted previously.

Newborn screening is conducted through the state newborn screening program, and protocols for ordering the screen vary by state. Contact information for each state's newborn screening program is available (http://genes-r-us.uthscsa.edu/resources/consumer/statemap.htm; Appendix 4).

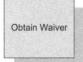

If parental permission is not obtained, parents or guardians should be asked to sign a waiver documenting their choice to decline newborn screening. A sample waiver form is included as Appendix 5; appropriate waiver forms should also be available through the state health department.

PCPs should flag the charts of any patients who have not been screened so that the lack of screening will be taken into account should any subsequent concerns emerge regarding the child's growth or development. The chart note should also prompt the pediatrician to return to the question of newborn screening with subsequent visits to determine whether parents have changed their minds.

Special Circumstances

- In cases in which newborn screening is delayed, the PCP should consult with the state newborn screening program regarding the availability and usefulness of the newborn screening protocol.

- In the case of preterm births, neonatal transfusion, and other circumstances in which screening is not ordered or a second specimen is required, the PCP should consult with a neonatal specialist.

APPENDIX 3.

Algorithm 2

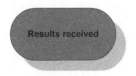

In the case of an out-of-range screening result, the pediatrician identified on the newborn screening card should be called by the state newborn screening program within the first week after birth. Normal results are often transmitted by mail; these may arrive before to the 2- to 4-week visit.

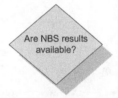

Delays or procedural failures at hospitals, state laboratories, or other facilities or within the newborn screening program may result in late or lost results. The PCP cannot assume a "no news is good news" approach with regard to newborn screening.

Office staff should check routinely for newborn screening results before the 2- to 4-week visit and pursue missing results in advance of that visit.

If newborn screening results are not available before the 2- to 4-week visit, the PCP should contact the state newborn screening program for the results at that time.

Special Circumstances

Newborn screening results may occasionally be sent to the wrong pediatrician. Physicians who receive results for patients no longer in their care should immediately contact the state newborn screening program and/or hospital to alert them that the PCP may not have received these results.

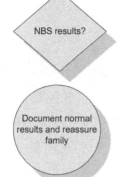

The state newborn screening program will report results as normal, unsatisfactory, or abnormal.

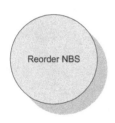

Normal newborn screening results should be noted in the infant's chart and shared with the parents or guardians. Keep in mind that newborn screening does not rule out congenital disorders that are not included in the panel and does not absolutely guarantee the absence of the disorders that are screened.

Special Circumstances

Currently, 9 states mandate a second screening, and 12 states allow it. If necessary, the PCP should order another newborn screening.

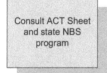

In instances where the specimen is unacceptable for testing, the infant's newborn screen must be reordered and a specimen must be obtained promptly.

If abnormal results are received, the PCP should access the ACT sheet specific to the disorder. The ACT sheet may be provided by the state newborn screening program or can be accessed at: www.acmg.net/resources/policies/ACT/condition-analyte-links.htm.

The most important actions to take are highlighted on the ACT sheets and include:

- When to contact the family;
- Whom to consult and whether an appointment is needed immediately;
- When the patient must be seen by the PCP;
- Whether further confirmatory testing is needed and what tests should be conducted;
- Whether treatment is necessary and what treatment to initiate;

- How to educate parents about the disorder;
- When findings need to be reported back to the newborn screening program.

In addition to following ACT sheet recommendations, the PCP should consult with the state newborn screening program.

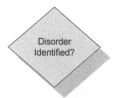

After an abnormal screening result is obtained, confirmatory testing and/or definitive consultation with subspecialists are required before a final diagnosis can be made.

Special Circumstances

In addition to true or false positive results, confirmatory tests may identify the child as a carrier of the disorder or may be of indeterminate result.

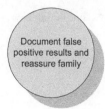

In the event that the initial positive result proves to be a false positive result, the PCP can provide reassurance to parents. Up to 20% of these parents will persist in their concerns about the health of their children for months or years after screening.

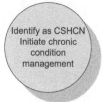

To lay the foundation for comprehensive and collaborative care, it is critical during this time of uncertainty that the parents and family of the neonate be provided with disorder-specific information and support as they await final clarification of the child's diagnosis and begin to plan for treatment and management. Frequent, specific, and supportive communication from the PCP will help to avoid confusion and build trust.

The parents and family of the neonate should be provided with disorder-specific information and support as they await final clarification of the child's diagnosis and begin to plan for treatment and management.

Any child in whom a significant medical disorder is diagnosed should be entered into the practice's registry for children with special health care needs, and chronic care management should be initiated. Chronic care management provides proactive care for children with special health care needs, including condition-related office visits, written care plans, explicit comanagement with specialists, appropriate patient education, and effective information systems for monitoring and tracking the child's disorder.

A subspecialist may provide substantial ongoing care for a child with a severe and complex disorder. However, the PCP retains the responsibility to provide a medical home, which is the central source of "family-centered, accessible, continuous, coordinated, comprehensive, compassionate, and culturally effective" care for the family, and the family should be encouraged to maintain their relationship with their PCP.

The complex nature of many disorders identified by newborn screening may require care by a team of medical subspecialists, therapists, nutritionists, and educators. Clearly defined roles may help to reduce redundancies of services and prevent fragmentation of care.

APPENDIX 4   CONTACT INFORMATION FOR STATE NEWBORN SCREENING PROGRAMS

State	Contact	Web Site	Telephone	E-mail
Alabama	Melissa Tucker, AuD, CCC-A, Director of Newborn Screening Program	www.adph.org/newbornscreening	(334) 206–2944	melissatucker@adph.state.al.us
Alaska	Stephanie Birch, RNC, BSN, MPH, MCH Title V and CSHCN Director	www.hss.state.ak.us/dph/wcfh/screening_testing.htm	(907) 334–2424	stephanie_birch@health.state.ak.us
Arizona	Jan Kerrigan, RN, Program Manager	www.aznewborn.com/index.htm	(602) 364–1409	kerrigij@azdhs.gov
Arkansas	Dianne Pettit, Newborn Screening Coordinator	www.healthyarkansas.com/services/services_ph2.html#Newborn	(501) 280–4145	dpettit@arkansas.gov
California	John E. Sherwin, PhD, NBS Director	www.dhs.ca.gov/pcfh/gdb/html/nbs/	(510) 231–1728	jsherwin@dhs.ca.gov
Colorado	Vickie Thomson, MA, Director for the Newborn Screening Program	www.cdphe.state.co.us/ps/hcp/nbms/index.html	(303) 692–2458	vickie.thomson@colorado.edu
Connecticut	Vine Samuels, Newborn Screening Supervisor	www.dph.state.ct.us/BCH/NBS/NBS.htm	(860) 509–8081	vine.samuels@po.state.ct.us
Delaware	Betsy Voss, Newborn Screening Program Director	www.dhss.delaware.gov/dhss/dph/chca/dphnsp1.html	(302) 741–2987	betsy.voss@state.de.us
District of Columbia	Michelle Sermon, Genetics Program Specialist	http://doh.dc.gov/doh/cwp/view,a,3,q,573233,dohNav_GID,1802,dohNav,%67C33200%67C3324%67C.asp	(202) 442–9162	michelle.sermon@dc.gov
Florida	Lois Taylor, Director, Florida Newborn Screening Program	www.cms-kids.com/InfantScrning.htm	(850) 245–4670	lois.taylor@doh.state.fl.us
Georgia	Mary Ann Henson, MSN, Genetics Program Manager	http://health.state.ga.us/programs/nsmscd/index.asp	(404) 657–6359	mahenson@dhr.state.ga.us
Hawaii	Christine Matsumoto, Newborn Metabolic Screening Program Coordinator	www.state.hi.us/health/family-child-health/genetics/genetics/nbshome.html	(808) 733–9069	chris.matsumoto@fhsd.health.state.hi.us
Idaho	Paige Fincher, Acting Manager	www.healthandwelfare.idaho.gov	(208) 334–4935	fincherp@idhw.state.id.us
Illinois	Claude-Alix Jacob, Deputy Director	www.idph.state.il.us/HealthWellness/genetics.htm	(217) 785–4093	claude.jacob@illinois.gov
Indiana	Iris Stone, Chief Nurse Consultant	www.in.gov/isdh/programs/nbs/NewbornScrSitemap.htm	(317) 233–1379	istone@isdh.in.gov
Iowa	Kimberly Noble Piper, State Genetics Coordinator	www.idph.state.ia.us/genetics/neonatal_parent_page.asp	(515) 281–6466	kpiper@idph.state.ia.us
Kansas	Melanie Warren, Follow-up Coordinator	www.kdheks.gov/newborn_screening	(785) 291–3363	mwarren@kdhe.state.ks.us
Kentucky	Sandy Fawbush, Nurse Administrator	http://chfs.ky.gov/dph/ach/ecd/newbornscreening.htm	(502) 564-3756, ext 3563	sandy.fawbush.ky.gov
Louisiana	Charles Myers, GSW, Program Administrator	www.dhh.louisiana.gov/offices/page.asp? ID = 263&Detail = 6302	(504) 219–4411	charlie@dhh.la.gov
Maine	John (Jack) A. Krueger, MSChE, Chief, Health and Environmental Testing Laboratory	www.maine.gov/dhhs/etl/newborn.htm	(207) 287–2727	john.a.krueger@maine.gov
Maryland	Susan Panning, NBS Director	www.fha.state.md.us/genetics/html/nbs_ndx.cfm	(410) 767–6730	panny.s.dhmh.state.md.us
Massachusetts	Roger Eaton, Director	www.umassmed.edu/nbs/index.aspx	(617) 983–6300	roger.eaton@umassmed.edu
Michigan	William Young, Newborn Screening Program Director	www.michigan.gov/mdch/0,1607,7-132-2942_4911_4916-64851---,00.html	(517) 335–8938	youngw@michigan.gov
Minnesota	Mark McCann, Supervisor, Newborn Screening Public Health Laboratory	www.health.state.mn.us/divs/fh/mcshn/nbshome.htm	(651) 201–5450; (651) 201–5471 (fax)	mark.mccann@state.mn.us
Mississippi	Beryl W. Polk, Director of Genetic Services	www.msdh.state.ms.us/msdhsite/index.cfm/41,0101,html	(601) 576–7619	bpolk@msdh.state.ms.us
Missouri	Sharmini V. Rogers, MD, BBS, MPH, Bureau Chief of Genetics and Healthy Childhood	www.dhss.mo.gov/NewbornScreening	(573) 751–6214	sharmini.rogers@dhss.mo.gov
Montana	Sib Clack, Newborn Screening Manager	www.dphhs.mt.gov/PHSD/family-health/newborn/newborn-screening.shtml	(406) 444–1216	sclack@mt.gov

APPENDIX 4 Continued

State	Contact	Telephone	Web Site	E-mail
Nebraska	Julie Miller, Program Manager	(402) 471-6733	www.hhs.state.ne.us/nsp	julie.miller@hhss.ne.gov
Nevada	[Vacant]		http://health.nv.gov/index.php	
New Hampshire	Marcia LaVochkin, Newborn Screening Program Coordinator	(603) 271-4225	www.dhhs.state.nh.us/DHHS/MCH/default.htm	mlavochkin@dhhs.state.nh.us
New Jersey	Mary Mickles, Program Manager of Newborn Screening and Genetics Services	(609) 292-1582	www.state.nj.us/health/fhs/nbs/index.shtml	mary.mickles@doh.state.nj.us
New Mexico	[Vacant]	(505) 841-2581	http://sld.state.nm.us/nms	
New York	Michele Caggana, MD, SCD FACNG Chief of Laboratory of Genetic Services	(518) 473-3854	www.wadsworth.org/newborn	mxc08@health.state.ny.us
North Carolina	Shu Chiang, Unit Supervisor Newborn Screening/Clinical Commissioner	(919) 733-3937	http://slph.state.nc.us/Newborn/default.asp	chu.chiang@ncmail.net
North Dakota	Barb Schweitzer, RN, Director of Newborn Screening	(701) 328-4538	www.ndmch.com/metabolic-screening/default.asp	bschweit@nd.gov
Ohio	William Becker, MD, Medical Director of Laboratory	(888) 634-5227	www.odh.ohio.gov/odhPrograms/phl/newbrn/nbrn1.aspx	william.becker@odh.ohio.gov
Oklahoma	Pam King, MPA, RN, Director of Genetics and State Genetics Coordinator	(405) 271-9444 ext 56737	www.health.state.ok.us/program/gp/index.html	pamk@health.ok.gov
Oregon	Cheryl Hermerath, Newborn Screening Program Manager	(503) 229-5882	http://oregon.gov/DHS/ph/nbs/index.shtml	cheryl.a.hermerath@state.or.us
Pennsylvania	M. Jeffery Shoemaker, PhD, Director	(610) 280-3464	www.dsf.health.state.pa.us/health/cwp/view.asp?a=167&q=202513	mshoemaker@state.pa.us
Puerto Rico	P.J.Santiago Borrero, Director of Hereditary Disease Program	(787) 754-3623		pjsantiago@centennial.net
Rhode Island	Ellen Amore, MS, Newborn Screening Program Manager	(401) 222-4601	www.health.ri.gov/genetics/newborn.php	ellena@doh.state.ri.us
South Carolina	Kathy Tomashitis, Pediatric Screening Follow-up Program, SC DHEC, Women and Children's Services	(803) 898-0619	www.scdhec.net/health/lab/analyt/newborn.htm	tomashk@dhec.sc.gov
South Dakota	Lucy Fossen, Newborn Screening Coordinator	(605) 773-2944	www.state.sd.us/doh/NewbornScreening	lucy.fossen@state.sd.us
Tennessee	Mitzi Lamberth, Newborn Screening Follow-up Program Director	(615) 262-6304	http://health.state.tn.us/womenshealth/NBS/index.htm	mitzi.lamberth@state.tn.us
Texas	David Martinez, Program Director	(512) 458-7111, ext 2216	www.dshs.state.tx.us/newborn/default.shtm	davidr.martinez@dshs.state.tx.us
Utah	Fay Keune, RN, Program Manager	(801) 584-8256	http://health.utah.gov/newbornscreening	fkeune@utah.gov
Vermont	Cynthia Ingham, Newborn Screening Program Chief	(802) 951-5180	http://healthvermont.gov/regs/newborn_screening_reg.aspx	cingham@vdh.state.vt.us
Virginia	Sharon K. Williams, RN, MS, Genetics Program Manager	(804) 864-7712	www.vahealth.org/PSGS/	sharonk.williams@vdh.virginia.gov
Washington	Mike Glass, Director	(206) 418-5470	www.doh.wa.gov/ehsphl/phl/newborn/default.htm	mike.glass@doh.wa.gov
West Virginia	Cathy Cummons, Newborn Screening Research Director	(304) 558-5388	www.wvdhhr.org/mcfh/icah/unlinked/newborn_screening.htm	cathycummons@wvdhhr.org
Wisconsin	Gary Hoffman, Newborn Screening Laboratory Manager	(608) 262-4692	www.slh.wisc.edu/newborn	hoffman@mail.slh.wis.edu
Wyoming	Shelly Gonzalez Sherry Long, Metabolic Records Analyst Nurse Consultant	(307) 777-7943; (307) 777-7948	http://wdh.state.wy.us/csh/index.asp	sgonza@state.wy.us; slong@state.wy.us

MCH indicates Maternal Child Health; CSHCN, children with special health care needs; NBS, newborn screening; SC DHEC, South Carolina Department of Health and Environmental Control.

THE AMERICAN ACADEMY OF PEDIATRICS STRONGLY RECOMMENDS NEWBORN SCREENING FOR ALL INFANTS

Refusal for Newborn Screening

Child's Name: _____ Child's Date of Birth: _____

Parent's/Legal Guardian's Name: _____

My child's doctor/nurse _____has advised me that my child (named above) should participate in the newborn screening program.

☐   As the parent or legal guardian of my child (named above), I choose to decline participation in my state's newborn screening program.

I have been provided information about newborn screening in my state and the importance of early identification of the diseases. I have had the opportunity to discuss these with my child's doctor or nurse, who has answered my questions regarding the recommended screening. I understand the following:

- The purpose of and the need for newborn screening.
- The risks and benefits of newborn screening.
- **If my child does not participate in newborn screening, the consequences of a late diagnosis of certain conditions can include mental retardation or death.**
- My child's doctor or nurse and the American Academy of Pediatrics strongly recommend that all newborn infants be screened for certain disorders.
- If my child has one of my state's screened conditions, failure to participate in newborn screening may endanger the health or life of my child.

Nevertheless, I have decided at this time to decline participation in the newborn screening program for my child, as indicated by checking the box above.

I acknowledge that I have read this document or it has been read to me in its entirety and I fully understand it.

Parent's/Legal Guardian's Signature _____ Date _____

Witness _____ Date _____

I have had the opportunity to re-discuss my decision not to participate in my state's newborn screening program and still decline the recommended participation.

Parent's initials _____ Date _____ Parent's initials _____ Date _____
Parent's initials _____ Date _____ Parent's initials _____ Date _____

LF\ 6014946.1

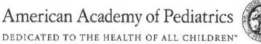

American Academy of Pediatrics
DEDICATED TO THE HEALTH OF ALL CHILDREN™

APPENDIX 5: DOCUMENTING REFUSAL TO HAVE INFANTS UNDERGO NEWBORN SCREENING

Despite the best efforts of health care professionals to educate parents and guardians about the need to have their infants undergo newborn screening and the importance of newborn screening in the early identification of certain diseases, some parents and guardians will decline to have their infants undergo newborn screening.

All parents and guardians should be informed about the purpose of and need for newborn screening, the risks and benefits of newborn screening, and the consequences of late diagnosis of certain conditions that would have been identified earlier through newborn screening. The use of this or a similar form that demonstrates the importance you place on newborn screening and focuses attention on the unnecessary risk for which a parent or guardian is accepting responsibility may, in some instances, induce a wavering parent or guardian to accept your recommendation.

Disclaimer. This form may be used as a template for such documentation, but it should not be used without obtaining legal advice from a qualified health care attorney about the use of the form in your practice. Moreover, completion of a form, in and of itself, never substitutes for good risk communication, nor would it provide absolute immunity from liability. For instances in which parents or guardians refuse newborn screening, health care professionals should take advantage of their ongoing relationship with the family and revisit the discussion on subsequent visits. Documentation in the medical chart of such follow-up discussions is strongly recommended, and the template, therefore, makes provision for this documentation.

This form may be duplicated or changed to suit your needs and your patients' needs and should be reviewed with your health care attorney before use. It will be available on the AAP Web[7] site (www.aap.org/bookstore).

TECHNICAL REPORT

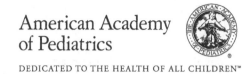

American Academy of Pediatrics

DEDICATED TO THE HEALTH OF ALL CHILDREN™

Newborn Screening for Biliary Atresia

Kasper S. Wang, MD, FAAP, FACS, THE SECTION ON SURGERY, THE COMMITTEE ON FETUS AND NEWBORN, THE CHILDHOOD LIVER DISEASE RESEARCH NETWORK

abstract

Biliary atresia is the most common cause of pediatric end-stage liver disease and the leading indication for pediatric liver transplantation. Affected infants exhibit evidence of biliary obstruction within the first few weeks after birth. Early diagnosis and successful surgical drainage of bile are associated with greater survival with the child's native liver. Unfortunately, because noncholestatic jaundice is extremely common in early infancy, it is difficult to identify the rare infant with cholestatic jaundice who has biliary atresia. Hence, the need for timely diagnosis of this disease warrants a discussion of the feasibility of screening for biliary atresia to improve outcomes. Herein, newborn screening for biliary atresia in the United States is assessed by using criteria established by the Discretionary Advisory Committee on Heritable Disorders in Newborns and Children. Published analyses indicate that newborn screening for biliary atresia by using serum bilirubin concentrations or stool color cards is potentially life-saving and cost-effective. Further studies are necessary to evaluate the feasibility, effectiveness, and costs of potential screening strategies for early identification of biliary atresia in the United States.

Biliary atresia is the most common cause of pediatric end-stage liver disease and the leading indication for pediatric liver transplantation.[1] Infants with biliary atresia develop jaundice and pale, acholic stools within the first few weeks after birth, secondary to fibroinflammatory obstruction of the extrahepatic bile ducts that drain bile from the liver into the intestines. Early diagnosis and successful surgical drainage of bile (the Kasai hepatic portoenterostomy) are associated with greater survival with the child's native liver. Lack of effective drainage inevitably results in liver failure within a year and death within 2 years without transplantation. Successful surgical drainage can, in most instances, prevent or delay the need for liver transplantation, which is associated with significant morbidities from requisite lifelong immunosuppression.[2–5] Unfortunately, because noncholestatic jaundice is extremely common in early infancy, it is difficult to identify the rare infant with cholestasis who has biliary atresia. Education regarding the importance of early identification of biliary atresia could be included in professional continuing education programs for primary care physicians. Thus, the need for timely

Technical reports from the American Academy of Pediatrics benefit from expertise and resources of liaisons and internal (AAP) and external reviewers. However, technical reports from the American Academy of Pediatrics may not reflect the views of the liaisons or the organizations or government agencies that they represent.

The guidance in this report does not indicate an exclusive course of treatment or serve as a standard of medical care. Variations, taking into account individual circumstances, may be appropriate.

All technical reports from the American Academy of Pediatrics automatically expire 5 years after publication unless reaffirmed, revised, or retired at or before that time.

www.pediatrics.org/cgi/doi/10.1542/peds.2015-3570

DOI: 10.1542/peds.2015-3570

PEDIATRICS (ISSN Numbers: Print, 0031-4005; Online, 1098-4275).

diagnosis of this disease warrants a discussion of the feasibility of screening for biliary atresia to improve outcomes.

The Discretionary Advisory Committee on Heritable Disorders in Newborns and Children, established in 2003, evaluates conditions nominated for inclusion in the Recommended Uniform Screening Panel and subsequently makes recommendations to the secretary of the US Department of Health and Human Services.[6] An external evidence review group informs the Advisory Committee on the direct and indirect evidence used to answer a series of key questions regarding the potential benefit of newborn screening for a condition. The Advisory Committee then grades the evidence in terms of the benefit of screening and feasibility of screening for the condition.[6-8] Herein, these key questions are used to inform a consensus among the authors of this report in the evaluation of newborn screening for biliary atresia in the United States.

Biliary atresia is an idiopathic cholangiopathy presenting with a

---

KEY QUESTION SET 1: DEFINING BILIARY ATRESIA AND THE EXTENT OF DISEASE

- Is there a case definition for biliary atresia that can be uniformly and reliably applied?
- What is the incidence and prevalence of biliary atresia?
- What is the natural history of biliary atresia, including the spectrum of severity and variations by key phenotypic or genotypic characteristics?

---

series of findings: (1) complete obstruction of extrahepatic bile ducts documented by cholangiography or bile duct histology, (2) proliferation of intrahepatic bile ducts on liver biopsy, and (3) marked intrahepatic fibrosis at an early age.[4] The reported incidence of biliary atresia ranges from 5 per 100 000 in the Netherlands to 32 per 100 000 live births in French Polynesia.[9] The incidence of biliary atresia is approximately 6.5 to 7.5 per 100 000 live births in the US mainland and 10.1 per 100 000 live births in Hawaii.

The natural history of biliary atresia explains why it is difficult to diagnose. Infants with biliary atresia generally appear healthy as newborns. They do, however, exhibit jaundice at birth or shortly thereafter and may be clinically indistinguishable from infants with nonconjugated or indirect hyperbilirubinemia, such as "physiological jaundice" and "breast milk–associated jaundice." Conditions causing conjugated or direct hyperbilirubinemia, which are much less common, include infections, such as toxoplasmosis, rubella, cytomegalovirus, herpes, and hepatitis B, and genetic conditions, such as Alagille syndrome, α-1 antitrypsin deficiency, cystic fibrosis, progressive familial intrahepatic cholestasis, mitochondrial hepatopathies, and bile acid synthesis defects. The diagnosis of biliary atresia should be considered for any infant with an elevated serum conjugated bilirubin concentration and pale or acholic stools. Because nearly half of all newborn infants exhibit jaundice in the early days of life, making a diagnosis other than physiologic jaundice or breast milk–associated jaundice is challenging. Thus, a late-stage diagnosis of biliary atresia is not uncommon.

The treatment of biliary atresia is the hepatic portoenterostomy, as originally described by Kasai in 1959. The operation involves excision of the extrahepatic biliary tree, with reestablishment of bile flow via a Roux-en-Y segment of intestine sewn directly to the liver at the portal plate.[1] Whereas all infants with biliary atresia not receiving the Kasai operation will need liver transplantation in the first 1 to 2 years of life, infants receiving the Kasai operation gain considerable benefit, and some avoid liver transplantation altogether. Ultimately, however, approximately 80% of all patients with biliary atresia will require liver transplantation by 10 years of age.[1] Patients with successful biliary drainage may develop cirrhosis more slowly, which can delay the need for liver transplantation into childhood or early adult life. This group of patients is generally healthier before the transplantation, has a larger pool of liver donors for the liver transplantation, and has a better postoperative course after liver transplantation. The most significant factor correlating with success of the Kasai operation is the infant's age at the time of surgery, with younger infants receiving the greatest benefit. The extent of intrahepatic fibrosis at the time of diagnosis is a key pathologic finding that correlates negatively with prognosis with treatment.[1,10] Clinical evidence of cirrhosis at diagnosis (ie, presence of ascites) correlates with poorer outcome after portoenterostomy.[1] Evidence of associated splenic malformations, such as asplenia or polysplenia, also is associated with poorer outcomes.[1,11]

Hence, there is a good case definition of biliary atresia, which is uniformly and reliably applied; the incidence is comparable to other diseases for which screening is performed, such as phenylketonuria and congenital adrenal hyperplasia; and early recognition and treatment contribute to improving transplant-free survival.

Two screening tests have been investigated: serum conjugated or direct bilirubin concentrations and stool color cards. Because the earliest

KEY QUESTION SET 2: MODALITIES AND POTENTIAL EFFECTIVENESS OF SCREENING FOR BILIARY ATRESIA

- What methods are available to screen newborn-infants for biliary atresia?
- What are the accuracy; the ability to distinguish early versus late onset cases; the sensitivity, specificity, and predictive values; the analytic and clinical validity; and the feasibility of implementing these methods for universal screening?
- What are the potential harms or risks of screening for biliary atresia?
- What is known about costs and cost-effectiveness of screening for biliary atresia? What pilot testing has taken place in population studies or clinical groups?

indicator of abnormality in biliary atresia is an increased conjugated bilirubin concentration, this is a logical test to investigate for universal screening, and several studies have found promising results. In 2003, Powell et al[12] studied a large community-based program in the United Kingdom wherein conjugated bilirubin concentrations were measured from blood samples in neonates younger than 28 days. Of 23 415 samples, conjugated bilirubin concentrations exceeded 18 µmol/L (1.05 mg/dL) in 3.8% of samples. The fraction of conjugated bilirubin relative to total bilirubin exceeded 20% in 16% of samples, and 107 samples (0.46%) exceeded both cutoffs. No infant with a normal test result had liver disease. Thus, this test had a sensitivity of 100%, a specificity of 99.59%, and a positive predictive value of 10%, which is low because of the rarity of clinical liver disease in neonates. Ultimately, 11 of 12 infants with abnormal results on repeat testing were diagnosed with liver disease, 2 of whom had biliary atresia. Although the authors concluded that serum conjugated

bilirubin concentration may be an effective marker for neonatal liver disease, the sensitivity and specificity of screening for biliary atresia may not be accurate, given that only 2 infants would be expected to have biliary atresia in the sample size used. Additional larger studies are, therefore, needed to validate these findings.

Harpavat et al[13] retrospectively studied whether elevated conjugated bilirubin concentration can be used as an early screening test for infants with biliary atresia. Of 61 infants with biliary atresia, 34 had had serum direct or conjugated bilirubin concentration measured within 96 hours of life, and all demonstrated elevated concentrations, which increased over the first 96 hours. The authors speculated that an elevated conjugated bilirubin concentration might be present in all infants with biliary atresia in the immediate postnatal period. In subsequent follow-up, the authors have validated this observation by identifying elevated conjugated bilirubin concentration shortly after birth in 32 of 32 infants cared for at their institution who were later diagnosed with biliary atresia (S. Harpavat, MD, PhD, personal communication, 2015). Thus, serum conjugated or direct bilirubin concentration could prove a valuable screening test for biliary atresia. Cutoffs for the upper limit of normal in young infants would need to be verified in each hospital laboratory. The test would also need to be accompanied by an aggressive educational program for health care providers for an understanding of age-related normal values, as the infants in the Harpavat et al[13] study who had an early abnormal conjugated bilirubin concentration did not come to medical attention any sooner than those who did not have neonatal conjugated or direct bilirubin tested. These observations, in conjunction with those of Powell et al,[12] indicate great potential for serum bilirubin determinations as a screening tool for biliary atresia.

The second potential screening test is the use of stool color cards. The first universal national screening program was implemented in Taiwan, where there is a relatively high incidence of biliary atresia (37/100 000 live births) and, therefore, great motivation to identify infants with biliary atresia early.[14] Parents of all newborn infants were given color cards that showed examples of normal and acholic stools and were asked to report the color of their infant's stool to their pediatrician. In this study, cards were returned for 65% of 119 973 infants. Ninety-four of these infants had acholic stools, and 29 (31%) were ultimately diagnosed with biliary atresia, 90% of whom were diagnosed before 60 days of age. In the Taiwanese population, the stool color card screening program had a sensitivity of 89.7%, a specificity of 99.9%, a positive predictive value of 28.6%, and a negative predictive value of 99.9% for identification of biliary atresia.[14] Positive results from the screening led to focused diagnostic evaluations. In subsequent analyses, the authors concluded that implementation of this screening program led to earlier diagnosis and earlier Kasai surgery (66% vs 49% at <60 days of age) and was associated with improved 3-year jaundice-free survival (57% vs 31.5%) compared with a cohort of historical controls.[15] Confounding this correlation, however, was the increased use of prophylactic antibiotic agents, which may have prevented cholangitis and improved outcomes, following the Kasai operation in Taiwan part of the way through the historical control time period. Given these encouraging observations, Argentina[16] and Switzerland[17] implemented similar nationwide stool color card screening and biliary atresia education programs.

Gu et al[18] recently reported the 19-year experience of Tochigi Prefecture in Japan with stool color card screening for biliary atresia. The authors reported a decrease in the mean age at the time of the Kasai procedure from 70.3 days to 59.7 days. Of the 34 infants in whom biliary atresia was diagnosed during the study period, 26 were identified via screening. Eight infants were not identified via screening at 1-month follow-up for a variety of reasons, including no action taken despite reporting of pale stool, loss to follow-up, and noncompliance with use of the stool color card. These patients underwent the Kasai procedure at a much later age than those who were identified and promptly worked up for biliary atresia (77.5 ± 20.4 days vs 54.3 ± 15.8 days; P = .002). Survival with native liver for the 34 identified infants was better at 5, 10, and 15 years (87.6%, 76.9%, and 48.5%, respectively) compared with historical controls. Through 2010, the stool color card program has since expanded to 16 other administrative divisions in Japan.

Thus, serum conjugated bilirubin concentrations and stool color cards both exhibit reasonable clinical validity as potential screening modalities for biliary atresia. In neither case is there significant clinical risk or harm to the infant undergoing screening. It could be proposed that blood be drawn for serum bilirubin determinations at the same time as for any other blood tests before discharge from the newborn nursery.

Biliary atresia is currently diagnosed by using a number of modalities. Infants with unexplained conjugated hyperbilirubinemia can undergo serologic testing, including antibody titers against infectious diseases, including toxoplasmosis, rubella, cytomegalovirus, herpes, hepatitis B, syphilis, Coxsackie virus, Epstein-Barr virus, varicella-zoster virus, and human parvovirus, all of which can be associated with jaundice. Ultrasonography of the liver can assess for the presence and size of the gallbladder and identify abnormal

---

KEY QUESTION SET 3: CURRENT METHODS OF TESTING FOR BILIARY ATRESIA

- What are the current methods and costs of diagnostic testing for biliary atresia and availability and capability of diagnostic centers?
- For treatment, does presymptomatic or early symptomatic treatment improve health outcomes, and if so, more than treatment after symptoms develop?

---

findings at the porta hepatis, as well as identify a choledochal cyst. Ultrasonography also can determine the presence of ascites, whether 1 or multiple spleens are present, and the echogenicity of the liver, which is potentially reflective of fibrosis. A technetium-labeled hepatobiliary iminodiacetic acid scan can be performed to determine whether bile drains into the gastrointestinal tract. Nonexcretion of radioisotope into the intestines after initial uptake by hepatocytes is consistent with biliary atresia but may also occur in other intrahepatic cholestatic diseases, and, thus, it is a nonspecific finding. Liver biopsy can be performed to assess for pathologic features of biliary atresia percutaneously under conscious sedation or via a laparotomy with a wedge liver biopsy under general anesthesia if there are greater concerns for bleeding given coagulopathy. Liver transient elastography and sonography are currently under investigation to determine extent of fibrosis noninvasively before surgery.[19] Ultimately, the diagnosis of biliary atresia is confirmed and the Kasai procedure is performed after direct intraoperative visual inspection and intraoperative cholangiography performed by a pediatric surgeon. Charges and costs for these tests and procedures vary widely, and there are insufficient data to determine the cost for diagnosis.

Early diagnosis and treatment is optimal for biliary atresia. All infants with biliary atresia initially exhibit jaundice. They eventually excrete acholic stools. As weeks pass and the liver becomes increasingly fibrotic, infants with biliary atresia will exhibit manifestations of portal hypertension with abdominal ascites and spider angiomata. Failure to thrive, fat-soluble vitamin deficiencies, and cachexia also can develop because of profound malabsorption. The Kasai operation is ideally performed before onset of portal hypertension.

Kasai portoenterostomy is well established as the treatment of biliary atresia. Success rates of biliary drainage after the Kasai operation range from 47% in the United States to 65% in Japan.[1,20] Numerous studies have demonstrated that early diagnosis and treatment with the Kasai operation are associated with better survival without liver transplantation. A retrospective analysis of 251 patients at a single center found that 10-year survival without transplantation was highest (73%) if age at time of surgery was <60 days and lowest (11%) if age at

---

KEY QUESTION SET 4: EFFECTIVENESS OF TREATMENT OF BILIARY ATRESIA

- What is known about the efficacy and effectiveness of treatment?
- What is the relationship between treatment timing and treatment outcomes?
- Is treatment standardized? What are the potential harms or risks of treatment?

---

time of surgery was >91 days.[20] Two other cohort studies similarly showed greatest success rates when surgical drainage was performed at <30 or <45 days of age.[21] More recently, a prospective study of 159 infants funded by the National Institutes of Health reported that performance of the Kasai procedure at <75 days was associated with greater transplant-free survival.[1] Delayed treatment by Kasai procedure is associated not only with progressive liver failure but also with impaired neurodevelopmental outcome and poor nutritional status.[22,23] Although early diagnosis is associated with improved outcomes after Kasai operation, diagnosis at the time of end-stage liver failure may occur.[1] Screening would enhance awareness of biliary atresia within the pediatric community.

Even a successful Kasai operation with reestablished flow of bile does not ensure cessation of fibrogenesis and prevention of end-stage liver failure. However, without a successful Kasai operation, progression to end-stage liver failure is more rapid and inevitable. Postoperatively, ascending cholangitis is a common complication. Lee et al[24] reported that 27 (64%) of 42 patients experienced at least 1 episode of cholangitis after Kasai operation. Most patients in their cohort experienced multiple episodes of cholangitis requiring hospitalization, with an average length of stay of 15 days. Ng et al[25] reported that 17% of 219 patients who retained their native livers at least 5 years after their Kasai operations had experienced an episode of cholangitis in the preceding year.

A screening test algorithm for biliary atresia has 1 clear goal: to identify affected infants early so they can receive an early Kasai operation and associated benefits, without placing an excessive burden on families and the health care system from false-positive results. Both screening options have advantages and disadvantages. Conjugated bilirubin measurements are widely available, easily interpretable, and inexpensive, with clear cutoffs for abnormal values. They do require blood to be drawn, as conjugated bilirubin concentrations are not measured by instruments measuring

KEY QUESTION SET 5: IMPLICATIONS OF SCREENING FOR BILIARY ATRESIA

- What incremental costs are associated with the use of the screening test in (state) newborn screening programs for biliary atresia?
- What are the costs of diagnosis and the failure to diagnose in the presymptomatic period?
- What is the availability of treatment and the costs associated with treatment?

transcutaneous bilirubin. This blood can be obtained at the time of heel stick for the state newborn screen or when blood is obtained for total bilirubin measurements before hospital discharge. Ongoing prospective studies will further address problems and solutions with conjugated bilirubin screening.

The stool color card, on the other hand, avoids drawing blood. The cost is very low for essentially a colored postcard (less than $0.06 per card); however, its interpretation is more subjective and requires pediatricians and parents to work together to address questions about stool color. In addition, stools become acholic over time, so there is no "start" or "stop" time for the screening. Rather, it is a continuous screen, in which stools are monitored for the first few months of life. In some countries, there is a 1-month well-child visit (eg, for administration of hepatitis B virus vaccine) at which time the stool color card results are captured, allowing for early diagnosis of biliary atresia. The lack of a consistent follow-up visit at 1 month in the United States creates a challenge. Finally, a referral process would need to be clearly developed to ensure that all infants with a positive screen undergo the next level of evaluation. Thus, issues under Key Question 5 are continuing to be addressed and vary depending on the screening modality used.

Because biliary atresia is the number 1 cause of pediatric end-stage liver disease and liver transplantation, a disproportionally large fraction of total health care expenditures is spent on this relatively rare but highly morbid disease.[4] It is important to note that this conclusion was based on extrapolations from adult data and, therefore, underestimates the true cost of care related to lifelong immunosuppression after transplantation in the pediatric population. Hence, preventing or delaying liver transplantation through an early diagnosis translates to reduced health care expenditures, as further documented by a series of pediatric studies, 2 of which are briefly summarized in the next paragraph.

Mogul et al[26] modeled the cost-effectiveness of screening using the stool color card in the United States. By using Markov modeling based on the Taiwan Health Bureau findings projected over 20 years, screening with the stool color card was associated with nearly 30 life-years gained, 11 fewer transplants, 3 fewer deaths, and a decrease in total costs of nearly $9 million. Moreover, the authors concluded that there was a greater than 97% likelihood that screening using stool color cards would result in a gain in life-years and a significant cost savings. Schreiber et al[27] conducted a prospective study in which infant stool color cards were distributed to more than 6000 families in the maternity ward of a Canadian women's hospital. The authors used a variety of strategies to follow up on the infant stool color, from voluntary return of the cards at 30 days of age to follow-up with family physicians or families by random phone survey. The authors estimated stool color card utilization at 60% to 94%. By using Markov modeling, the authors further estimated the cost of screening in the Canadian population at approximately $213 000, for a gain of

9.7 life-years. The authors concluded that screening for biliary atresia by using infant stool color cards was not only feasible, but also effective and cost-effective. Although both studies support the cost-effectiveness of stool color card screening for biliary atresia, it should be noted that both studies relied on extrapolations from results in Taiwan, which may or may not be applicable in North America. Thus, further cost-effectiveness analysis based on a North American pilot study using stool color cards is required before concluding a true cost benefit in the United States.

The cost-effectiveness of screening by using serum conjugated bilirubin concentrations has not yet been established. It is worth noting, however, that many newborn nurseries routinely determine serum bilirubin concentrations at birth. As Harpavat et al[13] noted, all infants who had serum bilirubin determinations performed and ultimately were diagnosed with biliary atresia had elevated conjugated bilirubin concentrations. It is, therefore, worth further investigation to determine the cost-effectiveness of conjugated bilirubin determinations during the first few days of life.

It is important to note, however, that there are "hidden" costs associated with screening for biliary atresia using stool color cards. These include the additional time required to explain biliary atresia screening to parents, which, if past is prologue, will likely be added to preventive services without being recognized as increased services by public and private payers. Also, these additional newborn screening interventions will generate increased office visits and phone calls from concerned parents bringing their "color cards" and possibly soiled diapers for follow-up evaluation by the pediatrician. Future research on cost-effectiveness will be required to consider all costs, including those that may be considered "hidden." Nonetheless, even though stool color card screening for biliary atresia has not yet been performed in North America, these cost-effectiveness modeling data are encouraging, and there is merit to pursuing pilot testing to confirm these analyses.

CONCLUSIONS

The natural history of biliary atresia is sufficiently well established. Early diagnosis is clearly associated with better outcomes for infants with biliary atresia. Outcomes after the Kasai operation in the United States could potentially be improved with early diagnosis. Stool color cards distributed to mothers on discharge would not only function as a screening tool but also for educating primary care physicians and parents, engendering awareness that there is an abnormal color to infant stool.

Newborn screening for conjugated hyperbilirubinemia requires additional analysis. The American Academy of Pediatrics already recommends newborn screening for hyperbilirubinemia. Many nurseries, however, use transcutaneous bilirubin measurements in lieu of serum bilirubin determinations, but thus far, only newborn serum conjugated hyperbilirubinemia has been correlated with the eventual diagnosis of biliary atresia, and the utility of newborn serum conjugated bilirubin screening for biliary atresia remains unknown.

At this point, there is not sufficient evidence to conclude with a high degree of certainty that newborn screening would provide significant benefit for biliary atresia. Pilot studies are necessary to evaluate the feasibility, effectiveness, and costs of potential screening strategies for early identification of biliary atresia in the United States.

LEAD AUTHOR

Kasper S. Wang, MD, FAAP, FACS

SECTION ON SURGERY EXECUTIVE COMMITTEE, 2014–2015

R. Lawrence Moss, MD, FAAP, Chairperson
Michael G. Caty, MD, FACS, FAAP
Andrew Davidoff, MD, FACS, FAAP
Mary Elizabeth Fallat, MD, FAAP
Kurt F. Heiss, MD, FAAP
George Holcomb III, MD, MBA, FAAP
Rebecka L. Meyers, MD, FAAP

STAFF

Vivian Thorne

KEY POINTS

- Biliary atresia is a rare disease with high morbidity and mortality for which the natural history is reasonably well understood.
- Early performance of the Kasai portoenterostomy with successful surgical drainage of bile is associated with better outcomes for infants with biliary atresia; therefore, educational programs for pediatricians and other pediatric care providers to increase awareness of biliary atresia may be helpful.
- Published analyses indicate that newborn screening for biliary atresia, either by measuring serum conjugated bilirubin concentrations or using stool color cards, is potentially of sufficient sensitivity and specificity to be cost-effective.
- Further studies are necessary to evaluate the feasibility, effectiveness, and costs of potential screening strategies for early identification of biliary atresia in the United States.

COMMITTEE ON FETUS AND NEWBORN, 2014–2015

Kristi L. Watterberg, MD, FAAP, Chairperson
Susan Aucott, MD, FAAP
William E. Benitz, MD, FAAP
James J. Cummings, MD, FAAP
Eric C. Eichenwald, MD, FAAP
Jay Goldsmith, MD, FAAP
Brenda B. Poindexter, MD, FAAP
Karen Puopolo, MD, FAAP
Dan L. Stewart, MD, FAAP
Kasper S. Wang, MD, FAAP

LIAISONS

CAPT Wanda D. Barfield, MD, MPH, FAAP — *Centers for Disease Control and Prevention*

James Goldberg, MD — *American College of Obstetricians and Gynecologists*

Thierry Lacaze, MD — *Canadian Pediatric Society*

Erin L. Keels, APRN, MS, NNP-BC — *National Association of Neonatal Nurses*

Tonse N. K. Raju, MD, DCH, FAAP — *National Institutes of Health*

STAFF

Jim Couto, MA

CHILDHOOD LIVER DISEASE RESEARCH NETWORK

Nanda Kerkar, MD
Saul J. Karpen, MD, PhD
Ronald J. Sokol, MD, FAASLD
Kathleen B. Schwarz, MD
Douglas B Mogul, MD, MPH
Sanjiv Harpavat, MD, PhD

REFERENCES

1. Superina R, Magee JC, Brandt ML, et al; Childhood Liver Disease Research and Education Network. The anatomic pattern of biliary atresia identified at time of Kasai hepatoportoenterostomy and early postoperative clearance of jaundice are significant predictors of transplant-free survival. *Ann Surg.* 2011; 254(4):577–585

2. Dharnidharka VR, Tejani AH, Ho PL, Harmon WE. Post-transplant lymphoproliferative disorder in the United States: young Caucasian males are at highest risk. *Am J Transplant.* 2002;2:993–998

3. Kelly DA. Strategies for optimizing immunosuppression in adolescent transplant recipients: a focus on liver transplantation. *Paediatr Drugs.* 2003; 5(3):177–183

4. Sokol RJ, Mack C, Narkewicz MR, Karrer FM. Pathogenesis and outcome of biliary atresia: current concepts. *J Pediatr Gastroenterol Nutr.* 2003;37(1):4–21

5. Marchetti P. New-onset diabetes after liver transplantation: from pathogenesis to management. *Liver Transpl.* 2005; 11(6):612–620

6. Calonge N, Green NS, Rinaldo P, et al. Committee report: Method for evaluating conditions nominated for population-based screening of newborns and children. *Genet Med.* 2010;12:153–159

7. Kemper AR, Green NS, Calonge N, et al. Decision-making process for conditions nominated to the Recommended Uniform Screening Panel: statement of the US Department of Health and Human Services Secretary's Advisory Committee on Heritable Disorders in Newborns and Children. *Genet Med.* 2014;16:183–187

8. Perrin JM, Knapp AA, Browning MF, et al. An evidence development process for newborn screening. *Genet Med.* 2010;12: 131–134

9. Chardot C. Biliary atresia. *Orphanet J Rare Dis.* 2006;1:28

10. Pape L, Olsson K, Petersen C, von Wasilewski R, Melter M. Prognostic value of computerized quantification of liver fibrosis in children with biliary atresia. *Liver Transpl.* 2009;15(8):876–882

11. Schwarz KB, Haber BH, Rosenthal P, et al; Childhood Liver Disease Research and Education Network. Extrahepatic anomalies in infants with biliary atresia: results of a large prospective North American multicenter study. *Hepatology.* 2013;58(5):1724–1731

12. Powell JE, Keffler S, Kelly DA, Green A. Population screening for neonatal liver disease: potential for a community-based programme. *J Med Screen.* 2003; 10(3):112–116

13. Harpavat S, Finegold MJ, Karpen SJ. Patients with biliary atresia have elevated direct/conjugated bilirubin levels shortly after birth. *Pediatrics.* 2011;128(6). Available at: www.pediatrics. org/cgi/content/full/128/6/e1428

14. Chen SM, Chang MH, Du JC, et al; Taiwan Infant Stool Color Card Study Group. Screening for biliary atresia by infant stool color card in Taiwan. *Pediatrics.* 2006;117(4):1147–1154

15. Lien TH, Chang MH, Wu JF, et al; Taiwan Infant Stool Color Card Study Group. Effects of the infant stool color card screening program on 5-year outcome of biliary atresia in Taiwan. *Hepatology.* 2011;53(1):202–208

16. Ramonet M. Stool color cards for screening for biliary atresia. BA Single Topic Conference. Bethesda, MD: National Institutes of Health 2006;September 12–13

17. Wildhaber BE, Majno P, Mayr J, et al. Biliary atresia: Swiss national study, 1994-2004. *J Pediatr Gastroenterol Nutr.* 2008;46(3):299–307

18. Gu YH, Yokoyama K, Mizuta K, et al. Stool color card screening for early detection of biliary atresia and long-term native liver survival: a 19-year cohort study in Japan. *J Pediatr.* 2015; 166(4):897–902.e1

19. Kim S, Kang Y, Lee MJ, Kim MJ, Han SJ, Koh H. Points to be considered when applying FibroScan S probe in children with biliary atresia. *J Pediatr Gastroenterol Nutr.* 2014;59(5):624–628

20. Ohi R, Nio M, Chiba T, Endo N, Goto M, Ibrahim M. Long-term follow-up after surgery for patients with biliary atresia. *J Pediatr Surg.* 1990;25(4):442–445

21. Serinet MO, Wildhaber BE, Broué P, et al. Impact of age at Kasai operation on its results in late childhood and adolescence: a rational basis for biliary atresia screening. *Pediatrics.* 2009; 123(5):1280–1286

22. Caudle SE, Katzenstein JM, Karpen SJ, McLin VA. Language and motor skills are impaired in infants with biliary atresia before transplantation. *J Pediatr.* 2010; 156:936–940, 940.e1

23. DeRusso PA, Ye W, Shepherd R, et al; Biliary Atresia Research Consortium. Growth failure and outcomes in infants with biliary atresia: a report from the Biliary Atresia Research Consortium. *Hepatology.* 2007;46(5):1632–1638

24. Lee JY, Lim LT, Quak SH, Prabhakaran K, Aw M. Cholangitis in children with biliary atresia: health-care resource utilisation. *J Paediatr Child Health.* 2014;50(3):196–201

25. Ng VL, Haber BH, Magee JC, et al. Medical status of 219 children with biliary atresia surviving long-term with their native livers: results from a North American multicenter consortium. *J Pediatr.* 2014;165:539–546.e2

26. Mogul D, Zhou M, Intihar P, Schwarz K, Frick K. Cost-effective analysis of screening for biliary atresia with the stool color card. *J Pediatr Gastroenterol Nutr.* 2015;60(1):91–98

27. Schreiber RA, Masucci L, Kaczorowski J, et al. Home-based screening for biliary atresia using infant stool colour cards: a large-scale prospective cohort study and cost-effectiveness analysis. *J Med Screen.* 2014;21(3):126–132

SECTION 3

High-Risk Newborn/ Prematurity

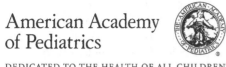

American Academy
of Pediatrics

DEDICATED TO THE HEALTH OF ALL CHILDREN™

Antenatal Counseling Regarding Resuscitation and Intensive Care Before 25 Weeks of Gestation

James Cummings, MD, FAAP, COMMITTEE ON FETUS AND NEWBORN

abstract

The anticipated birth of an extremely low gestational age (<25 weeks) infant presents many difficult questions, and variations in practice continue to exist. Decisions regarding care of periviable infants should ideally be well informed, ethically sound, consistent within medical teams, and consonant with the parents' wishes. Each health care institution should consider having policies and procedures for antenatal counseling in these situations. Family counseling may be aided by the use of visual materials, which should take into consideration the intellectual, cultural, and other characteristics of the family members. Although general recommendations can guide practice, each situation is unique; thus, decision-making should be individualized. In most cases, the approach should be shared decision-making with the family, guided by considering both the likelihood of death or morbidity and the parents' desires for their unborn child. If a decision is made not to resuscitate, providing comfort care, encouraging family bonding, and palliative care support are appropriate.

Clinical reports from the American Academy of Pediatrics benefit from expertise and resources of liaisons and internal (American Academy of Pediatrics) and external reviewers. However, clinical reports from the American Academy of Pediatrics may not reflect the views of the liaisons or the organizations or government agencies that they represent.

The guidance in this report does not indicate an exclusive course of treatment or serve as a standard of medical care. Variations, taking into account individual circumstances, may be appropriate.

All clinical reports from the American Academy of Pediatrics automatically expire 5 years after publication unless reaffirmed, revised, or retired at or before that time.

www.pediatrics.org/cgi/doi/10.1542/peds.2015-2336

DOI: 10.1542/peds.2015-2336

PEDIATRICS (ISSN Numbers: Print, 0031-4005; Online, 1098-4275).

INTRODUCTION

The anticipated birth of an extremely low gestational age (<25 weeks) infant presents many difficult questions for all involved, including whether to initiate resuscitation after delivery. Variations in practice continue to exist, driven in part by the unclear outcomes of these infants, individual bias with regard to these outcomes, the difficulty in communicating complex information to parents at an extremely stressful time, and the emotionally charged environment that typically exists around the impending delivery of an infant at the lower limits of viability.[1-9]

The topic of antenatal counseling at the borderline of viability (22–24 weeks of gestation) has been addressed in 2 American Academy of Pediatrics clinical reports.[10,11] Important factors in this area continue to evolve, including improved outcomes, changing attitudes of parents and physicians and other health care providers, and new approaches that facilitate communication with parents. The present revised clinical report includes new knowledge and understanding gained since the most recent report was published in 2009.

In February 2013, a workshop was convened by the Eunice Kennedy Shriver National Institute of Child Health and Human Development to discuss management and counseling issues surrounding periviable birth. An executive summary of this workshop was published concurrently in multiple journals in May 2014.[12–14] The intent of the present report was not to revisit issues that were thoroughly discussed at that workshop but to highlight key points relevant to counseling. In addition, whereas previous publications may have provided specific recommendations based on the anticipated gestational age, this statement emphasizes the limitations of that approach and the need to individualize counseling. This report also discusses factors important in communicating with prospective parents and presents ways to assist them with difficult decision-making. The goal of this report was to assist pediatric and obstetric care providers in effectively managing what remains one of the most difficult areas in perinatal medicine.

BACKGROUND

Some infants may be born at such an immature stage of development that the risk of death or severe long-term neurologic impairment is exceptionally high. Initiating resuscitation and offering life support to these newborn infants may be considered futile or not in the best interests of the child, but how to translate these concerns into clinical practice is unclear. Therefore, it is important that parents be involved in decision-making whenever possible. Ideally, shared decision-making and family-centered care should be the goals.

The primary goal of antenatal counseling in this situation is to allow parents to make an informed decision regarding intervention. In addition, counseling can provide parents with knowledge and support that will help them manage what will likely be a difficult aftermath. Effective counseling includes 3 key components: assessment of risks, communication of those risks, and ongoing support. In addition, factors that may influence decision-making need to be carefully considered.

OUTCOME ACCORDING TO GESTATIONAL AGE

Most countries, including the United States, continue to report that survival without significant neurologic sequelae is extremely rare in infants delivered before 23 weeks of gestation, even with full resuscitation and intensive care.[15–25] In addition, although improved outcomes for infants born beyond 23 weeks' gestation have been observed in many countries, most have not reported improvement in outcomes for infants delivered at 22 to 23 weeks of gestation.[15,16,19,22,23] Recent data, however, suggest that survival for infants born at less than 23 weeks' gestation can be improved if perinatal interventions (eg, antenatal steroids, operative deliveries for fetal distress, neonatal resuscitation) are made on the fetus' behalf.[26,27] Japan has recently reported intact survival rates for infants born alive at 22 weeks of gestation comparable to those born at 23 weeks of gestation, with overall survival rates of 33%.[28] A study in the United States found similar rates of survival among newborn infants born at 22 weeks' gestation.[29] Therefore, if survival were the only consideration, it would seem reasonable to offer resuscitation and intensive care to all infants born at or beyond 22 weeks of gestation. However, parents and health care providers have to struggle with other considerations, including the fact that

most surviving preterm infants born before 25 weeks' gestation will have some degree of neurodevelopmental impairment and possibly long-term problems involving other organ systems.[30] Infants born at 22 weeks' gestation have reported rates of moderate to severe neurodevelopmental impairment of 85% to 90%; for infants born at 23 weeks' gestation, these rates are not significantly lower.[29–32] The risk of permanent, severe neurodevelopmental and other special health care needs affect both the infant and the family and, for some parents, may outweigh the benefit of survival alone.[33–36]

LIMITATIONS OF GESTATIONAL AGE AS A PREDICTOR

Although gestational age is a strong determinant of outcome, 2 interrelated factors limit the use of gestational age as a predictor of outcome: the rate of fetal development during the early third trimester and the inaccuracy of gestational dating. Between 22 and 25 weeks of gestation, the fetus is in an extremely rapid stage of development of many organ systems essential for extrauterine survival. Thus, each additional day of gestation theoretically increases not only the chance of survival but also the chance for a healthy long-term outcome. However, in most situations, the physician cannot know the gestational age with this degree of precision. Wide variability in an individual woman's ovulatory cycle and vaginal bleeding during the first weeks of pregnancy can make pregnancy dating according to last menstrual period inaccurate. First-trimester fetal ultrasonographic examinations, which have become the gold standard of gestational age assessment,[37] typically use mathematical algorithms to report gestational age estimates not only by week but also by days, implying a degree of precision that does not actually exist. At best, fetal ultrasonographic dating is accurate within 8%, which translates to an accuracy of 4 to 5 days at 8 to 9 weeks of gestation but nearly 2 weeks at 24 weeks of gestation.[38] The most precise determination of gestational age occurs with assisted reproductive technologies, in which the date of fertilization or implantation may be accurately defined, giving a more precise date of conception. However, these technologies account for less than 2% of pregnancies.[39]

Despite the difficulty in using gestational age alone to predict outcome, it is generally agreed that only comfort care should be offered to infants born at less than 22 weeks of gestation and that resuscitation should be offered for infants born at or later than 25 weeks of gestation,[12–14,40–44] leaving a "gray zone" between 22 and 24 weeks of gestation, within which recommendations vary. However, a common thread shared by all these recommendations is that decisions in individual cases may be guided by considerations other than gestational age.

FACTORS OTHER THAN GESTATIONAL AGE THAT AFFECT OUTCOME

Many factors other than gestational age can affect pregnancy outcome. Preconception and pregnancy-related factors, such as maternal age, health, nutrition, substance use, and even genetics, may alter fetal growth and development and, hence, perinatal outcome. Significant complications during pregnancy (eg, chorioamnionitis, severe preeclampsia, intrauterine growth restriction, placental abruption) are known to affect neonatal outcomes. However, the degree to which any of these factors affects outcome independent of preterm birth is unclear.

Other factors, however, may be useful in refining our estimates of outcome based solely on gestational age. In

a large cohort of extremely preterm infants (22–25 weeks' gestation) from 19 perinatal centers across the country, several factors in addition to gestational age significantly affected neonatal survival and long-term neurodevelopmental outcome at 18 to 22 months; female gender, antenatal corticosteroids, singleton birth, and increased birth weight (per 100-g increments) were each significantly associated with improved outcomes.[45] Because the data in this study are now more than a decade old, its contemporary relevance may be limited. One recent study found survival rates and 18- to 22-month outcomes for infants born at 22 to 25 weeks' gestation to be significantly better than predicted by this model.[29] In addition, because these factors do not explain the marked variability in outcomes by center,[46] their applicability to a specific institutional environment is unclear. Nevertheless, such studies are valuable because they underscore the fact that gestational age should not be the only consideration in discussing prognosis with parents.

FACTORS THAT MAY INFLUENCE DECISION-MAKING

Attitudes of Health Care Providers

Both obstetric and neonatal care providers agree that some fetuses are too immature to warrant interventions solely aimed at improving neonatal outcome; these interventions include antenatal steroids, intervention for fetal distress, and delivery room resuscitation. However, there is no general agreement about the gestational age at which proactive management should occur.[4,47] Proactive institutional practices, particularly the use of antenatal steroids, are associated not only with improved outcomes in periviable infants but also improved outcomes in more mature infants.[48,49] Conversely, in institutions in which such infants are not fully supported

both before and after delivery (eg, not offering antenatal steroids but offering full resuscitation at birth), mortality rates for infants delivered before 25 weeks of gestation are increased.[4]

Physician attitudes regarding the appropriateness of resuscitation and intensive care are generally much more positive for infants born at 24 weeks of gestation compared with 22 weeks of gestation, but at any given gestational age, wide variation still exists. Data suggest that more experienced physicians tend to encourage shared decision-making with parents.[2] In addition, attitudes may be changing; whereas earlier studies suggested that obstetricians and neonatologists tended to overestimate morbidity and mortality rates for extremely preterm infants,[50] that no longer seems to be the case.[7,8]

Attitudes of Parents

Although outlooks can differ depending on background, most parents who have raised an extremely low gestational age survivor report only modest increases in stress and continue to support aggressive resuscitation for these infants.[51,52] Although survivors of extreme prematurity can have significant long-term health and developmental problems, former extremely preterm infants generally report better health outcomes than expected,[53,54] except perhaps during adolescence.[55] Even though parents report more health care–related concerns, they generally rate the health quality of life of their children fairly high.[56]

Although discussion of survival and long-term outcomes is important in counseling, many parents do not find quantitative predictions of death or morbidity to be central to their decision-making. Instead, religion, spirituality, and hope may be more important factors.[57,58] There are also cultural differences in terms of preferences for resuscitation of extremely preterm newborn infants, although these may reflect differences in institutional practices or resources.[59] Understanding the importance of parental values and experiences is essential to shared decision-making.[60,61]

Delivery Room Assessment

Given the uncertainty that surrounds the outcomes of these periviable infants, some physicians recommend a "wait-and-see" attitude, suggesting that a skilled resuscitator be present at the delivery to intervene should the infant appear "viable" at birth.[9] Indeed, this approach was suggested in an earlier edition of the *Textbook of Neonatal Resuscitation*.[62] However, such decision-making in the delivery room delays the initiation of resuscitation and is prone to error. For example, when experienced neonatologists viewed delivery room videos of extremely preterm births, their ability to predict survival was no better than a coin toss.[63] It is recommended, therefore, that decisions regarding resuscitation be well communicated and agreed on before the birth, if possible, and not be conditional on the newborn infant's appearance at birth. In rare circumstances, the newborn infant could be significantly more or less mature than anticipated, and this assessment could alter decisions made in the delivery room. Parents need to be informed of this possibility.

COMMUNICATION

When an extremely preterm birth is imminent, there is often little time to prepare the parents and to ascertain their wishes regarding resuscitation and subsequent neonatal intensive care. Optimal use of the limited time available, as well as the recognition and management of potential barriers to effective communication, will facilitate a beneficial discussion of anticipated outcomes and options.

Communication With Parents

The primary goal of antenatal counseling is to provide parents with information that will aid their decision-making. This counseling should include not only expected outcomes for the infant but also a discussion of available options (eg, comfort care). This communication needs to be sensitive to the religious, social, cultural, and ethnic diversity of the parents; in particular, for a parent with limited English proficiency, these discussions must include interpretation services, preferably face-to-face. Likewise, an appropriate interpreter may be needed for a parent who has limitations with hearing.

The value of providing statistical information during counseling is unclear, and there is evidence that this information is often misunderstood. Some authors have found that parents of extremely preterm infants who died after birth emphasize emotional and spiritual concerns as more important to their decision-making,[56] whereas others found that many parents preferred the use of statistics when receiving outcome information.[64] Regardless of the level of detail provided, it is important to realize that parents prefer to hear a range of outcomes rather than specific numbers.[60] Because outcomes of extreme prematurity vary widely among centers, institution-specific outcome data may be more applicable than group data from outside institutions. However, because institutional approaches can affect outcomes,[46] it should be recognized that applying only local data may create a self-fulfilling prophecy. In addition, the number of such infants born at a given institution may be so low that local data may be hard to interpret; therefore, using both local and outside data may be helpful in defining a range of outcomes.

Supplementing verbal information with written information improves parental knowledge of long-term outcomes and may reduce parental anxiety.[65] Visual aids, such as pictures, graphics, and short messages about resuscitation and complications associated with extreme preterm birth, enhance parental knowledge regarding survival and morbidities, although 1 study found that they did not seem to alter parental desire for resuscitation.[66] Also, although the use of visual aids improves the understanding of inexperienced parents, those who have previously had experience with a preterm birth gained little from the aids.[67] If written or other visual aids are used, the level of comprehension and literacy of the parent needs to be considered.

Regardless of the issues discussed and decisions made during initial counseling, ongoing support should be provided. Parents will benefit from additional discussion either before or after delivery, regardless of whether the newborn infant receives resuscitation or intensive care. Addressing parents' questions and concerns for a dying infant or the uncertain future of their extremely immature newborn infant will assist them during this difficult time.

Developing and Improving Communication Skills

In any institution, even those with training programs, the threatened birth of a periviable infant occurs infrequently enough that less experienced clinical staff and learners have limited opportunities to observe and to improve their communication skills. Therefore, when such an opportunity presents itself, an effort should be made to include these individuals in the process, with appropriate supervision. This involvement should be conducted in a manner that is respectful and not burdensome to the parents, and the roles of all present should be made clear. In addition to direct observation, simulated counseling sessions can mirror the real-life clinical situation and may assist individuals in developing and improving their communication skills.[68,69]

Communication Among Providers

Good communication among health care providers promotes optimal decision-making. Whenever possible, obstetricians and neonatologists should discuss each case together before, during, and after discussions with the prospective parents. In addition, with consultation from related service providers (eg, family support, social work, clinical ethics, palliative care, chaplaincy), health care institutions should develop policies and procedures that will not only frame discussions with parents but also inform staff and physicians.[70] Such guidance can be effectively used to counsel parents and to improve communication and consistency between service providers.[71]

A general approach to communication is suggested in the latest edition of the American Academy of Pediatrics/American Heart Association *Textbook of Neonatal Resuscitation*:

"Meeting with parents prior to a very high-risk birth is important for both the parents and the neonatal care providers. Both the obstetric provider and the provider who will care for the baby after birth should talk with the parents. Studies have shown that obstetric and neonatal perspectives are often different. If possible, such differences should be discussed prior to meeting with the parents so that the information presented is consistent. Sometimes, such as when the woman is in active labor, it may seem as if there is inadequate time for such discussions. However, it is better to have some discussion of potential issues, even if brief, with the baby's family than to wait until after the baby is born to initiate such conversations. Follow-up meetings can take place if the situation changes over subsequent hours and days."[43]

CONCLUSIONS

1. Fetal gestational age, as currently estimated, is an imprecise predictor of neonatal survival, but 22 weeks of gestation is generally accepted as the lower threshold of viability.

2. Although most infants delivered between 22 and 24 weeks' gestation will die in the neonatal period or have significant long-term neurodevelopmental morbidity, outcomes in individual cases are difficult to predict.

3. Outcomes of infants delivered at 22 to 24 weeks of gestation vary significantly from center to center.

4. Because of the uncertain outcomes for infants born at 22 to 24 weeks' gestation, it is reasonable that decision-making regarding the delivery room management be individualized and family centered, taking into account known fetal and maternal conditions and risk factors as well as parental beliefs regarding the best interest of the child.

5. Attitudes vary not only between providers and parents but also among physicians and staff. Ongoing interdisciplinary communication and written policies and procedures can promote consistent, timely, and effective counseling.

6. Optimal decision-making regarding the delivery room management can be promoted through joint discussions between the parents and both the obstetric and neonatal care providers whenever possible.

7. Factors to consider when communicating with parents include their ability to comprehend the situation, language preference, cultural and/or religious considerations, and family support structure. If the parent has limited English proficiency, an interpreter should be used. Visual aids and outcome data based on local institutional experience may be helpful when communicating concepts such as mortality and morbidity.

8. Optimal use of the limited time available, as well as the recognition and management of potential barriers to effective communication, will facilitate an effective discussion of anticipated outcomes and options.

9. Clinical learners may benefit from observing these prenatal counseling sessions. In addition, other educational tools, such as simulations, can be used to help them gain experience with such situations.

10. When a decision is made not to resuscitate a newborn infant, comfort care is appropriate, as is encouraging the family to spend time with the dying/deceased newborn infant. Providing religious, psychosocial, and/or palliative care support may assist families at this difficult time.

LEAD AUTHOR

James Cummings, MD, FAAP

COMMITTEE ON FETUS AND NEWBORN, 2014–2015

Kristi Watterberg, MD, FAAP, Chairperson
James Cummings, MD, FAAP
Eric Eichenwald, MD, FAAP
Brenda Poindexter, MD, FAAP
Dan L. Stewart, MD, FAAP
Susan W. Aucott, MD, FAAP
Karen M. Puopolo, MD, FAAP
Jay P. Goldsmith, MD, FAAP

FORMER COMMITTEE MEMBERS

Rosemarie Tan, PhD, MD
Jill Baley, MD
Richard Polin, MD

LIAISONS

William Benitz, MD, FAAP – *AAP Section on Perinatal Pediatrics*
Kasper S. Wang, MD, FACS, FAAP – *AAP Section on Surgery*
Thierry Lacaze, MD – *Canadian Pediatric Society*
Jeffrey L. Ecker, MD – *American College of Obstetricians and Gynecologists*
Tonse N. K. Raju, MD, DCH, FAAP – *National Institutes of Health*
Wanda Barfield, MD, MPH, FAAP – *Centers for Disease Control and Prevention*
Erin Keels, MS, APRN, NNP-BC – *National Association of Neonatal Nurses*

FORMER LIAISONS

Ann Jefferies, MD – *Canadian Pediatric Society*
Jeffrey Ecker, MD – *American College of Obstetricians and Gynecologists*

STAFF

Jim Couto, MA

REFERENCES

1. Arzuaga BH, Meadow W. National variability in neonatal resuscitation practices at the limit of viability. *Am J Perinatol.* 2014;31(6):521–528

2. Duffy D, Reynolds P. Babies born at the threshold of viability: attitudes of paediatric consultants and trainees in South East England. *Acta Paediatr.* 2011; 100(1):42–46

3. Gallagher K, Martin J, Keller M, Marlow N. European variation in decision-making and parental involvement during preterm birth. *Arch Dis Child Fetal Neonatal Ed.* 2014;99(3):F245–F249

4. Guinsburg R, Branco de Almeida MF, Dos Santos Rodrigues Sadeck L, et al; Brazilian Network on Neonatal Research. Proactive management of extreme prematurity: disagreement between obstetricians and neonatologists. *J Perinatol.* 2012;32(12):913–919

5. Kiefer AS, Wickremasinghe AC, Johnson JN, et al. Medical management of extremely low-birth-weight infants in the first week of life: a survey of practices in the United States. *Am J Perinatol.* 2009; 26(6):407–418

6. Martinez AM, Partridge JC, Yu V, et al. Physician counselling practices and decision-making for extremely preterm infants in the Pacific Rim. *J Paediatr Child Health.* 2005;41(4):209–214

7. Mulvey S, Partridge JC, Martinez AM, Yu VY, Wallace EM. The management of extremely premature infants and the perceptions of viability and parental counselling practices of Australian obstetricians. *Aust N Z J Obstet Gynaecol.* 2001;41(3):269–273

8. Ramsay SM, Santella RM. The definition of life: a survey of obstetricians and neonatologists in New York City hospitals regarding extremely premature births. *Matern Child Health J.* 2011;15(4): 446–452

9. Singh J, Fanaroff J, Andrews B, et al. Resuscitation in the "gray zone" of viability: determining physician preferences and predicting infant outcomes. *Pediatrics.* 2007;120(3): 519–526

10. MacDonald H; American Academy of Pediatrics. Committee on Fetus and Newborn. Perinatal care at the threshold of viability. *Pediatrics.* 2002;110(5): 1024–1027

11. Batton DG; Committee on Fetus and Newborn. Clinical report—antenatal counseling regarding resuscitation at an extremely low gestational age. *Pediatrics.* 2009;124(1):422–427

12. Raju TN, Mercer BM, Burchfield DJ, Joseph GF. Periviable birth: executive summary of a Joint Workshop by the Eunice Kennedy Shriver National Institute of Child Health and Human Development, Society for Maternal-Fetal Medicine, American Academy of Pediatrics, and American College of Obstetricians and Gynecologists. *J Perinatol.* 2014;34(5): 333–342

13. Raju TN, Mercer BM, Burchfield DJ, Joseph GF Jr. Periviable birth: executive summary of a joint workshop by the Eunice Kennedy Shriver National Institute of Child Health and Human Development, Society for Maternal-Fetal Medicine, American Academy of Pediatrics, and American College of Obstetricians and Gynecologists. *Am J Obstet Gynecol.* 2014;210(5):406–417

14. Raju TN, Mercer BM, Burchfield DJ, Joseph GF Jr. Periviable birth: executive summary of a joint workshop by the Eunice Kennedy Shriver National Institute of Child Health and Human Development, Society for Maternal-Fetal Medicine, American Academy of Pediatrics, and American College of Obstetricians and Gynecologists. *Obstet Gynecol.* 2014; 123(5):1083–1096

15. Donohue PK, Boss RD, Shepard J, Graham E, Allen MC. Intervention at the border of viability: perspective over a decade. *Arch Pediatr Adolesc Med.* 2009;163(10):902–906

16. Milligan DW. Outcomes of children born very preterm in Europe. *Arch Dis Child Fetal Neonatal Ed.* 2010;95(4):F234–F240

17. Pignotti MS, Berni R. Extremely preterm births: end-of-life decisions in European countries. *Arch Dis Child Fetal Neonatal Ed.* 2010;95(4):F273–F276

18. Stoll BJ, Hansen NI, Bell EF, et al; Eunice Kennedy Shriver National Institute of Child Health and Human Development Neonatal Research Network. Neonatal outcomes of extremely preterm infants from the NICHD Neonatal Research Network. *Pediatrics.* 2010;126(3):443–456

19. Swamy R, Mohapatra S, Bythell M, Embleton ND. Survival in infants live born at less than 24 weeks' gestation: the hidden morbidity of non-survivors. *Arch Dis Child Fetal Neonatal Ed.* 2010; 95(4):F293–F294

20. Berger TM, Bernet V, El Alama S, et al. Perinatal care at the limit of viability between 22 and 26 completed weeks of gestation in Switzerland. 2011 Revision of the Swiss recommendations. *Swiss Med Wkly.* 2011;141:w13280

21. Partridge JC, Sendowski MD, Martinez AM, Caughey AB. Resuscitation of likely nonviable infants: a cost-utility analysis after the Born-Alive Infant Protection Act. *Am J Obstet Gynecol.* 2012;206(1):49. e1–49.e10

22. Holtrop P, Swails T, Riggs T, De Witte D, Klarr J, Pryce C. Resuscitation of infants born at 22 weeks gestation: a 20-year retrospective. *J Perinatol.* 2013;33(3): 222–225

23. Seaton SE, King S, Manktelow BN, Draper ES, Field DJ. Babies born at the threshold of viability: changes in survival and workload over 20 years. *Arch Dis Child Fetal Neonatal Ed.* 2013;98(1):F15–F20

24. Boland RA, Davis PG, Dawson JA, Doyle LW; Victorian Infant Collaborative Study Group. Predicting death or major neurodevelopmental disability in extremely preterm infants born in Australia. *Arch Dis Child Fetal Neonatal Ed.* 2013;98(3):F201–F204

25. Institute of Medicine, Committee on Understanding Premature Birth and Assuring Healthy Outcomes. *Preterm Birth: Causes, Consequences, and Prevention.* Washington, DC: National Academies Press; 2007

26. Wilkinson D. The self-fulfilling prophecy in intensive care. *Theor Med Bioeth.* 2009;30(6):401–410

27. Salihu HM, Salinas-Miranda AA, Hill L, Chandler K. Survival of pre-viable preterm infants in the United States: a systematic review and meta-analysis. *Semin Perinatol.* 2013;37(6):389–400

28. Itabashi K, Horiuchi T, Kusuda S, et al. Mortality rates for extremely low birth weight infants born in Japan in 2005. *Pediatrics.* 2009;123(2):445–450

29. Kyser KL, Morriss FH Jr, Bell EF, Klein JM, Dagle JM. Improving survival of extremely preterm infants born between 22 and 25 weeks of gestation. *Obstet Gynecol.* 2012;119(4):795–800

30. Arnold C, Tyson JE. Outcomes following periviable birth. *Semin Perinatol.* 2014; 38(1):2–11

31. Ishii N, Kono Y, Yonemoto N, Kusuda S, Fujimura M; Neonatal Research Network, Japan. Outcomes of infants born at 22 and 23 weeks' gestation. *Pediatrics.* 2013;132(1):62–71

32. Moore GP, Lemyre B, Barrowman N, Daboval T. Neurodevelopmental outcomes at 4 to 8 years of children born at 22 to 25 weeks' gestational age: a meta-analysis. *JAMA Pediatr.* 2013; 167(10):967–974

33. Teisseyre N, Vanraet C, Sorum PC, Mullet E. The acceptability among lay persons and health professionals of actively ending the lives of damaged newborns. *Monash Bioeth Rev.* 2010;20(2): 14.1–14.24

34. Einarsdóttir J. Emotional experts: parents' views on end-of-life decisions for preterm infants in Iceland. *Med Anthropol Q.* 2009;23(1):34–50

35. Eichenwald EC, Chervenak FA, McCullough LB. Physician and parental decision making in newborn resuscitation. *Virtual Mentor.* 2008; 10(10):616–624

36. Rogoff M. In the absence of God: ethics in the modern hospital. *Neonatal Netw.* 2001;20(7):69–70

37. American Institute of Ultrasound Medicine, Committee on Obstetric Practice. Committee opinion no 611: method for estimating due date. *Obstet Gynecol.* 2014;124(4):863–866

38. Callen PW. The obstretric ultrasound examination. In: Callen P, ed. *Ultrasonography in Obstetrics and Gynecology.* 5th ed. Philadelphia, PA: Saunders Elsevier; 2008:3–25

39. Joshi N, Kissin D, Anderson JE, Session D, Macaluso M, Jamieson DJ. Trends and correlates of good perinatal outcomes in assisted reproductive technology. *Obstet Gynecol.* 2012;120(4):843–851

40. Nuffield Council on Bioethics. *Critical Care Decisions in Fetal and Neonatal Medicine: Ethical Issues.* London, England: Nuffield Council on Bioethics; 2006

41. Kattwinkel J, Perlman J, Aziz K, et al. Part 15: neonatal resuscitation: 2010 American Heart Association Guidelines for Cardiopulmonary Resuscitation and Emergency Cardiovascular Care. *Circulation.* 2010;122(18 suppl 3): S909–S919

42. Perlman JM, Wyllie J, Kattwinkel J, et al. Part 11: neonatal resuscitation: 2010 International Consensus on Cardiopulmonary Resuscitation and Emergency Cardiovascular Care Science With Treatment Recommendations. *Circulation.* 2010;122(16 suppl 2): S516–S538

43. American Academy of Pediatrics, American Heart Association. Lesson 9: ethics and care at the end of life. In: Kattwinkel J, ed. *Textbook of Neonatal Resuscitation.* 6th ed. Elk Grove Village, IL: American Academy of Pediatrics/ American Heart Association; 2011: 286–288

44. Jefferies AL, Kirpalani HM; Canadian Paediatric Society Fetus and Newborn Committee. Counselling and management for anticipated extremely preterm birth. *Paediatr Child Health.* 2012;17(8):443–446

45. Tyson JE, Parikh NA, Langer J, Green C, Higgins RD; National Institute of Child Health and Human Development Neonatal Research Network. Intensive care for extreme prematurity—moving beyond gestational age. *N Engl J Med.* 2008;358(16):1672–1681

46. Rysavy MA, Li L, Bell EF, et al. Unpacking the "center effect": patient- and hospital-level factors associated with improved outcomes in extremely preterm infants. Abstract presented at Pediatric Academic Societies Annual Meeting; May 3-6, 2014; Vancouver, British Columbia, Canada. Abstract 2014:E-PAS2014: 2850.2011. Available at: www. abstracts2view.com/pas/view.php?nu= PAS14L1_2850.1. Accessed January 19, 2015

47. Kariholu U, Godambe S, Ajitsaria R, et al; North-West London Perinatal Network. Perinatal network consensus guidelines on the resuscitation of extremely preterm infants born at <27 weeks' gestation. *Eur J Pediatr.* 2012;171(6): 921–926

48. Carlo WA, McDonald SA, Fanaroff AA, et al; Eunice Kennedy Shriver National Institute of Child Health and Human Development Neonatal Research Network. Association of antenatal corticosteroids with mortality and neurodevelopmental outcomes among infants born at 22 to 25 weeks' gestation. *JAMA.* 2011;306(21):2348–2358

49. Smith PB, Ambalavanan N, Li L, et al; Generic Database SubCommittee; Eunice Kennedy Shriver National Institute of Child Health, Human Development Neonatal Research Network. Approach to infants born at 22 to 24 weeks' gestation: relationship to outcomes of more-mature infants. *Pediatrics.* 2012;129(6). Available at: www.pediatrics.org/cgi/ content/full/129/6/e1508

50. Haywood JL, Goldenberg RL, Bronstein J, Nelson KG, Carlo WA. Comparison of perceived and actual rates of survival and freedom from handicap in premature infants. *Am J Obstet Gynecol.* 1994;171(2):432–439

51. Saigal S, Burrows E, Stoskopf BL, Rosenbaum PL, Streiner D. Impact of extreme prematurity on families of adolescent children. *J Pediatr.* 2000; 137(5):701–706

52. Schappin R, Wijnroks L, Uniken Venema MM, Jongmans MJ. Rethinking stress in parents of preterm infants: a meta-analysis. *PLoS One.* 2013;8(2):e54992

53. Hack M, Forrest CB, Schluchter M, et al. Health status of extremely low-birth-weight children at 8 years of age: child and parent perspective. *Arch Pediatr Adolesc Med.* 2011;165(10):922–927

54. Heinonen K, Pesonen AK, Lahti J, et al. Self- and parent-rated executive functioning in young adults with very low birth weight. *Pediatrics.* 2013;131(1). Available at: www.pediatrics.org/cgi/ content/full/131/1/e243

55. Wolke D, Chernova J, Eryigit-Madzwamuse S, Samara M, Zwierzynska K, Petrou S. Self and parent perspectives on health-related quality of life of adolescents born very preterm. *J Pediatr.* 2013;163(4):1020–1026.e2

56. Saigal S, Rosenbaum PL, Feeny D, et al. Parental perspectives of the health status and health-related quality of life

of teen-aged children who were extremely low birth weight and term controls. *Pediatrics*. 2000;105(3 pt 1): 569–574

57. Boss RD, Hutton N, Sulpar LJ, West AM, Donohue PK. Values parents apply to decision-making regarding delivery room resuscitation for high-risk newborns. *Pediatrics*. 2008;122(3): 583–589

58. Grobman WA, Kavanaugh K, Moro T, DeRegnier RA, Savage T. Providing advice to parents for women at acutely high risk of periviable delivery. *Obstet Gynecol*. 2010;115(5):904–909

59. Tucker Edmonds B, Fager C, Srinivas S, Lorch S. Racial and ethnic differences in use of intubation for periviable neonates. *Pediatrics*. 2011;127(5). Available at: www.pediatrics.org/cgi/content/full/127/5/e1120

60. Gaucher N, Payot A. From powerlessness to empowerment: mothers expect more than information from the prenatal consultation for preterm labour. *Paediatr Child Health*. 2011;16(10): 638–642

61. Janvier A, Barrington K, Farlow B. Communication with parents concerning withholding or withdrawing of life-sustaining interventions in neonatology. *Semin Perinatol*. 2014;38(1):38–46

62. American Academy of Pediatrics, American Heart Association. Lesson 9: ethics and care at the end of life. In: Kattwinkel J, ed. *Textbook of Neonatal Resuscitation*. 5th ed. Elk Grove Village, IL: American Academy of Pediatrics and the American Heart Association; 2006: 9.1–9.16

63. Manley BJ, Dawson JA, Kamlin CO, Donath SM, Morley CJ, Davis PG. Clinical assessment of extremely premature infants in the delivery room is a poor predictor of survival. *Pediatrics*. 2010; 125(3). Available at: www.pediatrics.org/cgi/content/full/125/3/e559

64. Paul DA, Epps S, Leef KH, Stefano JL. Prenatal consultation with a neonatologist prior to preterm delivery. *J Perinatol*. 2001;21(7):431–437

65. Muthusamy AD, Leuthner S, Gaebler-Uhing C, Hoffmann RG, Li SH, Basir MA. Supplemental written information improves prenatal counseling: a randomized trial. *Pediatrics*. 2012; 129(5). Available at: www.pediatrics.org/cgi/content/full/129/5/e1269

66. Kakkilaya V, Groome LJ, Platt D, et al. Use of a visual aid to improve counseling at the threshold of viability. *Pediatrics*. 2011;128(6). Available at: www.pediatrics.org/cgi/content/full/128/6/e1511

67. Guillén Ú, Suh S, Munson D, et al. Development and pretesting of a decision-aid to use when counseling parents facing imminent extreme premature delivery. *J Pediatr*. 2012; 160(3):382–387

68. Stokes TA, Watson KL, Boss RD. Teaching antenatal counseling skills to neonatal providers. *Semin Perinatol*. 2014;38(1): 47–51

69. Boss RD, Donohue PK, Roter DL, Larson SM, Arnold RM. "This is a decision you have to make": using simulation to study prenatal counseling. *Simul Healthc*. 2012; 7(4):207–212

70. Srinivas SK. Periviable births: communication and counseling before delivery. *Semin Perinatol*. 2013;37(6): 426–430

71. Kaempf JW, Tomlinson MW, Campbell B, Ferguson L, Stewart VT. Counseling pregnant women who may deliver extremely premature infants: medical care guidelines, family choices, and neonatal outcomes. *Pediatrics*. 2009; 123(6):1509–1515

CLINICAL REPORT   Guidance for the Clinician in Rendering Pediatric Care

American Academy
of Pediatrics

DEDICATED TO THE HEALTH OF ALL CHILDREN™

Apnea of Prematurity

Eric C. Eichenwald, MD, FAAP, COMMITTEE ON FETUS AND NEWBORN

abstract

Apnea of prematurity is one of the most common diagnoses in the NICU. Despite the frequency of apnea of prematurity, it is unknown whether recurrent apnea, bradycardia, and hypoxemia in preterm infants are harmful. Research into the development of respiratory control in immature animals and preterm infants has facilitated our understanding of the pathogenesis and treatment of apnea of prematurity. However, the lack of consistent definitions, monitoring practices, and consensus about clinical significance leads to significant variation in practice. The purpose of this clinical report is to review the evidence basis for the definition, epidemiology, and treatment of apnea of prematurity as well as discharge recommendations for preterm infants diagnosed with recurrent apneic events.

BACKGROUND

Apnea of prematurity is one of the most common diagnoses in the NICU. Despite the frequency of apnea of prematurity, it is unknown whether recurrent apnea, bradycardia, and hypoxemia in preterm infants are harmful. Limited data suggest that the total number of days with apnea and resolution of episodes at more than 36 weeks' postmenstrual age (PMA) are associated with worse neurodevelopmental outcome in preterm infants.[1,2] However, it is difficult to separate any potential adverse effects of apnea from the degree of immaturity at birth, because the incidence of apnea is inversely proportional to gestational age.[3] Research into the development of respiratory control in immature animals and preterm infants has facilitated our understanding of the pathogenesis and treatment of apnea of prematurity (Table 1). However, the lack of consistent definitions, monitoring practices, and consensus about clinical significance leads to significant variation in practice.[4–6] The purpose of this clinical report is to review the evidence basis for the definition, epidemiology, and treatment of apnea of prematurity as well as discharge recommendations for preterm infants diagnosed with recurrent apneic events.

DOI: 10.1542/peds.2015-3757

PEDIATRICS (ISSN Numbers: Print, 0031-4005; Online, 1098-4275).

To cite: Eichenwald EC and AAP COMMITTEE ON FETUS AND NEWBORN. Apnea of Prematurity. *Pediatrics*. 2016;137(1):e20153757

DEFINITION AND CLASSIFICATION

An apneic spell is usually defined as a cessation of breathing for 20 seconds or longer or a shorter pause accompanied by bradycardia (<100 beats per minute), cyanosis, or pallor. In practice, many apneic events in preterm infants are shorter than 20 seconds, because briefer pauses in airflow may result in bradycardia or hypoxemia. On the basis of respiratory effort and airflow, apnea may be classified as central (cessation of breathing effort), obstructive (airflow obstruction usually at the pharyngeal level), or mixed. The majority of apneic episodes in preterm infants are mixed events, in which obstructed airflow results in a central apneic pause, or vice versa.

EPIDEMIOLOGY AND TIME COURSE TO RESOLUTION

In an observational study, Henderson-Smart[3] reported that the incidence of recurrent apnea increased with decreasing gestational age. Essentially, all infants born at ≤28 weeks' gestation were diagnosed with apnea; beyond 28 weeks' gestation, the proportion of infants with apnea decreased, from 85% of infants born at 30 weeks' gestation to 20% of those born at 34 weeks' gestation. This relationship has important implications for NICU policy, because infants born at less than 35 weeks' gestation generally require cardiorespiratory monitoring after birth because of their risk of apnea. As expected with a developmental process, some infants born at 35 to 36 weeks' gestation may have respiratory control instability, especially when placed in a semiupright position.[7]

In Henderson-Smart's study, apneic spells stopped by 37 weeks' PMA in 92% of infants and by 40 weeks' PMA in more than 98% of infants.[3] The proportion of infants with apnea/ bradycardia events persisting beyond 38 weeks' PMA is higher in infants who were 24 to 26 weeks' gestational age at birth compared with those born at ≥28 weeks' gestation.[8] Infants with bronchopulmonary dysplasia may have delayed maturation of respiratory control, which can prolong apnea for as long as 2 to 4 weeks beyond term PMA.[8] In most infants, apnea of prematurity follows a common natural history, with more severe events that require intervention resolving first. Last to resolve are isolated, spontaneously resolving bradycardic events of uncertain clinical significance.[8]

Most studies examining the time course to resolution of apnea of prematurity have relied on nurses' recording of events in the medical record; however, several studies have shown a lack of correlation with electronically recorded events.[9,10] Standard NICU monitoring techniques are unable to detect events that are primarily obstructive in nature. With continuous electronic recording, it is evident that some preterm infants continue to have clinically unapparent apnea, bradycardia, and oxygen desaturation events even after discharge. The Collaborative Home Infant Monitoring Evaluation Study examined the occurrence of apnea/bradycardia events in >1000 preterm and healthy term infants monitored at home.[11] "Extreme events" (apnea >30 seconds and/or heart rate <60 beats per minute for >10 seconds) were observed most frequently in former preterm infants, decreasing dramatically until about 43 weeks' PMA. After 43 weeks' PMA, "extreme events" in both preterm and term infants were very rare.

Preterm infants with resolved apnea also may have clinically unapparent intermittent hypoxia events. In a recent study in former preterm infants after discontinuation of medical therapy for apnea, the mean number of seconds/hour of oxygen saturation less than 80% was 20.3 at 35 weeks' PMA, decreasing to 6.8 seconds/hour at 40 weeks' PMA.[12]

MONITORING FOR APNEA/ BRADYCARDIA

Most infants in NICUs are continuously monitored for heart rate, respiratory rate, and oxygen saturation. Cardiac alarms are most commonly set at 100 beats per minute, although lower alarm settings are acceptable in convalescent preterm infants. Apnea alarms are generally set at 20 seconds. However, apnea detection by impedance monitoring is potentially misleading. Impedance monitoring is prone to artifact attributable to body movement or cardiac activity and is unable to detect obstructive apnea. Practices differ as to when continuous oximetry is discontinued. In a study investigating the age at last recorded apnea and age at discharge from the hospital in 15 different NICUs, the duration of use of pulse oximetry was significantly different among hospital sites.[5] Later discontinuation of pulse oximetry was associated with a later PMA at recorded last apnea and longer length of stay, suggesting that oximetry may detect events that cardiorespiratory monitoring does not.

There are no data to suggest that a diagnosis of apnea of prematurity is

TABLE 1 Factors Implicated in the Pathogenesis of Apnea of Prematurity

Central Mechanisms	Peripheral Reflex Pathways
Decreased central chemosensitivity	Decreased carotid body activity
Hypoxic ventilatory depression	Increased carotid body activity
Upregulated inhibitory neurotransmitters	Laryngeal chemoreflex
Delayed central nervous system development	Excessive bradycardic response

associated with an increased risk of sudden infant death syndrome (SIDS) or that home monitoring can prevent SIDS in former preterm infants. Although infants born preterm have a higher risk of SIDS, epidemiologic and physiologic data do not support a causal link with apnea of prematurity. The mean PMA for SIDS occurrence for infants born between 24 and 28 weeks' gestation is estimated to be 47.1 weeks, compared with 53.5 weeks for term infants.[13] Apnea of prematurity resolves at a PMA before which most SIDS deaths occur; in the Collaborative Home Infant Monitoring Evaluation Study, extreme events in former preterm infants resolved by 43 weeks' PMA.[11] As such, routine home monitoring for preterm infants with resolved apnea of prematurity is not recommended. Cardiorespiratory monitoring after hospital discharge may be prescribed for some preterm infants with an unusually prolonged course of recurrent, extreme apnea. Current evidence suggests that if such monitoring is elected, it can be discontinued in most infants after 43 weeks' PMA unless indicated by other significant medical conditions.[14]

TREATMENTS

Xanthine Therapy

Methylxanthines have been the mainstay of pharmacologic treatment of apnea for decades. Adverse effects include tachycardia, emesis, and jitteriness. Both theophylline and caffeine are used, but caffeine citrate is preferred because of its longer half-life, higher therapeutic index, and lack of need for drug-level monitoring. Xanthines have multiple effects on respiration, including increased minute ventilation, improved carbon dioxide sensitivity, decreased periodic breathing, and decreased hypoxic depression of breathing. Their primary mechanism of action is thought to be blockade of inhibitory adenosine A_1 receptors, with resultant excitation of respiratory neural output, as well as blockade of excitatory adenosine A_{2A} receptors located on γ-aminobutyric acidergic neurons. Specific polymorphisms in the A_1 and A_{2A} adenosine receptor genes have been associated with a higher risk of apnea of prematurity as well as variability in response to xanthine therapy.[15] These observations may help explain apparent genetic susceptibility to apnea of prematurity, high concordance of its diagnosis in twins, and variability in response to xanthine therapy.[16]

The largest trial of caffeine citrate (Caffeine for Apnea of Prematurity Trial) randomly assigned 2006 infants with birth weights between 500 and 1250 g to caffeine or placebo in the first 10 postnatal days to prevent or treat apnea or to facilitate extubation.[17] Dosing of caffeine citrate in this study included a loading dose of 20 mg/kg followed by maintenance of 5 mg/kg per day, which could be increased to 10 mg/kg per day for persistent apnea. Caffeine-treated infants had a shorter duration of mechanical ventilation, lower incidence of bronchopulmonary dysplasia, and improved neurodevelopmental outcome at 18 months.[18] Differences in neurodevelopmental outcome were less evident at 5 years but favored the caffeine-treated subjects.[19] The study did not collect data on the frequency of apnea and therefore did not directly address the effect of caffeine on apnea; however, the data indicated that caffeine therapy, as used clinically in this trial, is safe and may have additional benefits by yet unknown mechanisms. However, the use of prophylactic caffeine solely for potential neurodevelopmental benefits requires additional study.

The optimal time to start caffeine therapy in infants at risk of apnea is not known. In infants >28 weeks' gestation who do not require positive pressure support, one reasonable approach would be to await the occurrence of apnea before initiating therapy.[20] In the Caffeine for Apnea of Prematurity Trial, earlier treatment with caffeine (<3 days) compared with later (≥3 days) was associated with a shorter duration of mechanical ventilation, although it is not clear whether infants started earlier on caffeine were assessed to be more likely to be extubated soon.[21] In a retrospective cohort study in 62 056 infants with very low birth weight discharged between 1997 and 2010, early caffeine therapy compared with later therapy was associated with a lower incidence of bronchopulmonary dysplasia (23.1% vs 30.7%; odds ratio: 0.68; 95% confidence interval: 0.69–0.80) as well as a shorter duration of mechanical ventilation (mean difference: 6 days; $P < .001$).[22] Further trials are needed to assess the safety and the potential benefits of early prophylactic caffeine in infants who require mechanical ventilation.

No trials have addressed when to discontinue xanthine treatment in preterm infants; however, timely discontinuation is advised to avoid unnecessary delays in discharge. Because of variability in when apnea resolves, the use of any specific gestational age may result in unnecessarily continuing therapy.[4,5,8] One approach might be a trial off therapy after a clinically significant apnea-free period (off positive pressure) of 5 to 7 days or 33 to 34 weeks' PMA, whichever comes first. However, there may be significant effects of caffeine on respiratory control in preterm infants with clinically resolved apnea. A recent study in preterm infants who had been treated with caffeine for apnea showed a decrease in the frequency of intermittent hypoxia episodes in those who received a prolonged course of therapy compared with a usual-care group.[12] Further study is necessary to determine the implications of this finding.

Nasal Continuous Positive Airway Pressure

Nasal continuous positive airway pressure (NCPAP) at pressures of 4 to 6 cm H_2O, usually in conjunction with treatment with a xanthine, is effective in reducing the frequency and severity of apnea in preterm infants.[23] It appears to work by splinting open the upper airway and decreasing the risk of obstructive apnea.[23] NCPAP may also decrease the depth and duration of oxygen desaturation during central apneas by helping maintain a higher end-expiratory lung volume. Limited evidence suggests that variable-flow continuous positive airway pressure (CPAP) devices may be more effective in the reduction in apnea events than conventional delivery systems for CPAP (ventilator or bubble CPAP).[24]

Humidified high-flow nasal cannula or nasal intermittent positive-pressure ventilation may be acceptable substitutes for NCPAP. However, larger studies that specifically examine the advantages and disadvantages of nasal intermittent positive-pressure ventilation and high-flow nasal cannula versus conventional NCPAP on the incidence and severity of recurrent apnea are needed.

Blood Transfusion

An increase in respiratory drive resulting from increased oxygen-carrying capacity, total content of oxygen in the blood, and increased tissue oxygenation is the proposed mechanism for red blood cell transfusions to reduce apnea of prematurity. Retrospective and prospective studies of the effects of blood transfusions on the incidence and severity of recurrent apnea in preterm infants are conflicting, perhaps because of a lack of blinding

of caregivers.[25,26] A recent study that used a novel computer algorithm to detect apnea, bradycardia, and oxygen desaturation in continuously recorded physiologic data from 67 preterm infants showed decreased apnea for the 3 days after blood transfusions compared with 3 days before.[27] These authors also reported that the probability of an apnea event in a 12-hour epoch was higher with a lower hematocrit, adjusted for PMA. These results suggest that anemia may increase the likelihood of apnea of prematurity and that blood transfusions may result in a short-term reduction in apnea. However, there are no data to indicate that blood transfusion results in any long-term reduction in apnea.

Gastroesophageal Reflux Treatment

Preterm infants have a hyperreactive laryngeal chemoreflex response that precipitates apnea when stimulated. In addition, almost all preterm infants show some degree of gastroesophageal reflux (GER). These 2 physiologic observations have led to speculation that GER can precipitate apnea in preterm infants and that pharmacologic treatment of GER might decrease the incidence or severity of apnea. Despite the frequent coexistence of apnea and GER in preterm infants, several studies examining the timing of reflux episodes in relation to apneic events indicate that they are rarely temporally related.[28,29] Additional data indicate that GER does not prolong or worsen concurrent apnea.[30] There is no evidence that pharmacologic treatment of GER with agents that decrease gastric acidity or that promote gastrointestinal motility decreases the risk of recurrent apnea in preterm infants.[31,32] Indeed, some studies have shown a coincident increase in recorded events with pharmacologic treatment of GER.[32] In addition, recent data suggest harmful effects (including an increased

incidence of necrotizing enterocolitis, late-onset sepsis, and death) of medications to reduce gastric acidity in preterm infants.[33]

DISCHARGE CONSIDERATIONS

Practice and management surrounding discharge decisions for infants with apnea of prematurity vary widely, but most physicians require infants to be apnea/bradycardia free for a period of time before discharge. In 1 survey, the majority of neonatologists (approximately 75%) required a 5- to 7-day observation period.[4] Common practice is to initiate this countdown period a few days after discontinuation of caffeine therapy (caffeine half-life, approximately 50–100 hours)[34] and to include only spontaneously occurring (ie, not feeding-related) events. Limited information exists about the recurrence of apnea or bradycardia after a specific event-free period. In a retrospective cohort of 1400 infants born at ≤34 weeks' gestation, Lorch et al[35] reported that a 5- to 7-day apnea-free period successfully predicted resolution of apnea in 94% to 96% of cases. However, the success rate was significantly lower for infants born at younger gestational ages. A 95% success rate threshold was 1 to 3 apnea-free days for infants born at ≥30 weeks' gestation, 9 days for those born at 27 to 28 weeks' gestation, and 13 days for infants born at <26 weeks' gestation. Similar gestational age effects were observed in another smaller retrospective study by Zupancic et al.[36] These results suggested that the specified event-free period need not be uniform for all infants, and shorter durations may be considered for older gestational ages. However, such recommendations are based on observed events, which may not be accurate, and the prescribed event-free periods do not preclude the possibility that a new circumstance (eg, intercurrent illness) may result in the re-emergence of apnea.

Discharge considerations are usually based on nursing observation and recording of apnea or bradycardia events, which may not always correlate with those events that are electronically recorded.[9,10] Preterm infants with a history of apnea who are otherwise deemed ready for discharge may have clinically unsuspected apnea, bradycardia, and/or hypoxemia events if archived continuous electronic recording is interrogated.[37] There is no evidence, however, that such events predict the recurrence of clinically significant events on discharge, SIDS, or the need for readmission to the hospital. As such, more intensive monitoring or pneumogram recordings in convalescent preterm infants approaching discharge may not be useful. However, standardizing the documentation and clinical approach to apnea within individual NICUs may reduce the variation in discharge timing.[38]

Infants born preterm may develop apnea and other signs of respiratory control instability with certain stresses, including general anesthesia and viral illnesses. Additional close monitoring in these situations may be indicated in preterm infants until 44 weeks' PMA, including former preterm infants readmitted for elective surgical procedures, such as hernia repair. In addition, the exacerbation of apnea has been reported in very preterm infants after their initial 2-month immunizations or ophthalmologic examinations, and rarely after the 4-month immunizations, while still in the NICU.[39]

CLINICAL IMPLICATIONS

1. Apnea of prematurity reflects immaturity of respiratory control. It generally resolves by 36 to 37 weeks' PMA in infants born at ≥28 weeks' gestation.

2. Infants born at <28 weeks' gestation may have apnea that persists to or beyond term gestation.

3. Individual NICUs are encouraged to develop policies for cardiorespiratory monitoring for infants considered at risk of apnea of prematurity.

4. Initial low heart rate alarms are most commonly set at 100 beats per minute. Lower settings for convalescent preterm infants older than 33 to 34 weeks' PMA may be reasonable.

5. Caffeine citrate is a safe and effective treatment of apnea of prematurity when administered at a 20-mg/kg loading dose and 5 to 10 mg/kg per day maintenance. Monitoring routine serum caffeine levels usually is not contributory to management. A trial off caffeine may be considered when an infant has been free of clinically significant apnea/bradycardia events off positive pressure for 5 to 7 days or at 33 to 34 weeks' PMA, whichever comes first.

6. Evidence suggests that GER is not associated with apnea of prematurity, and treatment of presumed or proven GER solely for the reduction in apnea events is not supported by currently available evidence.

7. Brief, isolated bradycardic episodes that spontaneously resolve and feeding-related events that resolve with interruption of feeding are common in convalescent preterm infants and generally need not delay discharge.

8. Individual units are encouraged to develop policies and procedures for caregiver assessment, intervention, and documentation of apnea/ bradycardia/desaturation events as well as the duration of the period of observation before discharge.

9. A clinically significant apnea event–free period before discharge of 5 to 7 days is commonly used, although a longer period may be suitable for infants born at less than 26 weeks' gestation. The specific event-free period may need to be individualized for some infants depending on the gestational age at birth and the nature and severity of recorded events.

10. Interrogation of electronically archived monitoring data may reveal clinically unsuspected events of uncertain significance. Such events do not predict subsequent outcomes, including recurrent clinical apnea or SIDS.

LEAD AUTHOR

Eric C. Eichenwald, MD, FAAP

COMMITTEE ON FETUS AND NEWBORN, 2014–2015

Kristi L. Watterberg, MD, FAAP, Chairperson
Susan Aucott, MD, FAAP
William E. Benitz, MD, FAAP
James J. Cummings, MD, FAAP
Eric C. Eichenwald, MD, FAAP
Jay Goldsmith, MD, FAAP
Brenda B. Poindexter, MD, FAAP
Karen Puopolo, MD, FAAP
Dan L. Stewart, MD, FAAP
Kasper S. Wang, MD, FAAP

LIAISONS

Wanda D. Barfield, MD, MPH, FAAP – *Centers for Disease Control and Prevention*
James Goldberg, MD – *American College of Obstetricians and Gynecologists*
Thierry Lacaze, MD – *Canadian Pediatric Society*
Erin L. Keels, APRN, MS, NNP-BC – *National Association of Neonatal Nurses*
Tonse N.K. Raju, MD, DCH, FAAP – *National Institutes of Health*

STAFF

Jim Couto, MA

REFERENCES

1. Janvier A, Khairy M, Kokkotis A, Cormier C, Messmer D, Barrington KJ. Apnea is associated with neurodevelopmental impairment in very low birth weight infants. *J Perinatol*. 2004;24(12):763–768

2. Pillekamp F, Hermann C, Keller T, von Gontard A, Kribs A, Roth B. Factors influencing apnea and bradycardia of prematurity—implications for neurodevelopment. *Neonatology*. 2007;91(3):155–161

3. Henderson-Smart DJ. The effect of gestational age on the incidence and duration of recurrent apnoea in newborn babies. *Aust Paediatr J*. 1981;17(4):273–276

4. Darnall RA, Kattwinkel J, Nattie C, Robinson M. Margin of safety for discharge after apnea in preterm infants. *Pediatrics*. 1997;100(5):795–801

5. Eichenwald EC, Blackwell M, Lloyd JS, Tran T, Wilker RE, Richardson DK. Inter-neonatal intensive care unit variation in discharge timing: influence of apnea and feeding management. *Pediatrics*. 2001;108(4):928–933

6. Eichenwald EC, Zupancic JA, Mao WY, Richardson DK, McCormick MC, Escobar GJ. Variation in diagnosis of apnea in moderately preterm infants predicts length of stay. *Pediatrics*. 2011;127(1). Available at: www.pediatrics.org/cgi/content/full/127/1/e53

7. Davis NL, Condon F, Rhein LM. Epidemiology and predictors of failure of the infant car seat challenge. *Pediatrics*. 2013;131(5):951–957

8. Eichenwald EC, Aina A, Stark AR. Apnea frequently persists beyond term gestation in infants delivered at 24 to 28 weeks. *Pediatrics*. 1997;100(3 pt 1):354–359

9. Razi NM, Humphreys J, Pandit PB, Stahl GE. Predischarge monitoring of preterm infants. *Pediatr Pulmonol*. 1999;27(2):113–116

10. Brockmann PE, Wiechers C, Pantalitschka T, Diebold J, Vagedes J, Poets CF. Under-recognition of alarms in a neonatal intensive care unit. *Arch Dis Child Fetal Neonatal Ed*. 2013;98(6):F524–F527

11. Ramanathan R, Corwin MJ, Hunt CE, et al; Collaborative Home Infant Monitoring Evaluation (CHIME) Study Group. Cardiorespiratory events recorded on home monitors: comparison of healthy infants with those at increased risk for SIDS. *JAMA*. 2001;285(17):2199–2207

12. Rhein LM, Dobson NR, Darnall RA, et al; Caffeine Pilot Study Group. Effects of caffeine on intermittent hypoxia in infants born prematurely: a randomized clinical trial. *JAMA Pediatr*. 2014;168(3):250–257

13. Malloy MH. Prematurity and sudden infant death syndrome: United States 2005-2007. *J Perinatol*. 2013;33(6):470–475

14. Committee on Fetus and Newborn, American Academy of Pediatrics. Apnea, sudden infant death syndrome, and home monitoring. *Pediatrics*. 2003;111(4 pt 1):914–917

15. Kumral A, Tuzun F, Yesilirmak DC, Duman N, Ozkan H. Genetic basis of apnoea of prematurity and caffeine treatment response: role of adenosine receptor polymorphisms. *Acta Paediatr*. 2012;101(7):e299–e303

16. Bloch-Salisbury E, Hall MH, Sharma P, Boyd T, Bednarek F, Paydarfar D. Heritability of apnea of prematurity: a retrospective twin study. *Pediatrics*. 2010;126(4). Available at: www.pediatrics.org/cgi/content/full/126/4/e779

17. Schmidt B, Roberts RS, Davis P, et al; Caffeine for Apnea of Prematurity Trial Group. Caffeine therapy for apnea of prematurity. *N Engl J Med*. 2006;354(20):2112–2121

18. Schmidt B, Roberts RS, Davis P, et al; Caffeine for Apnea of Prematurity Trial Group. Long-term effects of caffeine therapy for apnea of prematurity. *N Engl J Med*. 2007;357(19):1893–1902

19. Schmidt B, Anderson PJ, Doyle LW, et al; Caffeine for Apnea of Prematurity (CAP) Trial Investigators. Survival without disability to age 5 years after neonatal caffeine therapy for apnea of prematurity. *JAMA*. 2012;307(3):275–282

20. Schmidt B, Davis PG, Roberts RS. Timing of caffeine therapy in very low birth weight infants. *J Pediatr*. 2014;164(5):957–958

21. Davis PG, Schmidt B, Roberts RS, et al; Caffeine for Apnea of Prematurity Trial Group. Caffeine for Apnea of Prematurity Trial: benefits may vary in subgroups. *J Pediatr*. 2010;156(3):382–387

22. Dobson NR, Patel RM, Smith PB, et al. Trends in caffeine use and association between clinical outcomes and timing of therapy in very low birth weight infants. *J Pediatr*. 2014;164(5):992–998

23. Miller MJ, Carlo WA, Martin RJ. Continuous positive airway pressure selectively reduces obstructive apnea in preterm infants. *J Pediatr*. 1985;106(1):91–94

24. Pantalitschka T, Sievers J, Urschitz MS, Herberts T, Reher C, Poets CF. Randomised crossover trial of four nasal respiratory support systems for apnoea of prematurity in very low birthweight infants. *Arch Dis Child Fetal Neonatal Ed*. 2009;94(4):F245–F248

25. Valieva OA, Strandjord TP, Mayock DE, Juul SE. Effects of transfusions in extremely low birth weight infants: a retrospective study. *J Pediatr*. 2009;155(3):331–337

26. Westkamp E, Soditt V, Adrian S, Bohnhorst B, Groneck P, Poets CF. Blood transfusion in anemic infants with apnea of prematurity. *Biol Neonate*. 2002;82(4):228–232

27. Zagol K, Lake DE, Vergales B, et al. Anemia, apnea of prematurity, and blood transfusions. *J Pediatr*. 2012;161(3):417–421

28. Peter CS, Sprodowski N, Bohnhorst B, Silny J, Poets CF. Gastroesophageal

reflux and apnea of prematurity: no temporal relationship. *Pediatrics*. 2002;109(1):8–11

29. Poets CF. Gastroesophageal reflux and apnea of prematurity—coincidence, not causation [commentary on Corvaglia L et al. A thickened formula does not reduce apneas related to gastroesophageal reflux in preterm infants. Neonatology. 2013;103(2):98–102]. *Neonatology*. 2013;103(2):103–104

30. Di Fiore JM, Arko M, Whitehouse M, Kimball A, Martin RJ. Apnea is not prolonged by acid gastroesophageal reflux in preterm infants. *Pediatrics*. 2005;116(5):1059–1063

31. Wheatley E, Kennedy KA. Cross-over trial of treatment for bradycardia attributed to gastroesophageal reflux in preterm infants. *J Pediatr*. 2009;155(4):516–521

32. Kimball AL, Carlton DP. Gastroesophageal reflux medications in the treatment of apnea in premature infants. *J Pediatr*. 2001;138(3):355–360

33. Terrin G, Passariello A, De Curtis M, et al. Ranitidine is associated with infections, necrotizing enterocolitis, and fatal outcome in newborns. *Pediatrics*. 2012;129(1). Available at: www.pediatrics.org/cgi/content/full/129/1/e40

34. Charles BG, Townsend SR, Steer PA, Flenady VJ, Gray PH, Shearman A. Caffeine citrate treatment for extremely premature infants with apnea: population pharmacokinetics, absolute bioavailability, and implications for therapeutic drug monitoring. *Ther Drug Monit*. 2008;30(6):709–716

35. Lorch SA, Srinivasan L, Escobar GJ. Epidemiology of apnea and bradycardia resolution in premature infants. *Pediatrics*. 2011;128(2).

Available at: www.pediatrics.org/cgi/content/full/128/2/e366

36. Zupancic JA, Richardson DK, O'Brien BJ, Eichenwald EC, Weinstein MC. Cost-effectiveness analysis of predischarge monitoring for apnea of prematurity. *Pediatrics*. 2003;111(1):146–152

37. Barrington KJ, Finer N, Li D. Predischarge respiratory recordings in very low birth weight newborn infants. *J Pediatr*. 1996;129(6):934–940

38. Butler TJ, Firestone KS, Grow JL, Kantak AD. Standardizing documentation and the clinical approach to apnea of prematurity reduces length of stay, improves staff satisfaction, and decreases hospital cost. *Jt Comm J Qual Patient Saf*. 2014;40(6):263–269

39. Sánchez PJ, Laptook AR, Fisher L, Sumner J, Risser RC, Perlman JM. Apnea after immunization of preterm infants. *J Pediatr*. 1997;130(5):746–751

CLINICAL REPORT   Guidance for the Clinician in Rendering Pediatric Care

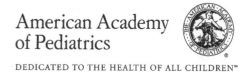

DEDICATED TO THE HEALTH OF ALL CHILDREN™

Diagnosis and Management of Gastroesophageal Reflux in Preterm Infants

Eric C. Eichenwald, MD, FAAP, COMMITTEE ON FETUS AND NEWBORN

abstract

Gastroesophageal reflux (GER), generally defined as the passage of gastric contents into the esophagus, is an almost universal phenomenon in preterm infants. It is a common diagnosis in the NICU; however, there is large variation in its treatment across NICU sites. In this clinical report, the physiology, diagnosis, and symptomatology in preterm infants as well as currently used treatment strategies in the NICU are examined. Conservative measures to control reflux, such as left lateral body position, head elevation, and feeding regimen manipulation, have not been shown to reduce clinically assessed signs of GER in the preterm infant. In addition, preterm infants with clinically diagnosed GER are often treated with pharmacologic agents; however, a lack of evidence of efficacy together with emerging evidence of significant harm (particularly with gastric acid blockade) strongly suggest that these agents should be used sparingly, if at all, in preterm infants.

Department of Pediatrics, Children's Hospital of Philadelphia, Philadelphia, Pennsylvania

Dr Eichenwald is the primary author of the policy and approved the final manuscript as submitted.

Clinical reports from the American Academy of Pediatrics benefit from expertise and resources of liaisons and internal (AAP) and external reviewers. However, clinical reports from the American Academy of Pediatrics may not reflect the views of the liaisons or the organizations or government agencies that they represent.

The guidance in this report does not indicate an exclusive course of treatment or serve as a standard of medical care. Variations, taking into account individual circumstances, may be appropriate.

All clinical reports from the American Academy of Pediatrics automatically expire 5 years after publication unless reaffirmed, revised, or retired at or before that time.

DOI: https://doi.org/10.1542/peds.2018-1061

Address correspondence to Eric C. Eichenwald, MD, FAAP. E-mail: eichenwald@email.chop.edu

PEDIATRICS (ISSN Numbers: Print, 0031-4005; Online, 1098-4275).

FINANCIAL DISCLOSURE: The author has indicated he has no financial relationships relevant to this article to disclose.

To cite: Eichenwald EC and AAP COMMITTEE ON FETUS AND NEWBORN. Diagnosis and Management of Gastroesophageal Reflux in Preterm Infants. *Pediatrics.* 2018;142(1):e20181061

INTRODUCTION

Gastroesophageal reflux (GER), generally defined as the passage of gastric contents into the esophagus,[1] is an almost universal phenomenon in preterm infants. The normal physiologic occurrence of GER in infants can be distinguished from pathologic GER disease, which includes troublesome symptoms or complications associated with GER.[2] GER occurs commonly in infants, in part because of relatively large volumes ingested during feeding and supine positioning, which frequently place the gastroesophageal junction in a liquid environment. Whether GER becomes clinically significant depends on both the quality (eg, degree of acidity) and quantity of reflux[3,4] as well as potential injury to the esophageal mucosa. GER is a common diagnosis in the NICU; however, there is as much as a 13-fold variation in its diagnosis and treatment across sites.[5,6] Preterm infants who are diagnosed with GER have longer hospital stays and higher hospital costs than infants without GER,[5,7,8] making it an important clinical phenomenon in the NICU.

GER in preterm infants is most often diagnosed and treated on the basis of clinical and behavioral signs rather than on specific testing to prove or disprove pathology,[6] and many infants continue to be treated after they are discharged from the hospital.[9] However, evidence that GER causes harm in preterm infants is scant.[10,11] Indeed, routine use of antireflux medications for the treatment of symptomatic GER in preterm infants was 1 of the therapies singled out as being of questionable value in the recent American Academy of Pediatrics (AAP) Choosing Wisely campaign.[12]

In this clinical report, the following will be reviewed: (1) the physiology of GER in preterm infants, (2) methods for its diagnosis, (3) evidence that it is associated with the signs frequently attributed to GER, and (4) the safety and efficacy of nonpharmacologic and pharmacologic therapy.

PHYSIOLOGY

The primary mechanism of GER in preterm infants is transient lower esophageal sphincter relaxation (TLESR). TLESR is an abrupt reflex decrease in lower esophageal sphincter (LES) pressure to levels at or below intragastric pressure, unrelated to swallowing. Preterm infants have dozens of episodes of TLESR each day,[13] many of which are associated with some degree of GER. As such, GER is a normal phenomenon in preterm infants, which is exacerbated by a pure liquid diet and age-specific body position.[3] In addition, the presence of an indwelling gastric tube through the esophageal sphincter increases the frequency of GER, presumably secondary to impaired closure of the LES.[14] Delayed gastric emptying does not appear to play a contributory role in GER in preterm infants, in that infants with symptomatic GER do not have delayed gastric emptying

compared with other infants.[15,16] However, GER is more common immediately after a feeding, likely because of gastric distension.[15] Body position also influences TLESR and GER in preterm infants. Infants placed in the right-side-down lateral position after a feeding have more TLESR episodes and liquid reflux compared with the left-side-down lateral position, despite gastric emptying being enhanced in the right lateral position.[17,18] Prone position also decreases episodes of GER versus supine position, likely because of more optimal positioning of the LES relative to the distended stomach.[17]

Mechanisms to protect the esophagus and airway from GER appear to be intact in the preterm infant. These include reflex forward peristalsis of the esophagus in response to distention from refluxate in the lower esophagus with closure of the upper esophageal sphincter to prevent refluxate reaching the pharynx. Despite these mechanisms, if refluxed material does reach the upper esophagus, the upper esophageal sphincter will reflexively open to allow the material into the pharynx, which results in the frequent episodes of "spitting" or emesis observed in infants.

DIAGNOSIS

Several methods have been used to diagnose GER in the preterm population, including contrast fluoroscopy, pH monitoring, and multichannel intraesophageal impedance (MII) monitoring. Although contrast fluoroscopy can be used to show episodes of reflux, it cannot be used to differentiate clinically significant GER from insignificant GER. Monitoring of pH in the lower esophagus has classically been used to diagnose GER in older children and adults. Reflux of acidic gastric contents results in transient periods of acidity in the

lower esophagus. Common measures obtained from pH probe monitoring include the total number of reflux episodes, the duration of the longest reflux episode, and the "reflux index" (RI), which is the percentage of the total recording time with an esophageal pH <4. In pH studies, an RI >7% is considered abnormal, an RI <3% considered normal, and RIs between 3% and 7% are considered indeterminate.[2] However, labeling a study "abnormal" does not prove that it is causing the symptoms in question.

Measurement of esophageal pH is not a reliable method to diagnose GER in preterm infants[19] because their stomach pH is rarely <4 owing to frequent milk feedings and a higher baseline pH. In addition, abnormal esophageal pH does not correlate well with symptom severity.[20] Other measures that have been investigated include the presence of pepsin in saliva[21] and the pH of oropharyngeal secretions.[22] Although these measures may correlate with acidic reflux, it is unknown whether they correlate with symptom severity.

Currently, the most accurate method for detecting GER is MII monitoring, which is frequently combined with simultaneous measurement of pH.[2] MII can be used to track the movement of fluids, solids, and air in the esophagus by measuring changes in electrical impedance between multiple electrodes along an esophageal catheter. MII can be used to discern whether a fluid bolus is traveling antegrade (swallow) or retrograde (reflux) in the esophagus and can be used to determine the height of the retrograde bolus. It is a reliable and reproducible technique for diagnosing GER in preterm infants[14] and can be combined with a pH sensor to determine if GER is acidic, mildly acidic, or alkaline. López-Alonso et al[23] measured 24-hour MII and pH in 26 healthy preterm infants with a median postmenstrual age of 32 weeks.

The median number of reflux episodes recorded in 24 hours was 71; 25.4% were acidic, 72.9% were weakly acidic, and 2.7% were alkaline. Of note, the gastric pH was higher than 4 for almost 70% of the recording time. Not surprisingly, periods of feeding were associated with a higher number of total reflux events per hour.

In practice, GER is diagnosed most often in infants on the basis of clinical and behavioral signs and/or response to a trial of pharmacologic or nonpharmacologic interventions.[6] Signs attributed to GER include feeding intolerance, poor growth, apnea, desaturation and bradycardia, and worsening pulmonary disease as well as nonspecific behavioral signs including arching, irritability, and apparent discomfort associated with feedings. There is no evidence, however, that these signs are temporally associated with measured GER episodes.[20,24,25] In 1 study of 40 preterm and 18 term infants evaluated with combined MII/pH testing for a clinical suspicion of GER, signs (including irritability, bradycardia and desaturations, or feeding intolerance) were rarely associated with documented reflux events.[20] In another study of 14 healthy preterm infants, Snel et al[24] recorded both esophageal pH and infant behaviors. General behavior scores did not change during esophageal acidification episodes. In addition, infants frequently demonstrated behaviors ascribed to GER (apparent discomfort, head retraction, and "mouthing") unrelated to pH-documented GER episodes. In these results, it is suggested that preterm infant behaviors commonly ascribed to reflux are, in reality, not associated with GER and that treatment should not be based solely on clinical signs.

GER IN THE PRETERM INFANT

Several clinical conditions are thought to be associated with GER in the preterm infant, although analyses are hampered because most cases of GER are diagnosed clinically.

Apnea, Desaturation, and Bradycardia

Preterm infants have a hyperreactive laryngeal response to chemoreceptor stimulation that precipitates apnea or bradycardia. In addition, as previously noted, almost all preterm infants have some GER. These 2 observations have led to speculation that GER can precipitate apnea, oxygen desaturation, and bradycardia episodes in preterm infants and that pharmacologic treatment of GER might decrease the incidence or severity of these events.[26] However, researchers examining the timing of reflux episodes in relation to apneic events have found that they are rarely temporally related[14,27] and that GER does not prolong or worsen apnea.[28] In 1 study, small amounts of normal saline were infused into the pharynx of sleeping preterm infants at term-equivalent age. The investigators found that swallow frequency increased, but apnea did not occur,[29] and they suggested that apnea is provoked when the larynx, not the pharynx, is stimulated. The larynx is not usually stimulated by reflux of small amounts of liquid. Finally, there is no evidence that pharmacologic treatment of GER with agents that decrease gastric acidity or promote gastrointestinal motility decrease the risk of recurrent apnea or bradycardia in preterm infants.[30,31]

Respiratory Disease and Bronchopulmonary Dysplasia

Proving a causal relationship between GER and respiratory symptoms in children has been difficult. Suggested methods of diagnostics, such as GER scintigraphy and the presence of lipid-laden macrophages in bronchoalveolar lavage, lack specificity[32] or correlate poorly with esophageal impedance and fail to differentiate reflux-related aspiration from primary aspiration from above.[33] In 1 study, children with a heterogeneous array of chronic lung problems who had documented GER had higher concentrations of pepsin and inflammatory interleukins in their bronchoalveolar lavage fluid than those without GER, suggesting microaspiration may contribute to their lung disease.[34]

It is not clear whether GER causes "silent" microaspiration in mechanically ventilated preterm infants that worsens lung disease, particularly in infants with developing or established bronchopulmonary dysplasia (BPD). In 1 study, it was reported that pepsin was detected in 93% of tracheal aspirates obtained from intubated preterm infants during the first postnatal month,[35] and in addition, that ventilated preterm infants who developed BPD had higher levels of tracheal aspirate pepsin than those who did not. In addition, these investigators reported that increased concentrations of pepsin were associated with increased severity of BPD[36] and speculated that chronic aspiration of gastric contents may contribute to the development of BPD. However, these results should be interpreted with caution because of emerging data on the low sensitivity and specificity of pepsin in bronchoalveolar lavage assays for the detection of GER-related aspiration.[37]

In contrast, Akinola et al[38] reported no relationship between the diagnosis of BPD and the clinical diagnosis of GER confirmed by esophageal pH monitoring.[38] In a small study comparing combined MII and pH monitoring in 12 infants with BPD and 34 without who were evaluated for clinical signs believed to be attributable to GER, infants with BPD had a similar number of documented reflux events as infants without BPD.[25] In both groups, fewer than 10% of the documented reflux events were temporally associated with reflux symptoms as assessed by nursing observation. However, infants with BPD were more likely to have "pH only events" (acidic pH in the lower esophagus without an associated MII determined reflux event), which were more often associated with symptoms, but at a low frequency (9% vs 4.9% in infants without BPD). Although infants with evolving BPD are more likely to have a diagnosis of and receive therapy for GER,[39] with these results, it is suggested that these infants do not have an increased incidence of symptomatic GER.

Feeding Problems

Some infants and children with GER may exhibit feeding problems, including feeding resistance, failure to thrive, or food aversion.[40,41] Although preterm infants may have frequent regurgitation, there is no evidence that this leads to poor growth or other nutritional difficulties.[7,42] Although preterm infants with a diagnosis of GER are sometimes treated with prokinetic agents to enhance gastric emptying,[6] there are no data to suggest that delayed gastric emptying is a physiologic mechanism for GER in this population.[15] As noted previously, other feeding-related behaviors in preterm infants often attributed to GER, including feeding-associated arching or irritability and oral feeding aversion, are not temporally associated with MII or lower pH documented reflux events and, thus, are not reliable markers of clinically significant reflux.[20,24]

TREATMENT

Although preterm infants frequently receive nonpharmacologic and pharmacologic therapy for GER, there is a paucity of data about the effect of treatment on symptoms or short- and long-term outcomes. Furthermore, the lack of randomized placebo-controlled trials of GER therapies in preterm infants makes it difficult to assess the efficacy of long-term therapy versus the expected natural history of GER. Despite the lack of data, in recent years, the use of antireflux medications both in the NICU and after discharge has substantially increased.[9,43]

Nonpharmacologic Management

Body Positioning

Body positioning is widely used as a conservative management approach to infants believed to have GER. Placing infants on a head-up angle is a common initial approach to management; however, head elevation is ineffective in reducing acid reflux in older infants. In addition, car seat placement was found to elicit worse acid GER in term infants.[44-46] This position has not been studied in preterm infants to prevent symptomatic GER, but there is no reason to expect the physiologic result would be different from term infants. Placing preterm infants in the left lateral versus right lateral position after feeding and in prone versus supine position may reduce TLESRs and reflux episodes.[15,17,18] However, although placement in the right lateral position may increase reflux episodes after feeding, van Wijk et al[18] showed that this position also enhanced gastric emptying. These authors suggested placing infants in the right lateral position immediately after feeding, followed in 1 hour by placing them in the left lateral position to decrease acid reflux. However, 1 small MII and pH study of term infants at a mean postnatal age of 13 weeks revealed that, despite a reduction in reflux episodes in the left lateral position, behavioral manifestations of reflux (crying and/or irritability) did not improve.[47] Thus, whether positioning techniques can reduce signs of GER in infants with reflux remains uncertain. Given that lateral and prone positioning also increase the risk of sudden infant death syndrome (SIDS),[48] the AAP and the North American Society for Pediatric Gastroenterology and Nutrition have concurred that infants with GER should be placed for sleep in the supine position, with the exception of the rare infants for whom the risk of death from GER is greater than the risk of SIDS.[2] The AAP Task Force on SIDS, after conferring with the authors of the North American Society for Pediatric Gastroenterology and Nutrition statement, provided additional guidance: "Examples of such upper airway disorders are those in which airway-protective mechanisms are impaired, including infants with anatomic abnormalities, such as type 3 or 4 laryngeal clefts, who have not undergone antireflux surgery."[48] Safe sleep approaches, including supine positioning on a flat and firm surface and avoidance of commercial devices designed to maintain head elevation in the crib, should be paramount as a model for parents of infants approaching discharge (ie, infants greater than 32 weeks' postmenstrual age) from the hospital.[49]

Feeding Strategies

If GER results from increased intragastric pressure, smaller-volume feedings given more frequently might result in fewer GER episodes. Omari et al[15] reported that feeding hourly, compared with feeding every 2 or 3 hours, resulted in fewer total GER episodes but more frequent acidic reflux episodes. Jadcherla et al[50] reported that longer feeding duration and slower milk flow rates were associated with fewer GER events, diagnosed by MII and pH study, although nutrient composition of expressed human milk may be compromised with this approach. No randomized trials have been used to compare the effects of continuous intragastric or transpyloric versus bolus intragastric tube feedings on GER symptom severity.[51]

Another feeding strategy has been to thicken feedings with agents including xanthan gum, starch, or rice cereal.[52] Unfortunately, in recent data, researchers have linked thickening with a xanthan gum product to late-onset necrotizing enterocolitis[53]; as such, it is recommended that xanthan gum or similar thickeners not be used in preterm or former preterm infants in the first year of life. Commercially available formula products that thicken on acidification in the stomach are not nutritionally appropriate for preterm infants. A systematic review of randomized controlled trials of thickened formulas in term infants with GER revealed that although these agents reduced episodes of regurgitation, they were ineffective in reducing acidic GER.[54] Only small trials of thickeners have been performed in the preterm population. In 1 trial of a starch-thickened preterm formula, the total number of GER episodes was unchanged compared with a standard formula feeding; however, total lower esophageal acid exposure was less with the thickened formula feeding. No assessment was made about whether the reduction in acid exposure had an effect on associated symptoms.[55]

In the data, it is suggested that elemental or extensively hydrolyzed protein formulas reduce gastrointestinal transit time and reduce symptoms in term infants with symptomatic GER.[56] These observations in term infants may be an overlap of signs of cow milk protein allergy and those attributed to GER, including vomiting, failure to thrive, and irritability.[57] In contrast, in small studies of preterm infants, although feeding with extensively hydrolyzed protein formula compared with standard formula or human milk resulted in fewer reflux episodes as measured by MII and pH study,[58,59] it did not reduce behavioral signs of GER.[59]

It is unclear what role cow milk protein allergy may play in preterm infants with signs of GER; a trial of extensively hydrolyzed protein-based formula may be reasonable in age-appropriate preterm infants with signs of severe reflux.

Pharmacologic Management

Prokinetic Agents

Prokinetic (promotility) agents include metoclopramide, domperidone, and erythromycin. Prokinetic agents have been widely used in older infants to reduce the symptoms of GER. These drugs appear to improve gastric emptying, reduce regurgitation, and enhance LES tone. None of these drugs has been shown to reduce GER symptoms in preterm infants,[60,61] and all have the potential for significant adverse effects, including a higher risk of infantile pyloric stenosis (erythromycin), cardiac arrhythmia (erythromycin), and neurologic side effects (domperidone and metoclopramide). Because of a lack of data about efficacy and a concerning safety profile, these drugs should not be used in preterm infants if the only indication is the treatment of GER.

Sodium Alginate

In older infants and children, researchers in several studies have revealed that alginate-containing formulations, which are frequently combined with sodium bicarbonate, may reduce the symptoms of GER.[61] In the presence of gastric acid, alginate formulations precipitate into a low-density viscous gel that acts as a physical barrier to the gastric mucosa; when combined with sodium bicarbonate (Gaviscon), a carbon dioxide foam forms, which preferentially is refluxed into the esophagus during GER events, protecting the lower esophagus from acidification. In preterm infants in small studies, sodium alginate preparations decreased the number of acidic GER episodes and

total esophageal acid exposure[62] and decreased the frequency of regurgitation.[63] However, the long-term safety of these preparations in preterm infants has not been evaluated.

Histamine-2 Receptor Blockers

Histamine-2 (H_2) receptor blockers (eg, ranitidine, famotidine) compete with histamine for the H_2 receptor in the parietal cells in the stomach, decreasing hydrochloric acid secretion and increasing intragastric pH. H_2 receptor blockers are frequently prescribed for infants in whom GER is clinically diagnosed[6,9] on the theory that these symptoms are secondary to acidic reflux into the lower esophagus. However, no researchers have assessed the efficacy of H_2 blockers on the symptom profile of preterm infants with presumed reflux. In addition, use of these drugs in preterm infants has been linked to an increased incidence of necrotizing enterocolitis in several studies[64] and a higher incidence of late-onset infections and death,[65] possibly resulting from alteration of the intestinal microbiome.[66]

Proton Pump Inhibitors

Proton pump inhibitors (PPIs) block the gastric proton pump, decreasing both basal and stimulated parietal cell acid secretion. PPIs in older children have been associated with a higher risk of gastric bacterial overgrowth, gastroenteritis, and community-acquired pneumonia.[67–69] PPIs are used less often than H_2 blockers in preterm infants but are used for similar indications.[9] Given their effect on gastric acid secretion, it is likely that PPIs would have similar potential adverse effects as H_2 blockers, although this has not been investigated. Although there is evidence that administration of PPIs will consistently maintain the stomach pH >4 in preterm infants, they are largely ineffective in relieving clinical signs of GER. In randomized double-blind placebo-controlled trials, both omeprazole and lansoprazole were ineffective in reducing GER signs in infants. In addition, lansoprazole was associated with a higher rate of adverse events.[70]

SUMMARY AND RECOMMENDATIONS

1. GER is almost universal in preterm infants. It is a physiologic process secondary to frequent TLESR, relatively large-volume liquid diet, and age-specific body positioning. As such, it is a normal developmental phenomenon that will resolve with maturation.

2. Pathologic GER occurs when reflux of acidic gastric contents causes injury to the lower esophageal mucosa. Although preterm infants do have some acidic GER episodes, most GER episodes in this population are only weakly acidic because of their lower gastric acidity and frequent milk feedings, making such esophageal injury unlikely to occur.

3. Signs commonly ascribed to GER in preterm infants include feeding intolerance or aversion, poor weight gain, frequent regurgitation, apnea, and desaturation and bradycardia and behavioral signs, including irritability and perceived postprandial discomfort. In the data, the temporal association of these perceived signs of GER with either acidic or nonacidic reflux episodes as measured by MII and pH is not supported, and the signs will usually improve with time without treatment.

4. Data regarding the possible association between worsening lung disease attributable to GER and microaspiration in mechanically ventilated preterm infants are sparse. Further studies to elucidate such an association and to assess the effect of GER treatment on the severity of lung disease are needed.

5. There is marked variability in the diagnosis and treatment of GER in preterm infants among NICUs, perhaps because the diagnosis is usually made by clinical assessment of signs and symptoms and/or a trial of nonpharmacologic or pharmacologic treatment rather than definitive tests.

6. Conservative measures to control reflux, such as left lateral body position, head elevation, and feeding regimen manipulation, have not been shown to reduce clinically assessed signs of GER in the preterm infant; for infants greater than 32 weeks' postmenstrual age, safe sleep approaches, including supine positioning on a flat and firm surface and avoidance of commercial devices designed to maintain head elevation in the crib, should be paramount as a model for parents of infants approaching discharge from the hospital.

7. Preterm infants with clinically diagnosed GER are often treated with pharmacologic agents; however, a lack of evidence of efficacy together with emerging evidence of significant harm (particularly with gastric acid blockade) strongly suggest that these agents should be used sparingly, if at all, in preterm infants.

LEAD AUTHOR

Eric C. Eichenwald, MD, FAAP

COMMITTEE ON FETUS AND NEWBORN, 2017–2018

James J. Cummings, MD, FAAP, Chairperson
Susan Wright Aucott, MD, FAAP
Eric C. Eichenwald, MD, FAAP
Jay P. Goldsmith, MD, FAAP
Ivan L. Hand, MD, FAAP
Sandra E. Juul, MD, PhD, FAAP
Brenda Bradley Poindexter, MD, MS, FAAP
Karen M. Puopolo, MD, PhD, FAAP
Dan L. Stewart, MD, FAAP

LIAISONS

RADM Wanda D. Barfield, MD, MPH, FAAP – *Centers for Disease Control and Prevention*
Thierry Lacaze, MD – *Canadian Paediatric Society*
Maria A. Mascola, MD – *American College of Obstetricians and Gynecologists*
Meredith Mowitz, MD, MS, FAAP – *Section on Neonatal-Perinatal Medicine*
Tonse N. K. Raju, MD, DCH, FAAP – *National Institutes of Health*

STAFF

Jim Couto, MA

ABBREVIATIONS

AAP: American Academy of Pediatrics
BPD: bronchopulmonary dysplasia
GER: gastroesophageal reflux
H_2: histamine-2
LES: lower esophageal sphincter
MII: multichannel intraesophageal impedance
PPI: proton pump inhibitor
RI: reflux index
SIDS: sudden infant death syndrome
TLESR: transient lower esophageal sphincter relaxation

FUNDING: No external funding.

POTENTIAL CONFLICT OF INTEREST: The author has indicated he has no potential conflicts of interest to disclose.

REFERENCES

1. Lightdale JR, Gremse DA; Section on Gastroenterology, Hepatology, and Nutrition. Gastroesophageal reflux: management guidance for the pediatrician. *Pediatrics*. 2013;131(5). Available at: www.pediatrics.org/cgi/content/full/131/5/e1684

2. Vandenplas Y, Rudolph CD, Di Lorenzo C, et al; North American Society for Pediatric Gastroenterology Hepatology and Nutrition; European Society for Pediatric Gastroenterology Hepatology and Nutrition. Pediatric gastroesophageal reflux clinical practice guidelines: joint recommendations of the North American Society for Pediatric Gastroenterology, Hepatology, and Nutrition (NASPGHAN) and the European Society for Pediatric Gastroenterology, Hepatology, and Nutrition (ESPGHAN). *J Pediatr Gastroenterol Nutr*. 2009;49(4):498–547

3. Poets CF. Gastroesophageal reflux: a critical review of its role in preterm infants. *Pediatrics*. 2004;113(2). Available at: www.pediatrics.org/cgi/content/full/113/2/e128

4. Poets CF, Brockmann PE. Myth: gastroesophageal reflux is a pathological entity in the preterm infant. *Semin Fetal Neonatal Med*. 2011;16(5):259–263

5. Jadcherla SR, Slaughter JL, Stenger MR, Klebanoff M, Kelleher K, Gardner W. Practice variance, prevalence, and economic burden of premature infants diagnosed with GERD. *Hosp Pediatr*. 2013;3(4):335–341

6. Dhillon AS, Ewer AK. Diagnosis and management of gastro-oesophageal reflux in preterm infants in neonatal intensive care units. *Acta Paediatr*. 2004;93(1):88–93

7. Khalaf MN, Porat R, Brodsky NL, Bhandari V. Clinical correlations in infants in the neonatal intensive care unit with varying severity of gastroesophageal reflux. *J Pediatr Gastroenterol Nutr*. 2001;32(1):45–49

8. Ferlauto JJ, Walker MW, Martin MS. Clinically significant gastroesophageal reflux in the at-risk premature neonate: relation to cognitive scores, days in the NICU, and total hospital charges. *J Perinatol*. 1998;18(6, pt 1):455–459

9. Slaughter JL, Stenger MR, Reagan PB, Jadcherla SR. Neonatal histamine-2 receptor antagonist and proton pump inhibitor treatment at United States children's hospitals. *J Pediatr*. 2016;174:63–70.e3

10. Golski CA, Rome ES, Martin RJ, et al. Pediatric specialists' beliefs about gastroesophageal reflux disease in premature infants. *Pediatrics*. 2010;125(1):96–104

11. Tighe M, Afzal NA, Bevan A, Hayen A, Munro A, Beattie RM. Pharmacological treatment of children with gastro-oesophageal reflux. *Cochrane Database Syst Rev*. 2014;(11):CD008550

12. Ho T, Dukhovny D, Zupancic JA, Goldmann DA, Horbar JD, Pursley DM. Choosing wisely in newborn medicine: five opportunities to increase value. *Pediatrics*. 2015;136(2). Available at: www.pediatrics.org/cgi/content/full/136/2/e482

13. Omari TI, Barnett C, Snel A, et al. Mechanisms of gastroesophageal reflux in healthy premature infants. *J Pediatr*. 1998;133(5):650–654

14. Peter CS, Sprodowski N, Bohnhorst B, Silny J, Poets CF. Gastroesophageal reflux and apnea of prematurity: no temporal relationship. *Pediatrics*. 2002;109(1):8–11

15. Omari TI, Barnett CP, Benninga MA, et al. Mechanisms of gastro-oesophageal reflux in preterm and term infants with reflux disease. *Gut*. 2002;51(4):475–479

16. Ewer AK, Durbin GM, Morgan ME, Booth IW. Gastric emptying and gastro-oesophageal reflux in preterm infants. *Arch Dis Child Fetal Neonatal Ed*. 1996;75(2):F117–F121

17. Corvaglia L, Rotatori R, Ferlini M, Aceti A, Ancora G, Faldella G. The effect of body positioning on gastroesophageal reflux in premature infants: evaluation by combined impedance and pH monitoring. *J Pediatr*. 2007;151(6):591–596, 596.e1

18. van Wijk MP, Benninga MA, Dent J, et al. Effect of body position changes on postprandial gastroesophageal reflux and gastric emptying in the healthy premature neonate. *J Pediatr*. 2007;151(6):585–590, 590.e1–e2

19. Mitchell DJ, McClure BG, Tubman TR. Simultaneous monitoring of gastric and oesophageal pH reveals limitations of conventional oesophageal pH monitoring in milk fed infants. *Arch Dis Child*. 2001;84(3):273–276

20. Funderburk A, Nawab U, Abraham S, et al. Temporal association between reflux-like behaviors and gastroesophageal reflux in preterm and term infants. *J Pediatr Gastroenterol Nutr*. 2016;62(4):556–561

21. Farhath S, He Z, Saslow J, et al. Detection of pepsin in mouth swab: correlation with clinical gastroesophageal reflux in preterm infants. *J Matern Fetal Neonatal Med*. 2013;26(8):819–824

22. James ME, Ewer AK. Acid oro-pharyngeal secretions can predict gastro-oesophageal reflux in preterm infants. *Eur J Pediatr*. 1999;158(5):371–374

23. López-Alonso M, Moya MJ, Cabo JA, et al. Twenty-four-hour esophageal impedance-pH monitoring in healthy preterm neonates: rate and characteristics of acid, weakly acidic, and weakly alkaline gastroesophageal reflux. *Pediatrics*. 2006;118(2). Available at: www.pediatrics.org/cgi/content/full/118/2/e299

24. Snel A, Barnett CP, Cresp TL, et al. Behavior and gastroesophageal reflux in the premature neonate. *J Pediatr Gastroenterol Nutr*. 2000;30(1):18–21

25. Nobile S, Noviello C, Cobellis G, Carnielli VP. Are infants with bronchopulmonary dysplasia prone to gastroesophageal reflux? A prospective observational study with esophageal pH-impedance monitoring. *J Pediatr*. 2015;167(2):279–285.e1

26. Eichenwald EC; Committee on Fetus and Newborn, American Academy of Pediatrics. Apnea of Prematurity. *Pediatrics*. 2016;137(1):e20153757

27. Poets CF. Gastroesophageal reflux and apnea of prematurity—coincidence, not causation. Commentary on L. Corvaglia et al.: a thickened formula does not reduce apneas related to

gastroesophageal reflux in preterm infants (Neonatology 2013;103;98-102). *Neonatology.* 2013;103(2):103–104

28. Di Fiore JM, Arko M, Whitehouse M, Kimball A, Martin RJ. Apnea is not prolonged by acid gastroesophageal reflux in preterm infants. *Pediatrics.* 2005;116(5):1059–1063

29. Page M, Jeffery HE. Airway protection in sleeping infants in response to pharyngeal fluid stimulation in the supine position. *Pediatr Res.* 1998;44(5):691–698

30. Wheatley E, Kennedy KA. Cross-over trial of treatment for bradycardia attributed to gastroesophageal reflux in preterm infants. *J Pediatr.* 2009;155(4):516–521

31. Kimball AL, Carlton DP. Gastroesophageal reflux medications in the treatment of apnea in premature infants. *J Pediatr.* 2001;138(3):355–360

32. Kazachkov MY, Muhlebach MS, Livasy CA, Noah TL. Lipid-laden macrophage index and inflammation in bronchoalveolar lavage fluids in children. *Eur Respir J.* 2001;18(5):790–795

33. Bar-Sever Z. Scintigraphic evaluation of gastroesophageal reflux and pulmonary aspiration in children. *Semin Nucl Med.* 2017;47(3):275–285

34. Starosta V, Kitz R, Hartl D, Marcos V, Reinhardt D, Griese M. Bronchoalveolar pepsin, bile acids, oxidation, and inflammation in children with gastroesophageal reflux disease. *Chest.* 2007;132(5):1557–1564

35. Farhath S, Aghai ZH, Nakhla T, et al. Pepsin, a reliable marker of gastric aspiration, is frequently detected in tracheal aspirates from premature ventilated neonates: relationship with feeding and methylxanthine therapy. *J Pediatr Gastroenterol Nutr.* 2006;43(3):336–341

36. Farhath S, He Z, Nakhla T, et al. Pepsin, a marker of gastric contents, is increased in tracheal aspirates from preterm infants who develop bronchopulmonary dysplasia. *Pediatrics.* 2008;121(2). Available at: www.pediatrics.org/cgi/content/full/121/2/e253

37. Abdallah AF, El-Desoky T, Fathi K, Elkashef WF, Zaki A. Clinical utility of bronchoalveolar lavage pepsin in diagnosis of gastroesophageal reflux among wheezy infants. *Can Respir J.* 2016;2016:9480843

38. Akinola E, Rosenkrantz TS, Pappagallo M, McKay K, Hussain N. Gastroesophageal reflux in infants < 32 weeks gestational age at birth: lack of relationship to chronic lung disease. *Am J Perinatol.* 2004;21(2):57–62

39. Fuloria M, Hiatt D, Dillard RG, O'Shea TM. Gastroesophageal reflux in very low birth weight infants: association with chronic lung disease and outcomes through 1 year of age. *J Perinatol.* 2000;20(4):235–239

40. Dellert SF, Hyams JS, Treem WR, Geertsma MA. Feeding resistance and gastroesophageal reflux in infancy. *J Pediatr Gastroenterol Nutr.* 1993;17(1):66–71

41. Mathisen B, Worrall L, Masel J, Wall C, Shepherd RW. Feeding problems in infants with gastro-oesophageal reflux disease: a controlled study. *J Paediatr Child Health.* 1999;35(2):163–169

42. Frakaloss G, Burke G, Sanders MR. Impact of gastroesophageal reflux on growth and hospital stay in premature infants. *J Pediatr Gastroenterol Nutr.* 1998;26(2):146–150

43. Malcolm WF, Gantz M, Martin RJ, Goldstein RF, Goldberg RN, Cotten CM; National Institute of Child Health and Human Development Neonatal Research Network. Use of medications for gastroesophageal reflux at discharge among extremely low birth weight infants. *Pediatrics.* 2008;121(1):22–27

44. Orenstein SR, Whitington PF, Orenstein DM. The infant seat as treatment for gastroesophageal reflux. *N Engl J Med.* 1983;309(13):760–763

45. Orenstein SR. Effects on behavior state of prone versus seated positioning for infants with gastroesophageal reflux. *Pediatrics.* 1990;85(5):765–767

46. Bagucka B, De Schepper J, Peelman M, Van de Maele K, Vandenplas Y. Acid gastro-esophageal reflux in the 10 degrees-reversed-Trendelenburg-position in supine sleeping infants. *Acta Paediatr Taiwan.* 1999;40(5):298–301

47. Loots C, Kritas S, van Wijk M, et al. Body positioning and medical therapy for infantile gastroesophageal reflux symptoms. *J Pediatr Gastroenterol Nutr.* 2014;59(2):237–243

48. Moon RY; Task Force on Sudden Infant Death Syndrome. SIDS and other sleep-related infant deaths: evidence base for 2016 updated recommendations for a safe infant sleeping environment. *Pediatrics.* 2016;138(5):e20162940

49. American Academy of Pediatrics Committee on Fetus and Newborn. Hospital discharge of the high-risk neonate. *Pediatrics.* 2008;122(5):1119–1126

50. Jadcherla SR, Chan CY, Moore R, Malkar M, Timan CJ, Valentine CJ. Impact of feeding strategies on the frequency and clearance of acid and nonacid gastroesophageal reflux events in dysphagic neonates. *JPEN J Parenter Enteral Nutr.* 2012;36(4):449–455

51. Richards R, Foster JP, Psaila K. Continuous versus bolus intragastric tube feeding for preterm and low birth weight infants with gastro-oesophageal reflux disease. *Cochrane Database Syst Rev.* 2014;(7):CD009719

52. Madhoun LL, Siler-Wurst KK, Sitaram S, Jadcherla SR. Feed-thickening practices in NICUs in the current era: variability in prescription and implementation patterns. *J Neonatal Nurs.* 2015;21(6):255–262

53. Beal J, Silverman B, Bellant J, Young TE, Klontz K. Late onset necrotizing enterocolitis in infants following use of a xanthan gum-containing thickening agent. *J Pediatr.* 2012;161(2):354–356

54. Horvath A, Dziechciarz P, Szajewska H. The effect of thickened-feed interventions on gastroesophageal reflux in infants: systematic review and meta-analysis of randomized, controlled trials. *Pediatrics.* 2008;122(6). Available at: www.pediatrics.org/cgi/content/full/122/6/e1268

55. Corvaglia L, Aceti A, Mariani E, et al. Lack of efficacy of a starch-thickened preterm formula on gastro-oesophageal reflux in preterm infants: a pilot study. *J Matern Fetal Neonatal Med.* 2012;25(12):2735–2738

56. Garzi A, Messina M, Frati F, et al. An extensively hydrolysed cow's milk formula improves clinical symptoms of gastroesophageal reflux and reduces the gastric emptying time in infants. *Allergol Immunopathol (Madr)*. 2002;30(1):36–41

57. Salvatore S, Vandenplas Y. Gastroesophageal reflux and cow milk allergy: is there a link? *Pediatrics*. 2002;110(5):972–984

58. Corvaglia L, Mariani E, Aceti A, Galletti S, Faldella G. Extensively hydrolyzed protein formula reduces acid gastro-esophageal reflux in symptomatic preterm infants. *Early Hum Dev*. 2013;89(7):453–455

59. Logarajaha V, Onga C, Jayagobib PA, et al. PP-15 the effect of extensively hydrolyzed protein formula in preterm infants with symptomatic gastro-oesophageal reflux. *J Pediatr Gastroenterol Nutr*. 2015;61(4):526

60. Hibbs AM, Lorch SA. Metoclopramide for the treatment of gastroesophageal reflux disease in infants: a systematic review. *Pediatrics*. 2006;118(2):746–752

61. Corvaglia L, Monari C, Martini S, Aceti A, Faldella G. Pharmacological therapy of gastroesophageal reflux in preterm infants. *Gastroenterol Res Pract*. 2013;2013:714564

62. Corvaglia L, Aceti A, Mariani E, De Giorgi M, Capretti MG, Faldella G. The efficacy of sodium alginate (Gaviscon) for the treatment of gastro-oesophageal reflux in preterm infants. *Aliment Pharmacol Ther*. 2011;33(4):466–470

63. Atasay B, Erdeve O, Arsan S, Türmen T. Effect of sodium alginate on acid gastroesophageal reflux disease in preterm infants: a pilot study. *J Clin Pharmacol*. 2010;50(11):1267–1272

64. Guillet R, Stoll BJ, Cotten CM, et al; National Institute of Child Health and Human Development Neonatal Research Network. Association of H2-blocker therapy and higher incidence of necrotizing enterocolitis in very low birth weight infants. *Pediatrics*. 2006;117(2). Available at: www.pediatrics.org/cgi/content/full/117/2/e137

65. Terrin G, Passariello A, De Curtis M, et al. Ranitidine is associated with infections, necrotizing enterocolitis, and fatal outcome in newborns. *Pediatrics*. 2012;129(1). Available at: www.pediatrics.org/cgi/content/full/129/1/e40

66. Gupta RW, Tran L, Norori J, et al. Histamine-2 receptor blockers alter the fecal microbiota in premature infants. *J Pediatr Gastroenterol Nutr*. 2013;56(4):397–400

67. Wang K, Lin HJ, Perng CL, et al. The effect of H2-receptor antagonist and proton pump inhibitor on microbial proliferation in the stomach. *Hepatogastroenterology*. 2004;51(59):1540–1543

68. Laheij RJ, Sturkenboom MC, Hassing RJ, Dieleman J, Stricker BH, Jansen JB. Risk of community-acquired pneumonia and use of gastric acid-suppressive drugs. *JAMA*. 2004;292(16):1955–1960

69. Canani RB, Cirillo P, Roggero P, et al; Working Group on Intestinal Infections of the Italian Society of Pediatric Gastroenterology, Hepatology and Nutrition (SIGENP). Therapy with gastric acidity inhibitors increases the risk of acute gastroenteritis and community-acquired pneumonia in children. *Pediatrics*. 2006; 117(5). Available at: www.pediatrics.org/cgi/content/full/117/5/e817

70. Orenstein SR, Hassall E, Furmaga-Jablonska W, Atkinson S, Raanan M. Multicenter, double-blind, randomized, placebo-controlled trial assessing the efficacy and safety of proton pump inhibitor lansoprazole in infants with symptoms of gastroesophageal reflux disease. *J Pediatr*. 2009; 154(4):514–520.e4

POLICY STATEMENT   Organizational Principles to Guide and Define the Child Health
Care System and/or Improve the Health of all Children

American Academy
of Pediatrics

DEDICATED TO THE HEALTH OF ALL CHILDREN™

Donor Human Milk for the High-Risk Infant: Preparation, Safety, and Usage Options in the United States

COMMITTEE ON NUTRITION, SECTION ON BREASTFEEDING, COMMITTEE ON FETUS AND NEWBORN

abstract

The use of donor human milk is increasing for high-risk infants, primarily for infants born weighing <1500 g or those who have severe intestinal disorders. Pasteurized donor milk may be considered in situations in which the supply of maternal milk is insufficient. The use of pasteurized donor milk is safe when appropriate measures are used to screen donors and collect, store, and pasteurize the milk and then distribute it through established human milk banks. The use of nonpasteurized donor milk and other forms of direct, Internet-based, or informal human milk sharing does not involve this level of safety and is not recommended. It is important that health care providers counsel families considering milk sharing about the risks of bacterial or viral contamination of nonpasteurized human milk and about the possibilities of exposure to medications, drugs, or herbs in human milk. Currently, the use of pasteurized donor milk is limited by its availability and affordability. The development of public policy to improve and expand access to pasteurized donor milk, including policies that support improved governmental and private financial support for donor milk banks and the use of donor milk, is important.

DOI: 10.1542/peds.2016-3440

PEDIATRICS (ISSN Numbers: Print, 0031-4005; Online, 1098-4275).

Copyright © 2017 by the American Academy of Pediatrics

FINANCIAL DISCLOSURE: The authors have indicated they do not have a financial relationship relevant to this article to disclose.

FUNDING: No external funding.

POTENTIAL CONFLICT OF INTEREST: The authors have indicated they have no potential conflicts of interest to disclose.

To cite: AAP COMMITTEE ON NUTRITION, AAP SECTION ON BREASTFEEDING, AAP COMMITTEE ON FETUS AND NEWBORN. Donor Human Milk for the High-Risk Infant: Preparation, Safety, and Usage Options in the United States. Pediatrics. 2017;139(1):e20163440

INTRODUCTION

Human milk provides health benefits for all newborn infants but is of particular importance for high-risk infants, especially those born with very low birth weight (<1500 g). Donor human milk also can be beneficial to supplement the mother's own milk when necessary. The evidence to support the use of donor human milk has been reviewed,[1–6] and recent studies[7–9] support health benefits for its use in infants with a birth weight <1500 g, especially in decreasing rates of necrotizing enterocolitis.

Donor milk banks represent a safe and effective approach to obtaining, pasteurizing, and dispensing human milk for use in NICUs and other settings. However, accessibility to donor milk in the United States continues to be substantially limited in terms of supply, cost, and distribution. Because of these limitations, some parents have chosen to exchange human milk that is not pasteurized or handled by an established milk bank with each other (milk sharing). This report reviews the preparation, safety, and usage options for donor human milk in the United States.

PREPARATION OF DONOR HUMAN MILK, PASTEURIZATION, AND DISTRIBUTION

The number of human milk banks in the United States is increasing. Currently, there are 20 donor milk banks in the United States and 4 in Canada that pasteurize milk as part of a professional organization for supporters of nonprofit human milk banking, the Human Milk Banking Association of North America (HMBANA); 7 others are in various stages of planning and development (www.hmbana.org). In addition, several commercial (for-profit) human milk banks collect, pasteurize, and distribute donor human milk but are not part of HMBANA.

Donor Human Milk Collection

HMBANA has established policies for donor human milk collection, as do commercial human milk banks.[10] These have been described in the literature[1,2] and in the policies usually found on the Web sites of the individual milk banks. Guidelines for donors include completion of a health screen, blood serologic testing, and detailed instructions on collecting, storing, and shipping milk.[10] In contrast, direct milk sharing or other forms of milk collection and distribution are extremely variable in the screening of donors and the methods of milk storage and transportation.

Pasteurization

Several methods may be used to pasteurize donor human milk,

and these have been reviewed extensively.[1,3,11] The Holder pasteurization method uses heating at 62.5°C for 30 minutes and is the primary method used by HMBANA milk banks. One commercial milk bank, Medolac Laboratories (Lake Oswego, OR), uses a different thermal pasteurization system.

Distribution

In the United States and Canada, most donor milk is distributed by established milk banks to NICUs. Each milk bank and/or processing center has policies, including cost-related guidelines, for this distribution. The distribution of donor milk may be subject to federal or state guidelines in some situations, but at the time of this publication, there are no restrictions on the use of pasteurized donor human milk in any state in the United States.

Frozen donor human milk is distributed by using shipping guidelines established by the milk banks. Receiving hospitals are provided guidance related to temperature and other storage conditions for the milk, and these may be subject to state and local regulations. Hospitals that use frozen donor human milk must have properly regulated freezers and other methods for handling and tracking donor milk.

SAFETY

Human milk is a biological product; therefore, whether from an infant's own mother or a donor mother, there will always be concerns about contamination. Possible contaminants are infectious agents, including both bacteria and viruses, and contamination with other substances, most notably toxic components in the environment (eg, pesticides, mercury, medications, drugs, or herbs).

Although a detailed description of each of these is beyond the scope of

this statement, the processes used in pasteurization of donor human milk are highly effective in removing viral infectious contaminants.[10-14] Human milk banks vary in their approach to bacterial screening of incoming milk, but postpasteurization bacteriologic cultures are performed routinely. Published data[10,11] have revealed a very low or unmeasurable level of infectious contaminants. Families and caregivers may be reassured that, at the time of this publication, there are no reported cases of pasteurized donor human milk causing an infection with hepatitis viruses or HIV and that the likelihood of this type of infection occurring in a neonate given donor human milk is extremely small.

With regard to noninfectious contaminants, although these can be difficult to completely eliminate, the pooling process with donor milk makes it very unlikely that these will represent a significant exposure risk. An exception to this is cow milk protein, which is present in the milk of mothers who include dairy in their diet. The contamination of human milk purchased via the Internet with cow milk (up to a 10% dilution of the human milk) has recently been reported.[15]

In contrast, informal direct milk sharing without pasteurization exposes infants to a range of possible risks, including bacterial contamination[16] and viral transmission, including cytomegalovirus, hepatitis viruses, and HIV.[17] Individual screening is performed by some Internet-based groups that organize direct milk sharing, but these are neither consistently applied nor documented. Furthermore, even with serologic blood testing, infectious complications remain a significant risk in unpasteurized milk.

Because direct milk sharing is often arranged by using milk from a single donor mother, other contaminants, such as medications or drugs, may be a higher risk than with pooled milk products. It is unknown what effects paying women for milk might have on these risks.

Growth Issues

Early studies in the use of donor human milk for small preterm infants showed relatively slow growth. More recent studies[18-20] showed improved growth outcomes, which may be attributable both to a greater availability of donor milk with higher nutrient content and to widely used strategies for fortifying donor milk. However, these are retrospective cohort studies, and further studies are needed. Strategies for fortifying donor human milk include both commercial human milk–based and cow milk protein–based fortifiers. Both types of fortifiers have been shown to lead to appropriate growth, and the use of donor human milk does not need to be limited on the basis of growth concerns in most high-risk infants. Growth monitoring is always paramount for infants, and human milk fortification is needed for all infants with very low birth weight.

Loss of Nutrients and Antiinflammatory Properties

The process of pasteurization destroys cells, such neutrophils and stem cells, and affects macronutrients and antiinflammatory factors. In addition, pasteurization can eliminate bacterial strains with probiotic properties. Substantial evidence describing these losses is available.[21-25] Bioactive components of human milk, including lactoferrin and immunoglobulins, are substantially decreased by pasteurization, but there is much less effect on macro- or micronutrients, including vitamins.[22,23] Overall, the benefits of improved feeding tolerance and clinical outcomes support the concept that some nutrient losses of bioactive components should not limit the use of donor human milk or preclude

its pasteurization before use. Donor human milk may have a lower protein and energy content than the milk of mothers of preterm infants, in addition to lost bile salt–dependent lipase activity, which may affect fortification strategies and growth. Alternative sterilization methods to preserve innate bioactive properties and to decrease the cost of preparing donor milk need investigation.

The principal goal for infants with very low birth weight is the provision of the mother's own milk, with donor human milk as a bridge or support while the mother's milk is made available or increasing in volume. It is important to encourage and assist mothers to pump or express and provide their own milk whenever possible and at the maximum volume possible. Although the use of donor human milk has not been shown to decrease the frequency or volume of mother's own milk to NICU patients,[9,23,26,27] vigilance and education are needed regarding the superiority of mother's own milk relative to donor human milk.

USAGE

Infants <1500 g Birth Weight

The supply of donor human milk currently available in the United States and Canada is less than optimal. Although a goal of providing donor milk to supplement the mother's milk for all preterm infants has been described,[5] this goal may not be achievable for a period of time; thus, prioritization may be needed for infants weighing <1500 g. Relatively few data are available on whether this would include small for gestational age infants, such as those who are >32 to 33 weeks' postmenstrual age at birth who also weigh <1500 g; but, in general, the primary guide for use is birth weight, not gestational age, in prioritizing donor milk use.

There are no clear guidelines for discontinuing the use of donor human milk in an infant <1500 g birth weight when the volume of mother's milk is not adequate. A range of postmenstrual ages from 32 to 36 weeks is commonly used in the United States, because this range covers the highest risk period for necrotizing enterocolitis. Further research is needed to clarify the optimal timing of discontinuing donor human milk. Breastfeeding should be encouraged during hospitalization for these infants to enhance the likelihood of successful breastfeeding after hospital discharge.[28]

Other Intestinal Diseases

Fewer data are available regarding the use of donor human milk in other high-risk infants, including infants with abdominal wall defects, such as gastroschisis or omphalocele, and other conditions, such as congenital heart disease. Nonetheless, some infants with these conditions or other neonatal disorders may benefit from donor human milk either because of a direct effect on intestinal growth or improved feeding tolerance.[29] In these cases, payers may expect documentation of intolerance to specialized infant formulas and the medical necessity for donor human milk before providing payment for human milk at home or in the hospital.

Outpatient (Home) Versus Hospital Distribution

The vast majority of donor human milk distributed from HMBANA milk banks is distributed to hospitals for internal use in NICU patients. However, in some cases, donor human milk may be provided for home use from HMBANA milk banks.[1] In cases of limited supply, health care providers, such as community pediatricians and neonatologists, can work together to establish priority for such use relative to local NICU needs. A pediatrician/

neonatal clinician generally will need to be involved in ordering and supervising the use of donor milk in any outpatient setting. Clear documentation as to the reason for the use of donor human milk at home is recommended.

OTHER POLICY ISSUES

Cost Reimbursement

A major limitation in the use of donor human milk is the cost of providing this milk to hospitals or to families. Reimbursement for donor milk is inconsistent between states and often between sources of payment. Health care providers can advocate for the development of public and local hospital policies to enhance the availability and affordability of donor human milk on the basis of evidence. Resources from the American Academy of Pediatrics and other groups can also assist those involved in the care of neonates in this discussion.

The use of donor human milk in appropriate high-risk infants is consistent with good health care for these infants.[30,31] Policies are needed to provide high-risk infants access to donor human milk on the basis of documented medical necessity, not financial status.

Federal and State Regulation of Milk Banks and Donor Milk Sharing

Legal issues exist regarding the regulation of donor human milk banks on both a state and national level. Federal or state guidelines are needed regarding the preparation, handling, and transfer of human milk as well as the operation of donor human milk banks and would be best accomplished via formal regulation by the US Food and Drug Administration with oversight by the Centers for Disease Control and Prevention.

Families of high-risk infants should be fully informed about the current state of research regarding the benefits of using human milk to decrease the risks of complications such as necrotizing enterocolitis. This discussion may include appropriate warnings about risks related to infectious complications when human milk is shared or distributed outside of established milk banks. Neonatologists and other health care providers should advocate for policies of full disclosure of the risks and benefits related to direct or informal milk sharing without pasteurization. Hospitals should develop standards such that all human milk given to infants meets appropriate standards for preparation and distribution and that pasteurization of all donor human milk occurs.

SUMMARY OF KEY POINTS

1. Although a mother's own milk is always preferred, donor human milk may be used for high-risk infants when the mother's milk is not available or the mother cannot provide milk. Priority should be given to providing donor human milk to infants <1500 g birth weight.

2. Human milk donors should be identified and screened by using methods such as those currently used by HMBANA milk banks or other established commercial milk banks.

3. Donor milk should be pasteurized according to accepted standards. Postpasteurization testing should be performed according to internal quality-control guidelines.

4. Health care providers should discourage families from direct human milk sharing or purchasing human milk from the Internet because of the increased risks of bacterial or viral contamination of nonpasteurized milk and the possibility of exposure to medications, drugs, or other substances, including cow milk protein.

5. The use of donor human milk in appropriate high-risk infants should not be limited by an individual's ability to pay. Policies are needed to provide high-risk infants access to donor human milk on the basis of documented medical necessity, not financial status.

LEAD AUTHORS

Steven A. Abrams, MD, FAAP
Susan Landers, MD, FAAP
Lawrence M. Noble, MD, FAAP
Brenda B. Poindexter, MD, FAAP

COMMITTEE ON NUTRITION, 2015–2016

Stephen Daniels, MD, PhD, FAAP, Chairperson
Mark Corkins, MD, FAAP
Sarah de Ferranti, MD, FAAP
Neville H. Golden, MD, FAAP
Jae H. Kim, MD, PhD, FAAP
Sheela N. Magge, MD, MSCE, FAAP
Sarah Jane Schwarzenberg, MD, FAAP

LIAISONS

Carrie L. Assar, PharmD, MS – *Food and Drug Administration*
Jeff Critch, MD – *Canadian Pediatric Society*
Van Hubbard, MD, PhD – *National Institutes of Health*
Kelley Scanlon, PhD – *Centers for Disease Control and Prevention*
Valery Soto, MS, RD, LD – *US Department of Agriculture*

STAFF

Debra Burrowes, MHA

SECTION ON BREASTFEEDING EXECUTIVE COMMITTEE, 2015–2016

Joan Younger Meek, MD, MS, RD, FAAP, Chairperson
Margreete G. Johnston, MD, MPH, FAAP
Mary Ellen O'Connor, MD, MPH, FAAP
Lisa M. Stellwagen, MD, FAAP
Jennifer Peelen Thomas, MD, MPH, FAAP
Julie L. Ware, MD, FAAP
Richard J. Schanler, MD, FAAP, Immediate Past Chair

STAFF

Ngozi Onyema-Melton, MPH

COMMITTEE ON FETUS AND NEWBORN, 2015–2016

Kristi L. Watterberg, MD, FAAP, Chairperson
Susan Wright Aucott, MD, FAAP

William E. Benitz, MD, FAAP
James J. Cummings, MD, FAAP
Eric C. Eichenwald, MD, FAAP
Jay P. Goldsmith, MD, FAAP
Brenda B. Poindexter, MD, MS, FAAP
Karen M. Puopolo, MD, PhD, FAAP
Dan L. Stewart, MD, FAAP

LIAISONS

Erin L. Keels, APRN, MS, NNP – *National Association of Neonatal Nurses*
Thierry Lacaze, MD – *Canadian Pediatric Society*
Maria A. Mascola – *American College of Obstetricians and Gynecologists*
Tonse N.K. Raju, MD, FAAP – *National Institutes of Health*

STAFF

Jim R. Couto, MA

ABBREVIATION

HMBANA: Human Milk Banking Association of North America

REFERENCES

1. Landers S, Hartmann BT. Donor human milk banking and the emergence of milk sharing. *Pediatr Clin North Am.* 2013;60(1):247–260

2. Arslanoglu S, Ziegler EE, Moro GE; World Association of Perinatal Medicine Working Group on Nutrition. Donor human milk in preterm infant feeding: evidence and recommendations. *J Perinat Med.* 2010;38(4):347–351

3. Arslanoglu S, Corpeleijn W, Moro G, et al; ESPGHAN Committee on Nutrition. Donor human milk for preterm infants: current evidence and research directions. *J Pediatr Gastroenterol Nutr.* 2013;57(4):535–542

4. Bertino E, Giuliani F, Baricco M, et al. Benefits of donor milk in the feeding of preterm infants. *Early Hum Dev.* 2013;89(suppl 2):S3–S6

5. Quigley M, McGuire W. Formula versus donor breast milk for feeding preterm or low birth weight infants. *Cochrane Database Syst Rev.* 2014;4:CD002971

6. Section on Breastfeeding. Breastfeeding and the use of human milk. *Pediatrics.* 2012;129(3). Available

at: www.pediatrics.org/cgi/content/full/129/3/e827

7. Sullivan S, Schanler RJ, Kim JH, et al. An exclusively human milk-based diet is associated with a lower rate of necrotizing enterocolitis than a diet of human milk and bovine milk-based products. *J Pediatr.* 2010;156(4):562–7.e1

8. Cristofalo EA, Schanler RJ, Blanco CL, et al. Randomized trial of exclusive human milk versus preterm formula diets in extremely premature infants. *J Pediatr.* 2013;163(6):1592–1595, e1

9. Kantorowska A, Wei JC, Cohen RS, Lawrence RA, Gould JB, Lee HC. Impact of donor milk availability on breast milk use and necrotizing enterocolitis rates. *Pediatrics.* 2016;137(3):e20153123

10. Human Milk Banking Association of North America. *Guidelines for Establishment and Operation of a Donor Human Milk Bank.* 16th ed. Fort Worth, TX: Human Milk Banking Association of North America; 2011

11. Czank C, Prime DK, Hartmann B, Simmer K, Hartmann PE. Retention of the immunological proteins of pasteurized human milk in relation to pasteurizer design and practice. *Pediatr Res.* 2009;66(4):374–379

12. Landers S, Updegrove K. Bacteriological screening of donor human milk before and after Holder pasteurization. *Breastfeed Med.* 2010;5(3):117–121

13. Terpstra FG, Rechtman DJ, Lee ML, et al. Antimicrobial and antiviral effect of high-temperature short-time (HTST) pasteurization applied to human milk. *Breastfeed Med.* 2007;2(1):27–33

14. de Segura AG, Escuder D, Montilla A, et al. Heating-induced bacteriological and biochemical modifications in human donor milk after holder pasteurisation. *J Pediatr Gastroenterol Nutr.* 2012;54(2):197–203

15. Keim SA, Kulkarni MM, McNamara K, et al. Cow's milk contamination of human milk purchased via the Internet. *Pediatrics.* 2015;135(5). Available at: www.pediatrics.org/cgi/content/full/135/5/e1157

16. Keim SA, Hogan JS, McNamara KA, et al. Microbial contamination of

human milk purchased via the Internet. *Pediatrics.* 2013;132(5). Available at: www.pediatrics.org/cgi/content/full/132/5/e1227

17. Lindemann PC, Foshaugen I, Lindemann R. Characteristics of breast milk and serology of women donating breast milk to a milk bank. *Arch Dis Child Fetal Neonatal Ed.* 2004;89(5):F440–F441

18. Colaizy TT, Carlson S, Saftlas AF, Morriss FH Jr. Growth in VLBW infants fed predominantly fortified maternal and donor human milk diets: a retrospective cohort study. *BMC Pediatr.* 2012;12:124–133

19. Rochow N, Fusch G, Choi A, et al. Target fortification of breast milk with fat, protein, and carbohydrates for preterm infants. *J Pediatr.* 2013;163(4):1001–1007

20. Hair AB, Hawthorne KM, Chetta KE, Abrams SA. Human milk feeding supports adequate growth in infants ≤ 1250 grams birth weight. *BMC Res Notes.* 2013;6:459–467

21. García-Lara NR, Vieco DE, De la Cruz-Bértolo J, Lora-Pablos D, Velasco NU, Pallás-Alonso CR. Effect of Holder pasteurization and frozen storage on macronutrients and energy content of breast milk. *J Pediatr Gastroenterol Nutr.* 2013;57(3):377–382

22. García-Lara NR, Escuder-Vieco D, García-Algar O, De la Cruz J, Lora D, Pallás-Alonso C. Effect of freezing time on macronutrients and energy content of breastmilk. *Breastfeed Med.* 2012;7(4):295–301

23. Silvestre D, Miranda M, Muriach M, Almansa I, Jareño E, Romero FJ. Antioxidant capacity of human milk: effect of thermal conditions for the pasteurization. *Acta Paediatr.* 2008;97(8):1070–1074

24. Wada Y, Lönnerdal B. Bioactive peptides released from in vitro digestion of human milk with or without pasteurization. *Pediatr Res.* 2015;77(4):546–553

25. Coscia A, Peila C, Bertino E, et al. Effect of Holder pasteurisation on human milk glycosaminoglycans. *J Pediatr Gastroenterol Nutr.* 2015;60(1):127–130

26. Delfosse NM, Ward L, Lagomarcino AJ, et al. Donor human milk largely

replaces formula-feeding of preterm infants in two urban hospitals. *J Perinatol.* 2013;33(6):446–451

27. Arslanoglu S, Moro GE, Bellù R, et al. Presence of human milk bank is associated with elevated rate of exclusive breastfeeding in VLBW infants. *J Perinat Med.* 2013;41(2):129–131

28. Meier PP, Engstrom JL, Patel AL, Jegier BJ, Bruns NE. Improving the use of human milk during and after the NICU stay. *Clin Perinatol.* 2010;37(1):217–245

29. Kohler JA Sr, Perkins AM, Bass WT. Human milk versus formula after gastroschisis repair: effects on time to full feeds and time to discharge. *J Perinatol.* 2013;33(8):627–630

30. Parker MG, Barrero-Castillero A, Corwin BK, Kavanagh PL, Belfort MB, Wang CJ. Pasteurized human donor milk use among US level 3 neonatal intensive care units. *J Hum Lact.* 2013;29(3):381–389

31. Perrine CG, Scanlon KS. Prevalence of use of human milk in US advanced care neonatal units. *Pediatrics.* 2013;131(6):1066–1071

American Academy
of Pediatrics
DEDICATED TO THE HEALTH OF ALL CHILDREN™

"Late-Preterm" Infants: A Population at Risk

Guidance for the Clinician in Rendering Pediatric Care

William A. Engle, MD, Kay M. Tomashek, MD, Carol Wallman, MSN, and the Committee on Fetus and Newborn

ABSTRACT

Late-preterm infants, defined by birth at 34⁶/₇ through 36⁶/₇ weeks' gestation, are less physiologically and metabolically mature than term infants. Thus, they are at higher risk of morbidity and mortality than term infants. The purpose of this report is to define "late preterm," recommend a change in terminology from "near term" to "late preterm," present the characteristics of late-preterm infants that predispose them to a higher risk of morbidity and mortality than term infants, and propose guidelines for the evaluation and management of these infants after birth.

INTRODUCTION

Infants born at 34⁶/₇ through 36⁶/₇ weeks' gestation, or "late-preterm" infants, are often the size and weight of some term infants (born at 37⁰/₇–41⁶/₇ weeks' gestation). Because of this fact, late-preterm infants may be treated by parents, caregivers, and health care professionals as though they are developmentally mature and at low risk of morbidity. They are often managed in newborn level 1 (basic) nurseries or remain with their mother after birth.[1]

Late-preterm infants are physiologically and metabolically immature.[2–8] As a consequence, late-preterm infants are at higher risk than are term infants of developing medical complications that result in higher rates of mortality and morbidity during the birth hospitalization.[6–8] In addition, late-preterm infants have higher rates of hospital readmission during the neonatal period than do term infants.[2,4,7–9] During the last 15 years, the proportion of all US births that were late preterm increased from 7.3% in 1990 to 9.1% in 2005.[10] In 2005, late-preterm births accounted for more than 70% of all preterm births (<37 weeks' gestation), or approximately 377 000 infants.[10–12] In fact, much of the increase in the preterm birth rate in recent years can be attributed to increases in late-preterm births.[12,13]

The reason for the increase in late-preterm births during the last decade is not well understood. One hypothesis is that it may be attributable, in part, to increased use of reproductive technologies and, as a result, an increase in multifetal pregnancies.[11,14–16] Another hypothesis is that advances in obstetric practice have led to an increase in surveillance and medical interventions during pregnancy.[11,14–17] As a result, fetuses considered to be at risk of stillbirth, including those with intrauterine growth restriction, fetal anomalies, and intrapartum asphyxia, may be identified earlier, which results in more deliveries at 34 to 36 weeks' gestation. For example, between 1989 and 2003, the use of electronic fetal monitoring and prenatal ultrasonography increased substantially from 68.1% to 85.4% and 47.6% to 67%, respectively.[10] Rates of labor induction and cesarean delivery also in-

www.pediatrics.org/cgi/doi/10.1542/peds.2007-2952

doi:10.1542/peds.2007-2952

All clinical reports from the American Academy of Pediatrics automatically expire 5 years after publication unless reaffirmed, revised, or retired at or before that time.

The guidance in this report does not indicate an exclusive course of treatment or serve as a standard of medical care. Variations, taking into account individual circumstances, may be appropriate.

Key Words
late preterm, near-term, moderate preterm, morbidity, mortality, readmission

PEDIATRICS (ISSN Numbers: Print, 0031-4005; Online, 1098-4275). Copyright © 2007 by the American Academy of Pediatrics

TABLE 1 Statistical and Conventional Definitions of Weeks of Gestation, Completed Weeks of Gestation, Late Preterm Gestation, and Term Gestation

	Gestation, wk	Gestation, Completed Weeks[a]							
Fraction of week[b]		0/7	1/7	2/7	3/7	4/7	5/7	6/7	
Statistical day[c]	0	0	1	2	3	4	5	6	1
Medical Convention day[d]		1	2	3	4	5	6	7	
	1	7	8	9	10	11	12	13	2
		8	9	10	11	12	13	14	
	33	231	232	233	234	235	236	237	34
		232	233	234	235	236	237	238	
	34	238	239	240	241	242	243	244	35
		239	240	241	241	243	244	245	
	35	245	246	247	248	249	250	251	36
		246	247	248	249	250	251	252	
	36	252	253	254	255	256	257	258	37
		253	254	255	256	257	258	259	
	37	259	260	261	262	263	264	265	38
		260	261	262	263	264	265	266	
	38	266	267	268	269	270	271	272	39
		267	268	269	270	271	272	273	
	39	273	274	275	276	277	278	279	40
		274	275	276	277	278	279	280	
	40	280	281	282	283	284	285	286	41
		281	282	283	284	285	286	287	
	41	287	288	289	290	291	292	293	42
		288	289	290	291	292	293	294	
	42	294	295	296	297	298	299	300	43
		295	296	297	298	299	300	301	

Late-preterm gestation is defined by medical convention as 34⁰/₇ weeks (239 days) through and including 36⁶/₇ weeks (259 days) after the beginning of the mother's last normal menstrual period. This is indicated in days with a red background. For comparison, term gestation spans from 37⁰/₇ weeks (260 days) through and including 41⁶/₇ weeks (294 days) after the beginning of the mother's last normal menstrual period, which is indicated in days with an aqua background.

[a] Completed week of gestation indicates the number of 7-day intervals that have passed since the beginning of the mother's last normal menstrual period. For example, the first completed week occurs after 1 seven-day interval (0⁶/₇th week or 7 days) has passed. The 37th completed week occurs after 37 seven-day intervals (36⁶/₇ weeks or 259 days) have passed.

[b] Fraction of a week indicates the days of each gestational week as a fraction. For example, the first day of gestation is the first day of the mother's 36⁰/₇th week of gestation and ends on the 36⁶/₇th week of gestation.

[c] Statistical day indicates that the first day of the mother's last menstrual period begins as day 0 and is not complete until the beginning of day 1.

[d] This statistical view of gestational age differs by 1 day from the conventional medical count of days, which indicates that the first day of the mother's last menstrual period begins as day 1. This important difference is indicated by the statistically defined days that have a gray background and conventionally defined days having no background or a red or aqua background.

creased during the last decade.[10,11] It is important to note, however, that the increased intensity of care provided to pregnant women has been accompanied by significant reductions in stillbirths, perinatal mortality, and births beyond 40 weeks' gestation.[11,14]

It is important to understand why these infants are being born early as well as the unique problems that this growing population of infants may experience. A clearer understanding of the underlying risk factors, associated etiologies, and their relative effects on delivery at 34⁰/₇

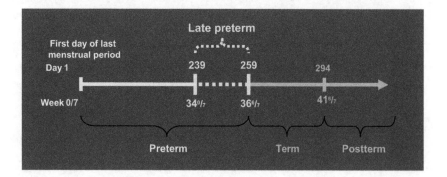

FIGURE 1
Late-preterm definition.

through 36⁶/₇ weeks' gestation on the mother and fetus is needed to develop interventions to prevent unnecessary late-preterm births and to improve the management of infants who are born late preterm. Thus, additional research is needed to determine the gestational age at delivery that optimally balances the risk of fetal morbidity or death against risks associated with late-preterm birth for both the mother and the fetus.

The purpose of this report is to define "late preterm," recommend a change in terminology to "late preterm" from the previously used "near term," describe the medical complications and health risks commonly encountered by late-preterm infants, suggest guidelines to identify and manage these complications and risks during the birth hospitalization and after discharge, and identify gaps in knowledge concerning the medical and developmental outcomes of these infants.

DEFINITION OF LATE PRETERM

The gestational age attributed to a newborn infant can be confusing, because the first day of a mother's last normal menstrual period is counted as either day 0 or day 1 depending on whether a statistical or conventional medical definition, respectively, is used. This difference in definition of gestational age accounts for a 1-day variation among data systems when determining the chronologic age of a newborn infant on the first day after birth (Table 1). The day of birth is counted as day 1 when using the conventional medical definition and day 0 when using the statistical definition. The use of conventional medical terminology is illustrated in the definitions of gestational age recommended by the American Academy of Pediatrics, the American College of Obstetricians and Gynecologists, and the World Health Organization.[18–20] For example, "preterm" is defined as birth that occurs on or before the end of the last day of the 37th completed week (ie, 36⁶/₇ weeks' gestation) after the onset of the mother's last menstrual period, which equates to 259 days in common medical terminology. The statistical definition for the last day of the 37th completed week of gestation is 258 days. Understanding these definitions is complicated further by financial systems that define the first day of age as delivery before

12:00 AM (midnight) and the subsequent day beginning immediately after 12:00 AM.

The use of the term "completed week" is also confusing. Completed weeks of gestation are defined by the number of 7-day intervals after the first day of the last menstrual period (Table 1).[5,20] For example, the end of the 37th completed week of gestation is 36⁶/₇ weeks' gestation, because 37 seven-day intervals (259 days) have transpired. To further clarify, the end of the 37th completed week is not 37⁶/₇ weeks' gestation; the beginning of the 38th week of gestation is designated as 37⁰/₇ weeks' gestation (260 days).[5,20]

A variety of terms have been used to describe preterm infants born at a number of different intervals between 32 and 37 weeks' gestation ("late preterm," "near term," "marginally preterm," "moderately preterm," "minimally preterm," and "mildly preterm").[2,6,12,21] In contrast, preterm, term, and postterm are mutually exclusive categories that have each been defined precisely according to week and day of gestation (counting the first day as day 1) by the American Academy of Pediatrics, the American College of Obstetricians and Gynecologists, and the World Health Organization (Fig 1).[18,19] As previously described, "preterm" is defined as a birth that occurs on or before the end of the last day of the 37th week (259th day) after the onset of the mother's last menstrual period. "Term" is defined as a birth that occurs on the first day (260th day) of the 38th week through the end of the last day of the 42nd week (294th day) after the onset of the last menstrual period (Table 1). "Postterm" describes the birth of an infant that occurs on or after the first day (295th day) of the 43rd week after the onset of the last menstrual period.

The 2005 workshop "Optimizing Care and Outcome of the Near-Term Pregnancy and the Near-Term Newborn Infant" sponsored by the National Institutes of Health recommended that infants born at 34⁰/₇ through 36⁶/₇ weeks' gestation after the onset of the mother's last menstrual period be referred to as late preterm to emphasize that these infants are preterm and, as such, are at risk of immaturity-related medical complications (Tables 2 and 3).[5] Furthermore, use of the term "near term," which connotes that the infant is almost term and,

TABLE 2   Late-Preterm Infants and the Most Frequent Complications of Prematurity During the Birth Hospitalization

Outcome During Initial Birth Hospitalization	Late-Preterm Morbidity		Term Morbidity		OR (95% CI)	P
	No.	%	No.	%		
Feeding difficulties						
Wang et al[2] (35–36⁶/₇ wk)	29	32.2	7	7.4	—	—
Hypoglycemia						
Wang et al[2] (35–36⁶/₇ wk)	14	15.6	5	5.3	3.30 (1.1–12.2)	.028
Jaundice						
Wang et al[2] (35–36⁶/₇ wk)	49	54.4	36	37.9	1.95 (1.04–3.67)	.027
Temperature instability						
Wang et al[2] (35–36⁶/₇ wk)	9	10.0	0	0.0	Infinite	.0012
Apnea						
Henderson-Smart[38] (34–35⁶/₇ wk)	—	7.0	—	<0.1	—	—
Merchant et al[42] (35–36⁶/₇ wk)	6	12.0	0	0.0	12.0 (4.5–24.3)	.0267
Wang et al[2] (35–36⁶/₇ wk)	4	4.0	0	0.0		.054
Respiratory distress						
Escobar et al[24] (34–36⁶/₇ wk)	345	10.7	975	2.7	—	—
Gilbert et al[70] (34–36⁶/₇ wk)	1167	3.6	843	0.8	—	—
Rubaltelli et al[33] (34–36⁶/₇ wk)	314	9.6	359	0.6	—	—
Wang et al[2] (35–36⁶/₇ wk)	26	28.9	4	4.2	9.14 (2.9–37.8)	.00001
Received intravenous infusion						
Wang et al[2] (35–36⁶/₇ wk)	24	26.7	5	5.3	6.48 (2.3–22.9)	.0007
Underwent sepsis evaluation						
Wang et al[2] (35–36⁶/₇ wk)	33	36.7	12	12.6	3.97 (1.8–9.2)	.00015
Received mechanical ventilation						
Gilbert et al[70] (34–36⁶/₇ wk)	1103	3.4	950	0.9	—	—

OR indicates odds ratio; CI, confidence interval; —, data not reported.

therefore, almost fully mature, should be discouraged, because it might lead health care professionals to underestimate the inherent risks to these infants.[5,20]

Workshop members acknowledged that the definition of "late preterm" was arbitrary.[5] The day after the end of the 34th completed week of gestation (ie, 239th day or 34⁰/₇ weeks' gestation after the onset of the mother's last menstrual period) was recommended as the lower limit, because it is frequently used as a cutoff point for obstetric decision-making, as a criterion for admission to a level 2 or 3 NICU, and for epidemiologic and clinical research. The upper limit of gestational age for prematurity was previously established as 36⁶/₇ weeks' gestation (259th day after the onset of the mother's last menstrual period). Thus, it was recommended that this same upper limit be applied to the late-preterm category of infants.

DEVELOPMENTAL AND PHYSIOLOGIC IMMATURITY OF LATE-PRETERM INFANTS

Late-preterm infants have not been studied frequently, and understanding of the developmental biology and mechanisms of disease experienced by these infants is largely incomplete.[2,5,7,8,22–30] Management strategies, therefore, are based on general principles, clinical experience, and extrapolation from knowledge of very preterm and term infants. Recently, descriptive studies that detailed the epidemiology, medical problems, and risk of

mortality experienced by late-preterm infants have stimulated interest in exploring the comparative biology and basic mechanisms of disease in these infants.[2–8] Several important factors that may predispose late-preterm infants to medical conditions associated with immaturity, such as respiratory distress, apnea, temperature instability, hypoglycemia, hyperbilirubinemia, and poor feeding, are reviewed briefly in this report. However, a comprehensive review of the physiologic and functional deficits that predispose late-preterm infants to these conditions is beyond the scope of this report.[5]

After birth, infants with fetal lung structure and immature functional capacity are at greatest risk of respiratory distress, need for oxygen and positive-pressure ventilation, and admission for intensive care.[2,31–33] From 34⁰/₇ through 36⁶/₇ weeks' gestation, terminal respiratory units of the lung evolve from alveolar saccules lined with both cuboidal type II and flat type I epithelial cells (terminal sac period) to mature alveoli lined primarily with extremely thin type I epithelial cells (alveolar period).[34,35] During the alveolar period, pulmonary capillaries also begin to bulge into the space of each terminal sac, and adult pool sizes of surfactant are attained.[36] Functionally, this immature lung structure may be associated with delayed intrapulmonary fluid absorption, surfactant insufficiency, and inefficient gas exchange.[24,25]

Apnea occurs more frequently among late-preterm infants than term infants. The incidence of apnea in

TABLE 3 Late-Preterm Infants and Rates of Readmission to the Hospital After the Birth Hospitalization

Description of Comparison Groups by Study	Readmitted to Hospital[a]		Required Hospital Care[b]		Adjusted OR (95% CI)
	No.	%	No.	%	
All NICU survivors from 6 Kaiser Permanente hospitals, N = 6054 (Escobar et al[66])					
<33 wk, all LOS	20	3.4	—	—	1.88 (1.10–3.21)
33–36 wk, LOS < 96 h	31	5.7	—	—	2.94 (1.87–4.62)
33–36 wk, LOS ≥ 96 h	26	2.2	—	—	1.13 (0.69–1.84)
Term, LOS ≥ 96 h	32	2.8	—	—	1.31 (0.83–2.05)
Term, LOS < 96 h	56	2.2	—	—	Reference
One half of all births >34 wk born in UK northern region, N = 11406 (Oddie et al[4])					
35–37 wk	37	6.3	—	—	1.72 (1.15–2.57)
>40 wk	57	2.4	—	—	0.70 (0.51–0.95)
38–40 wk	178	3.4	—	—	Reference
All newborns surviving to discharge at 7 Kaiser Permanente hospitals, N = 33 276 (Escobar et al[3])					
<34 wk (100% in NICU)	26	3.0	—	—	0.96 (0.57–1.62)
34–36 wk, in NICU ≥ 24 h					0.89 (0.54–1.46)
34–36 wk, in NICU < 24 h					1.31 (0.41–4.21)
34–36 wk, never in NICU					3.10 (2.38–4.02)
All 34- to 36-wk infants	94	4.4	—	—	
≥37 wk, in NICU ≥ 24 h					0.79 (0.52–1.21)
≥37 wk, in NICU < 24 h					1.43 (0.73–2.81)
≥37 wk, never in NICU					Reference
All ≥37-wk infants	618	2.0	—	—	
All Massachusetts newborns discharged early after vaginal delivery, N = 25 324 (Tomashek et al[8])					
34–36 wk	35	3.5	—	—	1.8 (1.3, 2.5)[c]
37–41 wk	489	2.0	—	—	Reference
34–36 wk	—	—	43	4.3	1.5 (1.1, 2.0)[c]
37–41 wk	—	—	648	2.7	Reference

OR, odds ratio; CI, confidence interval; LOS, length of stay; UK, United Kingdom; —, data not reported.

[a] Readmitted to hospital within 2 weeks after birth hospitalization discharge (Escobar et al[3,66]) and within first 28 days of life (Oddie et al[4] and Tomashek et al[8]).

[b] Required hospital care includes hospital inpatient readmission and observational stay visit during neonatal period.

[c] Shown are relative risks with confidence limits.

late-preterm infants is reported to be between 4% and 7%,[28,31,37,38] compared with less than 1% to 2% at term.[38,39] It is notable that the frequency of apneic events at term was determined by using data from cardiopulmonary monitoring of healthy infants in their homes. Apneic events were inapparent to caregivers and resolved spontaneously. The predisposition to apnea in late-preterm infants is associated with several underlying factors including increased susceptibility to hypoxic respiratory depression, decreased central chemosensitivity to carbon dioxide, immature pulmonary irritant receptors, increased respiratory inhibition sensitivity to laryngeal stimulation, and decreased upper airway dilator muscle tone.[31,38,40–42] It is also suspected that late-preterm infants may be at higher risk of centrally mediated apnea, because their central nervous systems are developmentally immature (ie, fewer sulci and gyri, less myelin) and their brains are approximately two thirds the size of a term infant's brain.[30]

Little is known about cardiovascular physiology and pathobiology in late-preterm infants; it is generally believed that structural and functional immaturity restricts the amount of cardiovascular reserve that is available during times of stress.[43,44] Immature cardiovascular function also may complicate recovery of the late-preterm infant with respiratory distress because of delayed ductus arteriosus closure and persistent pulmonary hypertension.[45]

An infant's response to cold exposure after birth is related to gestational age and is affected by the physical size, the amount of mature brown and white adipose tissue, and maturity of the hypothalamus.[46–48] Brown-fat accumulation and maturation and concentrations of hormones responsible for brown-fat metabolism (eg, prolactin, leptin, norepinephrine, triiodothyronine, cortisol) peak at term.[49,50] Thus, late-preterm infants have less white adipose tissue for insulation, and they cannot generate heat from brown adipose tissue as effectively as infants born at term. In addition, late-preterm infants are likely to lose heat more readily than term infants, because they have a larger ratio of surface area to weight and are smaller in size.

Hypoglycemia may affect fasting newborn infants of all gestational ages because of insufficient metabolic responses to the abrupt loss of the maternal glucose supply after birth.[51-55] The incidence of hypoglycemia is inversely proportional to gestational age. Within the first 12 to 24 hours after birth, concentrations of enzymes that are essential for hepatic gluconeogenesis and hepatic ketogenesis rapidly increase. Thereafter, hypoglycemia typically resolves. Preterm infants are at increased risk of developing hypoglycemia after birth, because they have immature hepatic glycogenolysis and adipose tissue lipolysis, hormonal dysregulation, and deficient hepatic gluconeogenesis and ketogenesis. Blood glucose concentrations among preterm infants typically decrease to a nadir 1 to 2 hours after birth and remain low until metabolic pathways can compensate or exogenous sources of glucose are provided.[51,54] Carbohydrate metabolism among late-preterm infants is not well understood. However, immature glucose regulation likely occurs in late-preterm infants, because hypoglycemia that requires glucose infusion during the initial birth hospitalization occurs more frequently than in term infants.[2]

Jaundice and hyperbilirubinemia occur more commonly and are more prolonged among late-preterm infants than term infants, because late-preterm infants have delayed maturation and a lower concentration of uridine diphosphoglucuronate glucuronosyltransferase.[21,56] Late-preterm infants are 2 times more likely than term infants to have significantly elevated bilirubin concentrations and higher concentrations 5 and 7 days after birth.[21]

Late-preterm infants also have immature gastrointestinal function[57,58] and feeding difficulties that predispose them to an increase in enterohepatic circulation, decreased stool frequency, dehydration, and hyperbilirubinemia.[59-68] Feeding during the birth hospitalization may be transiently successful but not sustained after discharge. Feeding difficulties in late-preterm infants that are associated with relatively low oromotor tone, function, and neural maturation also predispose these infants to dehydration and hyperbilirubinemia.[30,67-69]

MORBIDITY AND MORTALITY AMONG LATE-PRETERM INFANTS

Late-preterm infants are at increased risk of neonatal morbidity compared with term infants. During the initial birth hospitalization, late-preterm infants are 4 times more likely than term infants to have at least 1 medical condition diagnosed and 3.5 times more likely to have 2 or more conditions diagnosed.[2] Late-preterm infants are more likely than term infants to be diagnosed during the birth hospitalization with temperature instability,[2] hypoglycemia,[2] respiratory distress,[2,24,33,70,71] apnea,[38,42] jaundice,[2] and feeding difficulties[2] (Table 2). During the first

month after birth, late-preterm infants are also more likely than term infants to develop hyperbilirubinemia[21,60,72,73] and to be readmitted for hyperbilirubinemia[3,59,64] and non–jaundice-related diagnoses such as feeding difficulties and "rule-out sepsis."[3]

Some of the reported increase in morbidity among late-preterm infants may be attributable to observation and detection bias, because a clinician's threshold to monitor late-preterm infants for medical complications may be lower than their threshold for term infants. For example, a hospital-based study found that late-preterm infants were evaluated for possible sepsis 3 times as often as term infants, and the majority of evaluated late-preterm infants received antibiotic treatment, whereas term infants did not.[2] However, studies have also found that late-preterm infants are at increased risk of developing more severe illness than term infants.[2,24,70] One study of all California singleton live births who survived to 1 year of age found that infants born at 34 to 36 weeks' gestation were 3 to 9 times more likely to require mechanical ventilation than infants born at 38 weeks' gestation.[70] Late-preterm infants are also more likely than term infants to have longer initial hospital stays and to be admitted to the NICU.[2,3,33,70] One large cohort study found that 88% of infants born at 34 weeks' gestation, 54% of infants born at 35 weeks' gestation, 25% of infants born at 36 weeks' gestation, 12% of infants born at 37 weeks' gestation, and 2.6% of infants born at 38 through 40 weeks' gestation were admitted to a NICU.[3]

Severity of illness is also reflected in the increased risk of mortality among late-preterm infants compared with term infants in the United States.[6,10] In 2002, the neonatal mortality rate (deaths among infants 0–27 days' chronologic age) for late-preterm infants was 4.6 times higher than the rate for term infants (4.1 vs 0.9 per 1000 live births, respectively). This difference in neonatal mortality has widened slightly since 1995, when there was a fourfold difference in rates between late-preterm and term infants (4.8 vs 1.2 per 1000 live births, respectively). The infant mortality rate was also higher among late-preterm infants than term infants in 2002 (7.7 vs 2.5 per 1000 live births, respectively). This threefold difference has remained relatively constant since 1995, at which time the infant mortality rate was 9.3 per 1000 live births among late-preterm infants and 3.1 per 1000 live births among term infants.

Several case-control studies designed to evaluate risk factors for neonatal hospital readmission after the birth hospitalization have identified late-preterm birth as a significant risk factor.[62,63,65,68,74] Studies that compared neonatal hospital readmission rates among late-preterm infants and other groups of infants, including term infants, have found that late-preterm infants are more likely to be readmitted than are term infants (Table 3).[3,4,8,24,59] A large study in the United Kingdom found that infants born at 35 through 37 weeks' gestation were

1.7 times more likely to be readmitted during the neonatal period than were infants born at 38 through 40 weeks' gestation (adjusted odds ratio: 1.7; 95% confidence interval: 1.2–2.6).[4] A retrospective cohort study of all newborn infants who survived to discharge at 7 hospitals within a large managed care organization found that 4.4% of all late-preterm infants were readmitted within 2 weeks after the birth hospitalization, compared with 3.0% of infants less than 34 weeks' gestation and 2.0% of infants born at or after 37 weeks' gestation.[3] Late-preterm infants who were never admitted to the NICU were at the highest risk of rehospitalization. This study also found that having a home visit or a scheduled outpatient visit within 72 hours after discharge was associated with a decreased risk of rehospitalization. In addition, a population-based study found that late-preterm infants who were not admitted to the NICU after birth were 2 to 3 times more likely than term infants to be rehospitalized for hyperbilirubinemia.[59]

Late-preterm infants with short NICU stays may be at increased risk of hospital readmission after the birth hospitalization compared with all other NICU survivors. A study that assessed outcomes among all newborn infants discharged alive from 6 NICUs within a large managed care organization found that preterm infants of 33 to 36 weeks' gestation with a hospital stay of less than 4 days had higher hospital readmission rates than all other groups, including the most preterm group.[66] The reason for readmission for the majority of these late-preterm infants was jaundice (71%), followed by suspected sepsis (20%) and feeding difficulties (16%).

Late-preterm infants who are discharged early (<2-night hospital stay) from the hospital after a vaginal delivery may be at increased risk of neonatal morbidity compared with term infants who are discharged early.[8] A population-based study that compared rates of postdischarge neonatal morbidity between singleton late-preterm and term infants who were discharged early found that 4.3% and 2.7% of infants, respectively, were either readmitted or had an observational stay; 3.5% and 2.0%, respectively, were readmitted. Jaundice and infection accounted for 77.1% of readmissions among late-preterm infants and 60.3% of readmissions among term infants. In this study, breastfed late-preterm infants were 1.8 times more likely to require hospital-related care and 2.2 times more likely to be readmitted than breastfed term infants. In contrast, there was no difference in need for subsequent hospital-related care or readmission between nonbreastfed late-preterm and term infants.

Several factors have been identified to be associated with an increased risk of hospital readmission, an observational hospital stay, or severe morbidity among late-preterm infants. A population-based cohort study of healthy, singleton late-preterm infants delivered vaginally in Massachusetts hospitals between 1998 and 2002 found that 6.1% received hospital care after the birth hospitalization or died during the neonatal period.[7] Risk factors for requiring hospital care or experiencing morbidity included being the first born, being breastfed at discharge, having a mother who had labor and delivery complications, being a recipient of public insurance at delivery, or being of Asian/Pacific Island descent.[7,9]

Although it is known that late-preterm infants are at increased risk compared with term infants for infant mortality, morbidity during the initial birth hospitalization, and neonatal morbidity that requires hospital readmission, the long-term health consequences of being born late preterm are not yet known.[75] Small clinical reports that compared late-preterm infants with term infants suggested a higher risk of cerebral palsy,[76] speech disorders,[77,78] neurodevelopmental handicaps,[78] behavioral abnormalities,[79] and competence (behavioral, scholastic, social, and global).[75,79–81] Given that late-preterm infants are born before their nervous systems have fully developed, large population studies that evaluate long-term neurodevelopmental and behavioral outcomes of these children are needed.[75]

The emotional, personal, and financial costs to individuals, family, and society associated with late-preterm births have not been sufficiently described.[82] A conservative estimate for the long-term medical, educational, and productivity costs associated with the birth of all infants before 37 weeks' gestation is approximately $51 600 for each infant or a total cost of $26.2 billion in 2005 dollars. Individual late-preterm infants, on average, require fewer financial and other resources than infants who are born more preterm. However, the total resources and costs associated with late-preterm birth are likely to be a relatively substantial part of the total cost of all preterm births, because the population of late-preterm infants is significantly larger than the population of infants who are born before 34 weeks' gestation.

Collaborative counseling by neonatal and obstetric clinicians about fetal, neonatal, and maternal outcomes is warranted when maternal or fetal conditions indicate the necessity for late-preterm birth. The obstetric clinician can discuss the indications for the delivery and the risks inherent in delaying delivery. The neonatal clinician can provide the family with gestational age-specific outcome information and help prepare the family for the newborn infant's anticipated course in the nursery. Collaborative counseling allows the family to be fully informed and to participate in decision-making. Under emergent conditions, the time to provide such counseling may not exist.

SUMMARY

1. Late-preterm infants are immature.

    a. Infants born at 34 $^{0/7}$ through 36 $^{6/7}$ weeks' gestation (239–259 days since the first day of the last

8. A feeding plan has been developed and is understood by the family.[86]

9. A risk assessment for the development of severe hyperbilirubinemia has been performed and appropriate follow-up has been arranged.[88]

10. Physical examinations of the infant reveal no abnormalities that require continued hospitalization.[85]

11. There is no evidence of active bleeding at the circumcision site for at least 2 hours.[85]

12. Maternal and infant test results are available and have been reviewed, including blood test results for maternal syphilis and hepatitis B surface-antigen status; cord or infant blood type and direct Coombs test results, as clinically indicated; and results of screenings performed in accordance with state regulations, including screening for HIV infection.[85,92]

13. Initial hepatitis B vaccine has been administered or an appointment has been scheduled for its administration, and the importance of immunizations has been stressed.[85]

14. Metabolic and genetic screenings have been performed in accordance with state requirements. If a newborn screening is performed before 24 hours of milk feeding, a system for repeating the screening must be in place in accordance with state policy.[93]

15. A car safety seat study completed by a trained professional to observe for apnea, bradycardia, or oxygen desaturation has been passed.[94]

16. Hearing assessment has been performed and the results have been documented in the medical chart. Results have been discussed with family or caregivers. If follow-up is needed, follow-up plans have been outlined.[95]

17. Family, environmental, and social risk factors have been assessed. When risk factors are identified, the discharge should be delayed until they are resolved or a plan to safeguard the infant is in place. Such risk factors may include but are not limited to:

    a. untreated parental substance use or positive toxicology test results in the mother or newborn infant;

    b. history of child abuse or neglect;

    c. mental illness in a parent in the home;

    d. lack of social support, particularly for single, first-time mothers;

    e. homelessness, particularly during this pregnancy;

    f. ongoing or established risk of domestic violence; or

    g. adolescent mother, particularly if other risk factors are present.[85]

18. The mother and caregivers have received information or training or have demonstrated competency in the following:

    a. infant's hospital course and current condition;

    b. expected pattern of urine and stool frequency for the breastfeeding or formula-fed neonate (verbal and written instruction is recommended);

    c. umbilical cord, skin, and newborn genital care;

    d. hand hygiene, especially as a means to reduce the risk of infection;

    e. use of a thermometer to assess an infant's axillary temperature;

    f. assessment and provision of appropriate layers of clothing;

    g. identification of common signs and symptoms of illness, such as hyperbilirubinemia, sepsis, and dehydration;

    h. assessment for jaundice;

    i. provision of a safe sleep environment, including positioning the infant on his or her back during sleep[96];

    j. newborn safety issues including car safety seat use, need for smoke/fire alarms, and hazards of secondhand tobacco smoke and environmental pollutants;

    k. appropriate responses to a complication or an emergency; and

    l. sibling interactions and appropriate inclusion in care responsibilities.

COMMITTEE ON FETUS AND NEWBORN, 2006–2007
Ann R. Stark, MD, Chairperson
David H. Adamkin, MD
Daniel G. Batton, MD
Edward F. Bell, MD
Vinod K. Bhutani, MD
Susan E. Denson, MD
Gilbert I. Martin, MD
Kristi L. Watterberg, MD
William Engle, MD

LIAISONS
Keith J. Barrington, MD
    Canadian Paediatric Society
Gary D. V. Hankins, MD
    American College of Obstetricians and Gynecologists
Tonse N. K. Raju, MD
    National Institutes of Health
Kay M. Tomashek, MD
    Centers for Disease Control and Prevention

Carol Wallman, MSN
National Association of Neonatal Nurses and
Association of Women's Health, Obstetric and
Neonatal Nurses

STAFF

Jim Couto, MA

REFERENCES

1. Stark AR; American Academy of Pediatrics, Committee on Fetus and Newborn. Levels of neonatal care [published correction appears in *Pediatrics*. 2005;115:1118]. *Pediatrics*. 2004;114: 1341–1347

2. Wang ML, Dorer DJ, Fleming MP, Catlin EA. Clinical outcomes of near-term infants. *Pediatrics*. 2004;114:372–376

3. Escobar GJ, Greene JD, Hulac P, et al. Rehospitalisation after birth hospitalisation: patterns among infants of all gestations. *Arch Dis Child*. 2005;90:125–131

4. Oddie SJ, Hammal D, Richmond S, Parker L. Early discharge and readmission to hospital in the first month of life in the Northern Region of the UK during 1998: a case cohort study. *Arch Dis Child*. 2005;90:119–124

5. Raju TN, Higgins RD, Stark AR, Leveno KJ. Optimizing care and outcome for late-preterm (near-term) gestations and for late-preterm infants: a summary of the workshop sponsored by the National Institutes of Health and Human Development. *Pediatrics*. 2006;118:1207–1214

6. Kramer MS, Demissie K, Yang H, Platt RW, Sauvé R, Liston R. The contribution of mild and moderate preterm birth to infant mortality. Fetal and Infant Health Study Group of the Canadian Perinatal Surveillance System. *JAMA*. 2000;284:843–849

7. Shapiro-Mendoza CK, Tomashek KM, Kotelchuck M, Barfield W, Weiss J, Evans S. Risk factors for neonatal morbidity and mortality among "healthy" late preterm newborns. *Semin Perinatol*. 2006;30:54–60

8. Tomashek KM, Shapiro-Mendoza CK, Weiss J, et al. Early discharge among late preterm and term newborns and risk of neonatal mortality. *Semin Perinatol*. 2006;30:61–68

9. Paul IM, Lehman EB, Hollenbeak CS, Maisels MJ. Preventable newborn readmissions since passage of the Newborns' and Mothers' Health Protection Act. *Pediatrics*. 2006;118:2349–2358

10. Martin JA, Hamilton BE, Sutton PD, Ventura SJ, Menacker F, Munson ML. Births: final data for 2003. *Natl Vital Stat Rep*. 2005;54(2):1–116

11. Davidoff MJ, Dias T, Damus K, et al. Changes in the gestational age distribution among U.S. singleton births: impact on rates of late preterm birth, 1992–2002 [published correction appears in *Semin Perinatol*. 2006;30:313]. *Semin Perinatol*. 2006;30:8–15

12. Martin JA, Park MM. Trends in twin and triplet births: 1980–97. *Natl Vital Stat Rep*. 1999;47(24):1–16

13. Joseph KS, Allen AC, Dodds L, Vincer MJ, Armson BA. Causes and consequences of recent increases in preterm birth among twins. *Obstet Gynecol*. 2001;98:57–64

14. Hankins GD, Longo M. The role of stillbirth prevention and late preterm (near-term) births. *Semin Perinatol*. 2006;30:20–23

15. Sibai BM. Preeclampsia as a cause of preterm and late preterm (near-term) births. *Semin Perinatol*. 2006;30:16–19

16. Moutquin JM. Classification and heterogeneity of preterm birth. *BJOG*. 2003;110:30–33

17. Linhart Y, Bashiri A, Maymon E, et al. Congenital anomalies are an independent risk factor for neonatal morbidity and perinatal mortality in preterm birth. *Eur J Obstet Gynecol Reprod Biol*. 2000;90:43–49

18. American Academy of Pediatrics; American College of Obste-

tricians and Gynecologists. *Guidelines for Perinatal Care*. Gilstrap LC, Oh W, eds. 5th ed. Elk Grove Village, IL: American Academy of Pediatrics; American College of Obstetricians and Gynecologists; 2002

19. World Health Organization. Sexual and reproductive health. Available at: www.who.int/reproductive-health. Accessed June 1, 2005

20. Engle WA. A recommendation for the definition of "late-preterm" (near-term) and the birth weight-gestational age classification system. *Semin Perinatol*. 2006;30:2–7

21. Sarici SU, Serdar MA, Korkmaz A, et al. Incidence, course, and prediction of hyperbilirubinemia in near-term and term newborns. *Pediatrics*. 2004;113:775–780

22. Seubert DE, Stetzer BP, Wolfe HM, Treadwell MC. Delivery of the marginally preterm infant: what are the minor morbidities? *Am J Obstet Gynecol*. 1999;181:1087–1091

23. Laptook A, Jackson GL. Cold stress and hypoglycemia in the late preterm ("near-term") infant: impact on nursery of admission. *Semin Perinatol*. 2006;30:24–27

24. Escobar GJ, Clark RH, Greene JD. Short-term outcomes of infants born at 35 and 36 weeks gestation: we need to ask more questions. *Semin Perinatol*. 2006;30:28–33

25. Jain L, Eaton DC. Physiology of fetal lung fluid clearance and the effect of labor. *Semin Perinatol*. 2006;30:34–43

26. Ward RM. Drug disposition in the late preterm ("near-term") newborn. *Semin Perinatol*. 2006;30:48–51

27. Clapp DW. Developmental regulation of the immune system. *Semin Perinatol*. 2006;30:69–72

28. Hunt CE. Ontogeny of autonomic regulation in late preterm infants born at 34–37 weeks postmenstrual age. *Semin Perinatol*. 2006;30:73–76

29. Neu J. Gastrointestinal maturation and feeding. *Semin Perinatol*. 2006;30:77–80

30. Kinney HC. The near-term (late pre-term) human brain and risk for periventricular leukomalacia: a review. *Semin Perinatol*. 2006;30:81–88

31. Arnon, S, Dolfin T, Litmanovitz I, Regev R, Bauer S, Fejgin M. Preterm labour at 34–36 weeks of gestation: should it be arrested? *Paediatr Perinat Epidemiol*. 2001;15:252–256

32. Avery ME, Mead J. Surface properties in relation to atelectasis and hyaline membrane disease. *AMA J Dis Child*. 1959;97: 517–523

33. Rubaltelli FF, Bonafe L, Tangucci M, Spagnolo A, Dani C. Epidemiology of neonatal acute respiratory disorders. *Biol Neonate*. 1998;74:7–15

34. Jobe AH. The respiratory system. Part 1: lung development and maturation. In: Martin RJ, Fanaroff AA, Walsh MC, eds. *Fanaroff and Martin's Neonatal-Perinatal Medicine*. 8th ed. Philadelphia, PA: Mosby Elsevier; 2006:1069–1194

35. Post M. Lung development: pulmonary structure and function. In: Gluckman PD, Heymann MA, eds. *Pediatrics and Perinatology: The Scientific Basis*. 2nd ed. New York, NY: Oxford University Press; 1996:797–800

36. Hawgood S. Alveolar region: pulmonary structure and function. In: Gluckman PD, Heymann MA, eds. *Pediatrics and Perinatology: The Scientific Basis*. 2nd ed. New York, NY: Oxford University Press; 1996:814–819

37. Henderson-Smart DJ, Pettigrew AG, Campbell DJ. Clinical apnea and brain-stem neural function in preterm infants. *N Engl J Med*. 1983;308:353–357

38. Henderson-Smart DJ. The effect of gestational age on the incidence and duration of recurrent apnoea in newborn babies. *Aust Paediatr J*. 1981;17:273–276

39. Ramanathan R, Corwin MJ, Hunt CE, et al. Cardiorespiratory events recorded on home monitors: comparison of healthy infants with those at increased risk for SIDS. *JAMA*. 2001;285: 2199–2207

40. Curzi-Dascalova L, Christova-Gueorguieva E. Respiratory pauses in normal prematurely born infants: a comparison with full-term newborns. *Biol Neonate.* 1983;44:325–332

41. Miller MJ, Fanaroff AA, Martin RJ. The respiratory system. Part 5: respiratory disorders in preterm and term infants. In: Martin RJ, Fanaroff AA, Walsh MC, eds. *Fanaroff and Martin's Neonatal-Perinatal Medicine.* 8th ed. Philadelphia, PA: Mosby Elsevier; 2006:1122–1146

42. Merchant JR, Worwa C, Porter S, Coleman JM, deRegnier RA. Respiratory instability of term and near-term healthy newborn infants in car safety seats. *Pediatrics.* 2001;108:647–652

43. Lee LA, Kimball TR, Daniels SR, Khoury P, Meyer RA. Left ventricular mechanics in the preterm infant and their effect on the measurement of cardiac performance. *J Pediatr.* 1992;120:114–119

44. Zahka KG. The cardiovascular system. Part 4: principles of neonatal cardiovascular hemodynamics. In: Martin RJ, Fanaroff AA, Walsh MC, eds. *Fanaroff and Martin's Neonatal-Perinatal Medicine.* 8th ed. Philadelphia, PA: Mosby Elsevier; 2006:1211–1215

45. Randala M, Eronen M, Andersson S, Pohjavuori M, Pesonen E. Pulmonary artery pressure in term and preterm neonates. *Acta Paediatr.* 1996;85:1344–1347

46. Hammarlund K, Sedin G. Transepidermal water loss in newborn infants. VI. Heat exchange with the environment in relation to gestational age. *Acta Paediatr Scand.* 1982;71:191–196

47. Sinclair JC. Management of the thermal environment. In: Sinclair JC, Bracken MB, eds. *Effective Care of the Newborn Infants.* New York, NY: Oxford University Press; 1992:40–58

48. Sedin G. Physical environment. Part 1: the thermal environment of the newborn infant. In: Martin RJ, Fanaroff AA, Walsh MC, eds. *Fanaroff and Martin's Neonatal-Perinatal Medicine.* 8th ed. Philadelphia, PA: Mosby Elsevier; 2006:585–597

49. Stephenson T, Budge H, Mostyn A, Pearce S, Webb R, Symonds ME. Fetal and neonatal adipose tissue maturation: a primary site of cytokine and cytokine-receptor action. *Biochem Soc Trans.* 2001;29:80–85

50. Symonds ME, Mostyn A, Pearce S, Budge H, Stephenson T. Endocrine and nutritional regulation of fetal adipose tissue development. *J Endocrinol.* 2003;179:293–299

51. Stanley CA, Pallotto EK. Disorders of carbohydrate metabolism. In: Taeusch HW, Ballard RA, Gleason CA, eds. *Avery's Diseases of the Newborn.* 8th ed. Philadelphia, PA: Elsevier Saunders; 2005:1410–1422

52. Cornblath M, Ichord R. Hypoglycemia in the neonate. *Semin Perinatol.* 2000;24:136–149

53. Ward Platt M, Deshpande S. Metabolic adaptation at birth. *Semin Fetal Neonatal Med.* 2005;10:341–350

54. Kalhan SC, Parimi PS. Metabolic and endocrine disorders. Part 1: disorders of carbohydrate metabolism. In: Martin RJ, Fanaroff AA, Walsh MC, eds. *Fanaroff and Martin's Neonatal-Perinatal Medicine.* 8th ed. Philadelphia, PA: Mosby Elsevier; 2006:1467–1491

55. Canadian Paediatric Society, Fetus and Newborn Committee. Screening guidelines for newborns at risk for low blood glucose. *Paediatr Child Health.* 2004;9:723–729

56. Kawade N, Onishi S. The prenatal and postnatal development of UDP-glucuronyltransferase activity towards bilirubin and the effect of premature birth on this activity in the human liver. *Biochem J.* 1981;196:257–260

57. Beserth CL. Developmental anatomy and physiology of the gastrointestinal tract. In: Taeusch HW, Ballard RA, Gleason CA, eds. *Avery's Diseases of the Newborn.* 8th ed. Philadelphia, PA: Elsevier Saunders; 2005:1071–1085

58. al Tawil Y, Berseth CL. Gestational and postnatal maturation of duodenal motor responses to intragastic feeding. *J Pediatr.* 1996;129:374–381

59. Bhutani VK, Johnson LH, Maisels MJ, et al. Kernicterus: epidemiological strategies for its prevention through systems-based approaches. *J Perinatol.* 2004;24:650–662

60. Newman TB, Escobar GJ, Gonzales VM, Armstrong MA, Gardner MN, Folck BF. Frequency of neonatal bilirubin testing and hyperbilirubinemia in a large health maintenance organization [published correction appears in *Pediatrics.* 2001;1:126]. *Pediatrics.* 1999;104:1198–1203

61. Hall RT, Simon S, Smith MT. Readmission of breastfed infants in the first 2 weeks of life. *J Perinatol.* 2000;20:432–437

62. Maisels MJ, Kring E. Length of stay, jaundice, and hospital readmission. *Pediatrics.* 1998;101:995–998

63. Maisels MJ, Newman TB. Jaundice in full-term and near-term babies who leave the hospital within 36 hours: the pediatrician's nemesis. *Clin Perinatol.* 1998;25:295–302

64. Brown AK, Damus K, Kim MH, et al. Factors relating to readmission of term and near-term neonates in the first two weeks of life. Early Discharge Survey Group of the Health Professional Advisory Board of the Greater New York Chapter of the March of Dimes. *J Perinat Med.* 1999;27:263–275

65. Soskolne EI, Schumacker R, Fyock C, Young ML, Schork A. The effect of early discharge and other factors on readmission rates of newborns. *Arch Pediatr Adolesc Med.* 1996;150:373–379

66. Escobar GJ, Joffe S, Gardner MN, Armstrong MA, Folck BF, Carpenter DM. Rehospitalization in the first two weeks after discharge from the neonatal intensive care unit. *Pediatrics.* 1999;104(1). Available at: www.pediatrics.org/cgi/content/full/104/1/e2

67. Johnson D, Jin Y, Truman C. Early discharge of Alberta mothers post-delivery and the relationship to potentially preventable newborn readmissions. *Can J Public Health.* 2002;93:276–280

68. Geiger AM, Petitti DB, Yao JF. Rehospitalisation for neonatal jaundice: risk factors and outcomes. *Paediatr Perinat Epidemiol.* 2001;15:352–358

69. Escobar GJ, Gonzales V, Armstrong MA, Folck B, Xiong B, Newman TB. Rehospitalization for neonatal dehydration: a nested case-control study. *Arch Pediatr Adolesc Med.* 2002;156:155–161

70. Gilbert WM, Nesbitt TS, Danielsen B. The cost of prematurity: quantification by gestational age and birth weight. *Obstet Gynecol.* 2003;102:488–492

71. Dani C, Reali MF, Bertini G, Wiechmann L, et al. Risk factors for the development of respiratory distress syndrome and transient tachypnoea in newborn infants. Italian Group of Neonatal Pulmonology. *Eur Respir J.* 1999;14:155–159

72. Newman TB, Liljestrand P, Escobar GJ. Infants with bilirubin levels of 30 mg/dL or more in a large managed care organization. *Pediatrics.* 2003;111:1303–1311

73. Chou SC, Palmer RH, Ezhuthachan S, et al. Management of hyperbilirubinemia in newborns: measuring performance by using a benchmarking model. *Pediatrics.* 2003;112:1264–1273

74. Grupp-Phelan J, Taylor JA, Liu LL, Davis RL. Early newborn hospital discharge and readmission for mild and severe jaundice. *Arch Pediatr Adolesc Med.* 1999;153:1283–1288

75. Adams-Chapman I. Neurodevelopmental outcome of the late preterm infant. *Clin Perinatol.* 2006;33:947–964

76. Himmelmann K, Hagberg G, Beckung E, Hagberg B, Uvebrant P. The changing panorama of cerebral palsy in Sweden. IX. Prevalence and origin in the birth-year period 1995–1998. *Acta Paediatr.* 2005;94:287–294

77. Pietz J, Peter J, Graf R, et al. Physical growth and neurodevelopmental outcome of nonhandicapped low-risk children born preterm. *Early Hum Dev.* 2004;79:131–143

78. Holmqvist P, Ragefalk C, Svenningsen NW. Low risk vaginally born preterm infants: a four year psychological and neurodevelopmental follow-up study. *J Perinat Med.* 1987;15:61–72

79. McCormick MC, Workman-Daniels K, Brooks-Gunn J. The

behavioral and emotional well-being of school-age children with different birth weights. *Pediatrics.* 1996;97:18–25

80. Huddy CL, Johnson A, Hope PL. Educational and behavioural problems in babies of 32–35 weeks gestation. *Arch Dis Child Fetal Neonatal Ed.* 2001;85:F23–F28

81. Gray RF, Indurkhya A, McCormick MC. Prevalence, stability, and predictors of clinically significant behavior problems in low birth weight children at 3, 5, and 8 years of age. *Pediatrics.* 2004;114:736–743

82. Institute of Medicine, Committee on Understanding Premature Birth and Assuring Healthy Outcomes. *Preterm Birth: Causes, Consequences, and Prevention.* Behrman RE, Butler AS, eds. Washington, DC: National Academies Press; 2007

83. American Academy of Pediatrics; American College of Obstetricians and Gynecologists. Care of the neonate. In: Gilstrap LC, Oh W, eds. *Guidelines for Perinatal Care.* 5th ed. Elk Grove Village, IL: American Academy of Pediatrics; American College of Obstetricians and Gynecologists; 2002:187–235

84. Engle WA; American Academy of Pediatrics, Committee on Fetus and Newborn. Age terminology during the perinatal period. *Pediatrics.* 2004;114:1362–1364

85. American Academy of Pediatrics, Committee on Fetus and Newborn. Hospital stay for healthy term newborns. *Pediatrics.* 2004;113:1434–1436

86. Wight NE. Breastfeeding the borderline (near-term) preterm infant. *Pediatr Ann.* 2003;32:329–336

87. Academy of Breastfeeding Medicine. Clinical protocol #10: breastfeeding the near-term infant (35 to 37 weeks gestation). Available at: www.bfmed.org/ace-files/protocol/near_term.pdf. Accessed June 4, 2007

88. American Academy of Pediatrics, Subcommittee on Hyperbilirubinemia. Management of hyperbilirubinemia in the newborn infant 35 or more weeks of gestation [published correction appears in *Pediatrics.* 2004;114:1138]. *Pediatrics.* 2004;114:297–316

89. Neifert MR. Prevention of breastfeeding tragedies. *Pediatr Clin North Am.* 2001;48:273–297

90. Gartner LM, Morton J, Lawrence RA, et al. Breastfeeding and the use of human milk. *Pediatrics.* 2005;115:496–506

91. Jensen D, Wallace S, Kelsay P. LATCH: a breastfeeding charting system and documentation tool. *J Obstet Gynecol Neonatal Nurs.* 1994;23:27–32

92. American Academy of Pediatrics; American College of Obstetricians and Gynecologists. Human immunodeficiency virus screening. *Pediatrics.* 1999;104:128

93. American Academy of Pediatrics; American College of Obstetricians and Gynecologists. Hospital discharge of the high-risk neonate: proposed guidelines. *Pediatrics.* 1998;102:411–417

94. American Academy of Pediatrics, Committee on Injury and Poison Prevention and Committee on Fetus and Newborn. Safe transportation of premature and low birth weight infants. *Pediatrics.* 1996;97:758–760

95. American Academy of Pediatrics, Task Force on Newborn and Infant Hearing. Newborn and infant hearing loss: detection and intervention. *Pediatrics.* 1999;103:527–530

96. American Academy of Pediatrics, Task Force on Sudden Infant Death Syndrome. The changing concept of sudden infant death syndrome: diagnostic coding shifts, controversies regarding the sleeping environment, and new variables to consider in reducing risks. *Pediatrics.* 2005;116:1245–1255

American Academy
of Pediatrics
DEDICATED TO THE HEALTH OF ALL CHILDREN™

POLICY STATEMENT

Noninitiation or Withdrawal of Intensive Care for High-Risk Newborns

Committee on Fetus and Newborn

Organizational Principles to Guide and Define the Child Health Care System and/or Improve the Health of All Children

ABSTRACT

Advances in medical technology have led to dilemmas in initiation and withdrawal of intensive care of newborn infants with a very poor prognosis. Physicians and parents together must make difficult decisions guided by their understanding of the child's best interest. The foundation for these decisions consists of several key elements: (1) direct and open communication between the health care team and the parents of the child with regard to the medical status, prognosis, and treatment options; (2) inclusion of the parents as active participants in the decision process; (3) continuation of comfort care even when intensive care is not being provided; and (4) treatment decisions that are guided primarily by the best interest of the child.

INTRODUCTION

As medical technology has advanced, outcomes for high-risk newborn infants have greatly improved. With advanced technology, such as assisted ventilation, it is now possible to keep some terminally or severely ill or extremely preterm infants alive for long periods of time. The result of such treatment is that dying may be prolonged or the infant may survive with profound neurologic or other debilitating problems.[1-3] The treatment of infants should be based on what is perceived to be in their best interest. Parents and health care professionals often confront difficult treatment decisions when faced with the care of a severely ill, extremely preterm, or terminally ill infant, in part because the effects of treatment decisions on the infant's outcome are not always predictable. In these circumstances, there is no ethical distinction between noninitiation and withdrawal of life-sustaining treatment.

THE TREATMENT DILEMMA

If intensive treatment uniformly resulted in survival with an acceptable quality of life for infants at risk, it would be the obvious choice for all severely ill infants. This outcome, of course, does not always occur. If intensive treatment is not provided to very ill infants, most of them will die, but some may survive with significant neurodevelopmental disability, perhaps in part because specific treatments were withheld. The following dilemma, therefore, exists: intensive treatment of all severely ill infants may result in prolongation of dying accompanied by significant discomfort for the infant or in survival with unacceptable quality of life; on the other hand, nonintensive treatment may result in increased mortality and morbidity. Either approach risks undesired and unpredictable results.

www.pediatrics.org/cgi/doi/10.1542/peds.2006-3180

doi:10.1542/peds.2006-3180

All policy statements from the American Academy of Pediatrics automatically expire 5 years after publication unless reaffirmed, revised, or retired at or before that time.

Key Words
treatment, resuscitation, withdrawal, newborn, neonate

PEDIATRICS (ISSN Numbers: Print, 0031-4005; Online, 1098-4275). Copyright © 2007 by the American Academy of Pediatrics

STRATEGY FOR CARE

For infants with poor prognosis, decisions about treatment should be made jointly by the health care team and the infant's family on the basis of the infant's physiologic maturity; the infant's medical condition, including any serious birth defects or medical complications; and the probabilities of death and severe disability based on the best available data.[4]

The types of decisions can be divided into 3 categories on the basis of prognosis[5]:

1. When early death is very likely and survival would be accompanied by high risk of unacceptably severe morbidity, intensive care is not indicated.

2. When survival is likely and risk of unacceptably severe morbidity is low, intensive care is indicated.

3. There may be cases that fall within these first 2 categories in which the prognosis is uncertain but likely to be very poor and survival may be associated with a diminished quality of life for the child; in these cases, parental desires should determine the treatment approach.

Whenever possible, discussion between the physician and parents should begin before the birth of a child with anticipated poor prognosis.[6] The obstetric care provider and the health care professional who will care for the infant after birth should collaborate in communicating with the expecting parents before the birth of the child. Such dialogue helps to ensure that appropriate care is provided for the individual infant on the basis of the infant's condition and prognosis at the time of birth. Sometimes, as when the woman is in active labor, it may seem that there is inadequate time for such a discussion. Nevertheless, it is essential that the meeting be conducted promptly and with great empathy. Follow-up meetings can take place if the situation changes over subsequent hours and days. Despite efforts to the contrary, an infant with a poor prognosis is sometimes born quickly, before the physicians can converse with the parents about the plan for treatment of the infant after birth. In such cases, the physician must use his or her judgment on behalf of the infant in deciding whether to initiate resuscitation of the infant until the parents can be involved in the decision. In making these decisions, the physician should err on the side of resuscitating the infant if the appropriate course is uncertain.

Once intensive care is initiated, the infant is continuously reevaluated, and the prognosis is reassessed on the basis of the best available information in conjunction with the physician's best medical judgment. This approach places significant responsibility on the physician and health care team to evaluate the benefits to and burdens on the infant with continuing intensive care. The family of the infant must be kept fully informed of the infant's evolving status and prognosis. The physician and family must be involved together in major decisions that ultimately could alter the infant's outcome.[7] Unless circumstances dictate otherwise, one physician should be designated as the spokesperson for the health care team and should discuss treatment options with the family and communicate decisions to the full health care team. When there is more than one valid approach to treatment, the physician should present these options to the family for their consideration and opinion. When the health care team is unable to agree on a treatment strategy, the physician, serving as the team leader, should attempt to resolve existing differences by using an independent medical consultant or consulting with the hospital bioethics committee.

The physician spokesperson must recognize that the parents' view of their child's status and the treatment choices is influenced by how the information is presented by the physician.[8] This recognition imposes a special obligation on the physician to present prognostic information in a frank and balanced way without coercion. The physician spokesperson must be sensitive to the parents' concerns and desires, which are often based on a complex combination of values and influences derived from their cultural, religious, educational, social, and ethnic backgrounds. The physician's role is to present the treatment options to the parents and provide guidance as needed. The parents' role is to participate actively in the decision-making process. Decisions to continue, limit, or stop intensive care must be based only on the best interest of the infant and not on the financial status of the parents or the financial interests of the physicians, the hospital, or any third-party payer.

The important role of the parents in decision-making must be respected. However, the physician's first responsibility is to the patient. The physician is not obligated to provide inappropriate treatment or to withhold beneficial treatment at the request of the parents. Treatment that is harmful, of no benefit, or futile and merely prolonging dying should be considered inappropriate. The physician must ensure that the chosen treatment, in his or her best medical judgment, is consistent with the best interest of the infant.

When there is conflict or disagreement between the recommendations of the physician and the desires of the infant's parents, continued discussion will often lead to agreement. If the disagreement continues, one option is to consult with the hospital bioethics committee. Another option is for the physician and family to seek another physician who is willing to provide care for the infant in the manner desired by the family. This disagreement between the physician and the family may result in the involvement of the court system. If this occurs, the physician should continue to serve as an advocate for the infant. Involvement of the court system is adversarial by nature and should be considered the last possible choice in resolution, to be used only in the case of irreconcilable differences of opinion, and it should be avoidable in nearly all cases.

RECOMMENDATIONS

1. Decisions about noninitiation or withdrawal of intensive care should be made by the health care team and the parents of a high-risk infant working together. This approach requires honest and open communication. Ongoing evaluation of the condition and prognosis of the high-risk infant is essential, and the physician, as the spokesperson for the health care team, must convey this information accurately and openly to the parents of the infant.

2. Parents should be active participants in the decision-making process concerning the treatment of severely ill infants.

3. Compassionate basic care to ensure comfort must be provided to all infants, including those for whom intensive care is not being provided.

4. The decision to initiate or continue intensive care should be based only on the judgment that the infant will benefit from the intensive care. It is inappropriate for life-prolonging treatment to be continued when the condition is incompatible with life or when the treatment is judged to be harmful, of no benefit, or futile.

COMMITTEE ON FETUS AND NEWBORN, 2005–2006

Ann R. Stark, MD, Chairperson
David H. Adamkin, MD
Daniel G. Batton, MD
*Edward F. Bell, MD
Vinod K. Bhutani, MD
Susan E. Denson, MD
William A. Engle, MD
Gilbert I. Martin, MD

LIAISONS

Keith J. Barrington, MD
    Canadian Paediatric Society

Gary D. V. Hankins, MD
    American College of Obstetricians and Gynecologists
Tonse N. K. Raju, MD, DCH
    National Institutes of Health
Kay M. Tomashek, MD, MPH
    Centers for Disease Control and Prevention
Carol Wallman, MSN, RNC, NNP
    National Association of Neonatal Nurses and
    Association of Women's Health, Obstetric and
    Neonatal Nurses

STAFF

Jim Couto, MA

*Lead author

REFERENCES

1. Saigal S, Stoskopf BL, Streiner DL, Burrows E. Physical growth and current health status of infants who were of extremely low birth weight and controls at adolescence. *Pediatrics.* 2001;108: 407–415
2. Hack M, Flannery DJ, Schluchter M, Cartar L, Borawski E, Klein N. Outcomes in young adulthood for very-low-birth-weight infants. *N Engl J Med.* 2002;346:149–157
3. Marlow N, Wolke D, Bracewell MA, Samara M; EPICure Study Group. Neurologic and developmental disability at six years of age after extremely preterm birth. *N Engl J Med.* 2005;352:9–19
4. McDonald H; American Academy of Pediatrics, Committee on Fetus and Newborn. Perinatal care at the threshold of viability. *Pediatrics.* 2002;110:1024–1027
5. American Heart Association, American Academy of Pediatrics. 2005 American Heart Association (AHA) guidelines for cardiopulmonary resuscitation (CPR) and emergency cardiovascular care (ECC) of pediatric and neonatal patients: neonatal resuscitation guidelines. *Pediatrics.* 2006;117(5). Available at: www.pediatrics.org/cgi/content/full/117/5/e1029
6. Paul DA, Epps S, Leef KH, Stefano JL. Prenatal consultation with a neonatologist prior to preterm delivery. *J Perinatol.* 2001;21: 431–437
7. McHaffie HE, Laing IA, Parker M, McMillan J. Deciding for imperilled newborns: medical authority or parental autonomy? *J Med Ethics.* 2001;27:104–109
8. Peerzada JM, Richardson DK, Burns JP. Delivery room decision-making at the threshold of viability. *J Pediatr.* 2004;145:492–498

SECTION 4

Respiratory Support

POLICY STATEMENT   Organizational Principles to Guide and Define the Child Health
Care System and/or Improve the Health of all Children

American Academy
of Pediatrics

DEDICATED TO THE HEALTH OF ALL CHILDREN™

The Apgar Score

AMERICAN ACADEMY OF PEDIATRICS COMMITTEE ON FETUS AND NEWBORN,
AMERICAN COLLEGE OF OBSTETRICIANS AND GYNECOLOGISTS COMMITTEE ON OBSTETRIC PRACTICE

abstract

The Apgar score provides an accepted and convenient method for reporting
the status of the newborn infant immediately after birth and the response to
resuscitation if needed. The Apgar score alone cannot be considered as
evidence of, or a consequence of, asphyxia; does not predict individual
neonatal mortality or neurologic outcome; and should not be used for that
purpose. An Apgar score assigned during resuscitation is not equivalent to
a score assigned to a spontaneously breathing infant. The American Academy
of Pediatrics and the American College of Obstetricians and Gynecologists
encourage use of an expanded Apgar score reporting form that accounts for
concurrent resuscitative interventions.

Also published in Obstetrics & Gynecology. Copyright October 2015 by
the American College of Obstetricians and Gynecologists, 409 12th
Street, SW, PO Box 96920, Washington, DC 20090-6920 and the American
Academy of Pediatrics, 141 Northwest Point Blvd, PO Box 927, Elk Grove
Village, IL 60009-0927. All rights reserved. ISSN 1074-861X

The American College of Obstetricians and Gynecologists Committee
Opinion no. 644: The Apgar score. Obstet Gynecol. 2015;125:XX–XX.
Accepted for publication Jul 22, 2015

www.pediatrics.org/cgi/doi/10.1542/peds.2015-2651

DOI: 10.1542/peds.2015-2651

PEDIATRICS (ISSN Numbers: Print, 0031-4005; Online, 1098-4275).

Copyright © 2015 by the American Academy of Pediatrics

INTRODUCTION

In 1952, Dr Virginia Apgar devised a scoring system that was a rapid
method of assessing the clinical status of the newborn infant at 1 minute
of age and the need for prompt intervention to establish breathing.[1]
Dr Apgar subsequently published a second report that included a larger
number of patients.[2] This scoring system provided a standardized
assessment for infants after delivery. The Apgar score comprises 5
components: (1) color; (2) heart rate; (3) reflexes; (4) muscle tone; and
(5) respiration. Each of these components is given a score of 0, 1, or 2.
Thus, the Apgar score quantitates clinical signs of neonatal depression,
such as cyanosis or pallor, bradycardia, depressed reflex response to
stimulation, hypotonia, and apnea or gasping respirations. The score is
reported at 1 minute and 5 minutes after birth for all infants, and at
5-minute intervals thereafter until 20 minutes for infants with a score less
than 7.[3] The Apgar score provides an accepted and convenient method for
reporting the status of the newborn infant immediately after birth and the
response to resuscitation if it is needed; however, it has been
inappropriately used to predict individual adverse neurologic outcome.

The purpose of the present statement was to place the Apgar score in its
proper perspective. This statement revises the 2006 College Committee
Opinion/American Academy of Pediatrics policy statement to include
updated guidance from the 2014 report *Neonatal Encephalopathy and
Neurologic Outcome* (second edition)[4] published by the American College

of Obstetricians and Gynecologists in collaboration with the American Academy of Pediatrics, along with new guidance on neonatal resuscitation. The guidelines of the Neonatal Resuscitation Program state that the Apgar score is useful for conveying information about the newborn infant's overall status and response to resuscitation. However, resuscitation must be initiated before the 1-minute score is assigned. Therefore, the Apgar score is not used to determine the need for initial resuscitation, what resuscitation steps are necessary, or when to use them.[3]

An Apgar score that remains 0 beyond 10 minutes of age may, however, be useful in determining whether continued resuscitative efforts are indicated because very few infants with an Apgar score of 0 at 10 minutes have been reported to survive with a normal neurologic outcome.[3,5,6] In line with this outcome, the 2011 Neonatal Resuscitation Program guidelines state that "if you can confirm that no heart rate has been detectable for at least 10 minutes, discontinuation of resuscitative efforts may be appropriate."[3]

The *Neonatal Encephalopathy and Neurologic Outcome* report defines a 5-minute Apgar score of 7 to 10 as reassuring, a score of 4 to 6 as moderately abnormal, and a score of 0 to 3 as low in the term infant and late-preterm infant.[4] In that report, an Apgar score of 0 to 3 at 5 minutes or more was considered a nonspecific sign of illness, which "may be one of the first indications of encephalopathy." However, a persistently low Apgar score alone is not a specific indicator for intrapartum compromise. Furthermore, although the score is widely used in outcome studies, its inappropriate use has led to an erroneous definition of asphyxia. Asphyxia is defined as the marked impairment of gas exchange, which, if prolonged, leads to progressive

hypoxemia, hypercapnia, and significant metabolic acidosis. The term asphyxia, which describes a process of varying severity and duration rather than an end point, should not be applied to birth events unless specific evidence of markedly impaired intrapartum or immediate postnatal gas exchange can be documented on the basis of laboratory test results.

LIMITATIONS OF THE APGAR SCORE

It is important to recognize the limitations of the Apgar score. It is an expression of the infant's physiologic condition at 1 point in time, which includes subjective components. There are numerous factors that can influence the Apgar score, including maternal sedation or anesthesia, congenital malformations, gestational age, trauma, and interobserver variability.[4] In addition, the biochemical disturbance must be significant before the score is affected. Elements of the score, such as tone, color, and reflex irritability, can be subjective and partially depend on the physiologic maturity of the infant. The score may also be affected by variations in normal transition. For example, lower initial oxygen saturations in the first few minutes need not prompt immediate supplemental oxygen administration; the Neonatal Resuscitation Program targets for oxygen saturation are 60% to 65% at 1 minute and 80% to 85% at 5 minutes.[3] The healthy preterm infant with no evidence of asphyxia may receive a low score only because of immaturity.[7,8] The incidence of low Apgar scores is inversely related to birth weight, and a low score cannot predict morbidity or mortality for any individual infant.[8,9] As previously stated, it is also inappropriate to use an Apgar score alone to diagnose asphyxia.

APGAR SCORE AND RESUSCITATION

The 5-minute Apgar score, and particularly a change in the score

between 1 minute and 5 minutes, is a useful index of the response to resuscitation. If the Apgar score is less than 7 at 5 minutes, the Neonatal Resuscitation Program guidelines state that the assessment should be repeated every 5 minutes for up to 20 minutes.[3] However, an Apgar score assigned during resuscitation is not equivalent to a score assigned to a spontaneously breathing infant.[10] There is no accepted standard for reporting an Apgar score in infants undergoing resuscitation after birth because many of the elements contributing to the score are altered by resuscitation. The concept of an assisted score that accounts for resuscitative interventions has been suggested, but the predictive reliability has not been studied. To correctly describe such infants and provide accurate documentation and data collection, an expanded Apgar score reporting form is encouraged (Fig 1). This expanded Apgar score may also prove useful in the setting of delayed cord clamping, in which the time of birth (ie, complete delivery of the infant), the time of cord clamping, and the time of initiation of resuscitation can all be recorded in the comments box.

The Apgar score alone cannot be considered to be evidence of or a consequence of asphyxia. Many other factors, including nonreassuring fetal heart rate–monitoring patterns and abnormalities in umbilical arterial blood gas results, clinical cerebral function, neuroimaging studies, neonatal electroencephalography, placental pathology, hematologic studies, and multisystem organ dysfunction, need to be considered in diagnosing an intrapartum hypoxic–ischemic event.[6] When a category I (normal) or category II (indeterminate) fetal heart rate tracing is associated with Apgar scores of 7 or higher at 5 minutes, a normal umbilical cord arterial blood pH ($\pm$1 SD), or both, it is not

Apgar Score Gestational age_____weeks

Sign	0	1	2	1 minute	5 minute	10 minute	15 minute	20 minute
Color	Blue or Pale	Acrocyanotic	Completely Pink					
Heart rate	Absent	<100 minute	>100 minute					
Reflex irritability	No Response	Grimace	Cry or Active Withdrawal					
Muscle tone	Limp	Some Flexion	Active Motion					
Respiration	Absent	Weak Cry; Hypoventilation	Good, Crying					
			Total					

Comments:		Resuscitation					
	Minutes	1	5	10	15	20
	Oxygen					
	PPV/NCPAP					
	ETT					
	Chest Compressions					
	Epinephrine					

FIGURE 1

Expanded Apgar score reporting form. Scores should be recorded in the appropriate place at specific time intervals. The additional resuscitative measures (if appropriate) are recorded at the same time that the score is reported by using a checkmark in the appropriate box. The comment box is used to list other factors, including maternal medications and/or the response to resuscitation between the recorded times of scoring. ETT, endotracheal tube; PPV/NCPAP, positive pressure ventilation/nasal continuous positive airway pressure.

consistent with an acute hypoxic–ischemic event.[4]

PREDICTION OF OUTCOME

A 1-minute Apgar score of 0 to 3 does not predict any individual infant's outcome. A 5-minute Apgar score of 0 to 3 correlates with neonatal mortality in large populations[11,12] but does not predict individual future neurologic dysfunction. Population studies have uniformly reassured us that most infants with low Apgar scores will not develop cerebral palsy. However, a low 5-minute Apgar score clearly confers an increased relative risk of cerebral palsy, reported to be as high as 20- to 100-fold over that of infants with a 5-minute Apgar score of 7 to 10.[9,13–15] Although individual risk varies, the population risk of poor neurologic outcomes also increases when the Apgar score is 3 or less at 10 minutes, 15 minutes, and 20 minutes.[16] When a newborn infant has an Apgar score of 5 or less at 5 minutes, umbilical arterial blood gas samples from a clamped section of the umbilical cord should be obtained, if possible.[17] Submitting the placenta for pathologic examination may be valuable.

OTHER APPLICATIONS

Monitoring of low Apgar scores from a delivery service may be useful. Individual case reviews can identify needs for focused educational programs and improvement in systems of perinatal care. Analyzing trends allows for the assessment of the effect of quality improvement interventions.

CONCLUSIONS

The Apgar score describes the condition of the newborn infant immediately after birth and, when properly applied, is a tool for standardized assessment.[18] It also provides a mechanism to record fetal-to-neonatal transition. Apgar scores do not predict individual mortality or adverse neurologic outcome. However, based on population studies, Apgar scores of less than 5 at 5 and 10 minutes clearly confer an increased relative risk of cerebral palsy, and the degree of abnormality correlates with the risk of cerebral palsy. Most infants with low Apgar scores, however, will not develop cerebral palsy. The Apgar score is affected by many factors, including gestational age, maternal

medications, resuscitation, and cardiorespiratory and neurologic conditions. If the Apgar score at 5 minutes is 7 or greater, it is unlikely that peripartum hypoxia–ischemia caused neonatal encephalopathy.

RECOMMENDATIONS

1. The Apgar score does not predict individual neonatal mortality or neurologic outcome and should not be used for that purpose.

2. It is inappropriate to use the Apgar score alone to establish the diagnosis of asphyxia. The term asphyxia, which describes a process of varying severity and duration rather than an end point, should not be applied to birth events unless specific evidence of markedly impaired intrapartum or immediate postnatal gas exchange can be documented.

3. When a newborn infant has an Apgar score of 5 or less at 5 minutes, umbilical arterial blood gas samples from a clamped section of the umbilical cord should be obtained. Submitting the placenta for pathologic examination may be valuable.

4. Perinatal health care professionals should be consistent in assigning an Apgar score during resuscitation; therefore, the American Academy of Pediatrics and the American College of Obstetricians and Gynecologists encourage use of an expanded Apgar score reporting form that accounts for concurrent resuscitative interventions.

AAP COMMITTEE ON FETUS AND NEWBORN, 2014–2015

Kristi L. Watterberg, MD, FAAP, Chairperson
Susan Aucott, MD, FAAP
William E. Benitz, MD, FAAP
James J. Cummings, MD, FAAP
Eric C. Eichenwald, MD, FAAP
Jay Goldsmith, MD, FAAP
Brenda B. Poindexter, MD, FAAP
Karen Puopolo, MD, FAAP
Dan L. Stewart, MD, FAAP
Kasper S. Wang, MD, FAAP

REFERENCES

1. Apgar V. A proposal for a new method of evaluation of the newborn infant. *Curr Res Anest Anal*. 1953;32(4):260–267

2. Apgar V, Holaday DA, James LS, Weisbrot IM, Berrien C. Evaluation of the newborn infant; second report. *J Am Med Assoc*. 1958;168(15):1985–1988

3. American Academy of Pediatrics and American Heart Association. *Textbook of Neonatal Resuscitation*. 6th ed. Elk Grove Village, IL: American Academy of Pediatrics and American Heart Association; 2011

4. American College of Obstetrics and Gynecology, Task Force on Neonatal Encephalopathy, American Academy of Pediatrics. *Neonatal Encephalopathy and Neurologic Outcome*. 2nd ed. Washington, DC: American College of Obstetricians and Gynecologists; 2014

5. Jain L, Ferre C, Vidyasagar D, Nath S, Sheftel D. Cardiopulmonary resuscitation of apparently stillborn infants: survival and long-term outcome. *J Pediatr*. 1991; 118(5):778–782

6. Kasdorf E, Laptook A, Azzopardi D, Jacobs S, Perlman JM. Improving infant outcome with a 10 min Apgar of 0. *Arch Dis Child Fetal Neonatal Ed*. 2015;100(2):F102–F105

7. Catlin EA, Carpenter MW, Brann BS IV, et al. The Apgar score revisited:

influence of gestational age. *J Pediatr*. 1986;109(5):865–868

8. Hegyi T, Carbone T, Anwar M, et al. The Apgar score and its components in the preterm infant. *Pediatrics*. 1998;101(1 pt 1):77–81

9. Ehrenstein V. Association of Apgar scores with death and neurologic disability. *Clin Epidemiol*. 2009;1:45–53

10. Lopriore E, van Burk GF, Walther FJ, de Beaufort AJ. Correct use of the Apgar score for resuscitated and intubated newborn babies: questionnaire study. *BMJ*. 2004;329(7458):143–144

11. Casey BM, McIntire DD, Leveno KJ. The continuing value of the Apgar score for the assessment of newborn infants. *N Engl J Med*. 2001;344(7):467–471

12. Li F, Wu T, Lei X, Zhang H, Mao M, Zhang J. The Apgar score and infant mortality. *PLoS One*. 2013;8(7):e69072

13. Moster D, Lie RT, Irgens LM, Bjerkedal T, Markestad T. The association of Apgar score with subsequent death and cerebral palsy: a population-based study in term infants. *J Pediatr*. 2001;138(6): 798–803

14. Nelson KB, Ellenberg JH. Apgar scores as predictors of chronic neurologic disability. *Pediatrics*. 1981;68(1):36–44

15. Lie KK, Grøholt EK, Eskild A. Association of cerebral palsy with Apgar score in low and normal birthweight infants: population based cohort study. *BMJ*. 2010;341:c4990

16. Freeman JM, Nelson KB. Intrapartum asphyxia and cerebral palsy. *Pediatrics*. 1988;82(2):240–249

17. Malin GL, Morris RK, Khan KS. Strength of association between umbilical cord pH and perinatal and long term outcomes: systematic review and meta-analysis. *BMJ*. 2010;340:c1471

18. Papile LA. The Apgar score in the 21st century. *N Engl J Med*. 2001;344(7): 519–520

CLINICAL REPORT Guidance for the Clinician in Rendering Pediatric Care

American Academy
of Pediatrics

DEDICATED TO THE HEALTH OF ALL CHILDREN™

Noninvasive Respiratory Support

James J. Cummings, MD, FAAP, Richard A. Polin, MD, FAAP, the COMMITTEE ON FETUS AND NEWBORN

abstract

Mechanical ventilation is associated with increased survival of preterm infants but is also associated with an increased incidence of chronic lung disease (bronchopulmonary dysplasia) in survivors. Nasal continuous positive airway pressure (nCPAP) is a form of noninvasive ventilation that reduces the need for mechanical ventilation and decreases the combined outcome of death or bronchopulmonary dysplasia. Other modes of noninvasive ventilation, including nasal intermittent positive pressure ventilation, biphasic positive airway pressure, and high-flow nasal cannula, have recently been introduced into the NICU setting as potential alternatives to mechanical ventilation or nCPAP. Randomized controlled trials suggest that these newer modalities may be effective alternatives to nCPAP and may offer some advantages over nCPAP, but efficacy and safety data are limited.

INTRODUCTION

Mechanical ventilation increases survival in preterm infants with respiratory failure; however, it is associated with an increased risk of bronchopulmonary dysplasia (BPD) and adverse neurodevelopmental outcomes.[1] Attempts to decrease lung injury by using gentler ventilation strategies and restricting oxygen use have resulted in only modest improvements in the incidence of BPD.[2] In 1987, Avery et al[3] published a small observational study suggesting that using continuous positive airway pressure (CPAP) as the primary mode of respiratory support reduced the need for supplemental oxygen at 28 days of life. More recent randomized clinical trials have demonstrated that, in comparison with prophylactic or early use of surfactant, the use of CPAP decreases the need for invasive mechanical ventilation and the combined outcome of death or BPD.[4,5] The most immature infants (24–25 weeks' gestational age) may benefit most from this strategy,[6] even though all randomized trials to date have shown a high rate of CPAP failure in these infants. CPAP has also been used to treat apnea of prematurity and is considered an evidence-based strategy to decrease postextubation failure.[7–10]

The search for ways to improve on CPAP in managing preterm infants with respiratory failure has identified 2 additional strategies of noninvasive ventilation: alternating nasal positive pressures, with

DOI: 10.1542/peds.2015-3758

Accepted for publication Oct 9, 2015

PEDIATRICS (ISSN Numbers: Print, 0031-4005; Online, 1098-4275).

Copyright © 2016 by the American Academy of Pediatrics

To cite: Cummings JJ, Polin RA, AAP the COMMITTEE ON FETUS AND NEWBORN. Noninvasive Respiratory Support. *Pediatrics.* 2016;137(1):e20153758

either nasal intermittent positive pressure ventilation (NIPPV) or bilevel nasal CPAP (BiPAP), and high-flow nasal cannula (HFNC). Numerous observational studies have investigated the utility of NIPPV or HFNC for a variety of neonatal disorders,[11-24] but only randomized clinical trials with direct comparisons to nasal CPAP (nCPAP) are used to inform this statement. It is important to note that when CPAP is used for comparison, the technologies used to provide positive pressure (ventilator or bubble CPAP) and the strategies used to decrease air-leak through the mouth (chin strap or pacifier) differ between studies.

NIPPV AND BIPAP

Technical Considerations

NIPPV most commonly uses a ventilator to provide intermittent breaths at peak inspiratory pressures and rates similar to those used for mechanical ventilation. NIPPV has also been used in combination with high frequency ventilation.[25] BiPAP systems provide sigh breaths with much lower pressures, longer inflation times (0.5–1.0 second for the higher nCPAP pressure), lower cycle rates (10–30 per minute), and small differences (<4 cm H_2O) between high and low nCPAP pressures. Randomized clinical trials of NIPPV in human newborn infants have used a wide range of set peak pressures (10–25 cm H_2O pressure) and ventilator rates (10–60 per minute), variable inflation times (0.3–0.5 seconds) and synchronized or nonsynchronized breaths. Both NIPPV and BiPAP are generally used in a nonsynchronized mode. Intermittent breaths are generally delivered through short binasal prongs, although masks[26] and long nasopharyngeal tubes[27] have been used.

Synchronization of breaths is difficult with NIPPV or BiPAP. A pneumatic capsule placed on the abdomen was used in the Infant Star ventilator to allow patient triggering, but this ventilator is no longer available. The Infant Flow Advance BiPAP device, which uses an abdominal trigger, is not approved for use in the United States. Other forms of synchronization using neurally adjusted ventilatory assistance,[28,29] flow triggering,[30] pressure triggering,[31] or respiratory inductance plethysmography[32,33] have not been investigated in large randomized trials.

Physiologic Principles

NIPPV offers the main physiologic advantage of CPAP (ie, stabilization of alveoli by positive airway pressure) and theoretically promotes better ventilation by delivering positive pressure breaths to the lower airways. In addition, NIPPV may trigger an augmented inspiratory reflex (Head's paradoxical reflex) in preterm infants. Data from surfactant-deficient piglets indicate that NIPPV results in less lung inflammation than synchronized intermittent mandatory ventilation.[34] The physiologic benefits of NIPPV may depend on whether the breaths are synchronized or nonsynchronized. Studies in preterm infants[30,32,35,36] indicate that, in comparison with CPAP, synchronized NIPPV decreased the work of breathing, improved thoracoabdominal asynchrony, increased tidal volumes and minute ventilation, and decreased carbon dioxide concentrations. Similarly, Ali et al[33] and Chang et al[37] found that synchronized NIPPV improved thoracoabdominal synchrony[33] and decreased inspiratory effort[33,37] but showed no benefit on tidal volume, minute ventilation, or P_{CO_2}. In contrast, Owen et al[38] found that nonsynchronized NIPPV increased the relative tidal volume by a modest 15% during inspiration, with no consistent effect during expiration. Pressure delivered during expiration slowed the respiratory rate (by prolonging expiration). NIPPV applied during apneic episodes increased tidal volumes only 5% of the time, suggesting the importance of synchronization of NIPPV with an open glottis.[38] Higher peak pressures did not consistently increase the likelihood of chest inflation. In addition, Owen et al[39] demonstrated that the pressure delivered to the inspiratory limb of the nasal prongs was highly variable and was highest and most variable when the infant was moving.[39] The variations in delivered pressure may reflect varying levels of resistance at the level of the glottis. Increasing the set peak inspiratory pressure did not consistently deliver a higher pressure to the infant, suggesting that a higher set pressure may not provide additional respiratory assistance.

Similar to the studies described previously, Miedema et al observed that nonsynchronized BiPAP (using the Infant Flow SiPAP system) did not increase tidal volumes or lower transcutaneous P_{CO_2} in stable preterm infants.[40] However, Migliori et al[40] (using a crossover design) demonstrated that nonsynchronized BiPAP compared with nCPAP in preterm infants 24 to 31 weeks' gestational age significantly improved ventilation and oxygenation in a 4-hour study.[41]

NIPPV for Apnea of Prematurity

Randomized studies of nonsynchronized NIPPV for apnea of prematurity included small numbers of infants, were mostly of short duration (Table 1), and have not revealed consistent benefit.[42-44] In the study by Ryan et al,[44] peak pressures were not transmitted to the chest wall, which is consistent with upper airway obstruction. There is very little evidence to support the effectiveness of NIPPV for apnea; however, a recent Cochrane review concluded, "NIPPV may be a useful method of augmenting the

TABLE 1 NIPPV or nCPAP for Apnea of Prematurity

Author[a] Year	Study Design	Gestational Age, wk	Study No.	Mode	Methylxanthines	End Point	Outcome
Ryan et al 1989[44]	Crossover trial: Infants allocated to CPAP or NIPPV for 6 h	26 ± 2	20	Nonsynchronized	Yes	Apnea events/h	No significant difference
Lin et al 1998[42]	Randomized clinical trial: Infants allocated to nCPAP or NIPPV for 4 h	27.6 (25–32)	34	Nonsynchronized	Yes	Apnea or bradycardia events/h	Significant reduction in apnea events with NIPPV ($P = .02$)
Pantalitschka et al 2009[43]	Crossover trial: Infants allocated to: Variable flow CPAP; Bubble CPAP; NIPPV; NIPPV + variable flow CPAP for 6 h	28 (24–32)	16	Nonsynchronized	No	Cumulative rate of bradycardia or desaturation episodes	Significant reduction with variable flow CPAP (with or without NIPPV). No benefit to bubble CPAP or NIPPV alone

[a] Refers to number in References.

beneficial effects of nCPAP in preterm infants with apnea that is frequent or severe. Additional safety and efficacy data are required before recommending NIPPV as a standard therapy for apnea."[9] No studies using synchronized NIPPV in infants with apnea have been performed.

NIPPV or nCPAP for Prevention of Postextubation Failure

NIPPV has been compared with nCPAP for prevention of postextubation failure in preterm infants[36,45–52] (Table 2).* The trial of Kirpalani included infants with respiratory distress syndrome (RDS; preintubation) and infants with RDS after extubation and permitted the use of ventilator-driven NIPPV (synchronized or nonsynchronized) and the use of bilevel devices. The study by O'Brien et al[51] used bilevel devices. The most recent Cochrane meta-analysis concluded that NIPPV decreased the risk of meeting respiratory failure criteria postextubation (relative risk [RR], 0.71; 95% confidence interval

---

* A study by Gao et al[47] is not included in Table 2, because it enrolled more mature infants. Similarly, the study of Ramanathan et al[54] is not included because infants randomly assigned to NIPPV were extubated sooner than those randomly assigned to nCPAP, who remained ventilated for a longer period of time.

[CI], 0.61–0.82) and the need for reintubation (RR, 0.76; 95% CI, 0.65–0.88).[7] Those benefits were more consistently observed in studies using synchronized NIPPV.

NIPPV or nCPAP for Management of Preterm Infants With RDS

The early use of CPAP with subsequent selective surfactant administration in extremely preterm infants results in lower rates of BPD/death when compared with prophylactic or early surfactant administration.[56] Furthermore, early initiation of CPAP may lead to a reduction in both the duration of mechanical ventilation and the need for postnatal corticosteroid therapy. NIPPV has been investigated as an alternative to CPAP for the acute management of infants with RDS (Table 3).[7,57–63]

Seven randomized trials have compared nCPAP with NIPPV for the initial management of infants with RDS (Table 3). All but 2 trials[50,64] enrolled infants >30 weeks' gestation, which is a population less likely to fail CPAP or develop BPD. Only 1 study was powered to detect a difference in the incidence of BPD, and none of the trials were blinded.[27,31,50,53–55,63,64]

Only 1 randomized trial has been published that limited enrollment to infants <30 weeks' gestation.[50] In this study, 1099 infants with RDS were

randomly assigned to receive NIPPV (ventilator-driven, synchronized, or nonsynchronized, or using a bilevel device) or nCPAP. Fifty-one percent of study infants were enrolled after extubation. The primary outcome was death before 36 weeks of postmenstrual age or survival with BPD (National Institute of Child Health and Human Development criteria or oxygen reduction test). The mean gestational age was 26 weeks; 38.4% of the NIPPV group died or survived with BPD (vs 36.7% of the nCPAP group [$P = .56$]). There were no differences in the duration of respiratory support or survival without BPD in infants randomly assigned to the NIPPV or nCPAP groups.

Safety of NIPPV

Most of the randomized trials summarized previously were small and not sufficiently powered to detect serious complications such as gastrointestinal tract perforation. Although abdominal distention has been observed, it has not been clinically significant. The rate of necrotizing enterocolitis is unaffected by use of NIPPV.[7] The capacity for NIPPV to cause nasal septum erosion/trauma has not been adequately studied but it is likely be similar to that observed with nCPAP.[50]

TABLE 2 NIPPV or nCPAP for Preterm Infants With RDS

Author[a] Year	Study Design	Mean Gestational Age, wk	Study No.	Mode	End Point	Methylxanthines or Surfactant	Outcome
Kugelman et al 2007[31]	Randomized	CPAP: 30.6; NIPPV: 31.1	86	Synchronized	Need for intubation	Methylxanthines (<40%). Surfactant as rescue therapy	NIPPV decreased need for intubation ($P < .05$) and BPD ($P < .05$)
Bisceglia et al 2007[53]	Randomized	CPAP: 30.6; NIPPV: 29.8	88	Nonsynchronized	Need for intubation	No methylxanthines; No surfactant	NIPPV decreased apnea episodes and duration of respiratory support, but no decrease in need for intubation
Kishore et al 2009[27]	Randomized	28–34	76	Nonsynchronized	Failure of noninvasive support	Aminophylline if birth wt <1000 g. Variable use of surfactant	NIPPV decreased failure rate at 48 h ($P = .024$) and 7 d ($P = .036$)
Meneses et al 2011[54]	Randomized	CPAP: 30.1; NIPPV: 29	200	Nonsynchronized	Need for mechanical ventilation in first 72 h	Methylxanthines in 100%. Surfactant as rescue therapy	No significant difference in need for ventilation
Shi et al 2014[55]	Randomized	CPAP: 34.2; NIPPV: 34.32	179 term and preterm	Nonsynchronized	Need for intubation	Surfactant as rescue therapy: 82%–83%	NIPPV decreased need for intubation in preterm infants ($P < .05$)
Kirpalani et al 2013[50]	Randomized	CPAP: 26.2; NIPPV: 26.1	1009	Synchronized and nonsynchronized	Death before 36 wk of postmenstrual age or survival with BPD	Caffeine: 82.9%; Surfactant ~20% (postrandomization)	No significant differences in survival or BPD

[a] Refers to number in References.

Biphasic nCPAP (BiPAP) Versus nCPAP

BiPAP is a form of noninvasive ventilation that provides 2 alternating levels of continuous positive airway pressure at set intervals using nasal prongs or a facemask. Two prospective randomized clinical trials have evaluated nCPAP versus BiPAP. Lista et al[65] randomly assigned 40 preterm infants with RDS and a mean gestational age of 30 weeks to receive synchronized BiPAP (Infant Flow) or nCPAP (Infant Flow) after surfactant administration and extubation. Infants randomly assigned to receive nCPAP had a significantly longer duration of respiratory support (mean ± SD:

TABLE 3 NIPPV or nCPAP for Prevention of Postextubation Failure

Author[a] Year	Study Design	Gestational Age, wk	Study No.	Synchronized or Nonsynchronized	End Point	Methylxanthines	Outcome
Khalaf et al 2001[48]	Randomized	CPAP: 27.6 NIPPV: 27.7	32	Synchronized	Extubation failure by 72 h	Aminophylline 100%	NIPPV increased success of extubation for 72 h ($P = .01$)
Friedlich et al 1999[47]	Randomized	CPAP: 27.6 NIPPV: 28.0	41	Synchronized	Extubation failure by 48 h	Aminophylline 82%–90%	NIPPV increased success of extubation ($P = .016$)
Barrington et al 2001[46]	Randomized	CPAP: 26.1 NIPPV: 26.1	54	Synchronized	Extubation failure	Aminophylline 100%	NIPPV increased success of extubation
Khorana et al 2008[49]	Randomized	CPAP: 29.25 NIPPV: 28.33	48	Nonsynchronized	Extubation failure by 7 d	Aminophylline 100%	Reintubation rate was not significantly different
Moretti et al 1999[36]	Randomized	CPAP: 27.1 NIPPV: 26.9	63	Synchronized	Extubation failure	Caffeine 100%	NIPPV increased success of extubation ($P < .01$)
Kirpalani et al 2013[50]	Randomized	CPAP: 26.2 NIPPV: 26.1	845	Synchronized and nonsynchronized	Respiratory failure after extubation	Caffeine 82.9%	Marginally decreased incidence of respiratory failure (RR, 0.86; 95% CI, 0.72–1.01)
O'Brien et al 2012[51]	Randomized	26^{0/7}–29^{6/7}	133	Nonsynchronized	Sustained extubation for 7 d	Caffeine 100%	Decreased need for ventilation at 7 d. No significant difference in rate of respiratory failure or need for reintubation

[a] Refers to number in References.

CPAP, 13.8 ± 8 days, versus BiPAP, 6.5 ± 4 days; $P = .027$). O'Brien et al[51] randomly assigned 128 infants (mean gestational age, 27 weeks) to receive nonsynchronized BiPAP (Infant flow) or nCPAP (Infant Flow) after extubation. The primary end point in this study, sustained extubation (≥7 days), was not different between groups. Retinopathy of prematurity (stage 2 or higher) was significantly more common in the BiPAP group, an observation that the authors could not explain.[51]

CONCLUSIONS

- In comparison with nCPAP, synchronized NIPPV decreases the frequency of postextubation failure.

- Studies using nonsynchronized NIPPV or BiPAP for postextubation failure are inconclusive.

- Data do not support the superiority of NIPPV/BiPAP (synchronized or nonsynchronized) over nCPAP for the management of infants with RDS.

- There is no published evidence of benefit of NIPPV or BiPAP for apnea of prematurity; however, there have been no published randomized trials using synchronized NIPPV or BiPAP.

- Further research is needed before recommending NIPPV or BiPAP over nCPAP for the management of infants with RDS or apnea.

HIGH-FLOW NASAL CANNULA

Technical Considerations

The commonly used term "high-flow nasal cannula" (HFNC) is somewhat oversimplified, because in clinical practice, much more than flow distinguishes HFNC from so-called low-flow nasal cannula (LFNC) devices. LFNCs are primarily used to deliver oxygen to infants with chronic lung disease (BPD) at flow rates <1 L/minute. Higher flows are reserved for older infants and children because of concerns about airway desiccation, mucosal injury, and airway obstruction.[66–68]

For the purpose of this report, any cannula that delivers gas at a flow >1 L/minute will be considered high flow. However, the term HFNC will specifically refer to the delivery of blended, heated, and humidified oxygen. This approximates the physiologic conditioning that is normally performed by the upper airway during spontaneous breathing in ambient air and maintains a healthy environment for the nasal mucosa.

Physiologic Principles

A key feature of HFNC is the preconditioning of the inspired gas. Because it normally takes metabolic energy for the body to warm and humidify the air we breathe, HFNC has the advantage of reducing resting energy expenditure.[69] Even though CPAP also uses warmed, humidified gas, an in vivo study revealed that the humidity of gas delivered by HFNC was significantly greater.[37] It is uncertain whether the increased humidity delivered by HFNC is clinically important.

The clinically reported respiratory benefits of HFNC primarily have been decreased work of breathing and reduced supplemental oxygen requirement. There are several proposed mechanisms of action to explain these findings, although none have been conclusively demonstrated in vivo.[69] These include the following: (1) reduction of inspiratory resistance[23]; (2) washout of nasopharyngeal dead space[70]; and (3) provision of positive airway distending pressure.[71,72]

Measurement of continuous distending pressure levels during HFNC use, both in vitro and in vivo, has produced variable results.[19,23,71–87] However, it is clear that under certain circumstances (tightly fitting nasal prongs, high flow rates, and closed mouth), HFNC can generate high nasopharyngeal airway pressures.[71,83] However, it is unlikely that excessive pressures with HFNC will occur if the manufacturers' recommendation to use prongs less than half the size of the nares is followed.

HFNC for Weaning From CPAP

There are no prospective, randomized studies of HFNC in preterm infants to facilitate weaning from CPAP. A recent matched-pair cohort study in 79 preterm infants ≤28 weeks' gestation compared weaning from nCPAP to LFNC versus HFNC and revealed that infants in the HFNC group weaned from nCPAP significantly sooner but had no difference in overall duration of respiratory support.[15]

HFNC After the INSURE Approach

One prospective trial has been conducted to determine whether HFNC can decrease reintubation after the INSURE (intubation–surfactant–extubation) procedure in preterm infants with RDS.[88] In this study, 45 infants (mean gestational age, 27.7 weeks) were randomly assigned to immediate extubation and placement on HFNC or maintained on mechanical ventilation and gradually weaned to extubation. Seventy percent (16 of 23) of the infants in the HFNC group did not require intubation, which suggests that HFNC might be an alternative to CPAP in preventing reintubation after INSURE.

HFNC Versus CPAP for Noninvasive Respiratory Support of Preterm Infants

Several prospective randomized trials have compared HFNC versus CPAP for the respiratory

TABLE 4 Prospective, Randomized Trials of HFNC Versus CPAP for Respiratory Support of Preterm Infants

Author[a] Year	GA, wk	HFNC, N	CPAP, N	HFNC, L/min	CPAP, cm H$_2$O	Failure Criteria	HFNC Failure[b]	CPAP Failure	P 2-tailed	Comments
Nair and Karna 2005[95]	27–34	13	15	5–6	5–6	Multiple[c]	2 (15)	2 (13)	1.0	Abstract only
Joshi et al 2008[91]	Mean=32.8	42	38	NS	NS	Intubation	8 (20)	11 (29)	.43	Abstract only
Lavizarri et al 2013[93]	29–36[6/7]	40	52	4–6	4–6	Intubation within 72 h	5 (13)	3 (6)	.29	Abstract only
Collins et al 2013[90]	<32	67	65	8	7 or 8	Multiple[c]	15 (22)	22 (34)	.14	
Manley et al 2013[94]	<32	152	151	5–6	7	Multiple[c]	52 (34)	39 (26)	.13	Noninferiority trial
Yoder et al 2013[96]	28–42	212	220	3–5	5–6	Intubation within 72 h	23 (11)	18 (8)	.34	Nasal trauma; HFNC: 9%; CPAP: 16% (P = .047)
Klingenberg et al 2014[92]	<34	10	10	5–6	4–5	EDIN discomfort scores	10.7 ± 3.3	11.1 ± 3.0	.35	Crossover trial with all infants crossing after 24 h
Osman et al 2014[97]	<35	23	37	2–8	4–6	PIPP[d]	4 (2–6)	10 (7–12)	<.01	Observational cross-sectional study
						Salivary cortisol	5 (4–6)	2 (1–2)	<.01	

GA, gestational age; NS, not specified; EDIN, Échelle de Douleur et d'Inconfort du Nouveau-né (French for newborn pain discomfort scale).

[a] Refers to number in References.

[b] Failure numbers are shown as N (%) or ±SD as scores (Klingenberg, Osman) or as levels (Osman).

[c] Criteria included a combination of decreased pH, increased P$_{CO_2}$, increased F$_{IO_2}$, and increased apnea/bradycardia episodes.

[d] PIPP, Premature Infant Pain Profile.[98]

management of preterm infants[89–96] (Table 4)[†]; 3 of these studies have been published only in abstract form.[91,93,95] Four studies compared HFNC versus CPAP as primary support only,[91–93,95] 2 of these compared HFNC versus CPAP for postextubation support,[90,94] and 1 study compared HFNC versus CPAP either as primary support or to reduce postextubation failure.[96]

In the 5 studies of primary support only, 3 compared the rate of respiratory failure, defined either by clinical worsening or the need for intubation, and revealed no differences.[91,93,95] Two additional studies did not assess respiratory failure, but compared pain and/or discomfort scores; an observational cross-sectional study in 60 preterm infants revealed that the application of HFNC was associated with less

[†] One study by Campbell et al,[91] although included in a recent meta-analysis of HFNC use,[99] is not included here, because the device used in that study did not deliver fully warmed and humidified gas.

pain compared with nCPAP,[97] whereas a randomized crossover study in 20 preterm infants revealed no differences during treatment.[92]

Collins et al[90] randomly assigned 132 mechanically ventilated preterm infants <32 weeks' gestational age to HFNC at 8 L/minute or nCPAP at either 7 or 8 cm H$_2$O, depending on supplemental oxygen requirement.[90] Treatment failure (predefined as a combination of acidosis, hypercarbia, oxygen requirement, and frequent apnea episodes) during the first 7 days postextubation was 22% (15 of 67) in the HFNC group and 34% (22 of 65) in the CPAP group (P = .14). The rate of reintubation within the first week was 10% (7 of 67) in the HFNC group and 12% (8 of 65) in the CPAP group (P = .79). Predefined nasal trauma scores (lower indicating less trauma) averaged 3.1 ± 7.2 in the HFNC group and 11.8 ± 10.7 in the CPAP group (P < .001).

Manley et al[94] randomly assigned 303 ventilated preterm infants (<32 weeks' gestational age) to HFNC at 5 to 6 L/minute (depending on

nasal prong size) or nCPAP at 7 cm H$_2$O after extubation.[94] Rescue therapy with CPAP for infants who failed HFNC was permitted, but the converse was not allowed. In addition, nonsynchronized NIPPV could be used at any time in the CPAP group or in any infant in the HFNC group who subsequently received CPAP. The incidence of treatment failure by predefined criteria was 34% in the HFNC group and 26% in the CPAP group (P = .13).[‡] The rate of reintubation was

[‡] Randomization was stratified by gestational age (<26 vs ≥26 weeks). Although not reaching statistical significance, there was a greater difference in failure rate between the treatment groups in the more immature stratum (81.3% in the HFNC group versus 61.3% in the CPAP group). This is consistent with a recent survey of neonatal intensive care nurses, the majority of whom believed that HFNC was less likely than nCPAP to prevent reintubation of infants of 24 to 26 weeks' gestational age.[98]

18% (27 of 152) in the HFNC group and 25% (38 of 151) in the CPAP group ($P = .12$). Nasal trauma was more common in the CPAP group ($P = .01$). The incidence of other serious adverse events was no different between groups.[99]

Yoder et al[96] randomly assigned 432 infants (gestational age range, 28–42 weeks) within 24 hours of birth, to avoid intubation ($n = 141$) or after mechanical ventilation ($n = 291$),[96] to receive either HFNC (3–5 L/minute flow, depending on weight) or nCPAP (5–6 cm H_2O), using a variety of devices. The nasal cannulas used in this trial allowed for an approximately 50% gap between each prong's outer diameter and the internal diameter of the respective naris, and free flow around the prongs was determined by periodic auscultation. Extubation failure, defined as reintubation within 72 hours, was 10.8% in the HFNC group and 8.2% in the CPAP group ($P = .34$). Intubation at any time occurred in 15.1% of infants in the HFNC group and 11.4% of infants in the CPAP group ($P = .25$). The incidence of nasal trauma was 9% in the HFNC group and 16% in the CPAP group ($P = .047$).

A Cochrane review published in 2011 concluded that there was insufficient evidence to establish the safety and effectiveness of HFNC compared with nCPAP.[100] However, at the time of that review, only 2 studies, both published only as abstracts, had been reported.[91,95] The 5 randomized clinical trials (with a total of 979 infants) reported after 2011 together suggested that HFNC is comparable to nCPAP in managing RDS or preventing postextubation failure and that HFNC causes less nasal trauma.

Miller et al[101] randomly assigned 40 ventilated preterm infants (26–29 weeks' gestational age) to 1 of 2 HFNC devices after initial extubation.[101] Infants were given a loading dose of caffeine and then extubated and placed on the HFNC device at 6 L/minute. The incidence of treatment failure, defined as the need for reintubation within 72 hours of initial extubation, was 18% (3 of 17) in 1 group and 9% (2 of 22) in the other ($P = .64$). The need for intubation within 7 days of initial extubation was 30% (5 of 17) in 1 group and 27% (6 of 22) in the other ($P = 1.0$).

Safety of HFNC

HFNC creates increased proximal airway pressure and, as with all forms of positive airway pressure, there is a risk of traumatic air dissection.[102,103] Pressure-relief valves incorporated into some HFNC devices may not be sufficient to avoid excessive pressure.[83] Careful attention should be given to the size of the prongs to allow an adequate leak between the prongs and the infant's nares, as well as the use of the lowest effective flow rates. No single randomized study to date has been sufficiently large to address safety concerns; however, recent studies of nearly 500 infants randomly assigned to HFNC in aggregate have suggested that the rate of air leak is comparable to that with nCPAP.

CONCLUSIONS

- HFNC devices used in preterm neonates should precondition inspiratory gases close to normal tracheal gas conditions (37°C and 100% relative humidity).
- HFNC devices that precondition the inspiratory gas mixture and deliver 2 to 8 L/minute flow may be an effective alternative to nCPAP for postextubation failure. However, more data are needed.

- HFNC may be associated with less nasal trauma than nCPAP, at HFNC flow rates up to 8 L/minute.
- HFNC may generate unpredictably high nasopharyngeal pressures and has potential for traumatic air dissection; careful attention to the size of the prongs, demonstration of an adequate air leak between the prongs and the nares, and use of the lowest clinically effective flow rates will reduce this risk.
- None of the published studies on HFNC have been sufficiently powered to determine the safety of HFNC.

LEAD AUTHORS

James J. Cummings, MD, FAAP
Richard A. Polin, MD, FAAP

COMMITTEE ON FETUS AND NEWBORN, 2014–2015

Kristi L. Watterberg, MD, FAAP, Chairperson
Brenda Poindexter, MD, FAAP
James J. Cummings, MD, FAAP
William E. Benitz, MD, FAAP
Eric C. Eichenwald, MD, FAAP
Brenda B. Poindexter, MD, FAAP
Dan L. Stewart, MD, FAAP
Susan W. Aucott, MD, FAAP
Jay P. Goldsmith, MD, FAAP
Karen M. Puopolo, MD, PhD, FAAP
Kasper S. Wang, MD, FAAP

PAST COMMITTEE ON FETUS AND NEWBORN MEMBER

Richard A. Polin MD, FAAP

LIAISONS

Tonse N. K. Raju, MD, DCH, FAAP – *National Institutes of Health*
CAPT. Wanda D. Barfield, MD, MPH, FAAP – *Centers for Disease Control and Prevention*
Erin L. Keels, APRN, MS, NNP-BC – *National Association of Neonatal Nurses*
Thierry Lacaze, MD – *Canadian Paediatric Society*
James Goldberg, MD – *American College of Obstetricians and Gynecologists*

CONSULTANT

Peter G. Davis, MD

STAFF

Jim R. Couto, MA

ABBREVIATIONS

BiPAP: bilevel nasal positive
      airway pressure
BPD: bronchopulmonary
      dysplasia
CI: confidence interval
CPAP: continuous positive airway
      pressure
HFNC: high-flow nasal cannula
LFNC: low-flow nasal cannula
nCPAP: nasal continuous positive
      airway pressure
NIPPV: nasal intermittent
      positive pressure
      ventilation
RDS: respiratory distress
      syndrome
RR: relative risk

REFERENCES

1. Natarajan G, Pappas A, Shankaran S, et al. Outcomes of extremely low birth weight infants with bronchopulmonary dysplasia: impact of the physiologic definition. *Early Hum Dev*. 2012;88(7):509–515

2. Berger TM, Fontana M, Stocker M. The journey towards lung protective respiratory support in preterm neonates. *Neonatology*. 2013;104(4):265–274

3. Avery ME, Tooley WH, Keller JB, et al. Is chronic lung disease in low birth weight infants preventable? A survey of eight centers. *Pediatrics*. 1987;79(1):26–30

4. Fischer HS, Bührer C. Avoiding endotracheal ventilation to prevent bronchopulmonary dysplasia: a meta-analysis. *Pediatrics*. 2013;132(5). Available at: www.pediatrics.org/cgi/content/full/132/5/e1351

5. Schmölzer GM, Kumar M, Pichler G, Aziz K, O'Reilly M, Cheung PY. Non-invasive versus invasive respiratory support in preterm infants at birth: systematic review and meta-analysis. *BMJ*. 2013;347(347):f5980

6. Carlo WA, Finer NN, Walsh MC, et al; SUPPORT Study Group of the Eunice Kennedy Shriver NICHD Neonatal Research Network. Target ranges of oxygen saturation in extremely preterm infants. *N Engl J Med*. 2010;362(21):1959–1969

7. Davis PG, Lemyre B, de Paoli AG, Kirpalani H. Nasal intermittent positive pressure ventilation (NIPPV) versus nasal continuous positive airway pressure (NCPAP) for preterm neonates after extubation. *Cochrane Database Syst Rev*. 2001; (3):CD003212

8. Henderson-Smart DJ, Subramaniam P, Davis PG. Continuous positive airway pressure versus theophylline for apnea in preterm infants. *Cochrane Database Syst Rev*. 2001; (4):CD001072 [Review]

9. Lemyre B, Davis PG, de Paoli AG. Nasal intermittent positive pressure ventilation (NIPPV) versus nasal continuous positive airway pressure (NCPAP) for apnea of prematurity. *Cochrane Database Syst Rev*. 2002; (1):CD002272

10. Miller MJ, Carlo WA, Martin RJ. Continuous positive airway pressure selectively reduces obstructive apnea in preterm infants. *J Pediatr*. 1985;106(1):91–94

11. Bhandari V, Finer NN, Ehrenkranz RA, et al; Eunice Kennedy Shriver National Institute of Child Health and Human Development Neonatal Research Network. Synchronized nasal intermittent positive-pressure ventilation and neonatal outcomes. *Pediatrics*. 2009;124(2):517–526

12. Bhandari V, Gavino RG, Nedrelow JH, et al. A randomized controlled trial of synchronized nasal intermittent positive pressure ventilation in RDS. *J Perinatol*. 2007;27(11):697–703

13. Cavari Y, Sofer S, Rozovski U, Lazar I. Non invasive positive pressure ventilation in infants with respiratory failure. *Pediatr Pulmonol*. 2012;47(10):1019–1025

14. de Jongh BE, Locke R, Mackley A, et al. Work of breathing indices in infants with respiratory insufficiency receiving high-flow nasal cannula and nasal continuous positive airway pressure. *J Perinatol*. 2014;34(1):27–32

15. Fernandez-Alvarez JR, Gandhi RS, Amess P, Mahoney L, Watkins R, Rabe H. Heated humidified high-flow nasal cannula versus low-flow nasal cannula as weaning mode from nasal CPAP in infants ≤28 weeks of gestation. *Eur J Pediatr*. 2014;173(1):93–98

16. Holleman-Duray D, Kaupie D, Weiss MG. Heated humidified high-flow nasal cannula: use and a neonatal early extubation protocol. *J Perinatol*. 2007;27(12):776–781

17. Jackson JK, Vellucci J, Johnson P, Kilbride HW. Evidence-based approach to change in clinical practice: introduction of expanded nasal continuous positive airway pressure use in an intensive care nursery. *Pediatrics*. 2003;111(4 pt 2). Available at: www.pediatrics.org/cgi/content/full/111/4/e542

18. Kulkarni A, Ehrenkranz RA, Bhandari V. Effect of introduction of synchronized nasal intermittent positive-pressure ventilation in a neonatal intensive care unit on bronchopulmonary dysplasia and growth in preterm infants. *Am J Perinatol*. 2006;23(4):233–240

19. Lampland AL, Plumm B, Meyers PA, Worwa CT, Mammel MC. Observational study of humidified high-flow nasal cannula compared with nasal continuous positive airway pressure. *J Pediatr*. 2009;154(2):177–182

20. Manzar S, Nair AK, Pai MG, et al. Use of nasal intermittent positive pressure ventilation to avoid intubation in neonates. *Saudi Med J*. 2004;25(10):1464–1467

21. Salama GSA, Alhadidi A, Ayyash FF, Khlefat A, Al Twall ES. Nasal SIMV as an initial mode of respiratory support for premature infants with RDS. An observational study. *Mid East J Med*. 2012;5(4):17–23

22. Santin R, Brodsky N, Bhandari V. A prospective observational pilot study of synchronized nasal intermittent positive pressure ventilation (SNIPPV) as a primary mode of ventilation in infants > or = 28 weeks with respiratory distress syndrome (RDS). *J Perinatol*. 2004;24(8):487–493

23. Saslow JG, Aghai ZH, Nakhla TA, et al. Work of breathing using high-flow nasal cannula in preterm infants. *J Perinatol*. 2006;26(8):476–480

24. Sun S, Tero R. Safety and efficacy of the Vapotherm 2000i in the

neonatal population. *Respir Care*. 2004;49(11):1384

25. Colaizy TT, Younis UM, Bell EF, Klein JM. Nasal high-frequency ventilation for premature infants. *Acta Paediatr*. 2008;97(11):1518–1522

26. Roberts CT, Davis PG, Owen LS. Neonatal non-invasive respiratory support: synchronised NIPPV, non-synchronised NIPPV or bi-level CPAP: what is the evidence in 2013? *Neonatology*. 2013;104(3):203–209

27. Sai Sunil Kishore M, Dutta S, Kumar P. Early nasal intermittent positive pressure ventilation versus continuous positive airway pressure for respiratory distress syndrome. *Acta Paediatr*. 2009;98(9):1412–1415

28. Terzi N, Piquilloud L, Rozé H, et al. Clinical review: Update on neurally adjusted ventilatory assist--report of a round-table conference. *Crit Care*. 2012;16(3):225

29. Lee J, Kim HS, Sohn JA, et al. Randomized crossover study of neurally adjusted ventilatory assist in preterm infants. *J Pediatr*. 2012;161(5):808–813

30. Moretti C, Giannini L, Fassi C, Gizzi C, Papoff P, Colarizi P. Nasal flow-synchronized intermittent positive pressure ventilation to facilitate weaning in very low-birthweight infants: unmasked randomized controlled trial. *Pediatr Int*. 2008;50(1):85–91

31. Kugelman A, Feferkorn I, Riskin A, Chistyakov I, Kaufman B, Bader D. Nasal intermittent mandatory ventilation versus nasal continuous positive airway pressure for respiratory distress syndrome: a randomized, controlled, prospective study. *J Pediatr*. 2007;150(5):521–526, 526.e1

32. Aghai ZH, Saslow JG, Nakhla T, et al. Synchronized nasal intermittent positive pressure ventilation (SNIPPV) decreases work of breathing (WOB) in premature infants with respiratory distress syndrome (RDS) compared to nasal continuous positive airway pressure (NCPAP). *Pediatr Pulmonol*. 2006;41(9):875–881

33. Ali N, Claure N, Alegria X, D'Ugard C, Organero R, Bancalari E. Effects of non-invasive pressure support ventilation (NI-PSV) on ventilation and respiratory effort in very low birth weight infants. *Pediatr Pulmonol*. 2007;42(8):704–710

34. Lampland AL, Meyers PA, Worwa CT, Swanson EC, Mammel MC. Gas exchange and lung inflammation using nasal intermittent positive-pressure ventilation versus synchronized intermittent mandatory ventilation in piglets with saline lavage-induced lung injury: an observational study. *Crit Care Med*. 2008;36(1):183–187

35. Kiciman NM, Andréasson B, Bernstein G, et al. Thoracoabdominal motion in newborns during ventilation delivered by endotracheal tube or nasal prongs. *Pediatr Pulmonol*. 1998;25(3):175–181

36. Moretti C, Gizzi C, Papoff P, et al. Comparing the effects of nasal synchronized intermittent positive pressure ventilation (nSIPPV) and nasal continuous positive airway pressure (nCPAP) after extubation in very low birth weight infants. *Early Hum Dev*. 1999;56(2-3):167–177

37. Chang HY, Claure N, D'ugard C, Torres J, Nwajei P, Bancalari E. Effects of synchronization during nasal ventilation in clinically stable preterm infants. *Pediatr Res*. 2011;69(1):84–89

38. Owen LS, Morley CJ, Dawson JA, Davis PG. Effects of non-synchronised nasal intermittent positive pressure ventilation on spontaneous breathing in preterm infants. *Arch Dis Child Fetal Neonatal Ed*. 2011;96(6):F422–F428

39. Owen LS, Morley CJ, Davis PG. Pressure variation during ventilator generated nasal intermittent positive pressure ventilation in preterm infants. *Arch Dis Child Fetal Neonatal Ed*. 2010;95(5):F359–F364

40. Miedema M, van der Burg PS, Beuger S, de Jongh FH, Frerichs I, van Kaam AH. Effect of nasal continuous and biphasic positive airway pressure on lung volume in preterm infants. *J Pediatr*. 2013;162(4):691–697

41. Migliori C, Motta M, Angeli A, Chirico G. Nasal bilevel vs. continuous positive airway pressure in preterm infants. *Pediatr Pulmonol*. 2005;40(5):426–430

42. Lin CH, Wang ST, Lin YJ, Yeh TF. Efficacy of nasal intermittent positive pressure ventilation in treating apnea of prematurity. *Pediatr Pulmonol*. 1998;26(5):349–353

43. Pantalitschka T, Sievers J, Urschitz MS, Herberts T, Reher C, Poets CF. Randomised crossover trial of four nasal respiratory support systems for apnoea of prematurity in very low birthweight infants. *Arch Dis Child Fetal Neonatal Ed*. 2009;94(4):F245–F248

44. Ryan CA, Finer NN, Peters KL. Nasal intermittent positive-pressure ventilation offers no advantages over nasal continuous positive airway pressure in apnea of prematurity. *Am J Dis Child*. 1989;143(10):1196–1198

45. Gao WW, Tan SZ, Chen YB, Zhang Y, Wang Y. [Randomized trail of nasal synchronized intermittent mandatory ventilation compared with nasal continuous positive airway pressure in preterm infants with respiratory distress syndrome]. *Zhongguo Dang Dai Er Ke Za Zhi*. 2010;12(7):524–526

46. Barrington KJ, Bull D, Finer NN. Randomized trial of nasal synchronized intermittent mandatory ventilation compared with continuous positive airway pressure after extubation of very low birth weight infants. *Pediatrics*. 2001;107(4):638–641

47. Friedlich P, Lecart C, Posen R, Ramicone E, Chan L, Ramanathan R. A randomized trial of nasopharyngeal-synchronized intermittent mandatory ventilation versus nasopharyngeal continuous positive airway pressure in very low birth weight infants after extubation. *J Perinatol*. 1999;19(6 pt 1):413–418

48. Khalaf MN, Brodsky N, Hurley J, Bhandari V. A prospective randomized, controlled trial comparing synchronized nasal intermittent positive pressure ventilation versus nasal continuous positive airway pressure as modes of extubation. *Pediatrics*. 2001;108(1):13–17

49. Khorana M, Paradeevisut H, Sangtawesin V, Kanjanapatanakul W, Chotigeat U, Ayutthaya JK. A randomized trial of non-synchronized Nasopharyngeal Intermittent Mandatory Ventilation (nsNIMV) vs. Nasal Continuous Positive Airway Pressure (NCPAP) in the prevention of extubation failure in pre-term < 1,500

grams. *J Med Assoc Thai.* 2008;91(3 suppl 3):S136–S142

50. Kirpalani H, Millar D, Lemyre B, Yoder BA, Chiu A, Roberts RS; NIPPV Study Group. A trial comparing noninvasive ventilation strategies in preterm infants. *N Engl J Med.* 2013;369(7):611–620

51. O'Brien K, Campbell C, Brown L, Wenger L, Shah V. Infant flow biphasic nasal continuous positive airway pressure (BP- NCPAP) vs. infant flow NCPAP for the facilitation of extubation in infants' ≤ 1,250 grams: a randomized controlled trial. *BMC Pediatr.* 2012;12:43

52. Ramanathan R, Sekar KC, Rasmussen M, Bhatia J, Soll RF. Nasal intermittent positive pressure ventilation after surfactant treatment for respiratory distress syndrome in preterm infants <30 weeks' gestation: a randomized, controlled trial. *J Perinatol.* 2012;32(5):336–343

53. Bisceglia M, Belcastro A, Poerio V, et al. A comparison of nasal intermittent versus continuous positive pressure delivery for the treatment of moderate respiratory syndrome in preterm infants. *Minerva Pediatr.* 2007;59(2):91–95

54. Meneses J, Bhandari V, Alves JG, Herrmann D. Noninvasive ventilation for respiratory distress syndrome: a randomized controlled trial. *Pediatrics.* 2011;127(2):300–307

55. Shi Y, Tang S, Zhao J, Shen J. A prospective, randomized, controlled study of NIPPV versus nCPAP in preterm and term infants with respiratory distress syndrome. *Pediatr Pulmonol.* 2014;49(7):673–678

56. Bahadue FL, Soll R. Early versus delayed selective surfactant treatment for neonatal respiratory distress syndrome. *Cochrane Database Syst Rev.* 2012;11(11):CD001456

57. Bancalari E, Claure N. The evidence for non-invasive ventilation in the preterm infant. *Arch Dis Child Fetal Neonatal Ed.* 2013;98(2):F98–F102

58. Bhandari V. Nasal intermittent positive pressure ventilation in the newborn: review of literature and evidence-based guidelines. *J Perinatol.* 2010;30(8):505–512

59. Bhandari V. Noninvasive respiratory support in the preterm infant. *Clin Perinatol.* 2012;39(3):497–511

60. Hutchison AA, Bignall S. Non-invasive positive pressure ventilation in the preterm neonate: reducing endotrauma and the incidence of bronchopulmonary dysplasia. *Arch Dis Child Fetal Neonatal Ed.* 2008;93(1):F64–F68

61. Mahmoud RA, Roehr CC, Schmalisch G. Current methods of non-invasive ventilatory support for neonates. *Paediatr Respir Rev.* 2011;12(3):196–205

62. Meneses J, Bhandari V, Alves JG. Nasal intermittent positive-pressure ventilation vs nasal continuous positive airway pressure for preterm infants with respiratory distress syndrome: a systematic review and meta-analysis. *Arch Pediatr Adolesc Med.* 2012;166(4):372–376

63. Tang S, Zhao J, Shen J, Hu Z, Shi Y. Nasal intermittent positive pressure ventilation versus nasal continuous positive airway pressure in neonates: a systematic review and meta-analysis. *Indian Pediatr.* 2013;50(4):371–376

64. Wood FE, Gupta S, Tin W, Sinha S. G170: randomised controlled trial of synchronised intermittent positive airway pressure (SiPAP) versus continuous positive airway pressure (CPAP) as a primary mode of respiratory support in preterm infants with respiratory distress syndrome. *Arch Dis Child.* 2013;98(supp1):A78

65. Lista G, Castoldi F, Fontana P, et al. Nasal continuous positive airway pressure (CPAP) versus bi-level nasal CPAP in preterm babies with respiratory distress syndrome: a randomised control trial. *Arch Dis Child Fetal Neonatal Ed.* 2010;95(2):F85–F89

66. Kopelman AE. Airway obstruction in two extremely low birthweight infants treated with oxygen cannulas. *J Perinatol.* 2003;23(2):164–165

67. Kopelman AE, Holbert D. Use of oxygen cannulas in extremely low birthweight infants is associated with mucosal trauma and bleeding,

and possibly with coagulase-negative staphylococcal sepsis. *J Perinatol.* 2003;23(2):94–97

68. Woodhead DD, Lambert DK, Clark JM, Christensen RD. Comparing two methods of delivering high-flow gas therapy by nasal cannula following endotracheal extubation: a prospective, randomized, masked, crossover trial. *J Perinatol.* 2006;26(8):481–485

69. Dysart K, Miller TL, Wolfson MR, Shaffer TH. Research in high flow therapy: mechanisms of action. *Respir Med.* 2009;103(10):1400–1405

70. Frizzola M, Miller TL, Rodriguez ME, et al. High-flow nasal cannula: impact on oxygenation and ventilation in an acute lung injury model. *Pediatr Pulmonol.* 2011;46(1):67–74

71. Locke RG, Wolfson MR, Shaffer TH, Rubenstein SD, Greenspan JS. Inadvertent administration of positive end-distending pressure during nasal cannula flow. *Pediatrics.* 1993;91(1):135–138

72. Sreenan C, Lemke RP, Hudson-Mason A, Osiovich H. High-flow nasal cannulae in the management of apnea of prematurity: a comparison with conventional nasal continuous positive airway pressure. *Pediatrics.* 2001;107(5):1081–1083

73. Arora B, Mahajan P, Zidan MA, Sethuraman U. Nasopharyngeal airway pressures in bronchiolitis patients treated with high-flow nasal cannula oxygen therapy. *Pediatr Emerg Care.* 2012;28(11):1179–1184

74. Collins CL, Holberton JR, König K. Comparison of the pharyngeal pressure provided by two heated, humidified high-flow nasal cannulae devices in premature infants. *J Paediatr Child Health.* 2013;49(7):554–556

75. Dani C, Pratesi S, Migliori C, Bertini G. High flow nasal cannula therapy as respiratory support in the preterm infant. *Pediatr Pulmonol.* 2009;44(7):629–634

76. de Klerk A. Humidified high-flow nasal cannula: is it the new and improved CPAP? *Adv Neonatal Care.* 2008;8(2):98–106

77. Haq I, Gopalakaje S, Fenton AC, McKean MC, J O'Brien C, Brodlie M. The evidence for high flow nasal cannula devices in infants. *Paediatr Respir Rev.* 2014;15(2):124–134

78. Hasan RA, Habib RH. Effects of flow rate and airleak at the nares and mouth opening on positive distending pressure delivery using commercially available high-flow nasal cannula systems: a lung model study. *Pediatr Crit Care Med.* 2011;12(1):e29–e33

79. Kubicka ZJ, Limauro J, Darnall RA. Heated, humidified high-flow nasal cannula therapy: yet another way to deliver continuous positive airway pressure? *Pediatrics.* 2008;121(1):82–88

80. Lee JH, Rehder KJ, Williford L, Cheifetz IM, Turner DA. Use of high flow nasal cannula in critically ill infants, children, and adults: a critical review of the literature. *Intensive Care Med.* 2013;39(2):247–257

81. Manley BJ, Dold SK, Davis PG, Roehr CC. High-flow nasal cannulae for respiratory support of preterm infants: a review of the evidence. *Neonatology.* 2012;102(4):300–308

82. Shaffer TH, Alapati D, Greenspan JS, Wolfson MR. Neonatal non-invasive respiratory support: physiological implications. *Pediatr Pulmonol.* 2012;47(9):837–847

83. Sivieri EM, Gerdes JS, Abbasi S. Effect of HFNC flow rate, cannula size, and nares diameter on generated airway pressures: an in vitro study. *Pediatr Pulmonol.* 2013;48(5):506–514

84. Spence KL, Murphy D, Kilian C, McGonigle R, Kilani RA. High-flow nasal cannula as a device to provide continuous positive airway pressure in infants. *J Perinatol.* 2007;27(12):772–775

85. Volsko TA, Fedor K, Amadei J, Chatburn RL. High flow through a nasal cannula and CPAP effect in a simulated infant model. *Respir Care.* 2011;56(12):1893–1900

86. Ward JJ. High-flow oxygen administration by nasal cannula for adult and perinatal patients. *Respir Care.* 2013;58(1):98–122

87. Wilkinson DJ, Andersen CC, Smith K, Holberton J. Pharyngeal pressure with high-flow nasal cannulae in premature infants. *J Perinatol.* 2008;28(1):42–47

88. Ovalle O, Gomez T, Troncoso G, Palacios J, Ortiz E. High flow nasal cannula after surfactant treatment for infant respiratory distress syndrome in preterm infants < 30 weeks [abstr]. *E-PAS.* 2005;57:3417. Available at: www.abstracts2view.com/pasall/view.php?nu=PAS5L1_1804. Accessed February 10, 2015

89. Campbell DM, Shah PS, Shah V, Kelly EN. Nasal continuous positive airway pressure from high flow cannula versus Infant Flow for Preterm infants. *J Perinatol.* 2006;26(9):546–549

90. Collins CL, Holberton JR, Barfield C, Davis PG. A randomized controlled trial to compare heated humidified high-flow nasal cannulae with nasal continuous positive airway pressure postextubation in premature infants. *J Pediatr.* 2013;162(5):949–954

91. Joshi R, Rajhans A, Patil S, Dominic S, Phadtare R, Devaskar U. High flow oxygen in neonatal respiratory failure: is it better than CPAP? [abstr]. *E-PAS.* 2008;63:3768.11. Available at: www.abstracts2view.com/pasall/view.php?nu=PAS08L1_2027. Accessed February 10, 2015

92. Klingenberg C, Pettersen M, Hansen EA, et al. Patient comfort during treatment with heated humidified high flow nasal cannulae versus nasal continuous positive airway pressure: a randomised cross-over trial. *Arch Dis Child Fetal Neonatal Ed.* 2014;99(2):F134–F137

93. Lavizzari A, Ciuffini F, Colnaghi M, et al. High flow nasal cannula versus nasal CPAP in the management of respiratory distress syndrome: preliminary data [abstr]. *E-PAS.* 2013:4515.262. Available at: www.abstracts2view.com/pasall/view.php?nu=PAS13L1_4515.262. Accessed February 10, 2015

94. Manley BJ, Owen LS, Doyle LW, et al. High-flow nasal cannulae in very preterm infants after extubation. *N Engl J Med.* 2013;369(15):1425–1433

95. Nair G, Karna P. Comparison of the effects of Vapotherm and nasal CPAP in respiratory distress in preterm infants [abstr]. *E-PAS.* 2005;57:2054. Available at: www.abstracts2view.com/pasall/view.php?nu=PAS5L1_1667. Accessed February 10, 2015

96. Yoder BA, Stoddard RA, Li M, King J, Dirnberger DR, Abbasi S. Heated, humidified high-flow nasal cannula versus nasal CPAP for respiratory support in neonates. *Pediatrics.* 2013;131(5). Available at: www.pediatrics.org/cgi/content/full/131/5/e1482

97. Osman M, Elsharkawy A, Abdel-Hady H. Assessment of pain during application of nasal-continuous positive airway pressure and heated, humidified high-flow nasal cannulae in preterm infants. *J Perinatol.* 2015;35(4):263–267 10.1038/jp.2014.206

98. Stevens B, Johnston C, Petryshen P, Taddio A. Premature Infant Pain Profile: development and initial validation. *Clin J Pain.* 1996;12(1):13–22

99. Roberts CT, Manley BJ, Dawson JA, Davis PG. Nursing perceptions of high-flow nasal cannulae treatment for very preterm infants. *J Paediatr Child Health.* 2014;50(10):806–810

100. Wilkinson D, Andersen C, O'Donnell CP, De Paoli AG. High flow nasal cannula for respiratory support in preterm infants. *Cochrane Database Syst Rev.* 2011; (5):CD006405

101. Miller SM, Dowd SA. High-flow nasal cannula and extubation success in the premature infant: a comparison of two modalities. *J Perinatol.* 2010;30(12):805–808

102. Hegde S, Prodhan P. Serious air leak syndrome complicating high-flow nasal cannula therapy: a report of 3 cases. *Pediatrics.* 2013;131(3). Available at: www.pediatrics.org/cgi/content/full/131/3/e939

103. Jasin LR, Kern S, Thompson S, Walter C, Rone JM, Yohannan MD. Subcutaneous scalp emphysema, pneumo-orbitis and pneumocephalus in a neonate on high humidity high flow nasal cannula. *J Perinatol.* 2008;28(11):779–781

CLINICAL REPORT   Guidance for the Clinician in Rendering Pediatric Care

American Academy
of Pediatrics

DEDICATED TO THE HEALTH OF ALL CHILDREN™

Oxygen Targeting in Extremely Low Birth Weight Infants

James J. Cummings, MD, FAAP, Richard A. Polin, MD, FAAP, COMMITTEE ON FETUS AND NEWBORN

abstract

The use of supplemental oxygen plays a vital role in the care of the critically ill preterm infant, but the unrestricted use of oxygen can lead to unintended harms, such as chronic lung disease and retinopathy of prematurity. An overly restricted use of supplemental oxygen may have adverse effects as well. Ideally, continuous monitoring of tissue and cellular oxygen delivery would allow clinicians to better titrate the use of supplemental oxygen, but such monitoring is not currently feasible in the clinical setting. The introduction of pulse oximetry has greatly aided the clinician by providing a relatively easy and continuous estimate of arterial oxygen saturation, but pulse oximetry has several practical, technical, and physiologic limitations. Recent randomized clinical trials comparing different pulse oximetry targets have been conducted to better inform the practice of supplemental oxygen use. This clinical report discusses the benefits and limitations of pulse oximetry for assessing oxygenation, summarizes randomized clinical trials of oxygen saturation targeting, and addresses implications for practice.

Clinical reports from the American Academy of Pediatrics benefit from expertise and resources of liaisons and internal (AAP) and external reviewers. However, clinical reports from the American Academy of Pediatrics may not reflect the views of the liaisons or the organizations or government agencies that they represent.

The guidance in this report does not indicate an exclusive course of treatment or serve as a standard of medical care. Variations, taking into account individual circumstances, may be appropriate.

All clinical reports from the American Academy of Pediatrics automatically expire 5 years after publication unless reaffirmed, revised, or retired at or before that time.

DOI: 10.1542/peds.2016-1576

PEDIATRICS (ISSN Numbers: Print, 0031-4005; Online, 1098-4275).

INTRODUCTION

The discovery of oxygen is attributed to Polish scientist Michal Sędziwój in 1604, and a series of observations by John Mayow, Carl Wilhelm Scheele, and Joseph Priestley established the necessity of oxygen for life. In the early 1940s, Wilson et al[1] demonstrated that the use of 70% oxygen reduced periodic breathing in preterm infants. In 1949, investigators studying breathing irregularities in newborn infants recommended using 40% to 50% oxygen for all preterm infants immediately after birth for as long as 1 month.[2]

In 1951, two physicians, Kate Campbell in Melbourne, Australia, and Mary Crosse in Birmingham, England, suggested that unrestricted use of oxygen was associated with an increased risk of retrolental fibroplasia (now called retinopathy of prematurity [ROP]).[3,4] Several small clinical studies during the next few years confirmed this suggestion and recommended restricted use of supplemental oxygen.[5–9] In those studies, there was a trend toward increased mortality in the oxygen-restricted

To cite: Cummings JJ, Polin RA, AAP COMMITTEE ON FETUS AND NEWBORN. Oxygen Targeting in Extremely Low Birth Weight Infants. *Pediatrics.* 2016;138(2):e20161576

infants, although it did not reach statistical significance.[5-7,9] Therefore, restricted oxygen use in preterm infants gained general acceptance, despite estimates of 16 additional deaths for every case of blindness prevented.[10]

Because measurement of arterial oxygen tension was not yet feasible clinically, none of the earlier studies of oxygen supplementation and ROP were able to correlate measures of blood or tissue oxygenation with increased risk of ROP. In 1977, a large, 5-center, prospective observational study could not demonstrate a correlation between high partial pressure of oxygen in arterial blood (Pao_2) and ROP but did find a strong association of ROP with cumulative supplemental oxygen exposure.[11] In 1987, a small randomized study of transcutaneous oxygen monitoring in infants with a birth weight <1300 g found a significantly lower rate of ROP in infants who were managed with continuous oxygenation measures versus standard intermittent oxygenation assessment.[12]

In the ensuing decades, numerous observational studies have indicated that the incidence of ROP and bronchopulmonary dysplasia could be reduced by restricted use of oxygen. In 2007, the *Guidelines for Perinatal Care* recommended an oxygen saturation range of 85% to 95%.[13] Recently completed randomized trials using nearly identical trial designs have now provided additional evidence regarding the effects of varying saturation targets in the NICU. The present clinical report discusses the benefits and limitations of pulse oximetry for assessing oxygenation, summarizes randomized clinical trials of oxygen saturation targeting, and addresses implications for practice.

PULSE OXIMETRY: ITS USES AND LIMITATIONS IN MONITORING OXYGEN DELIVERY

Principles of Pulse Oximetry

Pulse oximeters measure the differential absorption of red and infrared light by oxyhemoglobin and deoxyhemoglobin. In neonates and young infants, light is transmitted through a distal extremity and sensed by a detector placed on the opposite side of the extremity. Pulsatile blood flow results in fluctuations in blood volume, thereby changing the distance the light has to travel. Detecting this variable component of light transmission allows pulse oximeters to eliminate signals attributable to nonarterial blood elements, such as venous blood, skin, connective tissue, muscle, and bone, directly measuring the relative amounts of oxyhemoglobin and deoxyhemoglobin in arterial blood and reporting saturation (Spo_2).

Limitations of Pulse Oximetry for Monitoring Tissue Oxygenation

Device Limitations

Accuracy. The accuracy of pulse oximetry is determined by comparison of Spo_2 with the measured saturation of arterial blood (Sao_2). Most manufacturers report an SD of the difference between Spo_2 and actual Sao_2 of 3 points for neonates. However, because 1 SD on each side of the mean includes approximately 68% of the measurements, nearly one-third of the measurements will fall outside that range. For example, an Spo_2 reading of 88% could reflect an actual Sao_2 between 85% and 91% in 68% of infants but may fall outside a range of 82% to 94% in up to 5% of infants.

The accuracy of pulse oximetry also depends on the range of saturations being measured. Reports of increased inaccuracy at the lower ranges of saturation values commonly encountered in the NICU are of great concern. For oximetry saturation readings in the 85% to 89% range, early studies reported that actual arterial saturations were as much as 10 points lower.[14,15] These findings have been confirmed in the most recently developed devices using signal extraction technology to reduce motion artifact; in 1 study, 39% of oximeter readings in the 85% to 89% range had arterial saturations below that range, with 25% of those readings having an actual Sao_2 <80%.[16] This finding is consistent with a previous observation that using an 85% to 89% Spo_2 range resulted in Pao_2 values much lower than expected.[17] In addition, pulse oximeters are only calibrated down to 80%; saturations below this level are extrapolated and may therefore be subject to even greater error.

Averaging Times. Pulse oximeters do not give instantaneous readings of Spo_2 because aberrant signals can make the device response erratic. Modern devices use time-averaging (typically, from 2–16 seconds) over several heartbeats to smooth out the displayed readings. In general, longer averaging times result in a more stable value with fewer false alarms; however, longer averaging times are also less sensitive to brief deviations in saturation outside the targeted range. Longer averaging times not only reduce the detection of desaturations that are either brief (<30 seconds) or marked (<70%) but also overestimate the duration of some detected events by combining 2 or more shorter events.[18,19] Shorter averaging time will detect more events but result in more false alarms. Studies have not been able to demonstrate that averaging times alter the amount of time actually spent outside targeted ranges. However, a particular concern is the potential for delayed detection of hypoxemic events.

Pulse Oximeter Algorithms. Pulse oximeters do not measure oxygen saturation directly but derive

Spo_2 from an internal reference table generated from empirical measurements of Sao_2 in healthy adult subjects. No pulse oximeter uses calibration data derived from Sao_2 measurements in critically ill patients or even in well infants. Although the effect of age on pulse oximeter accuracy has not been studied, at least 1 study has shown that in critically ill adult patients, changes in Spo_2 tend to overestimate actual changes in Sao_2, and this discrepancy worsened with decreasing hemoglobin concentrations.[20]

Relationship Between Sao_2 and Pao_2

Oxygen delivery depends on 2 factors: oxygen content of the arterial blood and blood flow. Oxygen content is determined by hemoglobin-oxygen saturation and, to a much lesser extent, by dissolved oxygen; both hemoglobin saturation and dissolved content depend on the prevailing Pao_2. Although the relationship between Sao_2 and Pao_2 is reasonably linear at Sao_2 values <80%, the slope of that relationship changes at Sao_2 levels >80%, resulting in large changes in Pao_2 with small changes in Sao_2. This relationship is even more exaggerated in the presence of hemoglobin F, which shifts the oxyhemoglobin dissociation curve to the left. Given that Spo_2 is, at best, an estimate of Sao_2, Spo_2 measurements become poor predictors of actual Pao_2 levels, particularly when the infant is receiving supplemental oxygen.

Fetal Versus Adult Hemoglobin

Absent a history of intrauterine transfusion, all extremely low birth weight neonates have high concentrations (>95%) of hemoglobin F in their blood. Hemoglobin F has a higher affinity for oxygen than does hemoglobin A and enhances tissue oxygen delivery at lower Sao_2 levels. As the amount of hemoglobin A relative to hemoglobin F increases in the blood (eg, after a red blood cell transfusion), this ability diminishes. Because the absorption spectrum for hemoglobin F is similar to hemoglobin A, there is no effect on the correlation between Spo_2 and Sao_2.

Clinical Variables Affecting Oxygen Saturation Targeting

Few studies have examined ways to best target a specific oxygen saturation range in preterm infants. Manually maintaining oxygen saturation targets in a given range depends on several factors, including: (1) technology (ie, setting Spo_2 alarm limits); (2) personnel (bedside nurses); and (3) the clinical stability of the patient. Although automated, closed-loop systems of oxygen delivery have been developed, they are not approved for clinical use in the United States.[21]

Alarm Limits

Alarm limits must be distinguished from targets. Targets represent the clinical goal, and alarm limits are used to achieve that goal. In clinical practice, alarm limits typically are set at or slightly beyond the target range. Some monitoring systems allow the use of "alerts" or "soft" alarms, which are less disruptive (being either visual, or at a lower volume or frequency) but warn that a parameter is about to reach an alarm limit. In these cases, the alerts are set within the targets, and the alarm limits may be set wider.

From a human engineering perspective, there are 2 problems with the setting of alarm limits. First, the majority of alarms do not require intervention. Most are either false (eg, a displaced probe or electrode) or are so brief that an intervention is not required. Second, the sheer number of alarms that go off in a busy NICU in a single day can total in the thousands, leading to desensitization. Both issues can lead to disregard of alarms, either deliberately or unintentionally; this condition has been termed "alarm fatigue" and is one reason why providers change alarm limits from those ordered. Clucas et al[22] observed that in infants weighing <1500 g, the lower alarm limit was set correctly 91% of the time, but the upper alarm limit was set correctly only 23% of the time. This differential compliance with low versus high alarms could be attributable to an increased tendency for the high alarm limit to be reached, the assumption that hypoxemia is more detrimental than hyperoxemia, and/or the fact that many monitors automatically reset to a high alarm limit of 100% when first turned on.[23]

A balance must be struck between setting alarm limits too narrow (increasing the number of unnecessary alarms) or too wide (decreasing the safety margin for intervention). Studies have shown that matching the alarm limits with the target range is associated with more time spent within the target range.[24,25]

Personnel

In the multicenter COT (Canadian Oxygen Trial), study participants were maintained within the intended Spo_2 range between 68% and 79% of the time. Nurses from one of the centers identified several factors as important in targeting a specific saturation range, including: (1) education; (2) prompt response times; and (3) a favorable nurse-to-patient ratio.[26] Targets in the Canadian trial were achieved significantly more often than in other randomized studies,[25,27] even though those studies also used educational interventions and process algorithms.[24,28] Even in studies in which favorable nurse-to-patient ratios were believed to exist, infants spent 33% to 38% of the time outside their target ranges.[20,25] Maintaining infants in a given target range is an extremely labor-intensive process, as evidenced by studies showing that multiple manual adjustments per hour only achieved target ranges approximately 50% of the time.[29] Using a fully automated oxygen-controlling system improved targeting by 7% over manual control.[30]

An additional concern is that manual documentation of hyperoxemic and hypoxemic episodes results in significant underreporting of such events.[31,32] Better tracking of saturation targeting can be accomplished by using third-party data extraction technology[33] or by using the histogram feature available on some monitoring equipment.[27,34]

Stability of the Saturation Signal in Clinical Settings

Preterm infants who require respiratory support are at increased risk of straying outside desired oxygen saturation targets, particularly if they are receiving supplemental oxygen. Because these infants often have desaturations during routine care (eg, repositioning, feeding, suctioning), it was once common practice to increase supplemental oxygen just before delivering such care (ie, preoxygenation). Preoxygenation also has been used commonly during intubation or other invasive procedures. Such practices may be harmful.[35] Instead, oxygen saturation values should be monitored closely, with measures to increase oxygenation used only as needed to maintain Spo_2 within the target range.

RANDOMIZED CLINICAL TRIALS OF OXYGEN TARGETING

The optimal saturation range for preterm infants in the NICU has remained elusive for more than 70 years. Although studies performed more than 50 years ago suggested an increased mortality associated with restricted oxygen administration,[36] observational trials performed in the era of continuous Spo_2

monitoring suggest that mortality is unchanged, with target Spo_2 ranges as low as 70%.[37] In addition, data from the Vermont Oxford Network indicate that the incidences of ROP and bronchopulmonary dysplasia are lower when a lower oxygen saturation range is targeted.[38] However, because these were observational studies, no cause-and-effect relationship can be inferred.

The first published randomized controlled trial (RCT) of differential targeting of oxygen saturations was the STOP-ROP (Supplemental Therapeutic Oxygen for Prethreshold Retinopathy of Prematurity) trial, published in 2000.[39] This study randomized infants to treatment when they reached "prethreshold" ROP, at an average postnatal age of 10 weeks. In this multicenter trial, 649 infants with prethreshold ROP were randomized to a saturation range of 89% to 94% (conventional arm) or 96% to 99% (supplemental arm). Progression to threshold ROP was not significantly different between groups in the total population; however, significant benefit was observed for infants in the high oxygen saturation arm who did not have "plus disease" (abnormal dilation and tortuosity of posterior pole blood vessels). On the negative side, infants in the high-oxygen saturation arm experienced an increased length of supplemental oxygen therapy and more often received diuretics at 50 weeks' postmenstrual age.

A second RCT that randomized infants to treatment at a later postnatal age was the BOOST (Benefits of Oxygen Saturation Targeting) trial ($N = 358$ infants), which hypothesized that maintaining higher oxygen saturation target ranges (95%–98% vs 93%–96%) would improve growth and neurodevelopmental outcomes.[40] The pulse oximeters in both groups were modified to read a targeted value in the range of 93% to 96%.

The study reported no benefit to the higher saturation range but did find, similar to the STOP-ROP trial, that infants in the high-saturation arm had significant increases in length of oxygen therapy, supplemental oxygen at 36 weeks' corrected gestation, and home oxygen.

In 2003, an international meeting of clinical trials experts, statisticians, neonatologists, ophthalmologists, and developmental pediatricians was convened to harmonize the planned RCTs of different target saturation ranges to be able to conduct a prospective individual patient meta-analysis of the data after completion of the follow-up phase of the individual trials (NeOProM [Neonatal Oxygenation Prospective Meta-analysis]).[41] Investigators from all 3 planned studies agreed, including SUPPORT (Surfactant Positive Airway Pressure and Pulse Oximetry Trial), sponsored by the *Eunice Kennedy Shriver* National Institute for Child Health and Human Development; the BOOST-II United Kingdom, Australia, and New Zealand study groups; and the COT trial. Although there were small differences in study design and outcome measures (Table 1), the studies were similar in terms of the population enrolled, methods, interventions tested, and outcomes collected. All studies were masked by the use of pulse oximeters that read 3% above or below the infant's actual saturation value within the 85% to 95% range. Outside the range of study saturation values ($\leq$84% and $\geq$96%), true saturation values were displayed. The primary outcome of the NeOProM study was a composite of death or disability at 18 to 24 months of corrected age. It was estimated that 5000 infants would be needed to detect a 4% difference in the rate of death or disability.[42]

The first of these 3 RCTs to be published was SUPPORT.[43] In this study, infants between 24[0/7] weeks' and 27[6/7] weeks' gestational age

TABLE 1 RCTs of Differing Pulse Oximetry Targets

Study	Primary Outcome	Primary Outcome Results	Other Findings
STOP-ROP[39]	Rate of progression to threshold ROP (89%–94% vs 96%–99%) $N = 649$	No significant differences	• Higher saturation range exhibited worsening of chronic lung disease and longer duration of hospitalization
BOOST[40]	Growth and developmental outcomes (91%–94% vs 95%–98%) $N = 358$	No significant differences	• Higher saturation range required oxygen for a longer period of time, dependence on oxygen at 36 wk postmenstrual age, and need for home oxygen
SUPPORT[43,44]	Death, severe ROP, or both (85%–89% vs 91%–95%) $N = 1316$	No significant differences	• Severe ROP significantly more common in the higher Sa_{O_2} range • Increased mortality in the lower Sa_{O_2} range at 18–22 mo of corrected age • No significant difference in the composite outcome of death or neurodevelopmental impairment at 18–22 mo
BOOST II[45–48]	Death or neurodevelopmental impairment at 18–22 mo of corrected for prematurity (85%–89% vs 91%–95%) $N = 2448$	No significant differences in a pooled analysis of all 3 trials[47] No significant difference in individual trial analyses[46,48] In a post hoc analysis combining 2 of the 3 trials, the primary outcome occurred in 492 (48.1%) of 1022 in the lower target group versus 437 (43.1%) of 1013 in the higher target group (RR, 1.11 [95% CI, 1.01–1.23]; $P = .023$)[46]	• Change in oximeter algorithm during the study • Study stopped before complete enrollment • Severe ROP significantly more common in the higher Sa_{O_2} range • Significantly increased necrotizing enterocolitis at the lower saturation range • Significantly increased mortality at hospital discharge in the lower Sa_{O_2} range with the revised oximeter algorithm
COT[49]	Death before a corrected age of 18 mo or survival with ≥1 of the following: gross motor disability, cognitive or language delay, severe hearing loss, and bilateral blindness (85%–89% vs 91%–95%) $N = 1201$	No significant differences	• Change in oximeter algorithm during the study • No difference in mortality • Targeting the lower saturation range reduced the postmenstrual age at last use of oxygen therapy

COT, Canadian Oxygen Trial; BOOST, Benefits of Oxygen Saturation Targeting; STOP, Supplemental Therapeutic Oxygen for Prethreshold Retinopathy of Prematurity; SUPPORT, Surfactant Positive Airway Pressure and Pulse Oximetry Trial.

($N = 1316$) were randomized to the 2 different oxygen saturation ranges (85%–89% or 91%–95%) and also to either CPAP or intubation and surfactant, in a factorial design. Oxygen saturation targeting was initiated within 2 hours of birth. The primary outcome was a composite of severe ROP (defined as the presence of threshold retinopathy, need for surgical intervention, or the use of bevacizumab), death before discharge from the hospital, or both. The oximeters in SUPPORT used an older software algorithm that subsequently was updated for the other RCTs.

The composite primary outcome in SUPPORT did not differ significantly between the lower and the higher oxygen saturation groups (28.3% vs 32.1%; relative risk [RR], 0.90; 95% confidence interval [CI], 0.76–1.06). However, death before discharge from the NICU was significantly different, occurring in 19.9% of infants in the lower oxygen saturation group and 16.2% of infants in the higher oxygen saturation group (RR, 1.27; 95% CI, 1.01–1.60), with a number-needed-to-harm of 27. In contrast, the rate of severe ROP among survivors was 8.6% in the lower saturation group versus 17.9% in the higher saturation group (RR, 0.52 [95% CI, 0.37–0.73]), with a number-needed-to-benefit of 11.

At 18 to 22 months of corrected age, death or neurodevelopmental impairment occurred in 30.2% of infants in the lower oxygen saturation group and 27.5% of those in the higher oxygen saturation group (RR, 1.12 [95% CI, 0.94–1.32]).[44] Mortality remained significantly higher in the lower oxygen saturation group (22.1% vs 18.2%; RR, 1.25 [95% CI, 1.00–1.25]). No significant differences were detected in neurodevelopmental impairment, cerebral palsy, or blindness.

The next RCT published was BOOST-II, from the United Kingdom, Australia, and New Zealand.[45] Oxygen saturation targeting began in the first

24 hours of life but not as early as in the SUPPORT study. During these trials, investigators in the United Kingdom found that the standard oximeters (Masimo Corporation, Irvine, California) returned an unexpectedly low number of oxygen saturation values between 87% and 90%. They discovered that there was a shift-up in the oximeter calibration curve that caused values between 87% and 90% to read 1% to 2% higher. A new software algorithm was expected to improve oxygen saturation targeting, although that was not tested. The United Kingdom and Australian investigators began using oximeters with the new software approximately halfway through the trial. However, the New Zealand trial oximeters were not modified, because enrollment had already been completed. Of 2448 infants enrolled in BOOST-II, 1187 (48.5%) were monitored with oximeters incorporating the new software.

Because of the increased mortality in the lower oxygen saturation range in SUPPORT, the BOOST-II Data Safety and Monitoring Board conducted a safety analysis in December 2010.[50] In the 1187 infants monitored with the revised algorithm, those assigned to the lower target range had a significantly increased mortality rate at 36 weeks' gestational age (23.1% vs 15.9%; RR, 1.45 [95% CI, 1.15–1.84]). However, among the entire study population (N = 2448), there was no significant difference. The rate of ROP requiring treatment was reduced in the lower saturation group (10.6% vs 13.5%; RR, 0.79 [95% CI, 0.63–1.00]), and the rate of necrotizing enterocolitis requiring surgery or causing death was increased in that group (10.4% vs 8.0%; RR, 1.32 [95% CI, 1.02–1.68]). The rate of bronchopulmonary dysplasia was unaffected. Although a recent report combining outcomes for 2 of the 3 BOOST-II sites found a significant difference in the composite outcome of death or disability by 2 years of age in a post hoc analysis,[46] a pooled analysis from all 3 BOOST-II sites, as originally planned, showed no significant difference in this outcome between the 2 arms (46.8% in the lower vs 43.4% in the higher saturation group; P = .10).[47]

Two-year outcomes for the COT were published.[49] The primary outcome measure for this study was the rate of death (before 18 months of age) or survival with 1 or more disabilities (gross motor disability, severe hearing loss, bilateral blindness, and cognitive or language delay). Infants were randomly assigned to the lower saturation group or higher saturation group in the first 24 hours of life. Similar to BOOST-II, the calibration software for the oximeter was changed at the midpoint in the study. The number of infants enrolled was 1201, of whom 538 were monitored with oximeters using the new software. There was no difference in the primary composite outcome (51.6% in the lower vs 49.7% in the higher saturation range). Mortality was 16.6% in the 85% to 89% group and 15.3% in the 91% to 95% group. Infants in the lower saturation group had a shorter duration of supplemental oxygen but no changes in any other outcomes. Use of the revised oximeter software had no effect on the primary outcome or mortality.

Saugstad and Aune[51] published a systematic review of the 5 oxygen saturation trials. In total, 4911 infants were enrolled in the studies. At the time of this meta-analysis (in 2014), the composite outcome of death or severe neurosensory disability at 18 to 24 months of age was only available for SUPPORT and COT, and there was no difference in that composite outcome between groups. The RR of mortality using the original software in the BOOST-II and COT trials was 1.04 (95% CI, 0.88–1.22).

With the revised software (COT and BOOST-II United Kingdom and Australia), the RR of mortality in the lower saturation arm was 1.41 (95% CI, 1.14–1.74). For all 5 trials (SUPPORT; BOOST-II United Kingdom, Australia, and New Zealand; and COT), the risk of mortality was increased (RR, 1.18 [95% CI, 1.04–1.34]). Severe ROP was significantly reduced in the low saturation group (RR, 0.74 [95% CI, 0.59–0.92]), and the risk of necrotizing enterocolitis was increased (RR, 1.25 [95% CI, 1.05–1.49]). The rates of bronchopulmonary dysplasia, patent ductus arteriosus, and intraventricular hemorrhage grades 2 through 4 were not significantly different.

A more recent systematic review[52] of the 5 oxygen saturation trials concluded that although infants randomly assigned to the more liberal oxygen target ranges had higher survival rates (relative effect, 1.18 [95% CI, 1.03–1.36]) to discharge, the quality of evidence (assessed by using the Grading of Recommendations Assessment, Development and Evaluation approach[53]) for this estimate of effect was low for 1 or more of the following reasons: (1) the pulse oximeter algorithm was modified partway into the study; (2) the distribution of Spo_2 values did not achieve the planned degree of separation (the median Spo_2 in the 85% to 89% groups was >90%); (3) the BOOST-II trials were stopped prematurely on the basis of this outcome; and (4) the COT trial did not report on this outcome explicitly. In addition, although the investigators noted that necrotizing enterocolitis occurred less frequently in the higher saturation arms, there were no significant differences in bronchopulmonary dysplasia, ROP, hearing loss, or death or disability at 24 months of age.[52]

The mechanism(s) by which maintaining lower oxygen saturation levels might increase the risk of death is unclear, as the data from these trials suggest that tissue hypoxia was unlikely to be a factor.[23] In particular, in the SUPPORT trial, the proportion of infants with median oxygen saturations <85% was no different between the low and high saturation groups.[43] Conversely, a post hoc analysis from the SUPPORT trial found a disproportionally higher mortality rate in small-for-gestational-age infants in the lower oxygen saturation target group, suggesting a possible interaction[54]; if this observation can be confirmed in the other oxygen saturation trials, and more importantly in the individual patient analysis, it would suggest that small-for-gestational-age infants may be more vulnerable to lower oxygen saturations.

In the 5 RCTs discussed in this report, the degree to which individual infants may have been harmed or benefited by the oxygen saturation targets to which they were assigned is not clear.[55] Specifically, it would be helpful to know whether an individual infant's outcome correlated with the amount of time he or she spent within, above, or below the target oxygen saturation range. This information is particularly relevant to ROP because avoiding hypoxemic episodes may be as important as avoiding hyperoxemic episodes.[56–59] The preplanned individual patient meta-analysis of these trials (NeOProM) may shed some light on these critical questions.

CONCLUSIONS

Establishing a target range for oxygen saturation in infants of extremely low birth weight has both clinical and practical considerations, and the ideal target range remains an elusive goal. Nevertheless, data from several well-designed RCTs can inform practice. Pending additional data, including the individual patient meta-analysis (NeOProM), the following can be concluded:

1. The ideal physiologic target range for oxygen saturation for infants of extremely low birth weight is likely patient-specific and dynamic and depends on various factors, including gestational age, chronologic age, underlying disease, and transfusion status.

2. The ideal physiologic target range is a compromise among negative outcomes associated with either hyperoxemia (eg, ROP, bronchopulmonary dysplasia) or hypoxemia (eg, necrotizing enterocolitis, cerebral palsy, death). Recent RCTs suggest that a targeted oxygen saturation range of 90% to 95% may be safer than 85% to 89%, at least for some infants. However, the ideal oxygen saturation range for extremely low birth weight infants remains unknown.

3. Alarm limits are used to avoid potentially harmful extremes of hyperoxemia or hypoxemia. Given the limitations of pulse oximetry and the uncertainty that remains regarding the ideal oxygen saturation target range for infants of extremely low birth weight, these alarm limits could be fairly wide. Regardless of the chosen target, an upper alarm limit approximately 95% while the infant remains on supplemental oxygen is reasonable. A lower alarm limit will generally need to extend somewhat below the lower target, as it must take into account practical and clinical considerations, as well as the steepness of the oxygen saturation curve at lower saturations.

LEAD AUTHORS

James J. Cummings, MD, FAAP
Richard A. Polin, MD, FAAP

COMMITTEE ON FETUS AND NEWBORN, 2014–2015

Kristi L. Watterberg, MD, FAAP, Chairperson
Brenda Poindexter, MD, FAAP
James J. Cummings, MD, FAAP
William E. Benitz, MD, FAAP
Eric C. Eichenwald, MD, FAAP
Brenda B. Poindexter, MD, FAAP
Dan L. Stewart, MD, FAAP
Susan W. Aucott, MD, FAAP
Jay P. Goldsmith, MD, FAAP
Karen M. Puopolo, MD, PhD, FAAP
Kasper S. Wang, MD, FAAP

PAST COMMITTEE MEMBERS

Richard A. Polin, MD, FAAP
Waldemar A. Carlo, MD, FAAP

CONSULTANT

Waldemar A. Carlo, MD, FAAP

LIAISONS

Tonse N.K. Raju, MD, DCH, FAAP – *National Institutes of Health*
CAPT Wanda D. Barfield, MD, MPH, FAAP – *Centers for Disease Control and Prevention*
Erin L. Keels, APRN, MS, NNP-BC – *National Association of Neonatal Nurses*
Thierry Lacaze, MD – *Canadian Paediatric Society*
James Goldberg, MD – *American College of Obstetricians and Gynecologists*

STAFF

Jim R. Couto, MA

ABBREVIATIONS

CI: confidence interval
Pao_2: partial pressure of oxygen in arterial blood
ROP: retinopathy of prematurity
RR: relative risk
Sao_2: measured saturation of arterial blood
Spo_2: pulse oxygen saturation

FINANCIAL DISCLOSURE: The authors have indicated they do not have a financial relationship relevant to this article to disclose.

FUNDING: No external funding.

POTENTIAL CONFLICTS OF INTEREST: Dr Cummings is a consultant for ONY, Inc and Windtree Therapeutics (formerly Discovery Laboratories). Dr Polin is a consultant for Windtree Therapeutics and Fisher & Paykel.

REFERENCES

1. Wilson J, Long S, Howard P. Respiration of premature infants: response to variations of oxygen and to increased carbon dioxide in inspired air. *Am J Dis Child.* 1942;63(6):1080–1085

2. Howard PJ, Bauer AR. Irregularities of breathing in the newborn period. *Am J Dis Child.* 1949;77(5):592–609

3. Campbell K. Intensive oxygen therapy as a possible cause of retrolental fibroplasia; a clinical approach. *Med J Aust.* 1951;2(2):48–50

4. Crosse V. The problem of retrolental fibroplasia in the city of Birmingham. *Trans Ophthalmol Soc U K.* 1951;71:609–612

5. Lanman JT, Guy LP, Dancis J. Retrolental fibroplasia and oxygen therapy. *J Am Med Assoc.* 1954;155(3):223–226

6. Engle MA, Baker DH, Baras I, Freemond A, Laupus WE, Norton EW. Oxygen administration and retrolental fibroplasia. *AMA Am J Dis Child.* 1955;89(4):399–413

7. Kinsey VE. Retrolental fibroplasia; cooperative study of retrolental fibroplasia and the use of oxygen. *AMA Arch Opthalmol.* 1956;56(4):481–543

8. Patz A, Hoeck LE, De La Cruz E. Studies on the effect of high oxygen administration in retrolental fibroplasia. I. Nursery observations. *Am J Ophthalmol.* 1952;35(9):1248–1253

9. Weintraub DH, Tabankin A. Relationship of retrolental fibroplasia to oxygen concentration. *J Pediatr.* 1956;49(1):75–79

10. Bolton DP, Cross KW. Further observations on cost of preventing retrolental fibroplasia. *Lancet.* 1974;1(7855):445–448

11. Kinsey VE, Arnold HJ, Kalina RE, et al. PaO2 levels and retrolental fibroplasia: a report of the cooperative study. *Pediatrics.* 1977;60(5):655–668

12. Bancalari E, Flynn J, Goldberg RN, et al. Transcutaneous oxygen monitoring and retinopathy of prematurity. *Adv Exp Med Biol.* 1987;220:109–113

13. American Academy of Pediatrics and the American College of Obstetricians and Gynecologists. *Guidelines for Perinatal Care.* 6th ed. Elk Grove Village, IL: American Academy of Pediatrics; 2007

14. Brockway J, Hay WW Jr. Prediction of arterial partial pressure of oxygen with pulse oxygen saturation measurements. *J Pediatr.* 1998;133(1):63–66

15. Workie FA, Rais-Bahrami K, Short BL. Clinical use of new-generation pulse oximeters in the neonatal intensive care unit. *Am J Perinatol.* 2005;22(7):357–360

16. Rosychuk RJ, Hudson-Mason A, Eklund D, Lacaze-Masmonteil T. Discrepancies between arterial oxygen saturation and functional oxygen saturation measured with pulse oximetry in very preterm infants. *Neonatology.* 2012;101(1):14–19

17. Quine D, Stenson BJ. Arterial oxygen tension (Pao2) values in infants <29 weeks of gestation at currently targeted saturations. *Arch Dis Child Fetal Neonatal Ed.* 2009;94(1):F51–F53

18. Ahmed SJ, Rich W, Finer NN. The effect of averaging time on oximetry values in the premature infant. *Pediatrics.* 2010;125(1). Available at: www.pediatrics.org/cgi/content/full/125/1/e115

19. Vagedes J, Poets CF, Dietz K. Averaging time, desaturation level, duration and extent. *Arch Dis Child Fetal Neonatal Ed.* 2013;98(3):F265–F266

20. Perkins GD, McAuley DF, Giles S, Routledge H, Gao F. Do changes in pulse oximeter oxygen saturation predict equivalent changes in arterial oxygen saturation? *Crit Care.* 2003;7(4):R67

21. Claure N, Bancalari E. Automated closed loop control of inspired oxygen concentration. *Respir Care.* 2013;58(1):151–161

22. Clucas L, Doyle LW, Dawson J, Donath S, Davis PG. Compliance with alarm limits for pulse oximetry in

very preterm infants. *Pediatrics.* 2007;119(6):1056–1060

23. Sola A, Golombek SG, Montes Bueno MT, et al. Safe oxygen saturation targeting and monitoring in preterm infants: can we avoid hypoxia and hyperoxia? *Acta Paediatr.* 2014;103(10):1009–1018

24. Clarke A, Yeomans E, Elsayed K, et al. A randomised crossover trial of clinical algorithm for oxygen saturation targeting in preterm infants with frequent desaturation episodes. *Neonatology.* 2015;107(2):130–136

25. Hagadorn JI, Furey AM, Nghiem TH, et al; AVIOx Study Group. Achieved versus intended pulse oximeter saturation in infants born less than 28 weeks' gestation: the AVIOx study. *Pediatrics.* 2006;118(4):1574–1582

26. Armbruster J, Schmidt B, Poets CF, Bassler D. Nurses' compliance with alarm limits for pulse oximetry: qualitative study. *J Perinatol.* 2010;30(8):531–534

27. Lim K, Wheeler KI, Gale TJ, et al. Oxygen saturation targeting in preterm infants receiving continuous positive airway pressure. *J Pediatr.* 2014;164(4):730–736.e1

28. Ford SP, Leick-Rude MK, Meinert KA, et al. Overcoming barriers to oxygen saturation targeting. *Pediatrics.* 2006;118(suppl 2):S177–S186

29. van der Eijk AC, Dankelman J, Schutte S, Simonsz HJ, Smit BJ. An observational study to quantify manual adjustments of the inspired oxygen fraction in extremely low birth weight infants. *Acta Paediatr.* 2012;101(3):e97–e104

30. Waitz M, Schmid MB, Fuchs H, Mendler MR, Dreyhaupt J, Hummler HD. Effects of automated adjustment of the inspired oxygen on fluctuations of arterial and regional cerebral tissue oxygenation in preterm infants with frequent desaturations. *J Pediatr.* 2015;166(2):240–244.e1

31. Brockmann PE, Wiechers C, Pantalitschka T, Diebold J, Vagedes J, Poets CF. Under-recognition of

alarms in a neonatal intensive care unit. *Arch Dis Child Fetal Neonatal Ed.* 2013;98(6):F524–F527

32. Ruiz TL, Trzaski JM, Sink DW, Hagadorn JI. Transcribed oxygen saturation vs oximeter recordings in very low birth weight infants. *J Perinatol.* 2014;34(2):130–135

33. Cirelli J, McGregor C, Graydon B, James A. Analysis of continuous oxygen saturation data for accurate representation of retinal exposure to oxygen in the preterm infant. *Stud Health Technol Inform.* 2013;183:126–131

34. Bizzarro MJ, Li FY, Katz K, Shabanova V, Ehrenkranz RA, Bhandari V. Temporal quantification of oxygen saturation ranges: an effort to reduce hyperoxia in the neonatal intensive care unit. *J Perinatol.* 2014;34(1):33–38

35. Sola A, Saldeño YP, Favareto V. Clinical practices in neonatal oxygenation: where have we failed? What can we do? *J Perinatol.* 2008;28(suppl 1):S28–S34

36. Askie LM, Henderson-Smart DJ, Ko H. Restricted versus liberal oxygen exposure for preventing morbidity and mortality in preterm or low birth weight infants. *Cochrane Database Syst Rev.* 2009;(1):CD001077

37. Tin W, Milligan DW, Pennefather P, Hey E. Pulse oximetry, severe retinopathy, and outcome at one year in babies of less than 28 weeks gestation. *Arch Dis Child Fetal Neonatal Ed.* 2001;84(2):F106–F110

38. Payne NR, LaCorte M, Karna P, et al; Breathsavers Group, Vermont Oxford Network Neonatal Intensive Care Quality Improvement Collaborative. Reduction of bronchopulmonary dysplasia after participation in the Breathsavers Group of the Vermont Oxford Network Neonatal Intensive Care Quality Improvement Collaborative. *Pediatrics.* 2006;118(suppl 2):S73–S77

39. The STOP-ROP Multicenter Study Group. Supplemental Therapeutic Oxygen for Prethreshold Retinopathy of Prematurity (STOP-ROP), a randomized, controlled trial. I: primary outcomes. *Pediatrics.* 2000;105(2):295–310

40. Askie LM, Henderson-Smart DJ, Irwig L, Simpson JM. Oxygen-saturation targets and outcomes in extremely preterm infants. *N Engl J Med.* 2003;349(10):959–967

41. Cole CH, Wright KW, Tarnow-Mordi W, Phelps DL; Pulse Oximetry Saturation Trial for Prevention of Retinopathy of Prematurity Planning Study Group. Resolving our uncertainty about oxygen therapy. *Pediatrics.* 2003;112(6 pt 1):1415–1419

42. Askie LM, Brocklehurst P, Darlow BA, Finer N, Schmidt B, Tarnow-Mordi W; NeOProM Collaborative Group. NeOProM: Neonatal Oxygenation Prospective Meta-analysis Collaboration study protocol. *BMC Pediatr.* 2011;11(6):6

43. Carlo WA, Finer NN, Walsh MC, et al; SUPPORT Study Group of the Eunice Kennedy Shriver NICHD Neonatal Research Network. Target ranges of oxygen saturation in extremely preterm infants. *N Engl J Med.* 2010;362(21):1959–1969

44. Vaucher YE, Peralta-Carcelen M, Finer NN, et al; SUPPORT Study Group of the Eunice Kennedy Shriver NICHD Neonatal Research Network. Neurodevelopmental outcomes in the early CPAP and pulse oximetry trial. *N Engl J Med.* 2012;367(26):2495–2504

45. Stenson BJ, Tarnow-Mordi WO, Darlow BA, et al; BOOST II United Kingdom Collaborative Group; BOOST II Australia Collaborative Group; BOOST II New Zealand Collaborative Group. Oxygen saturation and outcomes in preterm infants. *N Engl J Med.* 2013;368(22):2094–2104

46. Tarnow-Mordi W, Stenson B, Kirby A, et al; BOOST-II Australia and United Kingdom Collaborative Groups. Outcomes of two trials of oxygen-saturation targets in preterm infants. *N Engl J Med.* 2016;374(8):749–760

47. Cummings JJ, Lakshminrusimha S, Polin RA. The BOOST trials and the pitfalls of post hoc analyses. *N Engl J Med.* 2016, In press

48. Darlow BA, Marschner SL, Donoghoe M, et al Randomized controlled trial of oxygen saturation targets in very preterm infants: two year outcomes. *J Pediatr.* 2014;165(1):30–35.e2

49. Schmidt B, Whyte RK, Asztalos EV, et al; Canadian Oxygen Trial (COT) Group. Effects of targeting higher vs lower arterial oxygen saturations on death or disability in extremely preterm infants: a randomized clinical trial. *JAMA.* 2013;309(20):2111–2120

50. Stenson B, Brocklehurst P, Tarnow-Mordi W; UK BOOST II trial; Australian BOOST II trial; New Zealand BOOST II trial. Increased 36-week survival with high oxygen saturation target in extremely preterm infants. *N Engl J Med.* 2011;364(17):1680–1682

51. Saugstad OD, Aune D. Optimal oxygenation of extremely low birth weight infants: a meta-analysis and systematic review of the oxygen saturation target studies. *Neonatology.* 2014;105(1):55–63

52. Manja V, Lakshminrusimha S, Cook DJ. Oxygen saturation target range for extremely preterm infants: a systematic review and meta-analysis. *JAMA Pediatr.* 2015;169(4):332–340

53. Guyatt GH, Oxman AD, Schünemann HJ, Tugwell P, Knottnerus A. GRADE guidelines: a new series of articles in the Journal of Clinical Epidemiology. *J Clin Epidemiol.* 2011;64(4):380–382

54. Walsh MC, Di Fiore JM, Martin RJ, Gantz M, Carlo WA, Finer N. Association of oxygen target and growth status with increased mortality in small for gestational age infants: further analysis of the Surfactant, Positive Pressure and Pulse Oximetry Randomized Trial. *JAMA Pediatr.* 2016;170(3):292–294

55. Bateman D, Polin RA. A lower oxygen-saturation target decreases retinopathy of prematurity but increases mortality in premature infants. *J Pediatr.* 2013;163(5):1528–1529

56. Thomas WJ, Rauser M, Dovich JA, Dustin L, Flaxel CJ. Oxygen saturation in premature infants at risk for threshold retinopathy of prematurity. *Eur J Ophthalmol.* 2011;21(2):189–193

57. Di Fiore JM, Bloom JN, Orge F, et al. A higher incidence of intermittent hypoxemic episodes is associated with severe retinopathy of prematurity. *J Pediatr.* 2010;157(1):69–73

58. Kaufman DA, Zanelli SA, Gurka MJ, Davis M, Richards CP, Walsh BK. Time outside targeted oxygen saturation range and retinopathy of prematurity. *Early Hum Dev.* 2014;90(suppl 2):S35–S40

59. York JR, Landers S, Kirby RS, Arbogast PG, Penn JS. Arterial oxygen fluctuation and retinopathy of prematurity in very-low-birth-weight infants. *J Perinatol.* 2004;24(2):82–87

ERRATA

Cummings JJ, Polin RA, COMMITTEE ON FETUS AND NEWBORN. Oxygen Targeting in Extremely Low Birth Weight Infants. *Pediatrics.* **2016;138(2):e20161576**

Errors occurred in the article by Cummings et al, titled "Oxygen Targeting in Extremely Low Birth Weight Infants" published in the August 2016 issue of *Pediatrics* (2016;138(2):e20161576; doi:10.1542/peds.2016-1576).

On page e6, under the section heading Randomized Clinical Trials of Oxygen Targeting, in paragraph 8, on lines 30-32, this reads: "a pooled analysis from all 3 BOOST-II sites, as originally planned, showed no significant difference in this outcome." This should have read: "a pooled analysis from all 3 BOOST-II sites showed no significant difference in this outcome."

On page e9, under References, reference # 47 reads: "Cummings JJ, Lakshminrusimha S, Polin RA. The BOOST trials and the pitfalls of post hoc analyses. *N Engl J Med* 2016, in press." This has been updated and should now read: "Cummings JJ, Lakshminrusimha S, Polin RA. Oxygen saturation targets in preterm infants [Letter to the Editor]. Reply: Tarnow-Mordi WO, Stenson B, Kirby A. *N Engl J Med* 2016;375(2):186-188."

doi:10.1542/peds.2016-2904

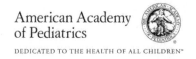

American Academy
of Pediatrics
DEDICATED TO THE HEALTH OF ALL CHILDREN™

Organizational Principles to Guide and Define the Child
Health Care System and/or Improve the Health of all Children

Policy Statement—Postnatal Corticosteroids to Prevent or Treat Bronchopulmonary Dysplasia

abstract

The purpose of this revised statement is to review current information on the use of postnatal glucocorticoids to prevent or treat bronchopulmonary dysplasia in the preterm infant and to make updated recommendations regarding their use. High-dose dexamethasone (0.5 mg/kg per day) does not seem to confer additional therapeutic benefit over lower doses and is not recommended. Evidence is insufficient to make a recommendation regarding other glucocorticoid doses and preparations. The clinician must use clinical judgment when attempting to balance the potential adverse effects of glucocorticoid treatment with those of bronchopulmonary dysplasia. *Pediatrics* 2010;126:800–808

INTRODUCTION

Chronic lung disease (CLD) after preterm birth, also known as bronchopulmonary dysplasia (BPD), a major morbidity of the very preterm infant, is remarkably resistant to therapeutic interventions and negatively affects neurodevelopmental outcomes.[1–4] In 2002, the American Academy of Pediatrics (AAP), in a policy statement regarding the use of postnatal corticosteroids for prevention or treatment of CLD in preterm infants, concluded that routine dexamethasone therapy for the prevention or treatment of CLD could not be recommended.[5] Instead, the AAP recommended that (1) use of dexamethasone for the prevention or treatment of CLD be limited to randomized, controlled trials (RCTs) with long-term follow-up, (2) alternative corticosteroids undergo further study, and (3) infants currently enrolled in RCTs of corticosteroids receive long-term neurodevelopmental follow-up. The statement added that outside the context of such trials, "the use of corticosteroids should be limited to exceptional clinical circumstances (eg, an infant on maximal ventilatory and oxygen support). In those circumstances, parents should be fully informed about the known short- and long-term risks and agree to treatment."[5]

Postnatal use of dexamethasone for BPD has decreased since the publication of the AAP statement; however, the incidence of BPD has not decreased.[6] Instead, several reports have suggested that the incidence or severity of BPD may have increased.[4,7,8] Moreover, results of additional clinical trials, meta-analyses, and follow-up studies have been published, warranting a review of the new information and revision of the statement. The objectives of this revised statement are to review data published since the 2002 AAP statement and to reexamine previous recommendations for the use of glucocorticoid therapy in view of new information.

COMMITTEE ON FETUS AND NEWBORN

KEY WORDS
bronchopulmonary dysplasia, preterm infant, glucocorticoid, dexamethasone, chronic lung disease

ABBREVIATIONS
CLD—chronic lung disease
BPD—bronchopulmonary dysplasia
AAP—American Academy of Pediatrics
RCT—randomized, controlled trial
CP—cerebral palsy

www.pediatrics.org/cgi/doi/10.1542/peds.2010-1534

doi:10.1542/peds.2010-1534

All policy statements from the American Academy of Pediatrics automatically expire 5 years after publication unless reaffirmed, revised, or retired at or before that time.

PEDIATRICS (ISSN Numbers: Print, 0031-4005; Online, 1098-4275).

LITERATURE REVIEW

Dexamethasone

Reviews and meta-analyses cited in the previous AAP statement indicated that dexamethasone may decrease mortality rates, facilitate extubation, and generally decrease the incidence of BPD but that it carries a significant risk for short- and long-term adverse effects, especially impairment of growth and neurodevelopment.[5,9–12] In recently updated systematic reviews, the Cochrane Collaboration continues to conclude that the benefits of dexamethasone therapy in the first week of life may not outweigh its many adverse effects.[13] In contrast, it concludes that treatment after the first postnatal week may reduce mortality rates without increasing adverse long-term neurodevelopmental outcomes, although long-term follow-up data remain limited.[14] Therefore, it has been suggested that "it appears prudent to reserve the

use of late corticosteroids to infants who cannot be weaned from mechanical ventilation and to minimize the dose and duration of any course of treatment."[14]

Two other systematic reviews have added different perspectives on dexamethasone and BPD. In the first review, a risk-weighted meta-analysis, the authors emphasized the importance of the a priori risk of death or BPD in different study populations.[15] In this analysis, the incidence of death or cerebral palsy (CP) was increased among dexamethasone-treated infants compared with placebo-treated infants in studies that enrolled patients at low risk (<35%) of BPD. In contrast, dexamethasone treatment decreased the risk of death or CP when infants at high risk of BPD (≥65%) were studied.[15] Thus, for infants at the highest risk of BPD, the beneficial effect of dexamethasone in reducing lung disease

seemed to outweigh its adverse effect of increasing the risk of CP. In the second meta-analysis, the authors compared outcomes for trials with different cumulative doses of dexamethasone and concluded that a higher cumulative dose improved rates of survival without BPD and did not increase adverse long-term effects.[16] However, 3 small individual RCTs that directly compared high versus low dexamethasone doses, variably defined, have revealed no differences in efficacy (Table 1).[17–19] These studies have generally been small and heterogeneous, which makes them difficult to compare.

The results of 3 RCTs that compared dexamethasone to placebo have been published since the previous AAP statement (Table 1); 1 was small and the other 2 were stopped early and are, therefore, underpowered.[20–22] One trial compared an early, short course

TABLE 1 RCTs of Dexamethasone to Prevent or Treat BPD Reported Since 2001

Study, No. of Centers	n	Eligibility Criteria (All on Mechanical Ventilation)	Dexamethasone Dosing Regimen	Outcome
McEvoy et al,[17] 1 center	62	500–1500 g BW; ≤32 wk gestation; 7–21 postnatal days	5 mg/kg per d tapered over 7 d vs 0.2 mg/kg tapered over 7 d	Rate of survival without BPD[a] 76% vs 73% (NS); no benefit to higher dose
Odd et al,[18] 1 center	33	≤1250 g BW; 1–3 wk of age	0.5 mg/kg per d tapered over 42 d vs "individualized" (same dose, shorter course)	Rate of survival without BPD: 24% vs 30% (NS); no difference in 18-mo outcomes
Malloy et al,[19] 1 center	16[b]	<1501 g BW; <34 wk gestation; <28 postnatal days	0.5 mg/kg per d tapered over 7 d vs 0.08 mg/kg per d for 7 d	Rate of survival without BPD: 11% vs 38% (NS); higher dose had more adverse effects, no apparent benefit
Walther et al,[20] 1 center	36	≥600 g BW; 24–32 wk gestation; 7–14 d postnatal age	0.2 mg/kg per d tapered over 14 d vs placebo	Rate of survival without BPD: 65% vs 47% (NS); extubation: 76% vs 42% (P < .05)
Anttila et al,[21] 6 centers	109[b]	500–999 g BW; ≤31 wk gestation; eligible at 4 h of age	0.25 mg/kg every 12 h × 4 doses vs placebo	Rate of survival without BPD: 58% vs 52% (NS)
Doyle et al,[22] 11 centers	70[b]	<1000 g BW; <28 wk gestation; >1 wk postnatal age	0.15 mg/kg per d tapered over 10 d vs placebo	Rate of survival without BPD: 14% vs 9% (NS); extubation: 60% vs 12% (odds ratio: 11.2 [95% confidence interval: 3.2–39.0])
Rozycki et al,[23] 1 center	61	650–2000 g BW; ≥ 14 d postnatal age	0.5 mg/kg per d tapered over 42 d vs inhaled beclomethasone at 3 different doses for 7 d followed by above-listed dexamethasone course, if still mechanically ventilated	Rate of survival without BPD: 53% vs 46% (NS); extubation by 7 d: 7 of 15 vs 6 of 46 (P < .01)

BW indicates birth weight; NS, not significant.
[a] BPD defined as receiving supplemental oxygen at 36 weeks postmenstrual age.
[b] Patient enrollment terminated early.

of dexamethasone to placebo and revealed no significant difference in mortality or BPD rates.[21] The other 2 trials evaluated the efficacy of a later, lower-dose course of dexamethasone for facilitating extubation, and the authors reported that significantly more dexamethasone-treated infants were successfully extubated during the treatment period.[20,22] Similar results were reported from an additional study that compared systemic dexamethasone to inhaled beclomethasone for extubation: significantly more dexamethasone-treated infants were successfully extubated within 7 days (Table 1).[23] These extubation trials were not powered to evaluate the effect of the treatment on rates of survival without BPD.

Many short-term adverse effects of dexamethasone therapy have been described; however, the main reason for the decline in its use is an adverse effect on neurodevelopment, particularly higher rates of CP. Since publication of the previous AAP statement, additional follow-up data on the adverse effects of dexamethasone have become available from RCTs (Table 2).[17,24–32] The heterogeneity of these reports makes it problematic to combine them meaningfully. Some studies revealed no adverse effects on neurodevelopmental outcomes at various ages, whereas others did. Most of the studies were small, which reduced their ability to either prove or disprove causation. Two RCTs that used low doses of dexamethasone revealed no significant increase in CP or other neurodevelopmental impairments when compared with placebo. Because only a total of 96 dexamethasone-treated infants were evaluated in these studies, the results must be interpreted with caution.[25,26]

Cohort studies of dexamethasone have revealed an association of its use with

TABLE 2 Neurodevelopmental Follow-up of Dexamethasone RCTs Reported After 2001

Study, Planned Age at Follow-up	Follow-up, % (No. of Infants Seen)	Treatment Start Time	Dexamethasone Dosing Regimen	Primary Neurodevelopmental Findings
McEvoy et al,[17] 1 y	66 (39)	At 7–21 d	High vs low dose: 7-d taper from 0.5 mg/kg per d vs 0.2 mg/kg per d	MDI < 70: 24% (high) vs 17% (low) (NS); CP: 10% vs 11% (NS)
Armstrong et al,[24] 18 mo chronological age	96 (64)	On day 7	42-d taper vs 3-d pulse	No difference in 18-mo outcomes No disability: 34% vs 31% (NS)
Doyle et al,[25] 2 y corrected age	98 (58)	After 7 d	0.15 mg/kg per d tapered over 10 d	Death or major disability: 46% vs 43% (NS); death or CP: 23% vs 37% (NS); CP: 14% vs 22% (NS); major disability 41% vs 31% (NS)
Stark et al,[26] 18–22 mo corrected age	74 (123)	On day 1	0.15 mg/kg per d tapered over 7 d	MDI < 70: 51% vs 43% (NS); PDI < 70: 30% vs 35% (NS); abnormal neurologic exam: 25% each group
Romagnoli et al,[27] 3 y	100 (30)	On day 4	0.5 mg/kg per d tapered over 1 wk	No differences in any parameter; CP: 9% vs 14% (NS)
Wilson et al,[28] 7 y	84 (127)	Before 3 d	4 groups: 0.5 mg/kg per d tapered over 12 d vs late (15 d) selective, vs inhaled early or late selective	No difference in cognitive, behavioral, CP, or combined outcomes
Yeh et al,[29] school age (mean: 8 y)	92 (146)	On day 1	0.5 mg/kg per d for 1 wk, then tapered for a total of 28 d	Treated children were shorter ($P = .03$), had smaller head circumference ($P = .04$), lower IQ scores ($P = .008$), and more significant disabilities (CP, IQ < 5th percentile, vision or hearing impairment): 39% vs 22% ($P = .04$)
O'Shea et al,[30] 4–11 y	89 (84)	On day 15–25	0.5 mg/kg per d tapered over 42 d vs placebo	Death or major NDI[a]: 47% vs 41% (NS); major NDI alone: 36% vs 14% ($P = .01$)
Gross et al,[31] 15 y	100 (22)	On day 14	0.5 mg/kg per d tapered over 42 d vs 18-d taper vs placebo	Intact survival (IQ > 70, normal neurologic exam, regular classroom): 69% vs 25% (18-d course) vs 18% (placebo) ($P < .05$)
Jones and the Collaborative Dexamethasone Trial Follow-up Group,[32] 13–17 y	95 (150)	At 2–12 wk	0.5 mg/kg per d for 7 d	No difference in moderate/severe disability (defined as IQ > 2 SDs < mean, CP, hearing or vision loss); CP: 24% vs 15% (relative risk: 1.58 [95% confidence interval: 0.81–3.07])

MDI indicates Bayley Mental Developmental Index; NS, not significant. PDI, Bayley Psychomotor Development Index; NDI, neurodevelopmental impairment.

[a] Major neurodevelopmental impairment included CP and/or an IQ score of <70.

impaired neurodevelopmental outcomes[3,4,33]; however, such an association cannot be construed as definitive evidence of harm. A clinician's decision to use a therapy incorporates numerous undocumented factors and varies from one clinician to the next, which may seriously confound the interpretation of such studies. Patients who receive dexamethasone for BPD are likely to be perceived as having more severe respiratory disease than infants who are not treated; such infants may have worse overall outcomes regardless of dexamethasone therapy. Authors of small series have also reported that infants treated with dexamethasone have more abnormalities on MRI than those not treated; again, causation cannot be attributed in the absence of an RCT.[34,35] Two previously reported RCTs revealed more cranial ultrasound abnormalities in dexamethasone-treated infants compared with those treated with placebo, but the patient numbers were quite small.[36,37]

In summary, high daily doses of dexamethasone have been linked frequently to adverse neurodevelopmental outcomes, and this therapy is discouraged. Because an increase in adverse neurodevelopmental outcomes in treatment studies that used low doses of dexamethasone has not been reported, further studies of low-dose dexamethasone to facilitate extubation are warranted.

Hydrocortisone

Results of 4 RCTs designed to evaluate the ability of early hydrocortisone therapy to improve rates of survival without BPD have been published (Table 3).[38–41] These studies were based on the premise that extremely preterm infants may have immature adrenal gland function, predisposing them to a relative adrenal insufficiency and inadequate anti-inflammatory capability during the first several weeks of life.[42–46] In contrast to the heterogeneous nature of previous dexamethasone trials, these studies were similar in design, time of initiation, duration, and dose. The direction of effect favored the hydrocortisone-treated infants in all 4 studies, and a significant increase in rate of survival without BPD in the hydrocortisone-treated infants was reported for 2 of the studies. The largest trial ($n = 360$) did not reveal a significant benefit of hydrocortisone treatment in the overall study group; however, for infants exposed to prenatal inflammation ($n = 149$), identified before the trial as a specific group for analysis, hydrocortisone treatment resulted in a significant decrease in mortality rate and an increase in rate of survival without BPD.[39]

Patient enrollment was halted early in 3 of these 4 studies because of a significant increase in spontaneous gastrointestinal perforation discovered in the largest trial,[39] a complication also observed with early dexamethasone.[47,48] The perforations may have resulted from an interaction between high endogenous cortisol concentrations and indomethacin therapy in the first 48 hours; however, because administration of indomethacin was not randomized, this hypothesis remains to be tested.

Neurodevelopmental outcomes at 18 to 22 months' corrected age have been published for 3 of these trials, and no adverse effects of hydrocortisone treatment were found.[49,50] In the largest multicenter trial, the incidence of death or major neurodevelopmental impairment (52% [hydrocortisone-treated] vs 56% [placebo]), major neurodevelopmental impairment alone (39% vs 44%), and CP (16% vs 18%) were similar.[49] The only significant findings favored the hydrocortisone-treated group and included a decreased incidence of a Bayley Scales of Infant Development (2nd ed) Mental Developmental Index (MDI) 2 SDs below the mean (MDI < 70, 27% vs 37%;

TABLE 3 RCTs of Early Hydrocortisone to Prevent BPD

Study, No. of Centers	n	Population: Mechanically Ventilated Infants	Hydrocortisone Dosing Regimen	Rate of Survival Without BPD[a] HC vs Placebo, %
Watterberg et al,[38] 2 centers	40	500–999 g BW; <48 h postnatal age	0.5 mg/kg every 12 h for 9 d 0.25 mg/kg every 12 h for 3 d	60 vs 35 ($P = .04$)
Watterberg et al,[39] 9 centers	360[b]	500–999 g BW; <48 h postnatal age	0.5 mg/kg every 12 h for 12 d 0.25 mg/kg every 12 h for 3 d	35 vs 34 (aOR[c]: 1.20 [95% CI: 0.72–1.99])
Peltoniemi et al,[40] 3 centers	51[b]	501–1250 g BW; <36 h postnatal age	2.0 mg/kg per d tapered to 0.75 mg/kg per d over 10 d	64 vs 46 (OR: 1.48 [95% CI: 0.49–4.48])
Bonsante et al,[41] 2 centers	50[b]	500–1249 g BW; <48 h postnatal age	0.5 mg/kg every 12 h for 9 d; 0.25 mg/kg every 12 h for 3 d	64 vs 32 ($P < .05$)
Total	601	—	—	—

BW indicates birth weight; aOR, adjusted odds ratio; OR, odds ratio; CI, confidence interval.

[a] BPD was defined as receiving supplemental oxygen at 36 weeks' postmenstrual age.

[b] Study enrollment was terminated early because of concern for spontaneous gastrointestinal perforation.

[c] Adjusted for center, birth weight, risk factors (gender, "outborn" [infants who were born at an outlying institution and transported into the study center], white race, vaginal delivery, no prenatal steroids, hydrocortisone, and/or vasopressor support at study entry).

odds ratio: 0.47 [95% confidence interval: 0.25–0.87]) and a higher incidence of awareness of object permanence (an early test of working memory and prefrontal executive function) (89% vs 79%; odds ratio: 2.19 [95% confidence interval: 1.06–4.52]).

Two other RCTs have evaluated administration of hydrocortisone to preterm infants during the first week of life with the objective of reducing respiratory morbidity. The first, published in 1974, had the objective of decreasing the severity of respiratory distress syndrome.[51] The investigators used a much higher dose (25 mg/kg per day on the first day of postnatal life), which showed no effect on respiratory distress syndrome. The second, published in 2003, was based on the hypothesis that extremely preterm infants have immature sodium channels and, therefore, cannot clear their lung liquid after birth.[52] Triiodothyronine (T_3) was given together with hydrocortisone to stimulate maturation of the sodium channels. The medications were started within 5 hours of birth and given as a constant infusion for 7 days. The investigators enrolled 253 infants and found no difference in their primary outcome variables of death or ventilator dependence at 7 days and at 14 days. At 36 weeks' postmenstrual age, 47% of the treated survivors and 51% of the placebo group remained on oxygen.

Reports of hydrocortisone therapy given to facilitate extubation have been limited to cohort studies. In the first reported study, 25 infants treated with hydrocortisone at 1 hospital (5 mg/kg per day, tapered over 3 weeks) were compared with 25 untreated infants at the same hospital and additionally with a cohort of 23 infants treated with dexamethasone (0.5 mg/kg per day, tapered over 3 weeks) at a separate hospital.[53] The investigators found that hydrocortisone was as effective as

dexamethasone in weaning infants from the ventilator and in decreasing supplemental oxygen therapy, with fewer short-term adverse effects. Follow-up of these children at school age revealed no differences in neurodevelopmental outcomes between hydrocortisone-treated infants and their comparison group, whereas dexamethasone-treated infants more often had an abnormal neurologic examination and less favorable school performance than their comparison cohort.[53,54] Subsequently, several large cohort studies from the same institution reported that, although hydrocortisone-treated children were younger, smaller, and sicker than their untreated comparison groups, there were no adverse effects of hydrocortisone treatment on IQ, visual motor integration, memory testing, CP, or findings on MRI.[55–57] Investigators from this institution have also reported that neonatal dexamethasone but not hydrocortisone therapy resulted in long-lasting changes in hypothalamic-pituitary-adrenal axis and T-cell function.[58]

Other Glucocorticoids (Systemic or Inhaled)

Since the previous AAP statement, no RCTs of other systemic glucocorticoids, such as prednisone or methylprednisolone, to treat or prevent BPD have been published. No additional evidence has been published to support the efficacy of inhaled glucocorticoids to prevent or decrease the severity of BPD.[59,60]

DISCUSSION: DIFFERENCES BETWEEN DEXAMETHASONE AND HYDROCORTISONE

As described previously, many RCTs have shown adverse neurodevelopmental outcomes after postnatal dexamethasone treatment for BPD, but neither multicenter RCTs nor cohort studies have revealed adverse effects

on functional or structural neurologic outcomes after neonatal hydrocortisone therapy. One possible explanation for the observed differences between dexamethasone and hydrocortisone is the difference in effective glucocorticoid dose. Neonatal animal studies have consistently revealed adverse effects on brain growth after high doses of glucocorticoid,[61,62] and results of evaluation of 22 patients who received high-dose hydrocortisone in a study from the early 1970s were suggestive of harm.[63,64] High-dose dexamethasone (0.5 mg/kg per day) is equivalent to at least 15 to 20 mg/kg per day of hydrocortisone,[65] far higher than the doses of hydrocortisone given in the recent studies described previously. Low-dose dexamethasone (0.1–0.15 mg/kg per day) may be equivalent to 3 to 6 mg/kg per day of hydrocortisone; however, because of its much longer biological half-life, it could have a much higher relative potency.[66] Lowering the dose of dexamethasone may, therefore, decrease its adverse effects, as is suggested by the 2 studies of outcome after lower-dose dexamethasone therapy.[25,26]

Second, the observed differences in neurodevelopmental outcomes may result from the different effects of these agents on the hippocampus, an area of the brain critical to learning, memory, and spatial processing.[67,68] The hippocampus contains a high density of both mineralocorticoid and glucocorticoid receptors.[69,70] Hydrocortisone, which is identical to native cortisol, can bind to both classes of receptors. In contrast, dexamethasone binds only to glucocorticoid receptors, which, in animal models, has been shown to result in degeneration and necrosis of hippocampal neurons.[71,72] This effect of dexamethasone is blocked by simultaneous administration of corticosterone (the cortisol equivalent in the rat).[71] In humans, neonatal treatment with dexamethasone, but not hydrocortisone, has been shown to alter hippocampal synaptic plasticity and associative memory formation in later life.[73] Dexamethasone exposure has also been linked to decreased hippocampal volume in 1 cohort study,[74] but cohort studies of infants treated with hydrocortisone have revealed no decrease in hippocampal volume,[55] no adverse effect on hippocampal metabolism, and no adverse effect on memory at school age[57] when compared with a larger, more mature group of nontreated infants.

Whatever the underlying explanation(s) for the observed differences in short- and long-term outcomes may be, further RCTs are needed to answer the many remaining questions, including whether lower doses of dexamethasone can avoid previously observed adverse effects, whether hydrocortisone is efficacious for extubation, whether specific groups of infants may derive particular benefit from hydrocortisone therapy, and whether the incidence of spontaneous gastrointestinal perforation during early glucocorticoid administration can be decreased by avoiding concomitant indomethacin or ibuprofen therapy and/or by monitoring cortisol concentrations.

SUMMARY AND RECOMMENDATIONS

- BPD remains a major morbidity of the extremely preterm infant and is consistently associated with adverse effects on long-term outcomes, including neurodevelopment. Additional RCTs of postnatal glucocorticoids are warranted to optimize therapy and improve outcomes for these infants. Those who design such trials in the future should attempt to minimize the use of open-label glucocorticoid, which

has confounded analysis of most previous trials, and should include assessment of long-term pulmonary and neurodevelopmental outcomes.

- High daily doses of dexamethasone (approximately 0.5 mg/kg per day) have been shown to reduce the incidence of BPD but have been associated with numerous short- and long-term adverse outcomes, including neurodevelopmental impairment, and at present there is no basis for postulating that high daily doses confer additional therapeutic benefit over lower-dose therapy. **Recommendation: in the absence of randomized trial results showing improved short- and long-term outcomes, therapy with high-dose dexamethasone cannot be recommended.**

- Low-dose dexamethasone therapy (<0.2 mg/kg per day) may facilitate extubation and may decrease the incidence of short- and long-term adverse effects observed with higher doses of dexamethasone. Additional RCTs sufficiently powered to evaluate the effects of low-dose dexamethasone therapy on rates of survival without BPD, as well as on other short- and long-term outcomes, are warranted. **Recommendation: there is insufficient evidence to make a recommendation regarding treatment with low-dose dexamethasone.**

- Low-dose hydrocortisone therapy (1 mg/kg per day) given for the first 2 weeks of life may increase rates of survival without BPD, particularly for infants delivered in a setting of prenatal inflammation, without adversely affecting neurodevelopmental outcomes. Clinicians should be aware of a possible increased risk of isolated intestinal perforation associated with early concomitant treatment with inhibitors of prosta-

glandin synthesis. Further RCTs powered to detect effects on neurodevelopmental outcomes, aimed at targeting patients who may derive most benefit and developing treatment strategies to reduce the incidence of isolated intestinal perforation, are warranted. **Recommendation: early hydrocortisone treatment may be beneficial in a specific population of patients; however, there is insufficient evidence to recommend its use for all infants at risk of BPD.**

- Higher doses of hydrocortisone (3–6 mg/kg per day) instituted after the first week of postnatal age have not been shown to improve rates of survival without BPD in any RCT. RCTs powered to assess the effect of this therapy on short- and long-term outcomes are needed. **Recommendation: existing data are insufficient to make a recommendation regarding treatment with high-dose hydrocortisone.**

IMPLICATIONS FOR PRACTICE

Because available data are conflicting and inconclusive, clinicians must use their own clinical judgment to balance the adverse effects of BPD with the potential adverse effects of treatments for each individual patient. Very low birth weight infants who remain on mechanical ventilation after 1 to 2 weeks of age are at very high risk of developing BPD.[14] When considering corticosteroid therapy for such an infant, clinicians might conclude that the risks of a short course of glucocorticoid therapy to mitigate BPD is warranted.[15] This individualized decision should be made in conjunction with the infant's parents.

LEAD AUTHOR
Kristi L. Watterberg, MD

COMMITTEE ON FETUS AND NEWBORN, 2009–2010
Lu-Ann Papile, MD, Chairperson

David H. Adamkin, MD
Jill E. Baley, MD
Vinod K. Bhutani, MD
Waldemar A. Carlo, MD
Praveen Kumar, MD
Richard A. Polin, MD
Rosemarie C. Tan, MD, PhD
Kasper S. Wang, MD

Kristi L. Watterberg, MD

LIAISONS

Captain Wanda Denise Barfield, MD, MPH –
Centers for Disease Control and Prevention
William H. Barth Jr, MD – American College of
Obstetricians and Gynecologists
Ann L. Jefferies, MD – Canadian Paediatric
Society

Rosalie O. Mainous, PhD, RNC, NNP – National
Association of Neonatal Nurses
Tonse N. K. Raju, MD, DCH – National Institutes
of Health

STAFF

Jim Couto, MA

REFERENCES

1. Morley CJ, Davis PG, Doyle LW, Brion LP, Hascoet JM, Carlin JB; COIN Trial Investigators. Nasal CPAP or intubation at birth for very preterm infants. N Engl J Med. 2008;358(7):700–708

2. Walsh M, Laptook A, Kazzi SN, et al. National Institute of Child Health and Human Development Neonatal Research Network. A cluster-randomized trial of benchmarking and multimodal quality improvement to improve rates of survival free of bronchopulmonary dysplasia for infants with birth weights of less than 1250 grams. 2007; 119(5):876–890

3. Vohr BR, Wright LL, Poole WK, McDonald SA. Neurodevelopmental outcomes of extremely low birth weight infants <32 weeks' gestation between 1993 and 1998. Pediatrics. 2005;116(3):635–643

4. Kobaly K, Schluchter M, Minich N, et al. Outcomes of extremely low birth weight (<1 kg) and extremely low gestational age (<28 weeks) infants with bronchopulmonary dysplasia: effects of practice changes in 2000 to 2003. Pediatrics. 2008;121(1):73–81

5. American Academy of Pediatrics, Committee on Fetus and Newborn; Canadian Paediatric Society, Fetus and Newborn Committee. Postnatal corticosteroids to treat or prevent chronic lung disease in preterm infants. Pediatrics. 2002; 109(2):330–338

6. Walsh MC, Yao Q, Horbar JD, Carpenter JH, Lee SK, Ohlsson A. Changes in the use of postnatal steroids for bronchopulmonary dysplasia in 3 large neonatal networks. Pediatrics. 2006;118(5): Available at: www.pediatrics.org/cgi/content/full/118/5/e1328

7. Shinwell ES, Karplus M, Reich D, et al. Early postnatal dexamethasone treatment and increased incidence of cerebral palsy. Arch Dis Child Fetal Neonatal Ed. 2000;83(3): F177–F181

8. Yoder BA, Harrison M, Clark RH. Time-related changes in steroid use and bronchopulmonary dysplasia in preterm infants. Pediatrics. 2009;124(2):673–679

9. Barrington KJ. The adverse neurodevelopmental effects of postnatal steroids in the preterm infant: a systematic review of RCTs. BMC Pediatr. 2001;1:1

10. Halliday HL, Ehrenkranz RA, Doyle LW. Early postnatal (<96 hours) corticosteroids for preventing chronic lung disease in preterm infants. Cochrane Database Syst Rev. 2003; (1):CD001146

11. Halliday HL, Ehrenkranz RA, Doyle LW. Moderately early (7–14 days) postnatal corticosteroids for preventing chronic lung disease in preterm infants. Cochrane Database Syst Rev. 2003;(1):CD001144

12. Halliday HL, Ehrenkranz RA, Doyle LW. Delayed (>3 weeks) postnatal corticosteroids for chronic lung disease in preterm infants. Cochrane Database Syst Rev. 2003;(1): CD001145

13. Halliday HL, Ehrenkranz RA, Doyle LW. Early (<8 days) corticosteroids for preventing chronic lung disease in preterm infants. Cochrane Database Syst Rev. 2009;(1): CD001146

14. Halliday HL, Ehrenkranz RA, Doyle LW. Late (>7 days) postnatal corticosteroids for chronic lung disease in preterm infants. Cochrane Database Syst Rev. 2009;(1): CD001145

15. Doyle LW, Halliday HL, Ehrenkranz RA, Davis PG, Sinclair JC. Impact of postnatal systemic corticosteroids on mortality and cerebral palsy in preterm infants: effect modification by risk for chronic lung disease. Pediatrics. 2005;115(3):655–661

16. Onland W, Offringa M, De Jaegere AP, van Kaam AH. Finding the optimal postnatal dexamethasone regimen for preterm infants at risk of bronchopulmonary dysplasia: a systematic review of placebo-controlled trials. Pediatrics. 2009;123(1): 367–377

17. McEvoy C, Bowling S, Williamson K, McGaw P, Durand M. Randomized, double-blinded trial of low-dose dexamethasone: II. Functional residual capacity and pulmonary outcome in very low birth weight infants at risk for bronchopulmonary dysplasia. Pediatr Pulmonol. 2004;38(1)55–63

18. Odd DE, Armstrong DL, Teele RL, Kuschel CA, Harding JE. A randomized trial of two dexamethasone regimens to reduce side-effects

in infants treated for chronic lung disease of prematurity. J Paediatr Child Health. 2004;40(5–6):282–289

19. Malloy CA, Hilal K, Rizvi Z Weiss M Muraskas JK. A prospective, randomized, double-masked trial comparing low dose to conventional dose dexamethasone in neonatal chronic lung disease. Internet J Pediatr Neonatol. 2005; 5(1). Available at: www.ispub.com/ostia/index.php?xmlPrinter=true&xmlFilePath=journals/ijpn/vol5n1/dexamethasone.xml. Accessed March 16, 2010

20. Walther FJ, Findlay RD, Durand M. Adrenal suppression and extubation rate after moderately early low-dose dexamethasone therapy in very preterm infants. Early Hum Dev. 2003;74(1):37–45

21. Anttila E, Peltoniemi O, Haumont D, et al. Early neonatal dexamethasone treatment for prevention of bronchopulmonary dysplasia: randomised trial and meta-analysis evaluating the duration of dexamethasone therapy. Eur J Pediatr. 2005; 164(8):472–481

22. Doyle LW, Davis PG, Morley CJ, McPhee A, Carlin JB; DART Study Investigators. Low-dose dexamethasone facilitates extubation among chronically ventilator-dependent infants: a multicenter, international, randomized, controlled trial. Pediatrics. 2006; 117(1):75–83

23. Rozycki HJ, Byron PR, Elliott GR, Carroll T, Gutcher GR. Randomized controlled trial of three different doses of aerosol beclomethasone versus systemic dexamethasone to promote extubation in ventilated premature infants. Pediatr Pulmonol. 2003; 35(5):375–383

24. Armstrong DL, Penrice J, Bloomfield FH, Knight DB, Dezoete JA, Harding JE. Follow up of a randomised trial of two different courses of dexamethasone for preterm babies at risk of chronic lung disease. Arch Dis Child Fetal Neonatal Ed. 2002;86(2): F102–F107

25. Doyle LW, Davis PG, Morley CJ, McPhee A, Carlin JB; DART Study Investigators. Outcome at 2 years of age of infants from the DART study: a multicenter, international, randomized, controlled trial of low-dose

dexamethasone. *Pediatrics*. 2007;119(4): 716–721

26. Stark AR, Carlo W, Vohr BR, et al. NICHD Neonatal Research Network. Neurodevelopmental outcome and growth at 18–22 months [abstract]. *Pediatr Res*. 2001;49: 388A

27. Romagnoli C, Zecca E, Luciano R, Torrioli G, Tortorolo G. A three year follow up of preterm infants after moderately early treatment with dexamethasone. *Arch Dis Child Fetal Neonatal Ed*. 2002;87(1):F55–F58

28. Wilson TT, Waters L, Patterson CC, et al. Neurodevelopmental and respiratory follow-up results at 7 years for children from the United Kingdom and Ireland enrolled in a randomized trial of early and late postnatal corticosteroid treatment, systemic and inhaled. The Open Study of Early Corticosteroid Treatment. *Pediatrics*. 2006;117(6): 2196–2205

29. Yeh TF, Lin YJ, Lin HC, et al. Outcomes at school age after postnatal dexamethasone therapy for lung disease of prematurity. *N Engl J Med*. 2004;350(13):1304–1313

30. O'Shea TM, Washburn LK, Nixon PA, Goldstein DJ. Follow-up of a randomized, placebo-controlled trial of dexamethasone to decrease the duration of ventilator dependency in very low birth weight infants: neurodevelopmental outcomes at 4 to 11 years of age. *Pediatrics*. 2007; 120(3): 594–602

31. Gross SJ, Anbar RD, Mettelman BB. Follow-up at 15 years of preterm infants from a controlled trial of moderately early dexamethasone for the prevention of chronic lung disease. *Pediatrics*. 2005; 115(3):681–687

32. Jones RA; Collaborative Dexamethasone Trial Follow-up Group. Randomized, controlled trial of dexamethasone in neonatal chronic lung disease: 13- to 17-year follow-up study: I. Neurologic, psychological, and educational outcomes. *Pediatrics*. 2005;116(2):370–378

33. Wilson-Costello D, Walsh MC, Langer JC, et al; Eunice Kennedy Shriver National Institute of Child Health and Human Development Neonatal Research Network. Impact of postnatal corticosteroid use on neurodevelopment at 18 to 22 months' adjusted age: effects of dose, timing, and risk of bronchopulmonary dysplasia in extremely low birth weight infants. *Pediatrics*. 2009;123(3): Available at: www.pediatrics.org/cgi/content/full/123/3/e430

34. Murphy BP, Inder TE, Huppi PS, et al. Impaired cerebral cortical gray matter growth after treatment with dexamethasone for neonatal chronic lung disease. *Pediatrics*. 2001;107(2):217–221

35. Parikh NA, Lasky RE, Kennedy KA, et al. Postnatal dexamethasone therapy and cerebral tissue volumes in extremely low birth weight infants. *Pediatrics*. 2007;119(2): 265–272

36. O'Shea TM, Kothadia JM, Klinepeter KL, et al. Randomized placebo-controlled trial of a 42-day tapering course of dexamethasone to reduce the duration of ventilator dependency in very low birth weight infants: outcome of study participants at 1-year adjusted age. *Pediatrics*. 1999; 104(1 pt 1): 15–21

37. Noble-Jamieson CM, Regev R, Silverman M. Dexamethasone in neonatal chronic lung disease: pulmonary effects and intracranial complications. *Eur J Pediatr*. 1989;148(4): 365–367

38. Watterberg KL, Gerdes JS, Gifford KL, Lin HM. Prophylaxis against early adrenal insufficiency to prevent chronic lung disease in premature infants. *Pediatrics*. 1999;104(6): 1258–1263

39. Watterberg KL, Gerdes JS, Cole CH, et al. Prophylaxis of early adrenal insufficiency to prevent bronchopulmonary dysplasia: a multicenter trial. *Pediatrics*. 2004;114(6): 1649–1657

40. Peltoniemi O, Kari MA, Heinonen K, et al. Pretreatment cortisol values may predict responses to hydrocortisone administration for the prevention of bronchopulmonary dysplasia in high-risk infants. *J Pediatr*. 2005;146(5):632–637

41. Bonsante F, Latorre G, Iacobelli S, et al. Early low-dose hydrocortisone in very preterm infants: a randomized, placebo-controlled trial. *Neonatology*. 2007;91(4):217–221

42. Watterberg KL, Scott SM. Evidence of early adrenal insufficiency in babies who develop bronchopulmonary dysplasia. *Pediatrics*. 1995;95(1):120–125

43. Huysman MW, Hokken-Koelega AC, De Ridder MA, Sauer PJ. Adrenal function in sick very preterm infants. *Pediatr Res*. 2000; 48(5):629–633

44. Watterberg KL, Scott SM, Backstrom C, Gifford KL, Cook KL. Links between early adrenal function and respiratory outcome in preterm infants: airway inflammation and patent ductus arteriosus. *Pediatrics*. 2000; 105(2):320–324

45. Watterberg KL, Gerdes JS, Cook, KL. Impaired glucocorticoid synthesis in premature infants developing chronic lung disease. *Pediatr Res*. 2001;50(2):190–195

46. Nykänen P, Anttila E, Heinonen K, Hallman M, Voutilainen R. Early hypoadrenalism in premature infants at risk for bronchopulmo-

nary dysplasia or death. *Acta Paediatr*. 2007;96(11):1600–1605

47. Garland JS, Alex CP, Pauly TH, et al. A three-day course of dexamethasone therapy to prevent chronic lung disease in ventilated neonates: a randomized trial. *Pediatrics*. 1999;104(1 pt 1):91–99

48. Stark AR, Carlo WA, Tyson JE, et al; National Institute of Child Health and Human Development Neonatal Research Network. Adverse effects of early dexamethasone in extremely-low-birth-weight infants. *N Engl J Med*. 2001;344(2):95–101

49. Watterberg KL, Shaffer ML, Mishefske MJ, et al. Growth and neurodevelopmental outcomes after early low-dose hydrocortisone treatment in extremely low birth weight infants. *Pediatrics*. 2007;120(1):40–48

50. Peltoniemi OM, Lano A, Puosi R, et al; Neonatal Hydrocortisone Working Group. Trial of early neonatal hydrocortisone: two-year follow-up. *Neonatology*. 2009;95(3):240–247

51. Baden M, Bauer CR, Colle E, Klein G, Taeusch HW Jr, Stern L. A controlled trial of hydrocortisone therapy in infants with respiratory distress syndrome. *Pediatrics*. 1972; 50(4):526–534

52. Biswas S, Buffery J, Enoch H, Bland M, Markiewicz M, Walters D. Pulmonary effects of triiodothyronine (T3) and hydrocortisone (HC) supplementation in preterm infants less than 30 weeks gestation: results of the THORN trial—thyroid hormone replacement in neonates. *Pediatr Res*. 2003;53(1):48–56

53. van der Heide-Jalving M, Kamphuis PJ, van der Laan MJ, et al. Short- and long-term effects of neonatal glucocorticoid therapy: is hydrocortisone an alternative to dexamethasone? *Acta Paediatr*. 2003; 92(7): 827–835

54. Karemaker R, Heijnen CJ, Veen S, et al. Differences in behavioral outcome and motor development at school age after neonatal treatment for chronic lung disease with dexamethasone versus hydrocortisone. *Pediatr Res*. 2006;60(6):745–750

55. Lodygensky GA, Rademaker K, Zimine S, et al. Structural and functional brain development after hydrocortisone treatment for neonatal chronic lung disease. *Pediatrics*. 2005;116(1):1–7

56. Rademaker KJ, Uiterwaal CS, Groenendaal F, et al. Neonatal hydrocortisone treatment: neurodevelopmental outcome and MRI at school age in preterm-born children. *J Pediatr*. 2007;150(4):351–357

57. Rademaker KJ, Rijpert M, Uiterwaal CS, et al. Neonatal hydrocortisone treatment related to ^{1}H-MRS of the hippocampus and short-term memory at school age in pre-

term born children. *Pediatr Res.* 2006;59(2):309–313

58. Karemaker R, Kavelaars A, ter Wolbeek M, et al. Neonatal dexamethasone treatment for chronic lung disease of prematurity alters the hypothalamus-pituitary-adrenal axis and immune system activity at school age. *Pediatrics.* 2008;121(4): Available at: www.pediatrics.org/cgi/content/full/121/4/e870

59. Shah SS, Ohlsson A, Halliday H, Shah VS. Inhaled versus systemic corticosteroids for the treatment of chronic lung disease in ventilated very low birth weight preterm infants. *Cochrane Database Syst Rev.* 2007;(4):CD002057

60. Shah V, Ohlsson A, Halliday HL, Dunn MS. Early administration of inhaled corticosteroids for preventing chronic lung disease in ventilated very low birth weight preterm neonates. *Cochrane Database Syst Rev.* 2007;(4):CD001969

61. Howard E. Reductions in size and total DNA of cerebrum and cerebellum in adult mice after corticosterone treatment in infancy. *Exp Neurol.* 1968;22(2):191–208

62. Howard E, Benjamin JA. DNA, ganglioside and sulfatide in brains of rats given corticosterone in infancy, with an estimate of cell

loss during development. *Brain Res.* 1975;92(1):73–87

63. Taeusch HW Jr, Wang NS, Baden M, Bauer C, Stern L. A controlled trial of hydrocortisone therapy in infants with respiratory distress syndrome: II. Pathology. *Pediatrics.* 1973;52(6):850–854

64. Fitzhardinge PM, Eisen A, Lejtenyi C, Metrakos K, Ramsay M. Sequelae of early steroid administration to the newborn infant. *Pediatrics.* 1974;53(6):877–883

65. Williams GH, Dluhy RG. Diseases of the adrenal cortex. In:Fauci AS Braunwald E, Isselbacher KJ et al, eds. *Harrison's Principles of Internal Medicine.* 14th ed. New York, NY: McGraw-Hill; 1998:2035–2057

66. Meikle AW, Tyler FH. Potency and duration of action of glucocorticoids: effects of hydrocortisone, prednisone and dexamethasone on human pituitary-adrenal function. *Am J Med.* 1977;63(2):200–207

67. Goldman-Rakic PS. Development of cortical circuitry and cognitive function. *Child Dev.* 1987;58(3):601–622

68. Isaacs EB, Lucas A, Chong WK, et al. Hippocampal volume and everyday memory in children of very low birth weight. *Pediatr Res.* 2000;47(6):713–720

69. McEwen BS. The brain is an important target of adrenal steroid actions: a comparison of synthetic and natural steroids. *Ann N Y Acad Sci.* 1997;823:201–213

70. De Kloet ER, Vreugdenhil E, Oitzl MS, Joëls M. Brain corticosteroid receptor balance in health and disease. *Endocr Rev.* 1998; 19(3):269–301

71. Sloviter RS, Sollas AL, Neubort S. Hippocampal dentate granule cell degeneration after adrenalectomy in the rat is not reversed by dexamethasone. *Brain Res.* 1995;682(1–2):227–230

72. Hassan AH, von Rosenstiel P, Patchev VK, Holsboer F, Almeida OF. Exacerbation of apoptosis in the dentate gyrus of the aged rat by dexamethasone and the protective role of corticosterone. *Exp Neurol.* 1996;140(1):43–52

73. Huang CC, Lin HR, Liang YC, Hsu KS. Effects of neonatal corticosteroid treatment on hippocampal synaptic function. *Pediatr Res.* 2007;62(3):267–270

74. Thompson DK, Wood SJ, Doyle LW, et al. Neonate hippocampal volumes: prematurity, perinatal predictors, and 2-year outcome. *Ann Neurol.* 2008;63(5):642–651

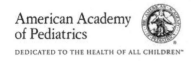

American Academy of Pediatrics

DEDICATED TO THE HEALTH OF ALL CHILDREN™

Organizational Principles to Guide and Define the Child
Health Care System and/or Improve the Health of all Children

POLICY STATEMENT

Respiratory Support in Preterm Infants at Birth

COMMITTEE ON FETUS AND NEWBORN

KEY WORDS
respiratory distress syndrome, preterm infant, neonate, surfactant, continuous positive airway pressure, bronchopulmonary dysplasia

ABBREVIATIONS
BPD—bronchopulmonary dysplasia
CI—confidence interval
CPAP—continuous positive airway pressure
INSURE—intubation, surfactant, and extubation
RDS—respiratory distress syndrome
RR—relative risk

www.pediatrics.org/cgi/doi/10.1542/peds.2013-3442

doi:10.1542/peds.2013-3442

PEDIATRICS (ISSN Numbers: Print, 0031-4005; Online, 1098-4275).

abstract

Current practice guidelines recommend administration of surfactant at or soon after birth in preterm infants with respiratory distress syndrome. However, recent multicenter randomized controlled trials indicate that early use of continuous positive airway pressure with subsequent selective surfactant administration in extremely preterm infants results in lower rates of bronchopulmonary dysplasia/death when compared with treatment with prophylactic or early surfactant therapy. Continuous positive airway pressure started at or soon after birth with subsequent selective surfactant administration may be considered as an alternative to routine intubation with prophylactic or early surfactant administration in preterm infants. *Pediatrics* 2014;133:171–174

BACKGROUND

Current practice guidelines in neonatology recommend administration of surfactant at or soon after birth in preterm infants with respiratory distress syndrome (RDS).[1] However, recent multicenter randomized controlled trials indicate that nasal continuous positive airway pressure (CPAP) may be an effective alternative to prophylactic or early surfactant administration.[2–8] Respiratory support is being achieved more frequently with CPAP and other less invasive approaches, such as the technique of intubation, surfactant, and extubation (INSURE).[9]

Experimental evidence documents that mechanical ventilation, particularly in the presence of surfactant deficiency, results in lung injury. Early randomized clinical trials demonstrated that surfactant administration in infants with established RDS decreased mortality, bronchopulmonary dysplasia (BPD), and pneumothorax.[10] Subsequent trials indicated that early selective administration of surfactant results in fewer pneumothoraces, less pulmonary interstitial emphysema, less BPD, and lower mortality compared with delayed selective surfactant therapy.[11] Trials of prophylactic administration of surfactant demonstrated decreased air leaks and mortality compared with selective surfactant therapy.[12] However, infants enrolled in these trials did not consistently receive early CPAP, an alternative therapy for the maintenance of functional residual capacity. Furthermore, control infants were intubated and mechanically ventilated without exogenous surfactant.

The INSURE strategy also resulted in fewer air leaks and shorter duration of ventilation when compared with later selective surfactant administration with continued ventilation. However, oxygen need and survival at 36 weeks' postmenstrual age or longer-term outcomes were not assessed in these trials.[13] It is also worth noting that the INSURE studies did not consistently use early CPAP in the control group. In fact, a recent large trial not included in this meta-analysis did not show a benefit of the INSURE strategy when compared with early CPAP.[7] The INSURE strategy may be more efficacious if an infant can be rapidly extubated. Studies in baboons have demonstrated an increase in the severity of pulmonary injury when extubation to CPAP is delayed, thus reducing the benefits of surfactant administration.[14] Decisions on extubation may have to be individualized, because some critically ill infants may not benefit from rapid extubation. Further research is needed to test the potential benefits of the INSURE strategy on important long-term outcomes. However, rapid extubation after surfactant administration may not be achievable or desirable in the most immature infants, and decisions to extubate should be individualized.

CPAP can be delivered by several noninvasive techniques such as nasal prongs, nasopharyngeal tube, or mask by using a water-bubbling system (bubble CPAP) or a ventilator. Although physician preference for bubble or ventilator CPAP is common, physiologic and clinical studies have been inconclusive. It is feasible to provide noninvasive nasal CPAP starting in the delivery room, even in extremely preterm infants (24–27 weeks' gestation), but the most immature infants had the highest risk of failure.[6] Noninvasive modes of ventilation, such as nasal intermittent ventilation, do not

appear to provide further benefits compared with CPAP.[15]

RANDOMIZED CONTROLLED TRIALS OF NASAL CPAP STARTING AT BIRTH

Recently published large, multicenter randomized controlled trials of prophylactic or early CPAP have enrolled very immature infants, a group that, in previous trials, benefited from surfactant treatment. The COIN (CPAP or INtubation) Trial of the Australasian Trial Network compared the effectiveness of nasal CPAP (8 cm of water pressure) to intubation and mechanical ventilation in preterm infants who were breathing spontaneously at 5 minutes after birth.[4] There was a trend for a lower rate of death or BPD in infants who received CPAP and used fewer corticosteroids postnatally. The mean duration of ventilation was shorter in the CPAP group (3 days in the CPAP group and 4 days in the ventilator group). However, the CPAP group had a higher rate of pneumothorax than the ventilator group (9% vs 3%; $P < .001$). Although surfactant therapy was not required for intubated infants, three-quarters of the intubation cohort received surfactant. Similarly, 46% of infants in the CPAP group required ventilator support, and 50% received surfactant. Therefore, the comparison was between early CPAP (with 50% of infants ultimately receiving surfactant) and intubation and ventilation, mostly but not always with surfactant administration.

The largest CPAP trial ($N = 1310$), the Surfactant Positive Pressure and Pulse Oximetry Randomized Trial (SUPPORT) conducted by the *Eunice Kennedy Shriver* National Institutes of Health and Human Development Neonatal Research Network investigators, was designed to evaluate nasal CPAP started immediately after birth by

using a limited-ventilation strategy compared with prophylactic surfactant therapy and ventilator support started within 60 minutes after birth by using a limited ventilation strategy in infants born at 24 to 27 weeks' gestation.[5] This trial used prospectively defined criteria for intubation and extubation. The rate of death or BPD in the CPAP group was 48% compared with 51% in the surfactant group (relative risk [RR]: 0.91; 95% confidence interval [CI]: 0.83–1.01; $P = .07$). Among infants born at 24 and 25 weeks' gestation, the death rate was lower in the CPAP group than in the surfactant group (20% vs 29%; RR: 0.68; 95% CI: 0.5–0.92; $P = .01$). Two-thirds of the infants in the CPAP group ultimately received surfactant. In addition, duration of mechanical ventilation was shorter (25 vs 28 days), and use of postnatal corticosteroid therapy was reduced in the CPAP group (7% vs 13%). The rate of air leaks did not differ between the groups, and there were no adverse effects of the CPAP strategy despite a reduction in the use of surfactant. This trial demonstrated that nasal CPAP started immediately after birth is an effective and safe alternative to prophylactic or early surfactant administration and may be superior. A follow-up study at 18 to 22 months' corrected age showed that death or neurodevelopmental impairment occurred in 28% of the infants in the CPAP group compared with 30% of those in the surfactant/ventilation group (RR: 0.93; 95% CI: 0.78–1.10; $P = .38$).[16] CPAP and the limited-ventilation strategy, rather than intubation and surfactant, resulted in less respiratory morbidity by 18 to 22 months' corrected age.[17]

The Vermont Oxford Network Delivery Room Management Trial randomly assigned infants born at 26 to 29 weeks' gestation to 1 of 3 treatment groups: prophylactic surfactant and continued ventilation, prophylactic surfactant and extubation to CPAP, or CPAP (without surfactant).[7] There were no statistically significant differences between the 3 groups, but when compared with the prophylactic surfactant group, the RR of BPD or death was 0.83 (95% CI: 0.64–1.09) for the CPAP group and 0.78 (95% CI: 0.59–1.03) for the INSURE group.

Other trials have compared early CPAP with prophylactic or early surfactant administration. The CURPAP[2] and Colombian Network[3] trials did not demonstrate a difference in the rate of BPD between the 2 treatment strategies. Moreover, in the Colombian Network trial,[3] infants randomly assigned to prophylactic CPAP had a higher risk of pneumothorax (9%) than infants randomly assigned to INSURE (2%). Infants in the South American Neocosur Network trial were randomly assigned to early CPAP (with rescue using an INSURE strategy) or oxygen hood (with rescue using mechanical ventilation).[8] The early CPAP strategy (and selective of INSURE, if needed) reduced the need for mechanical ventilation and surfactant.

Standard but diverse CPAP systems have been used in these and other large randomized controlled trials reviewed, including bubble CPAP and ventilator CPAP. A detailed description of the practical aspects of using CPAP systems are beyond the scope of this statement but are available in the published literature.[18,19]

Preterm infants are frequently born precipitously in hospitals without the capability of CPAP. CPAP can be provided with a bag and mask or other comparable devices in these circumstances. However, special expertise is necessary because CPAP may not be easy to use without specific training. Safe transport before delivery may be preferable depending on clinical circumstances.

Thus, care should be individualized on the basis of the capabilities of health workers in addition to the patient's condition.

A meta-analysis of prophylactic surfactant versus prophylactic stabilization with CPAP and subsequent selective surfactant administration in preterm infants showed that prophylactic administration of surfactant compared with stabilization with CPAP and selective surfactant administration was associated with a higher risk of death or BPD (RR: 1.12; 95% CI: 1.02–1.24; $P <$ .05).[11] The previously reported benefits of prophylactic surfactant could no longer be demonstrated.

It is notable that infants as immature as 24 weeks' gestational age were enrolled in many of the trials. In a subgroup analysis in the SUPPORT trial, the most immature infants (born at 24 and 25 weeks' gestation) benefited the most from the CPAP strategy. Many extremely preterm infants can be managed with CPAP only; early application of nasal CPAP (without surfactant administration) was successful in 50% of infants weighing ≤750 g at birth in 1 retrospective review.[20]

Surfactant administration can be expensive, particularly in low-resource settings. Additionally, intubation and mechanical ventilation may not be possible or desirable in institutions with limited resources. CPAP provides an alternative for early respiratory support in resource-limited settings. Emerging evidence indicates that early CPAP is an effective strategy for respiratory support in extremely preterm infants, including very immature infants. CPAP appears to be at least as safe and effective as early surfactant therapy with mechanical ventilation.[9]

CONCLUSIONS

1. Based on a meta-analysis of prophylactic surfactant versus CPAP as well as on other trials of more selective early use of surfactant versus CPAP not included in the meta-analysis, the early use of CPAP with subsequent selective surfactant administration in extremely preterm infants results in lower rates of BPD/death when compared with treatment with prophylactic or early surfactant therapy (Level of Evidence: 1).

2. Preterm infants treated with early CPAP alone are not at increased risk of adverse outcomes if treatment with surfactant is delayed or not given (Level of Evidence: 1).

3. Early initiation of CPAP may lead to a reduction in duration of mechanical ventilation and postnatal corticosteroid therapy (Level of Evidence: 1).

4. Infants with RDS may vary markedly in the severity of the respiratory disease, maturity, and presence of other complications, and thus it is necessary to individualize patient care. Care for these infants is provided in a variety of care settings, and thus the capabilities of the health care team need to be considered.

RECOMMENDATION

1. Using CPAP immediately after birth with subsequent selective surfactant administration may be considered as an alternative to routine intubation with prophylactic or early surfactant administration in preterm infants (Level of Evidence: 1, Strong Recommendation).[21] If it is likely that respiratory support with a ventilator will be needed, early administration of surfactant followed by rapid extubation is preferable to prolonged ventilation (Level of Evidence: 1, Strong Recommendation).[21]

LEAD AUTHORS

Waldemar A. Carlo, MD, FAAP
Richard A. Polin, MD, FAAP

COMMITTEE ON FETUS AND NEWBORN, 2012–2013

Lu-Ann Papile, MD, FAAP, Chairperson
Richard A. Polin, MD, FAAP
Waldemar A. Carlo, MD, FAAP
Rosemarie Tan, MD, FAAP

Praveen Kumar, MD, FAAP
William Benitz, MD, FAAP
Eric Eichenwald, MD, FAAP
James Cummings, MD, FAAP
Jill Baley, MD, FAAP

LIAISONS

Tonse N. K. Raju, MD, FAAP — *National Institutes of Health*
CAPT Wanda Denise Barfield, MD, FAAP — *Centers for Disease Control and Prevention*

Erin Keels, MSN — *National Association of Neonatal Nurses*
Anne Jefferies, MD – *Canadian Pediatric Society*
Kasper S. Wang, MD, FAAP — *AAP Section on Surgery*
George Macones, MD — *American College of Obstetricians and Gynecologists*

STAFF

Jim Couto, MA

REFERENCES

1. Engle WA; American Academy of Pediatrics Committee on Fetus and Newborn. Surfactant-replacement therapy for respiratory distress in the preterm and term neonate. *Pediatrics*. 2008;121(2):419–432

2. Sandri F, Ancora G, Lanzoni A, et al. Prophylactic nasal continuous positive airways pressure in newborns of 28-31 weeks gestation: multicentre randomised controlled clinical trial. *Arch Dis Child Fetal Neonatal Ed*. 2004;89(5):F394–F398

3. Rojas MA, Lozano JM, Rojas MX, et al; Colombian Neonatal Research Network. Very early surfactant without mandatory ventilation in premature infants treated with early continuous positive airway pressure: a randomized, controlled trial. *Pediatrics*. 2009;123(1):137–142

4. Morley CJ, Davis PG, Doyle LW, Brion LP, Hascoet JM, Carlin JB; COIN Trial Investigators. Nasal CPAP or intubation at birth for very preterm infants. *N Engl J Med*. 2008;358(7):700–708

5. Finer NN, Carlo WA, Walsh MC, et al; SUPPORT Study Group of the Eunice Kennedy Shriver NICHD Neonatal Research Network. Early CPAP versus surfactant in extremely preterm infants. *N Engl J Med*. 2010;362(21):1970–1979

6. Finer NN, Carlo WA, Duara S, et al; National Institute of Child Health and Human Development Neonatal Research Network. Delivery room continuous positive airway pressure/positive end-expiratory pressure in extremely low birth weight infants: a feasibility trial. *Pediatrics*. 2004;114(3):651–657

7. Dunn MS, Kaempf J, de Klerk A, et al; Vermont Oxford Network DRM Study Group. Randomized trial comparing 3 approaches to the initial respiratory management of preterm neonates. *Pediatrics*. 2011;128(5). Available at: www.pediatrics.org/cgi/content/full/128/5/e1069

8. Tapia JL, Urzua S, Bancalari A, et al; South American Neocosur Network. Randomized trial of early bubble continuous positive airway pressure for very low birth weight infants. *J Pediatr*. 2012;161(1):75–80, e1

9. Pfister RH, Soll RF. Initial respiratory support of preterm infants: the role of CPAP, the INSURE method, and noninvasive ventilation. *Clin Perinatol*. 2012;39(3):459–481

10. Soll RF, McQueen MC. Respiratory distress syndrome. In: Sinclair JC, Bracken B, eds. *Effective Care of the Newborn Infant*. Oxford, United Kingdom: Oxford University Press; 1992:325–358

11. Bahadue FL, Soll R. Early versus delayed selective surfactant treatment for neonatal respiratory distress syndrome. *Cochrane Database Syst Rev*. 2012;11(11):CD001456

12. Rojas-Reyes MX, Morley CJ, Soll R. Prophylactic versus selective use of surfactant in preventing morbidity and mortality in preterm infants. *Cochrane Database Syst Rev*. 2012;3(3):CD000510

13. Stevens TP, Harrington EW, Blennow M, Soll RF. Early surfactant administration with brief ventilation vs. selective surfactant and continued mechanical ventilation for preterm infants with or at risk for respiratory distress syndrome. *Cochrane Database Syst Rev*. 2007;(4):CD003063

14. Thomson MA, Yoder BA, Winter VT, Giavedoni L, Chang LY, Coalson JJ. Delayed extubation to nasal continuous positive airway pressure in the immature baboon model of bronchopulmonary dysplasia: lung clinical and pathological findings. *Pediatrics*. 2006;118(5):2038–2050

15. Kirpalani H, Millar D, Lemyre B, Yoder B, Chiu A, Roberts R. Nasal intermittent positive pressure (NIPPV) does not confer benefit above nasal CPAP (nCPAP) in extremely low birth weight (ELBW) infants <1000 g BW—the NIPPV International Randomized Controlled Trial [abstract]. E-PAS2012:1675.1.Available at: www.abstracts2-view.com/pas/view.php?nu=PAS12L1_511. Accessed February 7, 2013

16. Vaucher YE, Peralta-Carcelen M, Finer NN, et al; SUPPORT Study Group of the Eunice Kennedy Shriver NICHD Neonatal Research Network. Neurodevelopmental outcomes in the early CPAP and pulse oximetry trial. *N Engl J Med*. 2012;367(26):2495–2504

17. Stevens TP, Finer NN, Carlo WA, et al. Respiratory outcomes of the early CPAP and pulse oximetry trial. In: Pediatric Academic Societies Annual Meeting; May 4–7, 2013; Washington, DC. Abstract

18. Polin RA, Sahni R. Continuous positive airway pressure: old questions and new controversies. *J Neo Peri Med*. 2008;1(1):1–10

19. Sahni R, Wung JT. Continuous positive airway pressure (CPAP). *Indian J Pediatr*. 1998;65(2):265–271

20. Ammari A, Suri M, Milisavljevic V, et al. Variables associated with the early failure of nasal CPAP in very low birth weight infants. *J Pediatr*. 2005;147(3):341–347

21. American Academy of Pediatrics Steering Committee on Quality Improvement and Management. Classifying recommendations for clinical practice guidelines. *Pediatrics*. 2004;114(3):874–877

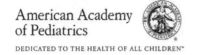

American Academy
of Pediatrics
DEDICATED TO THE HEALTH OF ALL CHILDREN™

Guidance for the Clinician in
Rendering Pediatric Care

CLINICAL REPORT

Surfactant Replacement Therapy for Preterm and Term Neonates With Respiratory Distress

abstract

Respiratory failure secondary to surfactant deficiency is a major cause of morbidity and mortality in preterm infants. Surfactant therapy substantially reduces mortality and respiratory morbidity for this population. Secondary surfactant deficiency also contributes to acute respiratory morbidity in late-preterm and term neonates with meconium aspiration syndrome, pneumonia/sepsis, and perhaps pulmonary hemorrhage; surfactant replacement may be beneficial for these infants. This statement summarizes the evidence regarding indications, administration, formulations, and outcomes for surfactant-replacement therapy. The clinical strategy of intubation, surfactant administration, and extubation to continuous positive airway pressure and the effect of continuous positive airway pressure on outcomes and surfactant use in preterm infants are also reviewed. *Pediatrics* 2014;133:156–163

INTRODUCTION

Surfactant replacement was established as an effective and safe therapy for immaturity-related surfactant deficiency by the early 1990s.[1] Systematic reviews of randomized, controlled trials confirmed that surfactant administration in preterm infants with established respiratory distress syndrome (RDS) reduces mortality, decreases the incidence of pulmonary air leak (pneumothoraces and pulmonary interstitial emphysema), and lowers the risk of chronic lung disease or death at 28 days of age (Table 1).[2–11] Subsequent trials indicated that prophylactic or early administration of surfactant resulted in fewer pneumothoraces, less pulmonary interstitial emphysema, and improved survival without bronchopulmonary dysplasia (BPD). However, recent randomized clinical trials indicate that the benefits of prophylactic surfactant are no longer evident in groups of infants when continuous positive airway pressure (CPAP) is used routinely.[5]

This clinical report updates a 2008 report from the American Academy of Pediatrics.[1] As in the previous report, a number of clinically important topics are reviewed surrounding use of surfactant, including prophylactic versus rescue replacement, preparations and administration techniques, the synergistic effects of surfactant and antenatal steroids, and surfactant therapy for respiratory disorders other than RDS. In addition, the effect of CPAP on RDS and surfactant replacement and the

Richard A. Polin, MD, FAAP, Waldemar A. Carlo, MD, FAAP, and COMMITTEE ON FETUS AND NEWBORN

KEY WORDS
surfactant, antenatal steroids, respiratory distress syndrome, meconium aspiration syndrome, neonatal pneumonia, neonatal sepsis, congenital diaphragmatic hernia, pulmonary hemorrhage, persistent pulmonary hypertension, preterm, term

ABBREVIATIONS
BPD—bronchopulmonary dysplasia
CI—confidence interval
CPAP—continuous positive airway pressure
ECMO—extracorporeal membrane oxygenation
INSURE—intubation, surfactant administration, and extubation
LOE—level of evidence
NNTB—number needed to benefit
RDS—respiratory distress syndrome
RR—relative risk
SP-B—surfactant protein B

The guidance in this report does not indicate an exclusive course of treatment or serve as a standard of medical care. Variations, taking into account individual circumstances, may be appropriate.

www.pediatrics.org/cgi/doi/10.1542/peds.2013-3443

doi:10.1542/peds.2013-3443

All clinical reports from the American Academy of Pediatrics automatically expire 5 years after publication unless reaffirmed, revised, or retired at or before that time.

PEDIATRICS (ISSN Numbers: Print, 0031-4005; Online, 1098-4275).

TABLE 1 Meta-analyses of Surfactant Replacement: Prophylaxis and Rescue Treatment With Animal-Derived and Synthetic Surfactant[2,3,8,11]

| Outcome | Prophylactic Surfactant | | Rescue Surfactant | |
| | Animal Derived | Synthetic | Animal Derived | Synthetic |
	N RR (95% CI)	N RR (95% CI)	N RR (95% CI)	N RR (95% CI)
Neonatal mortality	8 0.60 (0.47–0.77)	7 0.70 (0.58–0.85)	10 0.68 (0.57–0.82)	6 0.73 (0.61–0.88)
Pneumothorax	9 0.40 (0.29–0.54)	6 0.67 (0.50–0.90)	12 0.42 (0.34–0.52)	5 0.64 (0.55–0.76)
PIE	6 0.46 (0.36–0.59)	2 0.68 (0.50–0.93)	8 0.45 (0.37–0.55)	4 0.62 (0.54–0.71)
BPD[a]	8 0.91 (0.79–1.05)	4 1.06 (0.83–1.36)	12 0.95 (0.84–1.08)	5 0.75 (0.61–0.92)
BPD/death[a]	8 0.80 (0.72–0.88)	4 0.89 (0.77–1.03)	12 0.83 (0.77–0.90)	4 0.73 (0.65–0.83)

N, number; PIE, pulmonary interstitial emphysema.

[a] Defined at 28 d.

efficacy of the INSURE approach (intubation, surfactant administration, and extubation to CPAP) are reviewed.

PRETERM INFANTS AND SURFACTANT EFFECTIVENESS IN CLINICAL TRIALS

Surfactant trials have included infants born between 23 and 34 weeks' gestation and/or with birth weight between 500 and 2000 g.[1–12] The results of subgroup analyses from such studies indicated that surfactant therapy decreased mortality rates most effectively in infants born at less than 30 weeks' gestation or with birth weight <1250 g.[12] In addition, surfactant replacement reduced the incidence of pneumothorax, pulmonary interstitial emphysema, and the combined outcome of death or BPD, compared with no surfactant replacement[12]; these findings suggest that lung injury is mitigated after surfactant replacement. The incidence of other medical morbidities, such as BPD, intraventricular hemorrhage, necrotizing enterocolitis, health care–associated infections, retinopathy of prematurity, and patent ductus arteriosus, has not changed with surfactant replacement, but this may be attributable, in part, to the large reduction in mortality with surfactant replacement therapy.[13] The onset of clinical signs of patent ductus arteriosus may occur earlier, and the incidence of pulmonary hemorrhage, especially in infants born at less than 27 weeks' gestation, may be increased with surfactant therapy. Surfactant replacement is effective for larger and more mature preterm infants with established RDS.

PROPHYLACTIC VERSUS RESCUE SURFACTANT

A prophylactic, or preventive, surfactant strategy is defined as intubation and surfactant administration to infants at high risk of developing RDS for the primary purpose of preventing worsening RDS rather than treatment of established RDS; this has been operationalized in clinical studies as surfactant administration in the delivery room before initial resuscitation efforts or the onset of respiratory distress or, most commonly, after initial resuscitation but within 10 to 30 minutes after birth. This contrasts with a rescue or treatment surfactant strategy, in which surfactant is given only to preterm infants with established RDS. Rescue surfactant is most often administered within the first 12 hours after birth, when specified threshold criteria of severity of RDS are met.

The meta-analysis of studies conducted before routine application of CPAP demonstrated a lower mortality rate (relative risk [RR] 0.69; 95% confidence interval [CI] 0.56–0.85; number needed to benefit [NNTB] 20) and a decrease in the risk of air leak (RR 0.79; 95% CI 0.63–0.98) in preterm infants receiving prophylactic surfactant versus rescue surfactant.[14] However, when the studies that allowed for routine application of CPAP were included in the meta-analysis (National Institute of Child Health and Human Development SUPPORT Trial and Vermont Oxford Network Delivery Room Management Trial), the benefits of prophylactic surfactant on mortality (RR 0.89; 95% CI 0.76–1.04) and air leak (RR 0.86; 95% CI 0.71–1.04) could no longer be demonstrated.[5] Furthermore, infants receiving prophylactic surfactant had a higher incidence of BPD or death than did infants stabilized on CPAP (RR 1.12; 95% CI 1.02–1.24). Secondary analyses of studies that did or did not use CPAP to stabilize infants demonstrated a trend to a lower risk of intraventricular hemorrhage (RR 0.91; 95% CI 0.82–1.00) and severe intraventricular hemorrhage (RR 0.87; 95% CI 0.70–1.04) with prophylactic surfactant. That finding cannot be explained; however, there was considerable heterogeneity in the trials included in the meta-analysis. The risks of developing other complications of prematurity, such as retinopathy of prematurity, patent ductus arteriosus, and periventricular leukomalacia, were not significantly different.

When studies investigating infants born at <30 weeks' gestation were analyzed separately,[5] similar findings were noted. However, there was a trend for an increased risk of chronic lung disease in infants born at <30 weeks' gestation who received prophylactic surfactant (RR 1.13; 95% CI 1.00–1.28) and a significant increase in death or chronic lung disease (RR 1.13; 95% CI 1.02–1.25) with use of prophylactic surfactant.

EARLY VERSUS DELAYED SELECTIVE SURFACTANT TREATMENT OF RDS

Although there are no statistically significant benefits to prophylactic use of surfactant when compared with prophylactic CPAP, several studies have investigated whether administration of surfactant early in the course of respiratory insufficiency improves clinical outcomes. Early rescue is defined as surfactant treatment within 1 to 2 hours of birth, and late rescue is defined as surfactant treatment 2 or more hours after birth. A recent meta-analysis of early (within 2 hours) versus delayed surfactant treatment concluded that the risks of mortality (RR 0.84; 95% CI 0.74–0.95), air leak (RR 0.61; 95% CI 0.48–0.78), chronic lung disease (RR 0.69; 95% CI 0.55–0.86), and chronic lung disease or death (RR 0.83; 95% CI 0.75–0.91) were significantly decreased. There were no differences in other complications of prematurity.[7]

EARLY ADMINISTRATION OF SURFACTANT FOLLOWED BY BRIEF VENTILATION AND EXTUBATION TO CPAP (INSURE STRATEGY)

The INSURE strategy is widely used throughout the world. In randomized clinical trials performed before 2008, the INSURE approach, compared with rescue surfactant administration in infants with RDS, was associated with a significantly reduced need for mechanical ventilation (RR 0.67; 95% CI 0.57–0.79) and a reduced need for oxygen at 28 days.[6] In an analysis stratified by fraction of inspired oxygen requirement at study entry, a significantly higher frequency of patent ductus arteriosus was observed among infants in the rescue surfactant group, who required a fraction of inspired oxygen greater than 0.45 (RR 2.15; 95% CI 1.09–4.23). The Vermont Oxford Network Delivery Room Management Trial (*n* = 648) randomly assigned infants born at 26 to 29 weeks' gestation to 1 of 3 treatment groups: prophylactic surfactant and continued ventilation, prophylactic surfactant and rapid extubation to CPAP (INSURE), or nasal

CPAP without surfactant.[15] When compared with the group of infants receiving prophylactic surfactant and continued ventilation, the RR of death or BPD was 0.78 (95% CI 0.59–1.03) for the INSURE group and 0.83 (95% CI 0.64–1.09) for the CPAP group. However, in the nasal CPAP group, 48% were managed without intubation and 54% without surfactant treatment. A recent meta-analysis demonstrated that prophylactic surfactant (with rapid extubation to CPAP) was associated with a higher risk of death or BPD (RR 1.12; 95% CI 1.02–1.24; number needed to harm of 17) when compared with early stabilization with CPAP and selective surfactant administration.[5] In infants with birth weight ≥1250 g and mild to moderate RDS, elective intubation and administration of surfactant decreased the need for mechanical ventilation but had no effect on the duration of oxygen therapy, ventilator therapy, or hospital stay.[16]

ANIMAL-DERIVED VERSUS SYNTHETIC SURFACTANT

A wide variety of animal-derived and synthetic surfactants are available commercially (Table 2); both are beneficial as therapy for RDS in preterm infants. Animal-derived surfactants are modified or purified from bovine or porcine lungs. Treatment with animal-derived surfactants (beractant [Survanta; Abbvie Inc, North Chicago, IL], calfactant [Infasurf; ONY Inc, Amherst, NY], and poractant [Curosurf; Chiesi Farmaceutici, Parma, Italy]) has several advantages over first-generation, protein-free synthetic surfactants (eg, colfosceril palmitate [Exosurf; GlaxoSmithKline, Middlesex, UK]).[3] These include lower mortality rates (RR 0.86; 95% CI 0.76–0.98; number needed to harm of 40) and fewer pneumothoraces (RR 0.63; 95% CI 0.53–0.75; NNTB 22).[4] Animal-derived surfactants contain variable amounts

of surfactant protein B (SP-B). SP-B enhances the rate of adsorption of phospholipids at the air-water interface, is involved in the formation of tubular myelin, and has antiinflammatory properties. However, it is unclear whether significant differences in clinical outcomes exist among the available animal-derived products.

A synthetic surfactant (lucinactant) that contains a 21-amino acid peptide that mimics SP-B activity has recently been approved for the prevention and treatment of RDS in preterm infants.[18,19] When compared with animal-derived surfactant (beractant or poractant), lucinactant was shown to be equivalent.[18,19] Neonatal morbidities (intraventricular hemorrhage, periventricular leukomalacia, pulmonary hemorrhage, sepsis, patent ductus arteriosus, retinopathy of prematurity, necrotizing enterocolitis, and BPD) were not significantly different between preterm infants treated with animal-derived surfactants and those treated with synthetic surfactants.

SURFACTANT ADMINISTRATION

Surfactant administration strategies have been based on manufacturer guidelines for individual surfactants.[1] The dose of surfactant, frequency of administration, and treatment procedures have been modeled after research protocols. Furthermore, repeated doses of surfactants given at intervals for predetermined indications have decreased mortality and morbidity compared with placebo or single surfactant doses.[10] However, given the long half-life for surfactant in preterm infants with RDS,[20] redosing should not be needed more often than every 12 hours, unless surfactant is being inactivated by an infectious process, meconium, or blood. Dosing intervals shorter than 12 hours recommended by some manufacturers are not based on human pharmacokinetic data.

TABLE 2 Composition and Dosage of Surfactants[17]

Surfactant	Main Phospholipids	Proteins	Phospholipid Concentration	Suggested Dose	Phospholipid per Dose
Animal-derived					
Beractant (Survanta[a]) minced bovine lung extract	DPPC and PG	(<0.1%) SP-B and (1%) SP-C	25 mg/mL	4 mL/kg	100 mg/kg
Calfactant (Infasurf[b]) bovine calf lung lavage	DPPC and PG	(0.7%) SP-B and (1%) SP-C	35 mg/mL	3 mL/kg	105 mg/kg
Poractant (Curosurf[c]) minced porcine lung extract	DPPC and PG	(0.6%)SP-B and (1%) SP-C	80 mg/mL	2.5 mL/kg and	100-200 mg/kg
				1.25 mL/kg	100 mg/kg
Synthetic					
Colfosceril (Exosurf[d])	DPPC (100%)	None	13.5 mg/mL	5 mL/kg	67.5 mg/kg
Synthetic, protein analog					
Lucinactant (Surfaxin[e])	DPPC and POPG	KL4 peptide as SP-B	30 mg/mL	5.8 mL/kg	175 mg/kg

DPPC, dipalmitoyl phosphatidylcholine; PG, phosphatidylglycerol; POPG, palmitoyloleyl phosphatidylglycerol; SP-C, surfactant protein C.
[a] Abbvie Inc, North Chicago, IL.
[b] ONY Inc, Amherst, NY.
[c] Chiesi Farmaceutici, Parma, Italy.
[d] GlaxoSmithKline, Middlesex, UK.
[e] Discovery Laboratories, Warrington, PA.

Surfactant administration procedures may be complicated by transient airway obstruction, oxygen desaturation, bradycardia, and alterations in cerebral blood flow and brain electrical activity. The delivery of surfactant can also result in rapid improvement in lung volume, functional residual capacity, and compliance. Thus, expeditious changes in mechanical ventilator settings may be necessary to minimize the risks of lung injury and air leak. Clinicians with expertise in these procedures should be responsible for surfactant administration whenever surfactant is given.

Surfactant has traditionally been administered through an endotracheal tube either as bolus, in smaller aliquots,[21] or by infusion through an adaptor port on the proximal end of the endotracheal tube.[19] In an animal model, administration of surfactant as an intratracheal bolus while disconnected from the mechanical ventilator resulted in more uniform distribution than an infusion administered over 30 minutes through a side-hole adapter.[22] However, a small clinical trial of human preterm infants showed no significant differences in clinical outcomes between methods.[23] During surfactant administration, reflux into the endotracheal tube occurred more often when the infusion technique was used. Similar clinical outcomes were also found when surfactant was administered as a bolus or as a 1-minute infusion through a side-hole adapter.[24] Because data are conflicting and limited, the optimal method of surfactant administration in preterm infants has yet to be clearly proven. Additionally, there is insufficient evidence to recommend the optimal number of fractional doses of surfactant or what body position is best when surfactant is administered.

A number of alternatives to intratracheal administration of surfactant have been evaluated in clinical trials.[25–32] These include use of aerosolized surfactant preparations, laryngeal mask airway-aided delivery of surfactant, instillation of pharyngeal surfactant, and administration of surfactant using thin intratracheal catheters. Theoretically, each of these methods could allow administration of surfactant without intubation in spontaneously breathing infants. In a recent study, Göpel et al[25] randomized 220 preterm infants born at 26 to 28 weeks' gestation to receive either surfactant administered via a thin plastic catheter (using laryngoscopy) or surfactant administered as a rescue therapy. All infants were maintained on CPAP. The administration of surfactant through a thin plastic catheter significantly reduced the need for mechanical ventilation and decreased the need for oxygen therapy at 28 days. More data are needed to recommend any of the alternative techniques for surfactant administration.

SURFACTANT REPLACEMENT THERAPY FOR RESPIRATORY DISORDERS OTHER THAN RDS

Surfactant inactivation and secondary dysfunction may occur with conditions such as meconium aspiration syndrome, persistent pulmonary hypertension of the newborn, neonatal pneumonia, and pulmonary hemorrhage.[33,34] Surfactant administration techniques, surfactant dosage, patient populations, entry criteria, and study outcomes in the small randomized trials and case series of surfactant replacement in neonates with secondary surfactant deficiency vary considerably.[35–42]

Meconium aspiration syndrome with severe respiratory failure and persistent pulmonary hypertension may be complicated by surfactant inactivation. Surfactant replacement by bolus or slow infusion in infants with severe meconium aspiration syndrome improved oxygenation and reduced the need for extracorporeal membrane oxygenation (ECMO) (RR 0.64; 95% CI 0.46–0.91; NNTB 6).[35] Surfactant did not reduce mortality or decrease the frequency of air leaks (pneumothoraces or pulmonary interstitial emphysema). In a blinded randomized clinical trial of infants receiving ECMO, administration of surfactant shortened the duration of the ECMO. Notably, there were no infants with congenital diaphragmatic hernia in that study.[36]

Surfactant inactivation may be associated with pneumonia.[37,38] In a small randomized trial of surfactant rescue therapy, the subgroup of infants with sepsis showed improved oxygenation and a reduced need for ECMO compared with a similar group of control infants.[37] Newborn infants with pneumonia or sepsis receiving rescue surfactant also demonstrated improved gas exchange compared with infants without surfactant treatment. The number of neonates who received surfactant for sepsis and pneumonia in these clinical reports is small, and no recommendation can be made.

Surfactant treatment of pulmonary hemorrhage is plausible, because blood inhibits surfactant function. However, only a few retrospective and observational reports have documented the benefits of such therapy, and the magnitude of benefit remains to be established.[39]

Congenital diaphragmatic hernia may be associated with surfactant insufficiency.[40] Although measurements of disaturated phosphatidylcholine from lungs of infants with congenital diaphragmatic hernia show synthetic rates similar to those from infants without diaphragmatic hernia, pool sizes and kinetics are altered.[40] However, surfactant treatment of a large series of infants with congenital diaphragmatic hernia did not improve

outcomes. In fact, the need for ECMO, the incidence of chronic lung disease, and mortality rate were increased with surfactant administration.[41,42]

ANTENATAL STEROIDS AND SURFACTANT REPLACEMENT

Surfactant trials that proved efficacy were performed at a time when antenatal steroid therapy was given infrequently.[43] By the late 1990s, most mothers of preterm infants born at less than 30 weeks' gestation had received antenatal steroids (58% to 92%).[44–46] Antenatal steroids significantly reduce mortality (RR 0.62; 95% CI 0.51–0.77; NNTB 23), RDS (RR 0.65; 95% CI 0.47–0.75; NNTB 12), and surfactant use in preterm infants (RR 0.45; 95% CI 0.22–0.93; NNTB 9),[47] most consistently in those born between 28 and 34 weeks' gestation.

Results of observational studies and clinical trials have inferred that antenatal steroids may reduce the need for prophylactic and early rescue surfactant replacement in infants born after 27 to 28 weeks' gestation,[16,48] but no randomized, controlled trials have addressed this issue. In infants born at or earlier than 27 weeks' gestation, the incidence of RDS is not reduced after exposure to antenatal steroids; however, in a recently published study, death or neurodevelopment impairment at 18 to 22 months was significantly lower for infants who had been

exposed to antenatal steroids at 23 to 25 weeks' gestation.[49] Infants born before 32 weeks' gestation who received both antenatal steroids and postnatal surfactant were found on subgroup analyses to have significant reductions in mortality, severity of respiratory distress, and air leaks when compared with subgroups that received neither steroids nor surfactant, antenatal steroids only, or surfactant only.[50–52] This finding corroborates evidence from animal models of RDS that the combination of antenatal steroids and postnatal surfactant improves lung function more than either treatment alone.[53–55]

An important additional benefit of antenatal steroids is a reduction in risk of intraventricular hemorrhage, an advantage not found with surfactant replacement alone.[56] The effects of antenatal steroids on other neonatal morbidities, such as necrotizing enterocolitis and patent ductus arteriosus, have been inconsistent. However, antenatal steroids have not significantly decreased the incidence of BPD.[50,51]

CPAP AND SURFACTANT

Randomized clinical trials suggest that nasal CPAP is acceptable as an alternative to surfactant administration in preterm infants with RDS. A clinical report from the American Academy of Pediatrics, "Respiratory Support of the Preterm Infant," is forthcoming.[57]

TABLE 3 Levels of Evidence[58]

Recommendation LOE	LOE	Grade of Recommendation
Preterm infants born at <30 wk of gestation who need mechanical ventilation because of severe RDS should be given surfactant after initial stabilization.	1	Strong Recommendation
Using CPAP immediately after birth with subsequent selective surfactant administration should be considered as an alternative to routine intubation with prophylactic or early surfactant administration in preterm infants.	1	Strong Recommendation
Rescue surfactant may be considered for infants with hypoxic respiratory failure attributable to secondary surfactant deficiency (eg, meconium aspiration syndrome or sepsis/pneumonia).	2	Recommendation

SUMMARY OF SCIENCE

1. Surfactant replacement, given as prophylaxis or rescue treatment, reduces the incidence of RDS, air leaks, and mortality in preterm infants with RDS (level of evidence [LOE] 1).

2. Both animal-derived and newer synthetic surfactants with SP-B–like activity decrease acute respiratory morbidity and mortality in preterm infants with RDS (LOE 1).

3. Early rescue surfactant treatment (<2 hours of age) in infants with RDS decreases the risk of mortality, air leak, and chronic lung disease in preterm infants (LOE 1).

4. Early initiation of CPAP with subsequent selective surfactant administration in extremely preterm infants results in lower rates of BPD/death when compared with treatment with prophylactic surfactant therapy (LOE 1).

5. Surfactant replacement has not been shown to affect the incidence of neurologic, developmental, behavioral, medical, or educational outcomes in preterm infants (LOE 2).

6. Surfactant treatment improves oxygenation and reduces the need for ECMO without an increase in morbidity in neonates with meconium aspiration syndrome (LOE 2).

7. Surfactant treatment of infants with congenital diaphragmatic hernia does not improve clinical outcomes (LOE 2).

8. Antenatal steroids and postnatal surfactant replacement independently and additively reduce mortality, the severity of RDS, and air leaks in preterm infants (LOE 2).

CLINICAL IMPLICATIONS (TABLE 3)

1. Preterm infants born at <30 weeks' gestation who need mechanical ventilation because of severe RDS should be given surfactant after initial stabilization (Strong Recommendation).

2. Using CPAP immediately after birth with subsequent selective surfactant administration should be considered as an alternative to routine intubation with prophylactic or early surfactant administration in preterm infants (Strong Recommendation).

3. Rescue surfactant may be considered for infants with hypoxic respiratory failure attributable to secondary surfactant deficiency (eg, pulmonary hemorrhage, meconium aspiration syndrome, or sepsis/pneumonia) (Recommendation).

4. Preterm and term neonates who are receiving surfactant should be managed by nursery and transport personnel with the technical and clinical expertise to administer surfactant safely and deal with multisystem illness. Therefore, pediatric providers who are without expertise, or who are inexperienced or uncomfortable with surfactant administration or managing an infant who has received surfactant should wait for the transport team to arrive.

LEAD AUTHORS
Richard A. Polin, MD, FAAP
Waldemar A. Carlo, MD, FAAP

COMMITTEE ON FETUS AND NEWBORN, 2012–2013
Lu-Ann Papile, MD, FAAP, Chairperson
Richard A. Polin, MD, FAAP
Waldemar A. Carlo, MD, FAAP
Rosemarie Tan, MD, FAAP
Praveen Kumar, MD, FAAP
William Benitz, MD, FAAP
Eric Eichenwald, MD, FAAP
James Cummings, MD, FAAP
Jill Baley, MD, FAAP

CONSULTANT
Roger F. Soll, MD, FAAP

LIAISONS
Tonse N. K. Raju, MD, FAAP – *National Institutes of Health*
CAPT Wanda Denise Barfield, MD, FAAP – *Centers for Disease Control and Prevention*
Erin Keels, MSN – *National Association of Neonatal Nurses*
Anne Jefferies, MD – *Canadian Pediatric Society*
Kasper S. Wang, MD, FAAP – *AAP Section on Surgery*
George Macones, MD – *American College of Obstetricians and Gynecologists*

STAFF
Jim Couto, MA

DISCLOSURES
Dr Carlo is on the Mednax Board of Directors. Dr Polin is a consultant for Discovery Laboratories.

REFERENCES

1. Engle WA; American Academy of Pediatrics Committee on Fetus and Newborn. Surfactant-replacement therapy for respiratory distress in the preterm and term neonate. *Pediatrics.* 2008;121(2):419–432

2. Soll RF. Synthetic surfactant for respiratory distress syndrome in preterm infants. *Cochrane Database Syst Rev.* 2000;(2):CD001149

3. Seger N, Soll R. Animal derived surfactant extract for treatment of respiratory distress syndrome. *Cochrane Database Syst Rev.* 2009; (2):CD007836

4. Soll RF, Blanco F. Natural surfactant extract versus synthetic surfactant for neonatal respiratory distress syndrome. *Cochrane Database Syst Rev.* 2001;(2):CD000144

5. Rojas-Reyes MX, Morley CJ, Soll R. Prophylactic versus selective use of surfactant in preventing morbidity and mortality in preterm infants. *Cochrane Database Syst Rev.* 2012;3(3):CD000510

6. Stevens TP, Harrington EW, Blennow M, Soll RF. Early surfactant administration with brief ventilation vs. selective surfactant

and continued mechanical ventilation for preterm infants with or at risk for respiratory distress syndrome. *Cochrane Database Syst Rev.* 2007;(4):CD003063

7. Bahadue FL, Soll R. Early versus delayed selective surfactant treatment for neonatal respiratory distress syndrome. *Cochrane Database Syst Rev.* 2012;11(11):CD001456

8. Soll R, Ozek E. Prophylactic protein free synthetic surfactant for preventing morbidity and mortality in preterm infants. *Cochrane Database Syst Rev.* 2010;(1): CD001079

9. Pfister RH, Soll R, Wiswell TE. Protein-containing synthetic surfactant versus protein-free synthetic surfactant for the prevention and treatment of respiratory distress syndrome. *Cochrane Database Syst Rev.* 2009;(4):CD006180

10. Soll R, Ozek E. Multiple versus single doses of exogenous surfactant for the prevention or treatment of neonatal respiratory distress syndrome. *Cochrane Database Syst Rev.* 2009;(1):CD000141

11. Soll RF. Prophylactic natural surfactant extract for preventing morbidity and mortality in preterm infants. *Cochrane Database Syst Rev.* 2000;(2):CD000511

12. Suresh GK, Soll RF. Overview of surfactant replacement trials. *J Perinatol.* 2005;25 (suppl 2):S40–S44

13. Philip AG. Neonatal mortality rate: is further improvement possible? *J Pediatr.* 1995;126(3):427–433

14. Soll RF, Morley CJ. Prophylactic versus selective use of surfactant in preventing morbidity and mortality in preterm infants. *Cochrane Database Syst Rev.* 2001;(2): CD000510

15. Dunn MS, Kaempf J, de Klerk A, et al; Vermont Oxford Network DRM Study Group. Randomized trial comparing 3 approaches to the initial respiratory management of preterm neonates. *Pediatrics.* 2011;128(5). Available at: www.pediatrics.org/cgi/content/full/128/5/e1069

16. Escobedo MB, Gunkel JH, Kennedy KA, et al; Texas Neonatal Research Group. Early surfactant for neonates with mild to moderate respiratory distress syndrome: a multicenter, randomized trial. *J Pediatr.* 2004;144(6): 804–808

17. Moya F, Javier MC. Myth: all surfactants are alike. *Semin Fetal Neonatal Med.* 2011;16 (5):269–274

18. Sinha SK, Lacaze-Masmonteil T, Valls i Soler A, et al; Surfaxin Therapy Against Respiratory Distress Syndrome Collaborative Group. A multicenter, randomized, controlled trial of lucinactant versus poractant alfa among very premature infants at high risk for respiratory distress syndrome. *Pediatrics.* 2005;115(4):1030–1038

19. Moya F, Sinha S, Gadzinowski J, et al; SELECT and STAR Study Investigators. One-year follow-up of very preterm infants who received lucinactant for prevention of respiratory distress syndrome: results from 2 multicenter randomized, controlled trials. *Pediatrics.* 2007;119(6). Available at: www.pediatrics.org/cgi/content/full/119/6/e1361

20. Cogo PE, Facco M, Simonato M, et al. Pharmacokinetics and clinical predictors of surfactant redosing in respiratory distress syndrome. *Intensive Care Med.* 2011; 37(3):510–517

21. Kendig JW, Ryan RM, Sinkin RA, et al. Comparison of two strategies for surfactant prophylaxis in very premature infants: a multicenter randomized trial. *Pediatrics.* 1998;101(6):1006–1012

22. Ueda T, Ikegami M, Rider ED, Jobe AH. Distribution of surfactant and ventilation in surfactant-treated preterm lambs. *J Appl Physiol (1985).* 1994;76(1):45–55

23. Zola EM, Gunkel JH, Chan RK, et al. Comparison of three dosing procedures for administration of bovine surfactant to neonates with respiratory distress syndrome. *J Pediatr.* 1993;122(3):453–459

24. Valls-i-Soler A, López-Heredia J, Fernández-Ruanova MB, Gastiasoro E; Spanish Surfactant Collaborative Group. A simplified surfactant dosing procedure in respiratory distress syndrome: the "side-hole" randomized study. *Acta Paediatr.* 1997;86(7): 747–751

25. Göpel W, Kribs A, Ziegler A, et al; German Neonatal Network. Avoidance of mechanical ventilation by surfactant treatment of spontaneously breathing preterm infants (AMV): an open-label, randomised, controlled trial. *Lancet.* 2011;378(9803):1627–1634

26. Schmölzer GM, Agarwal M, Kamlin CO, Davis PG. Supraglottic airway devices during neonatal resuscitation: an historical perspective, systematic review and meta-analysis of available clinical trials. *Resuscitation.* 2013;84(6):722–730

27. Kribs A. How best to administer surfactant to VLBW infants? *Arch Dis Child Fetal Neonatal Ed.* 2011;96(4):F238–F240

28. Mehler K, Grimme J, Abele J, Huenseler C, Roth B, Kribs A. Outcome of extremely low gestational age newborns after introduction of a revised protocol to assist preterm infants in their transition to extrauterine life. *Acta Paediatr.* 2012;101(12): 1232–1239

29. Abdel-Latif ME, Osborn DA. Laryngeal mask airway surfactant administration for prevention of morbidity and mortality in preterm infants with or at risk of respiratory distress syndrome. *Cochrane Database Syst Rev.* 2011;(7):CD008309

30. Abdel-Latif ME, Osborn DA. Nebulised surfactant in preterm infants with or at risk of respiratory distress syndrome. *Cochrane Database Syst Rev.* 2012;(10):CD008310

31. Abdel-Latif ME, Osborn DA. Pharyngeal instillation of surfactant before the first breath for prevention of morbidity and mortality in preterm infants at risk of respiratory distress syndrome. *Cochrane Database Syst Rev.* 2011;(3):CD008311

32. Abdel-Latif ME, Osborn DA, Challis D. Intra-amniotic surfactant for women at risk of preterm birth for preventing respiratory distress in newborns. *Cochrane Database Syst Rev.* 2010;(1):CD007916

33. Finer NN. Surfactant use for neonatal lung injury: beyond respiratory distress syndrome. *Paediatr Respir Rev.* 2004;5(suppl A):S289–S297

34. Donn SM, Dalton J. Surfactant replacement therapy in the neonate: beyond respiratory distress syndrome. *Respir Care.* 2009;54(9): 1203–1208

35. El Shahed AI, Dargaville P, Ohlsson A, Soll RF. Surfactant for meconium aspiration syndrome in full term/near term infants. *Cochrane Database Syst Rev.* 2007;(3): CD002054

36. Lotze A, Knight GR, Martin GR, et al. Improved pulmonary outcome after exogenous surfactant therapy for respiratory failure in term infants requiring extracorporeal membrane oxygenation. *J Pediatr.* 1993;122(2):261–268

37. Tan K, Lai NM, Sharma A. Surfactant for bacterial pneumonia in late preterm and term infants. *Cochrane Database Syst Rev.* 2012;(2):CD008155

38. Vento GM, Tana M, Tirone C, et al. Effectiveness of treatment with surfactant in premature infants with respiratory failure and pulmonary infection. *Acta Biomed.* 2012;83(suppl 1):33–36

39. Aziz A, Ohlsson A. Surfactant for pulmonary haemorrhage in neonates. *Cochrane Database Syst Rev.* 2012;(7):CD005254

40. Cogo PE, Zimmermann LJ, Meneghini L, et al. Pulmonary surfactant disaturated-phosphatidylcholine (DSPC) turnover and pool size in newborn infants with congenital diaphragmatic hernia (CDH). *Pediatr Res.* 2003;54(5):653–658

41. Van Meurs K; Congenital Diaphragmatic Hernia Study Group. Is surfactant therapy beneficial in the treatment of the term newborn infant with congenital diaphragmatic hernia? *J Pediatr.* 2004;145(3):312–316

42. Lally KP, Lally PA, Langham MR, et al; Congenital Diaphragmatic Hernia Study Group. Surfactant does not improve survival rate in preterm infants with congenital diaphragmatic hernia. *J Pediatr Surg.* 2004;39(6):829–833

43. Wright LL, Horbar JD, Gunkel H, et al. Evidence from multicenter networks on the current use and effectiveness of antenatal corticosteroids in low birth weight infants. *Am J Obstet Gynecol.* 1995;173(1):263–269

44. Chien LY, Ohlsson A, Seshia MM, Boulton J, Sankaran K, Lee SK; Canadian Neonatal Network. Variations in antenatal corticosteroid therapy: a persistent problem despite 30 years of evidence. *Obstet Gynecol.* 2002;99(3):401–408

45. Horbar JD, Badger GJ, Carpenter JH, et al; Members of the Vermont Oxford Network. Trends in mortality and morbidity for very low birth weight infants, 1991-1999. *Pediatrics.* 2002;110(1 pt 1):143–151

46. St John EB, Carlo WA. Respiratory distress syndrome in VLBW infants: changes in management and outcomes observed by the NICHD Neonatal Research Network. *Semin Perinatol.* 2003;27(4):288–292

47. Roberts D, Dalziel S. Antenatal corticosteroids for accelerating fetal lung maturation for women at risk of preterm birth. *Cochrane Database Syst Rev.* 2006;(3): CD004454

48. Gortner L, Wauer RR, Hammer H, et al. Early versus late surfactant treatment in preterm infants of 27 to 32 weeks' gestational age: a multicenter controlled clinical trial. *Pediatrics.* 1998;102(5):1153–1160

49. Carlo WA, McDonald SA, Fanaroff AA, et al; Eunice Kennedy Shriver National Institute of Child Health and Human Development Neonatal Research Network. Association of antenatal corticosteroids with mortality and neurodevelopmental outcomes among infants born at 22 to 25 weeks' gestation. *JAMA.* 2011;306(21):2348–2358

50. Jobe AH, Mitchell BR, Gunkel JH. Beneficial effects of the combined use of prenatal corticosteroids and postnatal surfactant on preterm infants. *Am J Obstet Gynecol.* 1993;168(2):508–513

51. Kari MA, Hallman M, Eronen M, et al. Prenatal dexamethasone treatment in conjunction with rescue therapy of human surfactant: a randomized placebo-controlled multicenter study. *Pediatrics.* 1994;93(5):730–736

52. White A, Marcucci G, Andrews E, Edwards K, Long W; The American Exosurf Neonatal Study Group I and The Canadian Exosurf Neonatal Study Group. Antenatal steroids and neonatal outcomes in controlled clinical trials of surfactant replacement. *Am J Obstet Gynecol.* 1995;173(1):286–290

53. Seidner S, Pettenazzo A, Ikegami M, Jobe A. Corticosteroid potentiation of surfactant dose response in preterm rabbits. *J Appl Physiol (1985).* 1988;64(6):2366–2371

54. Ikegami M, Jobe AH, Seidner S, Yamada T. Gestational effects of corticosteroids and surfactant in ventilated rabbits. *Pediatr Res.* 1989;25(1):32–37

55. Gladstone IM, Mercurio MR, Devenny SG, Jacobs HC. Antenatal steroids, postnatal surfactant, and pulmonary function in premature rabbits. *J Appl Physiol (1985).* 1989;67(4):1377–1382

56. National Institutes of Health. Effect of corticosteroids for fetal maturation on perinatal outcomes. *NIH Consens Statement.* 1994;12(2):1–24

57. Carlo W, Polin RA; American Academy of Pediatrics, Committee on Fetus and Newborn. Respiratory support in preterm infants at birth. *Pediatrics.* In press

58. US Preventive Services Task Force. Grade definition recommendations after 2007. Available at: www.uspreventiveservices-taskforce.org/uspstf/grades.htm. Accessed June 7, 2013

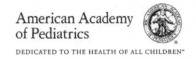

American Academy
of Pediatrics
DEDICATED TO THE HEALTH OF ALL CHILDREN™

Guidance for the Clinician in
Rendering Pediatric Care

CLINICAL REPORT

Use of Inhaled Nitric Oxide in Preterm Infants

abstract

Nitric oxide, an important signaling molecule with multiple regulatory effects throughout the body, is an important tool for the treatment of full-term and late-preterm infants with persistent pulmonary hypertension of the newborn and hypoxemic respiratory failure. Several randomized controlled trials have evaluated its role in the management of preterm infants ≤34 weeks' gestational age with varying results. The purpose of this clinical report is to summarize the existing evidence for the use of inhaled nitric oxide in preterm infants and provide guidance regarding its use in this population. *Pediatrics* 2014;133:164–170

INTRODUCTION

Nitric oxide (NO) is an important signaling molecule with multiple regulatory effects throughout the body. In perinatal medicine, inhaled nitric oxide (iNO) was initially studied for its pulmonary vasodilating effects in infants with pulmonary hypertension and has since become an important tool for the treatment of full-term and late-preterm infants with persistent pulmonary hypertension of the newborn and hypoxemic respiratory failure.[1] Inhaled NO also has multiple and complex systemic and pulmonary effects. In animal models of neonatal chronic lung disease, iNO stimulates angiogenesis, augments alveolarization, improves surfactant function, and inhibits proliferation of smooth muscle cells and abnormal elastin deposition.[2–6] Although the evidence for similar benefits in preterm infants is lacking, the off-label use of iNO in this population has escalated.[7] A study published in 2010 reported a sixfold increase (from 0.3% to 1.8%) in the use of iNO among infants born at less than 34 weeks' gestation between 2000 and 2008.[7] The greatest increase occurred among infants who were born at 23 to 26 weeks' gestation (0.8% to 6.6%). The National Institutes of Health convened a consensus panel in October 2010 to evaluate the evidence for safety and efficacy of iNO therapy in preterm infants. After reviewing the published evidence, the panel concluded that the available evidence does not support the use of iNO in early routine, early rescue, or later rescue regimens in the care of infants born at less than 34 weeks' gestation and that hospitals, clinicians, and the pharmaceutical industry should avoid marketing iNO for this group of infants.[8] An individual-patient data meta-analysis of 14 randomized controlled trials reached similar conclusions.[9] The purpose of this clinical report is to summarize the

Praveen Kumar MD, FAAP, and COMMITTEE ON FETUS AND NEWBORN

KEY WORDS
inhaled nitric oxide, preterm infants, hypoxic respiratory failure, bronchopulmonary dysplasia

ABBREVIATIONS
BPD—bronchopulmonary dysplasia
iNO—inhaled nitric oxide
NO—nitric oxide
NOCLD—Nitric Oxide Chronic Lung Disease study group

www.pediatrics.org/cgi/doi/10.1542/peds.2013-3444

doi:10.1542/peds.2013-3444

All clinical reports from the American Academy of Pediatrics automatically expire 5 years after publication unless reaffirmed, revised, or retired at or before that time.

PEDIATRICS (ISSN Numbers: Print, 0031-4005; Online, 1098-4275).

existing evidence for the use of iNO in preterm infants and provide guidance regarding its use in this population.

LITERATURE REVIEW

Use of iNO in Preterm Infants With Respiratory Failure

The benefits associated with iNO therapy in full-term and late-preterm infants with persistent pulmonary hypertension of the newborn and hypoxemic respiratory failure initiated interest in exploring whether iNO could reduce the rates of death and neonatal morbidities in more immature infants. Pilot studies reported short-term improvement in oxygenation with iNO, but no significant benefit was observed in mortality or other morbidities.[10–15] Subsequently, several randomized clinical trials were undertaken.[16–23] Table 1 outlines the study population, entry criteria, and dose and duration of iNO treatment and summarizes the outcomes for all published randomized controlled trials. Only 1 small trial of 40 patients reported a beneficial effect on survival (Table 1). Subgroup analyses of secondary outcomes have provided conflicting results. Post hoc analysis of the Neonatal Research Network study suggested that iNO therapy was associated with reduced rates of death and bronchopulmonary dysplasia (BPD) in infants with a birth weight greater than 1000 g, but higher mortality and increased risk of severe intracranial hemorrhage in infants weighing 1000 g or less at birth.[17] In contrast, another large multicenter US trial reported no significant difference in the primary outcome of death or BPD between treated and control groups; however, infants treated with iNO had fewer brain lesions (eg, grade 3 or 4 intracranial hemorrhage, periventricular leukomalacia, and/or ventriculomegaly) noted on cranial ultrasonography.[20] A European multicenter study reported that

infants randomized to iNO treatment had longer duration of ventilation, time on oxygen therapy, and length of hospital stay compared with the placebo group, although none of these results were statistically significant.[19]

Use of iNO in Preterm Infants to Improve the Rate of Survival Without BPD

Lung pathology in preterm infants with BPD is characterized by reduced numbers of large alveoli and abnormal pulmonary vasculature development. Surfactant deficiency, ventilator-induced lung injury, oxygen toxicity, and inflammation appear to play important roles in its pathogenesis.[26,27] In animal models of neonatal lung injury, iNO promotes angiogenesis, decreases apoptosis, and reduces lung inflammation and oxidant injury.[28–30] In an early study of iNO use in preterm infants, the incidence of BPD was reduced in treated infants who required ventilator support.[16] Of 3 subsequent large randomized trials designed to evaluate the effect of iNO therapy on survival without BPD,[20,24,25] 2 found no significant benefit[20,25] (Table 1). A third trial, which featured late treatment (7–21 days of age), a longer duration of drug exposure (25 days), and a higher cumulative dose, demonstrated a modest but statistically significant beneficial effect (44% iNO vs 37% placebo; $P = .042$).[24] A subgroup analysis showed that the beneficial effect was seen in infants enrolled between 7 and 14 days of age but not those enrolled between the ages of 15 and 21 days.[24]

EFFECTS OF INO THERAPY ON NEURODEVELOPMENTAL OUTCOME

Studies in animal models suggest that iNO may have direct beneficial effects on the brain through mechanisms involving the cerebral vasculature and/or neuronal maturation.[31,32] Other investigators have described a possible role

for intravascular NO-derived molecules in conserving and stabilizing NO bioactivity that may contribute to the regulation of regional blood flow and oxygen delivery.[33,34] Neurodevelopmental outcome has been reported for 6 clinical trials,[35–40] and of these, 1 noted a more favorable neurodevelopmental outcome at 1 year of age among the preterm cohort treated with iNO but no difference in the rate of cerebral palsy.[36]

EFFECTS OF INO THERAPY ON LONG-TERM PULMONARY OUTCOME OF SURVIVORS

In animal models, iNO decreases baseline airway resistance and may increase the rate of alveolarization.[2–6] To date, only 2 studies have reported respiratory outcomes of preterm infants treated with iNO.[41,42] In a telephone survey that included 456 infants in the Nitric Oxide Chronic Lung Disease (NOCLD) study group, the use of bronchodilators, inhaled steroids, systemic steroids, diuretics, and supplemental oxygen during the first year of life was less in the iNO-treated group, but there were no significant differences in the frequency of wheezing or the rate of rehospitalization. In the Inhaled Nitric Oxide Versus Ventilatory Support Without Inhaled Nitric Oxide multicenter trial, follow-up at 1 year of age showed no difference in maximal expiratory flow at functional residual capacity, wheezing, readmission rate, or use of respiratory medications.[42]

RESULTS OF META-ANALYSES OF STUDIES EVALUATING THE USE OF INO IN PRETERM INFANTS

Two published meta-analyses found no overall significant effect of iNO on the rate of mortality, BPD, intraventricular hemorrhage, or neurodevelopmental impairment.[43,44] In view of the limitations

TABLE 1 Randomized Controlled Trials of iNO in Preterm Infants

Author, Year	n	Gestational Age, wk	Birth Weight, g	Age at Enrollment	Entry Criteria	iNO Protocol	Primary Outcome	Study Results
Subhedar, 1997[11]	42	<32	—	96 h	Need for mechanical ventilation and high risk of developing CLD	20 ppm for at least first 2 h and then 5 ppm for 3–4 d	Death and/or CLD before discharge	No difference in primary outcome
Kinsella, 1999[12]	80	≤34	—	≤7 d	aAO₂ ratio <0.1 on 2 consecutive blood gases in first 7 d of life	5 ppm for 7–14 d	Survival	No difference in primary outcome; no difference in rate of IVH or CLD
The French-Belgian iNO Trial, 1999[13]	85	<33	—	<7 d	OI between 12.5 and 30.0 on 2 consecutive blood gases at least 1 h apart	10–20 ppm for a minimum of 2 h	OI reduction of ≥33% or at least 10 points	More treated infants achieved primary outcome; no difference in median OI at 2 h; no difference in survival or other outcomes
Srisuparp, 2002[15]	34	—	<2000	<72 h	OI ranging from >4 to >12 based on birth wt	20 ppm for 24–48 h and then 5 ppm for maximum of 7 d	Change in oxygenation	Improved oxygenation with treatment but no difference in survival or IVH
Schreiber, 2003[16]	207	<34	<2000	<72 h	Need for mechanical ventilation	10 ppm for first day then 5 ppm for 6 d	Death and survival without BPD at 36 wk postmenstrual age	Treatment associated with a decrease in the combined incidence of BPD and death; no difference in mortality alone
Van Meurs, 2005[17]	420	<34	401–1500	4–120 h; mean 26–28 h	OI ≥10 on 2 consecutive blood gases between 30 min and 12 h apart	5–10 ppm for maximum of 14 d	Incidence of death or BPD	No difference in primary outcome; no difference in rate of BPD, severe IVH, or PVL. Post hoc analyses: Decrease in primary outcome in cohort with birth weight >1000 g; higher rate of mortality and severe IVH in cohort with birth wt <1000 g
Hascoet, 2005[18]	145	<32	—	6–48 h	aAO₂ ratio <0.22	5 ppm for first h of treatment and further dosage were adjusted based on response; total duration of treatment not clearly defined but varied from 4 h in nonresponders to few days in responders	Intact survival at 28 d	No difference in primary outcome; iNO was an independent risk factor for the combined risk of death or brain lesion
Field, 2005[19]	108	<34	—	<28 d; median 1 d	Severe respiratory failure requiring assisted ventilation	5–40 ppm depending on patient response; total duration of treatment not clearly defined	Death or severe disability at 1 y corrected age; death or CLD	No difference in primary outcome
Kinsella, 2006[20]	793	≤34	500–1250	<48 h	Need for mechanical ventilation	5 ppm for maximum of 21 d	Death or BPD at 36 wk postmenstrual age	No difference in primary outcome but had a decreased risk of brain injury; decreased incidence of BPD in cohort with birth weight ≤1000 g
Dani, 2006[21]	40	<30	—	≤7 d	aAO₂ ratio <0.15	10 ppm for 4 h then 6 ppm until extubation	Death and BPD	Primary outcome less with iNO treatment

TABLE 1 Continued

Author, Year	n	Gestational Age, wk	Birth Weight, g	Age at Enrollment	Entry Criteria	iNO Protocol	Primary Outcome	Study Results
Ballard, 2006[24]	582	≤32	500–1250	7–21 d	Need for mechanical ventilation for lung disease between 7 and 21 d; infants with birth weight 500–799 g were eligible if requiring nasal CPAP	20 ppm for 48–96 h followed by 10, 5, and 2 ppm at weekly intervals, with a minimum treatment duration of 24 d	Survival without BPD at 36 wk of postmenstrual age	Improved survival without BPD at 36 wk postmenstrual age; post hoc analysis showed most benefit when iNO treatment was started between 7–14 d of age
Van Meurs, 2007[23]	29	<34	>1500	4–120 h; mean 24–25 h	OI ≥15 on 2 consecutive blood gases between 30 min and 12 h apart	5–10 ppm for maximum of 14 d	Incidence of death or BPD	No difference in primary outcome
Su and Chen, 2008[22]	65	<32	≤1500	Mean 2.5 d	OI ≥25	5–20 ppm based on patient response; treatment duration at physician discretion (mean duration 4.9 ± 2.3 d)	OI at 24 h after randomization	Improved oxygenation with iNO treatment; no difference in survival, CLD, IVH, PDA, ROP, or duration of intubation
Mercier, 2010[25]	800	<29	>500	First day of life	Need for surfactant or CPAP within 24 h of birth	5 ppm for minimum of 7 d and maximum of 21 d	Survival without BPD at 36 wk postmenstrual age	No difference in primary outcome; no difference in survival alone; no difference in BPD; no difference in brain injury

Dash indicates not part of enrollment criteria.

aAO₂, arterial-alveolar oxygen ratio; CLD, chronic lung disease; CPAP, continuous positive airway pressure; IVH, intraventricular hemorrhage; OI, oxygenation index; PDA, patent ductus arteriosus; PVL, periventricular leukomalacia; ROP, retinopathy of prematurity.

of meta-analysis using aggregate data from different trials and to identify any patient or treatment characteristics that might predict benefit, Askie et al[9] conducted an individual-patient data meta-analysis. Data from 3298 infants in 11 trials that included 96% of published data showed no statistically significant effect of iNO on the rate of death or chronic lung disease (relative risk 0.96; 95% confidence interval 0.92–1.01) or severe brain lesions on cranial imaging (relative risk 1.12; 95% confidence interval 0.98–1.28). There were no statistically significant differences in iNO effect according to any of the patient-level characteristics tested; however, the authors cautioned that they could not exclude the possibility of a small reduction in the combined outcome of death or chronic lung disease if a higher dose of iNO (20 ppm) was used after >7 days of age, as observed in the NOCLD study.[9,24]

COST-BENEFIT ANALYSES OF ROUTINE USE OF INO IN PRETERM INFANTS

Treatment with iNO is expensive and can add significantly to health care costs.[8] A retrospective economic evaluation using patient-level data from the NOCLD trial (the only trial showing clinical benefit) reported that the overall mean cost per infant for the initial hospitalization was similar in the treated and placebo groups; however, when iNO therapy was initiated between 7 and 14 days of age, there was a 71% probability that the treatment decreased costs and improved outcomes.[45] Cost-benefit analysis from 2 other studies failed to show any cost-benefit.[37,39] Among preterm infants in the Inhaled Nitric Oxide Versus Ventilatory Support Without Inhaled Nitric Oxide trial, there was no difference in resource use and cost of care through the 4-year assessment.[37] Using more robust research methodology, including data on postdischarge resource utilization and health-related quality of life evaluations, Watson et al[39] found that costs of care did not vary significantly by treatment arm through 1 year of age. Although quality-adjusted survival was slightly better with iNO therapy, the estimated incremental cost-effectiveness ratio was $2.25 million per quality-adjusted life year, with only a 12.9% probability that the incremental cost-effectiveness ratio would be less than $500 000 per quality-adjusted life year. Additionally, in subgroup analysis, total costs were significantly higher for the iNO-treated group in the smallest birth weight stratum (500–749 g).

SAFETY OF INO USE IN PRETERM INFANTS

The only information regarding the safety of iNO use in preterm infants is derived from the NOCLD trial.[46–49] The limited data suggest that iNO is safe and does not increase lung inflammation or oxidative stress.[46,48]

SUMMARY

1. The results of randomized controlled trials, traditional meta-analyses, and an individualized patient data meta-analysis study indicate that neither rescue nor routine use of iNO improves survival in preterm infants with respiratory failure (Evidence quality, A; Grade of recommendation, strong).[50]

2. The preponderance of evidence does not support treating preterm infants who have respiratory failure with iNO for the purpose of preventing/ameliorating BPD, severe intraventricular hemorrhage, or other neonatal morbidities (Evidence quality, A; Grade of recommendation, strong).

3. The incidence of cerebral palsy, neurodevelopmental impairment, or cognitive impairment in preterm infants treated with iNO is similar to that of control infants (Evidence quality, A).

4. The results of 1 multicenter, randomized controlled trial suggest that treatment with a high dose of iNO (20 ppm) beginning in the second postnatal week may provide a small reduction in the rate of BPD. However, these results need to be confirmed by other trials.

5. An individual-patient data meta-analysis that included 96% of preterm infants enrolled in all published iNO trials found no statistically significant differences in iNO effect according to any of the patient-level characteristics, including gestational age, race, oxygenation index, postnatal age at enrollment, evidence of pulmonary hypertension, and mode of ventilation.

6. There are limited data and inconsistent results regarding the effects of iNO treatment on pulmonary outcomes of preterm infants in early childhood.

LEAD AUTHOR
Praveen Kumar, MD, FAAP

COMMITTEE ON FETUS AND NEWBORN, 2012–2013
Lu-Ann Papile, MD, FAAP, Chairperson
Richard A. Polin, MD, FAAP
Waldemar A. Carlo, MD, FAAP
Rosemarie Tan, MD, FAAP
Praveen Kumar, MD, FAAP
William Benitz, MD, FAAP
Eric Eichenwald, MD, FAAP
James Cummings, MD, FAAP
Jill Baley, MD, FAAP

LIAISONS
Tonse N. K. Raju, MD, FAAP – *National Institutes of Health*
CAPT Wanda Denise Barfield, MD, FAAP – *Centers for Disease Control and Prevention*
Erin Keels, MSN – *National Association of Neonatal Nurses*
Anne Jefferies, MD – *Canadian Pediatric Society*
Kasper S. Wang, MD, FAAP – *AAP Section on Surgery*
George Macones, MD – *American College of Obstetricians and Gynecologists*

STAFF
Jim Couto, MA

REFERENCES

1. American Academy of Pediatrics, Committee on Fetus and Newborn. American Academy of Pediatrics. Committee on Fetus and Newborn. Use of inhaled nitric oxide. *Pediatrics*. 2000;106(2 pt 1):344–345

2. Lin YJ, Markham NE, Balasubramaniam V, et al. Inhaled nitric oxide enhances distal lung growth after exposure to hyperoxia in neonatal rats. *Pediatr Res*. 2005;58(1):22–29

3. McCurnin DC, Pierce RA, Chang LY, et al. Inhaled NO improves early pulmonary function and modifies lung growth and elastin deposition in a baboon model of neonatal chronic lung disease. *Am J Physiol Lung Cell Mol Physiol*. 2005;288(3): L450–L459

4. Ballard PL, Gonzales LW, Godinez RI, et al. Surfactant composition and function in a primate model of infant chronic lung disease: effects of inhaled nitric oxide. *Pediatr Res*. 2006;59(1):157–162

5. Bland RD, Albertine KH, Carlton DP, MacRitchie AJ. Inhaled nitric oxide effects on lung structure and function in chronically ventilated preterm lambs. *Am J Respir Crit Care Med*. 2005;172(7):899–906

6. Tang JR, Markham NE, Lin YJ, et al. Inhaled nitric oxide attenuates pulmonary hypertension and improves lung growth in infant rats after neonatal treatment with a VEGF receptor inhibitor. *Am J Physiol Lung Cell Mol Physiol*. 2004;287(2):L344–L351

7. Clark RH, Ursprung RL, Walker MW, Ellsbury DL, Spitzer AR. The changing pattern of inhaled nitric oxide use in the neonatal

intensive care unit. *J Perinatol.* 2010;30 (12):800–804

8. Cole FS, Alleyne C, Barks JD, et al. NIH Consensus Development Conference statement: inhaled nitric-oxide therapy for premature infants. *Pediatrics.* 2011;127(2): 363–369

9. Askie LM, Ballard RA, Cutter GR, et al; Meta-analysis of Preterm Patients on Inhaled Nitric Oxide Collaboration. Inhaled nitric oxide in preterm infants: an individual-patient data meta-analysis of randomized trials. *Pediatrics.* 2011;128(4):729–739

10. Skimming JW, Bender KA, Hutchison AA, Drummond WH. Nitric oxide inhalation in infants with respiratory distress syndrome. *J Pediatr.* 1997;130(2):225–230

11. Subhedar NV, Ryan SW, Shaw NJ. Open randomised controlled trial of inhaled nitric oxide and early dexamethasone in high risk preterm infants. *Arch Dis Child Fetal Neonatal Ed.* 1997;77(3):F185–F190

12. Kinsella JP, Walsh WF, Bose CL, et al. Inhaled nitric oxide in premature neonates with severe hypoxaemic respiratory failure: a randomised controlled trial. *Lancet.* 1999; 354(9184):1061–1065

13. The Franco-Belgium Collaborative NO Trial Group. Early compared with delayed inhaled nitric oxide in moderately hypoxaemic neonates with respiratory failure: a randomised controlled trial. *Lancet.* 1999; 354(9184):1066–1071

14. Truffert P, Llado-Paris J, Mercier JC, Dehan M, Bréart G; Franco-Belgian iNO Study Group. Early inhaled nitric oxide in moderately hypoxemic preterm and term newborns with RDS: the RDS subgroup analysis of the Franco-Belgian iNO Randomized Trial. *Eur J Pediatr.* 2003;162(9):646–647

15. Srisuparp P, Heitschmidt M, Schreiber MD. Inhaled nitric oxide therapy in premature infants with mild to moderate respiratory distress syndrome. *J Med Assoc Thai.* 2002; 85(suppl 2):S469–S478

16. Schreiber MD, Gin-Mestan K, Marks JD, Huo D, Lee G, Srisuparp P. Inhaled nitric oxide in premature infants with the respiratory distress syndrome. *N Engl J Med.* 2003;349 (22):2099–2107

17. Van Meurs KP, Wright LL, Ehrenkranz RA, et al; Preemie Inhaled Nitric Oxide Study. Inhaled nitric oxide for premature infants with severe respiratory failure. *N Engl J Med.* 2005;353(1):13–22

18. Hascoet JM, Fresson J, Claris O, et al. The safety and efficacy of nitric oxide therapy in premature infants. *J Pediatr.* 2005;146(3): 318–323

19. Field D, Elbourne D, Truesdale A, et al; INNOVO Trial Collaborating Group. Neonatal ventilation with inhaled nitric oxide versus ventilatory support without inhaled nitric oxide for preterm infants with severe respiratory failure: the INNOVO multicentre randomised controlled trial (ISRCTN 17821339). *Pediatrics.* 2005;115(4):926–936

20. Kinsella JP, Cutter GR, Walsh WF, et al. Early inhaled nitric oxide therapy in premature newborns with respiratory failure. *N Engl J Med.* 2006;355(4):354–364

21. Dani C, Bertini G, Pezzati M, Filippi L, Cecchi A, Rubaltelli FF. Inhaled nitric oxide in very preterm infants with severe respiratory distress syndrome. *Acta Paediatr.* 2006;95 (9):1116–1123

22. Su PH, Chen JY. Inhaled nitric oxide in the management of preterm infants with severe respiratory failure. *J Perinatol.* 2008; 28(2):112–116

23. Van Meurs KP, Hintz SR, Ehrenkranz RA, et al. Inhaled nitric oxide in infants >1500 g and <34 weeks gestation with severe respiratory failure. *J Perinatol.* 2007;27(6): 347–352

24. Ballard RA, Truog WE, Cnaan A, et al; NO CLD Study Group. Inhaled nitric oxide in preterm infants undergoing mechanical ventilation. *N Engl J Med.* 2006;355(4):343–353

25. Mercier JC, Hummler H, Durrmeyer X, et al; EUNO Study Group. Inhaled nitric oxide for prevention of bronchopulmonary dysplasia in premature babies (EUNO): a randomised controlled trial. *Lancet.* 2010;376(9738):346–354

26. Jobe AH, Bancalari E. Bronchopulmonary dysplasia. *Am J Respir Crit Care Med.* 2001; 163(7):1723–1729

27. Stenmark KR, Abman SH. Lung vascular development: implications for the pathogenesis of bronchopulmonary dysplasia. *Annu Rev Physiol.* 2005;67:623–661

28. Balasubramaniam V, Maxey AM, Morgan DB, Markham NE, Abman SH. Inhaled NO restores lung structure in eNOS-deficient mice recovering from neonatal hypoxia. *Am J Physiol Lung Cell Mol Physiol.* 2006; 291(1):L119–L127

29. Tang JR, Seedorf G, Balasubramaniam V, Maxey A, Markham N, Abman SH. Early inhaled nitric oxide treatment decreases apoptosis of endothelial cells in neonatal rat lungs after vascular endothelial growth factor inhibition. *Am J Physiol Lung Cell Mol Physiol.* 2007;293(5):L1271–L1280

30. Gutierrez HH, Nieves B, Chumley P, Rivera A, Freeman BA. Nitric oxide regulation of superoxide-dependent lung injury: oxidant-protective actions of endogenously produced and exogenously administered nitric oxide. *Free Radic Biol Med.* 1996;21(1):43–52

31. Zhang YT, Zhang DL, Cao YL, Zhao BL. Developmental expression and activity varia-

tion of nitric oxide synthase in the brain of golden hamster. *Brain Res Bull.* 2002;58(4): 385–389

32. Soygüder Z, Karadağ H, Nazli M. Neuronal nitric oxide synthase immunoreactivity in ependymal cells during early postnatal development. *J Chem Neuroanat.* 2004;27(1):3–6

33. Cannon RO, III, Schechter AN, Panza JA, et al. Effects of inhaled nitric oxide on regional blood flow are consistent with intravascular nitric oxide delivery. *J Clin Invest.* 2001;108(2):279–287

34. McMahon TJ, Moon RE, Luschinger BP, et al. Nitric oxide in the human respiratory cycle. *Nat Med.* 2002;8(7):711–717

35. Bennett AJ, Shaw NJ, Gregg JE, Subhedar NV. Neurodevelopmental outcome in high-risk preterm infants treated with inhaled nitric oxide. *Acta Paediatr.* 2001;90(5):573–576

36. Mestan KK, Marks JD, Hecox K, Huo D, Schreiber MD. Neurodevelopmental outcomes of premature infants treated with inhaled nitric oxide. *N Engl J Med.* 2005;353(1):23–32

37. Huddy CL, Bennett CC, Hardy P, et al; INNOVO Trial Collaborating Group. The INNOVO multicentre randomised controlled trial: neonatal ventilation with inhaled nitric oxide versus ventilatory support without nitric oxide for severe respiratory failure in preterm infants: follow up at 4–5 years. *Arch Dis Child Fetal Neonatal Ed.* 2008;93(6):F430–F435

38. Hintz SR, Van Meurs KP, Perritt R, et al; NICHD Neonatal Research Network. Neurodevelopmental outcomes of premature infants with severe respiratory failure enrolled in a randomized controlled trial of inhaled nitric oxide. *J Pediatr.* 2007;151(1): 16–22, 22.e1–e3

39. Watson RS, Clermont G, Kinsella JP, et al; Prolonged Outcomes After Nitric Oxide Investigators. Clinical and economic effects of iNO in premature newborns with respiratory failure at 1 year. *Pediatrics.* 2009; 124(5):1333–1343

40. Walsh MC, Hibbs AM, Martin CR, et al; NO CLD Study Group. Two-year neurodevelopmental outcomes of ventilated preterm infants treated with inhaled nitric oxide. *J Pediatr.* 2010;156(4):556–561.e1

41. Hibbs AM, Walsh MC, Martin RJ, et al. One-year respiratory outcomes of preterm infants enrolled in the Nitric Oxide (to prevent) Chronic Lung Disease trial. *J Pediatr.* 2008;153(4):525–529

42. Hoo AF, Beardsmore CS, Castle RA, et al; INNOVO Trial Collaborating Group. Respiratory function during infancy in survivors of the INNOVO trial. *Pediatr Pulmonol.* 2009;44(2):155–161

43. Barrington KJ, Finer N. Inhaled nitric oxide for respiratory failure in preterm infants.

Cochrane Database Syst Rev. 2010;(12): CD000509

44. Donohue PK, Gilmore MM, Cristofalo E, et al. Inhaled nitric oxide in preterm infants: a systematic review. *Pediatrics.* 2011;127(2). Available at: www.pediatrics.org/cgi/content/full/127/2/e414

45. Zupancic JA, Hibbs AM, Palermo L, et al; NO CLD Trial Group. Economic evaluation of inhaled nitric oxide in preterm infants undergoing mechanical ventilation. *Pediatrics.* 2009;124(5):1325–1332

46. Truog WE, Ballard PL, Norberg M, et al; Nitric Oxide (to Prevent) Chronic Lung Disease Study Investigators. Inflammatory markers and mediators in tracheal fluid of premature infants treated with inhaled nitric oxide. *Pediatrics.* 2007;119(4):670–678

47. Ballard PL, Merrill JD, Truog WE, et al. Surfactant function and composition in premature infants treated with inhaled nitric oxide. *Pediatrics.* 2007;120(2):346–353

48. Ballard PL, Truog WE, Merrill JD, et al. Plasma biomarkers of oxidative stress: relationship to lung disease and inhaled nitric oxide therapy in premature infants. *Pediatrics.* 2008;121(3):555–561

49. Posencheg MA, Gow AJ, Truog WE, et al; NO CLD Investigators. Inhaled nitric oxide in premature infants: effect on tracheal aspirate and plasma nitric oxide metabolites. *J Perinatol.* 2010;30(4):275–280

50. American Academy of Pediatrics Steering Committee on Quality Improvement and Management. Classifying recommendations for clinical practice guidelines. *Pediatrics.* 2004;114(3):874–877

SECTION 5

Infections/ Vaccinations

POLICY STATEMENT Organizational Principles to Guide and Define the Child Health Care System and/or Improve the Health of all Children

American Academy
of Pediatrics

DEDICATED TO THE HEALTH OF ALL CHILDREN™

Elimination of Perinatal Hepatitis B: Providing the First Vaccine Dose Within 24 Hours of Birth

COMMITTEE ON INFECTIOUS DISEASES, COMMITTEE ON FETUS AND NEWBORN

abstract

After the introduction of the hepatitis B vaccine in the United States in 1982, a greater than 90% reduction in new infections was achieved. However, approximately 1000 new cases of perinatal hepatitis B infection are still identified annually in the United States. Prevention of perinatal hepatitis B relies on the proper and timely identification of infants born to mothers who are hepatitis B surface antigen positive and to mothers with unknown status to ensure administration of appropriate postexposure immunoprophylaxis with hepatitis B vaccine and immune globulin. To reduce the incidence of perinatal hepatitis B transmission further, the American Academy of Pediatrics endorses the recommendation of the Advisory Committee on Immunization Practices of the Centers for Disease Control and Prevention that all newborn infants with a birth weight of greater than or equal to 2000 g receive hepatitis B vaccine by 24 hours of age.

DOI: https://doi.org/10.1542/peds.2017-1870

PEDIATRICS (ISSN Numbers: Print, 0031-4005; Online, 1098-4275).

Copyright © 2017 by the American Academy of Pediatrics

FINANCIAL DISCLOSURE: The authors have indicated they have no financial relationships relevant to this article to disclose.

FUNDING: No external funding.

POTENTIAL CONFLICT OF INTEREST: The authors have indicated they have no potential conflicts of interest to disclose.

To cite: AAP COMMITTEE ON INFECTIOUS DISEASES and AAP COMMITTEE ON FETUS AND NEWBORN. Elimination of Perinatal Hepatitis B: Providing the First Vaccine Dose Within 24 Hours of Birth. *Pediatrics.* 2017;140(3):e20171870

Approximately 1000 new cases of perinatal hepatitis B infection are identified annually in the United States.[1,2] Chronic hepatitis B infection occurs in up to 90% of infants infected with hepatitis B at birth or in the first year of life. When untreated, approximately 25% ultimately will die of hepatocellular carcinoma or liver cirrhosis. In the absence of postexposure prophylaxis at birth, the risk of perinatal transmission is substantial when an infant is born to a mother who is hepatitis B surface antigen (HBsAg) positive. The proportion of infants acquiring infection in this circumstance ranges from approximately 30% when mothers are hepatitis B e antigen (HBeAg) (a marker of infectivity) negative to approximately 85% when mothers are HBeAg positive. Because maternal HBeAg status frequently is unknown, the true risk to an individual newborn infant also generally is unknown. Postexposure prophylaxis is highly effective. Hepatitis B vaccine alone is 75% to 95% effective in preventing perinatal hepatitis B transmission when given within 24 hours of birth.[3,4] When postexposure prophylaxis with both hepatitis B vaccine and hepatitis B immune globulin (HBIG) is given, is timed appropriately, and is followed by completion of the infant hepatitis B immunization series, perinatal infection rates range from 0.7% to 1.1%.[5,6] These findings are the basis for the rationale for the current change in the recommendation regarding birth vaccination.

Prevention of perinatal transmission of hepatitis B is part of a national strategy for hepatitis B prevention that relies on testing all pregnant women for hepatitis B infection by testing women for HBsAg routinely during pregnancy and providing appropriate and timely prophylaxis to all newborn infants.[6] Appropriate prophylaxis consists of HBIG and/or hepatitis B vaccine, depending on the HBsAg status of the mother and the weight of the infant (Fig 1). The birth dose of hepatitis B vaccine is a critical safety net to protect infants born to hepatitis B–infected mothers not identified at the time of birth. The birth dose can prevent infection of infants born to infected mothers in situations in which the mother's results are never obtained, are misinterpreted, are falsely negative, are transcribed or reported to the infant care team inaccurately, or simply not communicated to the nursery. The Immunization Action Coalition reported greater than 500 such errors in perinatal hepatitis B prevention from 1999 to 2002.[7] The birth dose also provides protection to infants at risk from household exposure after the perinatal period. For infants born to HBsAg-negative mothers, the birth dose is the beginning of appropriate lifelong prophylaxis. Because the consequences of perinatally acquired hepatitis B are enduring and potentially fatal, the safety net of the birth dose is critically important. The incidence of new hepatitis B infections has increased in some states as a result of the opioid epidemic in the United States,[8] underscoring the urgency

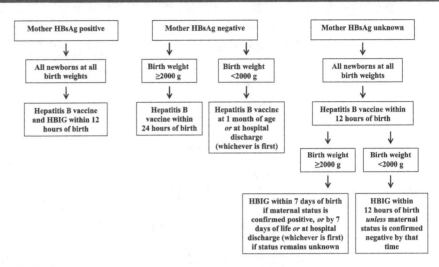

FIGURE 1
Administration of the birth dose of hepatitis B vaccine by maternal HBsAg status.

of improving perinatal prevention strategies.

Hepatitis B antiviral therapy now is offered during pregnancy to hepatitis B–infected women with high hepatitis B viral loads. Antiviral therapy started from 30 to 32 weeks' gestational age and continued until postpartum week 4 in the mother, in addition to newborn prophylaxis with hepatitis B vaccine and HBIG, has been associated with significantly reduced rates of perinatal hepatitis B virus transmission from highly viremic mothers.[9] There is no evidence, however, that maternal antenatal treatment alone without infant prophylaxis is sufficient to reduce the risk for perinatal transmission.[10]

The US Department of Health and Human Services has set a goal of 0 perinatal hepatitis B transmission in the United States by 2020.[6] Although 95% of infants born to infected women who are identified by the Centers for Disease Control and Prevention's Perinatal Hepatitis B Prevention Program do receive prophylaxis with HBIG and hepatitis B vaccine within 12 hours of birth, the overall hepatitis B immunization rate of newborn infants is suboptimal.[11] In 2005, the Centers for Disease Control and Prevention's Advisory Committee on

Immunization Practices (ACIP) issued hepatitis B vaccine recommendations that contained permissive language around administration of the birth dose of hepatitis B vaccine, allowing practitioners the option to delay this dose.[5] By 2014, a quality improvement study found that only 72% of infants received the birth dose of hepatitis B vaccine, which is less than the Healthy People 2020 target of 85%.[12] In October 2016, the ACIP rescinded the permissive language and instead stated the following: "For all medically stable infants weighing greater than or equal to 2000 grams at birth and born to HBsAg-negative mothers, the first dose of vaccine should be administered within 24 hours of birth. Only single-antigen hepatitis B vaccine should be used for the birth dose."[13,14]

RECOMMENDATIONS

The American Academy of Pediatrics Committee on Infectious Diseases and the Committee on Fetus and Newborn support removal of permissive language for delaying the birth dose of hepatitis B vaccine, endorse the recommendation of the ACIP for giving the birth dose within the first 24 hours of life in all medically stable infants weighing greater than or equal to 2000 g, and provide guidance for implementation.[15]

Vaccine Issues

After completion of a 3- or 4-dose hepatitis B vaccine series, 98% of healthy term infants achieve protective antibody concentrations. Protection may be lower in infants with birth weights less than 2000 g.[5] The optimal time to perform serologic testing to detect a vaccine response in infants is 1 to 2 months after the final dose of the hepatitis B vaccine series. Recommendations for postvaccination serologic testing of infants born to hepatitis B–infected mothers have been updated recently.[16] For infants born to HBsAg-positive mothers, postvaccination serologic testing by measuring hepatitis B surface antibody (anti-HBs) to document protection and HBsAg to rule out perinatal infection now is recommended at 9 to 12 months of age instead of 9 to 18 months. Infants who are HBsAg negative with anti-HBs levels less than 10 mIU/mL (nonprotective) require additional vaccine doses. The ACIP considered revaccination strategies in February 2017 and recommended that HBsAg-negative infants with anti-HBs levels less than 10 mIU/mL receive a single additional dose of hepatitis B vaccine and be retested for anti-HBs 1 to 2 months after that vaccine dose. If the anti-HBs level is still less than 10 mIU/mL, the infant should receive 2 additional doses of hepatitis B vaccine followed by retesting 1 to 2 months later. Infants with anti-HBs levels less than 10 mIU/mL after 2 3-dose series of hepatitis B vaccine are nonresponders, and available data do not suggest benefit from additional vaccinations. The ACIP noted that, on the basis of clinical circumstance or family preference, HBsAg-negative infants with anti-HBs levels less than 10 mIU/mL may be vaccinated instead with a second complete series followed by postvaccination testing 1 to 2 months after the final dose.

Hepatitis B vaccine is well tolerated in infants.[17,18] Commonly reported mild adverse events after hepatitis B vaccination in people of all ages from postmarketing surveillance data include pain (3%–29%), erythema (3%), swelling (3%), fever (1%–6%), and headache (3%). Safety of hepatitis B vaccines has been examined extensively; no evidence of a causal association between receipt of hepatitis B vaccine and neonatal sepsis or death, rheumatoid arthritis, Bell's palsy, autoimmune thyroid disease, hemolytic anemia in children, anaphylaxis, optic neuritis, Guillain-Barré syndrome, sudden-onset sensorineural hearing loss, or other chronic illnesses has been demonstrated through analysis of data from the Vaccine Safety Datalink.[5] Perinatal hepatitis B–prevention strategies are considered cost-effective, with a cost-effectiveness ratio of $2600 per quality-adjusted life-year.[19]

Implementation

The following are key steps for implementing appropriate administration of the birth dose of hepatitis B vaccine (see also Fig 1):

- Identify HBsAg-positive mothers before delivery and document maternal HBsAg status in infant records;

- Resolve unknown HBsAg status of mothers as soon as possible around delivery, and document maternal status in infant records;

- For all infants born to HBsAg-positive mothers, administer both hepatitis B vaccine and HBIG within 12 hours of birth, regardless of any maternal antenatal treatment with antiviral medications;

- For all infants with birth weight greater than or equal to 2000 g born to HBsAg-negative mothers, administer hepatitis B vaccine as a universal routine prophylaxis within 24 hours of birth;

- For all infants with birth weight less than 2000 g born to HBsAg-negative mothers, administer hepatitis B vaccine as a universal routine prophylaxis at 1 month of age or at hospital discharge (whichever is first);

- For all infants born to HBsAg-unknown mothers, administer hepatitis B vaccine within 12 hours of birth, and:

  o For infants with birth weight greater than or equal to 2000 g, administer HBIG by 7 days of age or by hospital discharge (whichever occurs first) if maternal HBsAg status is confirmed positive or remains unknown;

  o For infants with birth weight less than 2000 g, administer HBIG by 12 hours of birth unless maternal HBsAg status is confirmed negative by that time;

- Document infant vaccination accurately in birth hospital records and in the appropriate CDC Immunization Information Systems and state immunization registry. Review documentation accuracy periodically and address identified errors; and

- Develop procedures to educate all personnel involved in newborn care about recommendations for the birth dose of hepatitis B vaccine, including those personnel who provide care at planned home births.

COMMITTEE ON FETUS AND NEWBORN, 2016–2017

Kristi Watterberg, MD, FAAP, Chairperson
William Benitz, MD, FAAP
Ivan Hand, MD, FAAP
Eric Eichenwald, MD, FAAP
Brenda Poindexter, MD, FAAP
Dan L. Stewart, MD, FAAP
Susan W. Aucott, MD, FAAP
Karen M. Puopolo, MD, PhD, FAAP
Jay P. Goldsmith, MD, FAAP

LIAISONS

Kasper S. Wang, MD, FAAP – *American Academy of Pediatrics Section on Surgery*
Thierry Lacaze, MD – *Canadian Paediatric Society*
Maria Ann Mascola, MDD – *American College of Obstetricians and Gynecologists*
Tonse N.K. Raju, MD, DCH – *National Institutes of Health*
Wanda D. Barfield, MD, MPH, FAAP, RADM USPHS – *Centers for Disease Control and Prevention*
Erin Keels, MS, APRN, NNP-BC – *National Association of Neonatal Nurses*

STAFF

Jim Couto, MA

COMMITTEE ON INFECTIOUS DISEASES, 2016–2017

Carrie L. Byington, MD, FAAP, Chairperson
Yvonne A. Maldonado, MD, FAAP, Vice Chairperson
Elizabeth D. Barnett MD, FAAP
James D. Campbell, MD, FAAP
H. Dele Davies, MD, MS, MHCM, FAAP
Ruth Lynfield, MD, FAAP
Flor M. Munoz, MD, FAAP
Dawn Nolt, MD, MPH, FAAP
Ann-Christine Nyquist, MD, MSPH, FAAP
Sean O'Leary, MD, MPH, FAAP
Mobeen H. Rathore, MD, FAAP
Mark H. Sawyer, MD, FAAP
William J. Steinbach, MD, FAAP
Tina Q. Tan, MD, FAAP
Theoklis E. Zaoutis, MD, MSCE, FAAP

EX OFFICIO

David W. Kimberlin, MD, FAAP – *Red Book* Editor
Michael T. Brady, MD, FAAP – *Red Book* Associate Editor
Mary Anne Jackson, MD, FAAP – *Red Book* Associate Editor
Sarah S. Long, MD, FAAP – *Red Book* Associate Editor
Henry H. Bernstein, DO, MHCM, FAAP – *Red Book* Online Associate Editor
H. Cody Meissner, MD, FAAP – Visual *Red Book* Associate Editor

LIAISONS

Douglas Campos-Outcalt, MD, MPA – *American Academy of Family Physicians*
Amanda C. Cohn, MD, FAAP – *Centers for Disease Control and Prevention*
Karen M. Farizo, MD – *US Food and Drug Administration*
Marc Fischer, MD, FAAP – *Centers for Disease Control and Prevention*
Bruce G. Gellin, MD, MPH – *National Vaccine Program Office*
Richard L. Gorman, MD, FAAP – *National Institutes of Health*
Natasha Halasa, MD, MPH, FAAP – *Pediatric Infectious Diseases Society*

Joan L. Robinson, MD – *Canadian Paediatric Society*
Jamie Deseda-Tous, MD – *Sociedad Latinoamericana de Infectologia Pediatrica (SLIPE)*
Geoffrey R. Simon, MD, FAAP – *Committee on Practice Ambulatory Medicine*
Jeffrey R. Starke, MD, FAAP – *American Thoracic Society*

STAFF

Jennifer M. Frantz, MPH

ABBREVIATIONS

ACIP: Advisory Committee on Immunization Practices
Anti-HBs: hepatitis B surface antibody
HBeAg: hepatitis B e antigen
HBIG: hepatitis B immune globulin
HBsAg: hepatitis B surface antigen

REFERENCES

1. Centers for Disease Control and Prevention, Division of Viral Hepatitis. Surveillance for viral hepatitis—United States 2014. Revised September 26, 2016. Available at: https://www.cdc.gov/hepatitis/statistics/2014surveillance/. Accessed March 23, 2017

2. Ko SC, Fan L, Smith EA, Fenlon N, Koneru AK, Murphy TV. Estimated annual perinatal hepatitis b virus infections in the United States, 2000-2009. *J Pediatric Infect Dis Soc.* 2016;5(2):114–121

3. Beasley RP, Hwang LY, Lee GC, et al. Prevention of perinatally transmitted hepatitis B virus infections with hepatitis B immune globulin and hepatitis B vaccine. *Lancet.* 1983;2(8359):1099–1102

4. Lee C, Gong Y, Brok J, Boxall EH, Gluud C. Effect of hepatitis B immunisation in newborn infants of mothers positive for hepatitis B surface antigen: systematic review and meta-analysis. *BMJ.* 2006;332(7537):328–336

5. Mast EE, Margolis HS, Fiore AE, et al; Advisory Committee on Immunization Practices (ACIP). A comprehensive immunization strategy to eliminate transmission of hepatitis B virus infection in the United States: recommendations of the Advisory Committee on Immunization Practices (ACIP) part 1: immunization of infants, children, and adolescents. *MMWR Recomm Rep.* 2005;54(RR-16):1–31

6. US Department of Health and Human Services. Action plan for the prevention, care, & treatment of viral hepatitis. Updated 2014–2016. Available at: https://www.hhs.gov/sites/default/files/viral-hepatitis-action-plan.pdf. Accessed March 23, 2017

7. Immunization Action Coalition. Reducing medical errors: case reports. Available at: www.immunize.org/protect-newborns/guide/chapter2/case-reports.pdf. Accessed March 23, 2017

8. Harris AM, Iqbal K, Schillie S, et al. Increases in acute hepatitis b virus infections — Kentucky, Tennessee, and West Virginia, 2006–2013. *MMWR Morb Mortal Wkly Rep.* 2016;65(3):47–50

9. Pan CQ, Duan Z, Dai E, et al; China Study Group for the Mother-to-Child Transmission of Hepatitis B. Tenofovir to prevent hepatitis B transmission in mothers with high viral load. *N Engl J Med.* 2016;374(24):2324–2334

10. Chen HL, Lee CN, Chang CH, et al; Taiwan Study Group for the Prevention of Mother-to-Infant Transmission of HBV (PreMIT Study); Taiwan Study Group for the Prevention of Mother-to-Infant Transmission of HBV PreMIT Study. Efficacy of maternal tenofovir disoproxil fumarate in interrupting mother-to-infant transmission of hepatitis B virus. *Hepatology.* 2015;62(2):375–386

11. Schillie S, Walker T, Veselsky S, et al. Outcomes of infants born to women infected with hepatitis B. *Pediatrics.* 2015;135(5). Available at: www.pediatrics.org/cgi/content/full/135/5/e1141

12. Hill HA, Elam-Evans LD, Yankey D, Singleton JA, Kolasa M. National, state, and selected local area vaccination coverage among children aged 19-35 months - United States, 2014. *MMWR Morb Mortal Wkly Rep.* 2015;64(33):889–896

13. Kim DK, Riley LE, Harriman KH, Hunter P, Bridges CB. Advisory Committee on Immunization Practices Recommended Immunization Schedule for Adults Aged 19 Years or Older — United States, 2017. . *MMWR Morb Mortal Wkly Rep.* 2017; 66(5);136–138

14. US Department of Health and Human Services, Centers for Disease Control and Prevention. Advisory committee on immunization practices. summary report. 2016. Available at: https://www.cdc.gov/vaccines/acip/meetings/downloads/min-archive/min-2016-10.pdf. Accessed May 3, 2017

15. Committee on Infectious Diseases. Recommended childhood and adolescent immunization schedule—United States, 2017. *Pediatrics.* 2017;139(3):e20164007

16. Schillie S, Murphy TV, Fenlon N, Ko S, Ward JW. Update: shortened interval for postvaccination serologic testing of infants born to hepatitis B-infected mothers. *MMWR Morb Mortal Wkly Rep.* 2015;64(39):1118–1120

17. Eriksen EM, Perlman JA, Miller A, et al. Lack of association between hepatitis B birth immunization and neonatal death: a population-based study from the vaccine safety datalink project. *Pediatr Infect Dis J.* 2004;23(7):656–662

18. Lewis E, Shinefield HR, Woodruff BA, et al; Vaccine Safety Datalink Workgroup. Safety of neonatal hepatitis B vaccine administration. *Pediatr Infect Dis J.* 2001;20(11):1049–1054

19. Barbosa C, Smith EA, Hoerger TJ, et al. Cost-effectiveness analysis of the national perinatal hepatitis B prevention program. *Pediatrics.* 2014;133(2):243–253

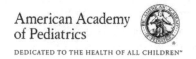

American Academy
of Pediatrics
DEDICATED TO THE HEALTH OF ALL CHILDREN™

TECHNICAL REPORT

Epidemiology and Diagnosis of Health Care–Associated Infections in the NICU

abstract

Health care–associated infections in the NICU are a major clinical problem resulting in increased morbidity and mortality, prolonged length of hospital stays, and increased medical costs. Neonates are at high risk for health care–associated infections because of impaired host defense mechanisms, limited amounts of protective endogenous flora on skin and mucosal surfaces at time of birth, reduced barrier function of neonatal skin, the use of invasive procedures and devices, and frequent exposure to broad-spectrum antibiotics. This statement will review the epidemiology and diagnosis of health care–associated infections in newborn infants. *Pediatrics* 2012;129:e1104–e1109

Richard A. Polin, MD, Susan Denson, MD, Michael T. Brady, MD, the COMMITTEE ON FETUS AND NEWBORN, and the COMMITTEE ON INFECTIOUS DISEASES

KEY WORDS
antibiotics, health care–associated infection, neonate, newborn, NICU, nosocomial infection

ABBREVIATIONS
CDC—Centers for Disease Control and Prevention
CPAP—continuous positive airway pressure

INTRODUCTION

Health care–associated infections are infections acquired in the hospital while receiving treatment of other conditions. They are common occurrences in patients of all ages and are estimated to result in 2 million infections, 90 000 deaths, and $28 to $45 billion in excess health care costs annually.[1,2] In the Pediatric Prevention Network national point prevalence survey, 11.2% of NICU patients had a health care–associated infection on the day of the survey.[3] Although there are no recent estimates of the cost of health care–associated infections in the NICU, Payne et al[4] estimated that health care–associated bloodstream infections added almost $100 million to the cost of treating infants with birth weights from 500 to 1499 g in 1999 dollars. Because this finding represented the excess costs associated with only one type of infection in one gestational age cohort, it provides just a glimpse of the financial impact of health care–associated infections in the NICU. This financial estimate does not include the potential morbidity and mortality concerns for the infant and the effect that the prolonged hospital stay has on the family and resource utilization within the hospital. Reducing health care–associated infections in the NICU would have benefits to infants, families, and the health care delivery system. The purpose of this technical report was to review the epidemiology and diagnosis of health care–associated infections in the NICU. A companion policy statement addresses strategies for the prevention of health care–associated infections.

EPIDEMIOLOGY

Newborn infants hospitalized in a NICU have host factors that not only make them more vulnerable to acquisition of health care–associated

www.pediatrics.org/cgi/doi/10.1542/peds.2012-0147

doi:10.1542/peds.2012-0147

PEDIATRICS (ISSN Numbers: Print, 0031-4005; Online, 1098-4275).

infections but also increase their risk of developing more serious illnesses. Whether an infant is born preterm or at term, many components of their innate and adaptive immune systems exhibit diminished function when compared with older children and adults. Infants with birth weights less than 1500 g (very low birth weight) have rates of health care–associated infections 3 times higher than those who weigh greater than 1500 g at birth. However, the increased susceptibility to infection in infants of very low birth weight is multifactorial and related to both the developmental deficiencies in the innate and adaptive immune systems and a greater likelihood of a critical illness requiring invasive monitoring and procedures. Furthermore, the immunologic deficiencies can be exacerbated by the critical nature of many of the illnesses affecting newborn infants.[5]

Colonization of mucous membranes and the skin occurs rapidly after birth. Newborn infants delivered vaginally are colonized with maternal bacteria acquired from the birth canal. In most instances, those organisms do not cause invasive disease; however, in critically ill newborn infants, this colonization can potentially lead to systemic infection when skin or mucosal surfaces are compromised. The stratum corneum of the skin is poorly developed before 26 weeks' gestation, and ill neonates are at increased risk of developing skin and mucosal injury (eg, by suctioning or invasive procedures), allowing invasive bacteria access to deeper tissues or vascular spaces. Furthermore, mucosal surfaces and skin of infants in the NICU are more likely to be colonized with Gram-negative enteric rods, staphylococci, enterococci, and Candida species. NICU-acquired microbes are more likely to be pathogenic and resistant because of frequent exposure of hospitalized infants to antibiotic agents.

Data describing the epidemiology and incidence of health care–associated infections in NICUs can be obtained from 4 sources: (1) the National Healthcare Safety Network (previously known as the National Nosocomial Infections Surveillance system) at the Centers for Disease Control and Prevention (CDC); (2) the Pediatric Prevention Network at the National Association of Children's Hospitals and Related Institutions; (3) the Vermont Oxford Network; and (4) the National Institute for Child Health and Human Development Neonatal Research Network.

In addition to preterm birth,[6,7] risk factors associated with an increased rate of health care–associated infections include the presence of invasive devices (intravascular catheters, endotracheal tubes, orogastric tubes, urinary catheters, and drains), exposure to broad-spectrum antibiotic agents, parenteral nutrition,[8] overcrowding and poor staffing ratios, administration of steroids and histamine$_2$-receptor antagonists, and acuity of underlying illness. Furthermore, the lower the birth weight, the more invasive technology is used.[6,7]

Parenteral nutrition is commonly administered to the sickest infants through central venous catheters or peripherally inserted central catheters. The relationship between central line use and increased risk of infection has been demonstrated in multiple studies[9–11]; administration of lipids may be an independent risk factor for bacterial or fungal sepsis.[10]

The most common type of health care–associated infection within the NICU is a catheter-associated bloodstream infection.[3] Within the first 30 days after birth, coagulase-negative Staphylococcus species, Staphylococcus aureus, Enterococcus species, and Gram-negative enteric bacteria are the most common etiologic agents. After 30 days of age, coagulase-negative Staphylococcus species remain the most common

pathogens; however, fungi, particularly Candida species and Malassezia furfur, have been noted with increasing frequency.[3] Central-line–related infections are, in large part, a result of problems with poor technique at the time of placement and ongoing care of the catheter site. Data suggest that the hub is a common source of contamination and subsequent infection.[12] Not surprisingly, the occurrence of catheter-associated bloodstream infections is highly related to the duration of catheter use and the number of times the catheter or hub is entered or opened.

Health care–associated lower respiratory tract infections and ventilator-associated pneumonia are of extreme importance for hospitalized infants because of their frequency and potential severity. Health care–associated pneumonia represents 6.8% to 32.3% of health care–associated infections in the NICU and is the second most frequent hospital-acquired infection in critically ill neonates.[7,13,14] The most recent National Healthcare Safety Network data indicate a pooled mean rate of ventilator-associated pneumonia from 0.7 to 2.2 per 1000 ventilator days.[7] However, rates varied among NICUs, with 90% of NICUs reporting rates between 2.1 and 7.3 per 1000 ventilator days. Variations in incidence likely reflect, in part, difficulty in making this diagnosis in infants with chronic lung disease. As with most health care–associated infections, birth weight and gestational age correlate inversely with the incidence of ventilator-associated pneumonia. Many of the risk factors for the development of health care–associated pneumonia in NICU patients are similar to those previously identified in adult patients, such as prolonged duration of mechanical ventilation, severe underlying cardiopulmonary disease, prolonged intravenous alimentation, and previous thoracoabdominal surgery.

Most bacterial health care–associated lower respiratory tract infections occur by aspiration of bacteria that colonize the oropharynx or the upper gastrointestinal tract. On rare occasions, health care–associated pneumonias may result from contiguous spread or a primary infection at a distant site. Under normal circumstances, the filtration system of the upper airway and the mucociliary clearance system of the large airways protect the lower respiratory tract from bacteria that may be present in the patient's environment or that reside in the upper respiratory tract. Endotracheal tubes bypass these initial host barrier defense mechanisms, providing direct access of bacteria and other pathogens to the lower respiratory tract. Uncuffed endotracheal tubes provide even easier access of microorganisms to the lower respiratory tract.[15–17] The aspiration of contaminated materials may be obvious or, more commonly, may be subclinical.[15–18] By using pepsin as a marker for aspiration, microaspiration has been detected in up to 92.8% of ventilated neonates.[18,19] Methylxanthines and bronchopulmonary dysplasia increase the frequency of microaspiration. Microaspiration is also more frequent in infants with severe bronchopulmonary dysplasia compared with those with moderate bronchopulmonary dysplasia.[18,19] Neonates who have either impaired swallowing mechanisms or anatomic abnormalities that prevent adequate protection of their airway are also at increased risk of aspiration.[15,16,20]

Dense bacterial polysaccharide biofilm can coat the endotracheal tubes, and polymicrobial flora become embedded into this film. Endotracheal suctioning can dislodge these aggregates of bacteria, providing a large bacterial inoculum directly into lower airways. Nasal continuous positive airway pressure (CPAP) does not bypass many of the protective barriers, does not require endotracheal suctioning, and reduces mechanical disruption of respiratory mucosa. This likely explains the lower risk of health care–associated pneumonia in neonates using nasal CPAP versus those treated with endotracheal intubation (1.8 vs 12.8 per 1000 nasal CPAP or ventilator days).[21] However, CPAP has been associated with an increased risk of Gram-negative infections.[22]

Skin and soft tissue infections are commonly observed in NICU patients. Neonates, especially those born preterm, have fragile skin, which is easily traumatized. Cellulitis, abscesses, and skin abrasions are frequently noted at sites of percutaneous puncture (lancets and scalp electrodes), in diaper or bandage areas, and at surgical incision sites. S aureus is by far the most common microorganism responsible for all skin and soft tissue infections in the NICU. The recent emergence of methicillin-resistant S aureus, both endemic health care–associated and community-associated strains, has made management of these infections complicated. Gram-negative enteric rods and yeasts are less commonly associated with skin and soft tissue infections than S aureus, but they are associated with surgical procedures, particularly those affecting the gastrointestinal tract.

DIAGNOSIS OF CENTRAL LINE–ASSOCIATED BLOODSTREAM INFECTIONS

The presence of a central venous catheter is a major risk factor for bloodstream infection. Coagulase-negative staphylococci are responsible for nearly 50% of catheter-related bloodstream infections. Other pathogens include Gram-negative organisms (~20%), S aureus (4% to 9%), Enterococcus species (3% to 5%), and Candida species (~10%).[23] Coagulase-negative staphylococci are skin commensals; therefore, interpretation of a blood culture result positive for this organism is difficult. The diagnosis is made even more problematic by the nonspecific signs of sepsis in the neonate. It is noteworthy that the databases of the National Healthcare Safety Network, Vermont Oxford Network, and the National Institute for Child Health and Human Development Network include infants with a single positive blood culture and clinical signs as "proven cases" of central line–associated bloodstream infection. Although many experts recommend obtaining both central line and peripheral blood cultures when evaluating neonatal patients for central line–associated bloodstream infection, a single blood culture sample is commonly obtained. In those situations, it may be difficult to determine whether the coagulase-negative Staphylococcus is the responsible pathogen or a contaminant, and the clinician will need to make a judgment on the basis of the laboratory data and response to treatment. The Infectious Diseases Society of America recommends that paired samples be drawn from the catheter and a peripheral vein (level of evidence: A-II).[24] Although this action may not be possible for all neonates, paired samples should be obtained whenever feasible. Neonates with a suspected central line–associated bloodstream infection should be treated with broad-spectrum antibiotic agents to cover both Gram-positive and Gram-negative pathogens. An algorithm for interpreting a positive blood culture result for coagulase-negative staphylococci is shown in Fig 1.

DIAGNOSIS OF HEALTH CARE–ASSOCIATED PNEUMONIA

Health care–associated pneumonia can have adverse clinical consequences, both from the infection itself and from

Clinical Signs and Symptoms of Sepsis

Draw *central and peripheral blood cultures* and begin broad-spectrum antibiotics

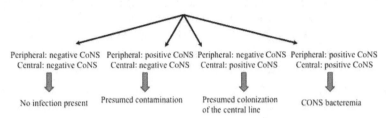

FIGURE 1

Algorithm for interpreting a positive blood culture result for coagulase-negative staphylococci (CONS).

its therapies. Health care–associated pneumonias in infants may result in increased exposure to broad-spectrum antibiotic agents, need for reintubation, increased duration of assisted ventilation, increased length and cost of hospitalization, secondary infections including sepsis, and even death.

The optimal method of diagnosing health care–associated pneumonia in neonates remains to be established. In neonates with underlying pulmonary disease, it may be difficult to differentiate between preexisting lung disease and health care–associated pneumonia or tracheitis. In general, the diagnosis of health care–associated pneumonia is made on the basis of evidence of respiratory decompensation with new and persistent infiltrates on a chest radiograph. Clinical signs suggesting that a health care–associated bacterial pneumonia has developed in an infant receiving mechanical ventilation include changes in the patient's respiratory status that are unexplained by other events and a significant increase in the quantity and quality of respiratory secretions. However, signs such as fever, leukocytosis, and changes in the quality and quantity of tracheobronchial secretions may occur for reasons other than the development of a health care–associated lower respiratory tract infection. Unfortunately, relying on clinical changes and chest radiographic findings for the diagnosis in a NICU

setting may overestimate the true incidence of health care–associated pneumonia. Infants with atelectasis, congenital heart disease, bronchopulmonary dysplasia, pulmonary hemorrhage, pulmonary edema, and surgical procedures affecting the chest may have radiographic changes that are similar to changes seen with pneumonia. The National Healthcare Safety Network and CDC definition requires at least 48 hours of mechanical ventilation accompanied by new and persistent radiographic infiltrates after the initiation of mechanical ventilation. In addition to these criteria, infants younger than 1 year old must exhibit worsening gas exchange and at least 3 of the following: (1) temperature instability with no other recognized cause; (2) leukopenia (white blood cell count $<4000/mm^3$); (3) change in the character of sputum or increased respiratory secretions or suctioning requirements; (4) apnea, tachypnea, nasal flaring, or grunting; (5) wheezing, rales, rhonchi, or cough; or (6) bradycardia (<100 beats/min) or tachycardia (>170 beats/min).[25] Baltimore,[26] however, has pointed out that the CDC definitions were developed for epidemiologic surveillance and have not been validated for clinical diagnosis.

Laboratory tests, such as Gram stain or bacterial culture, documenting the presence of inflammation and pathogenic microorganisms in lower respiratory

tract secretions may be helpful in establishing the presence of a health care–associated lower respiratory tract infection. However, in most cases, presence of bacteria in specimens obtained by suctioning the endotracheal tube represents colonization rather than an invasive infection, even when the culture is obtained immediately after intubation. In addition, the correlation between culture results obtained from endotracheal suction specimens and those from samples obtained directly from the lungs, pleural cavity, or blood is poor.[27,28]

When it is likely that a health care–associated bacterial pneumonia is present, a number of procedures can assist in establishing the etiologic agent. A Gram stain of a specimen obtained by suctioning through the endotracheal tube can provide evidence of an inflammatory (and potentially infectious) process in the lower respiratory tract.[29] The presence of an abundance of polymorphonuclear neutrophils or a significant increase in polymorphonuclear neutrophils from a previous Gram stain of the same secretions, regardless of the presence of a predominant bacterial organism, is supportive evidence that pneumonia is present but also may represent tracheitis. The presence of a single organism obtained by culture that is consistent with an organism identified on the Gram stain increases the likelihood that this agent is causally related to the health care–associated bacterial pneumonia.[29]

Numerous efforts have been made to develop techniques for obtaining specimens from the lower respiratory tract that can identify the bacteria responsible for the health care–associated pneumonia without interference by upper airway contamination. Transtracheal aspiration, transthoracic needle aspiration and biopsy, and bronchoscopy have been used in older children and adults to obtain samples directly from the lower respiratory tract, but these procedures are generally contraindicated in neonates. Moreover, there is a high rate of false-positive results in children who have underlying pulmonary conditions that might be confused with pneumonia by their clinical and radiographic appearances.

Bronchoalveolar lavage is a reliable method for obtaining lower respiratory tract secretion samples in older children and adults.[30–32] However, its role in diagnosing ventilator-associated pneumonia in older children and adults has not been established, and experience in preterm infants is limited. In intubated neonates, tracheal aspirates may provide information similar to that which can be obtained by bronchoalveolar lavage. However, for neonates with rapidly progressing lower respiratory tract disease or in whom a diagnosis is not established with routine tracheal aspirate, a bronchoalveolar lavage may be indicated (if technically feasible).[33–35] The aspirated fluid can be centrifuged, and the pellet can be examined immediately for bacteria (Gram stain or acridine orange) and fungi (KOH or Calcofluor). Cultures and other molecular diagnostic testing (eg, direct fluorescent antibody assay, polymerase chain reaction assay) can be performed for aerobic bacteria, fungi, and viruses. The differential count of white blood cells from bronchoalveolar lavage fluid may also be helpful. Infants with bacterial or fungal infections are more likely to have a high proportion of granulocytes in bronchoalveolar lavage fluid.[33,36]

Isolation of the same bacterial pathogen from the blood and the lower respiratory tract usually confirms that this organism is the agent responsible for the health care–associated pneumonia. However, only approximately 2% to 5% of patients with health care–associated bacterial pneumonia have positive blood cultures.[36]

LEAD AUTHORS
Richard A. Polin, MD
Susan Denson, MD
Michael T. Brady, MD

COMMITTEE ON FETUS AND NEWBORN, 2011–2012
Lu-Ann Papile, MD, Chairperson
Jill E. Baley, MD
Waldemar A. Carlo, MD
James J. Cummings, MD
Praveen Kumar, MD
Richard A. Polin, MD
Rosemarie C. Tan, MD, PhD
Kristi L. Watterberg, MD

LIAISONS
CAPT Wanda D. Barfield, MD, MPH – *Centers for Disease Control and Prevention*
Ann L. Jefferies, MD – *Canadian Pediatric Society*
George A. Macones, MD – *American College of Obstetricians and Gynecologists*
Rosalie O. Mainous, PhD, APRN, NNP-BC – *National Association of Neonatal Nurses*
Tonse N. K. Raju, MD, DCH – *National Institutes of Health*
Kasper S. Wang, MD – *AAP Section on Surgery*

STAFF
Jim Couto, MA

COMMITTEE ON INFECTIOUS DISEASES, 2011–2012
Michael T. Brady, MD, Chairperson
Carrie L. Byington, MD
H. Dele Davies, MD
Kathryn M. Edwards, MD
Mary P. Glode, MD

Mary Anne Jackson, MD
Harry L. Keyserling, MD
Yvonne A. Maldonado, MD
Dennis L. Murray, MD
Walter A. Orenstein, MD
Gordon E. Schutze, MD
Rodney E. Willoughby, MD
Theoklis E. Zaoutis, MD

LIAISONS
Marc A. Fischer, MD – *Centers for Disease Control and Prevention*
Bruce Gellin, MD – *National Vaccine Program Office*
Richard L. Gorman, MD – *National Institutes of Health*
Lucia Lee, MD – *Food and Drug Administration*
R. Douglas Pratt, MD – *Food and Drug Administration*
Jennifer S. Read, MD – *National Vaccine Program Office*
Joan Robinson, MD – *Canadian Pediatric Society*
Marco Aurelio Palazzi Safadi, MD – *Sociedad Latinoamericana de Infectologia Pediatrica (SLIPE)*
Jane Seward, MBBS, MPH – *Centers for Disease Control & Prevention*
Jeffrey R. Starke, MD – *American Thoracic Society*
Geoffrey Simon, MD – *Committee on Practice Ambulatory Medicine*
Tina Q. Tan, MD – *Pediatric Infectious Diseases Society*

EX OFFICIO
Carol J. Baker, MD – Red Book *Associate Editor*
Henry H. Bernstein, DO – Red Book *Associate Editor*
David W. Kimberlin, MD – Red Book *Associate Editor*
Sarah S. Long, MD – Red Book *Online Associate Editor*
H. Cody Meissner, MD – Visual Red Book *Associate Editor*
Larry K. Pickering, MD – Red Book *Editor*

CONSULTANT
Lorry G. Rubin, MD

STAFF
Jennifer Frantz, MPH

REFERENCES

1. Centers for Disease Control (CDC). Public health focus: surveillance, prevention, and control of nosocomial infections. *MMWR Morb Mortal Wkly Rep.* 1992;41(42):783–787

2. Stone PW. Economic burden of healthcare-associated infections: an American perspective. *Expert Rev Pharmacoecon Outcomes Res.* 2009;9(5):417–422

3. Sohn AH, Garrett DO, Sinkowitz-Cochran RL, et al; Pediatric Prevention Network. Prevalence of nosocomial infections in neonatal intensive care unit patients: results from

the first national point-prevalence survey. *J Pediatr.* 2001;139(6):821–827

4. Payne NR, Carpenter JH, Badger GJ, Horbar JD, Rogowski J. Marginal increase in cost and excess length of stay associated with nosocomial bloodstream infections in surviving very low birth weight infants. *Pediatrics.* 2004;114(2):348–355

5. Krause PJ, Herson VC, Boutin-Lebowitz J, et al. Polymorphonuclear leukocyte adherence and chemotaxis in stressed and healthy neonates. *Pediatr Res.* 1986;20(4):296–300

6. Goldmann DA, Durbin WA Jr, Freeman J. Nosocomial infections in a neonatal intensive care unit. *J Infect Dis.* 1981;144(5):449–459

7. Edwards JR, Peterson KD, Mu Y, et al. National Healthcare Safety Network (NHSN) report: data summary for 2006 through 2008, issued December 2009. *Am J Infect Control.* 2009;37(10):783–805

8. Wilson DC, Cairns P, Halliday HL, Reid M, McClure G, Dodge JA. Randomised controlled trial of an aggressive nutritional regimen in sick very low birthweight infants. *Arch Dis Child Fetal Neonatal Ed.* 1997;77(1):F4–F11

9. Johnson-Robbins LA, el-Mohandes AE, Simmens SJ, Keiser JF. Staphylococcus epidermidis sepsis in the intensive care nursery: a characterization of risk associations in infants < 1,000 g. *Biol Neonate.* 1996;69(4):249–256

10. Freeman J, Goldmann DA, Smith NE, Sidebottom DG, Epstein MF, Platt R. Association of intravenous lipid emulsion and coagulase-negative staphylococcal bacteremia in neonatal intensive care units. *N Engl J Med.* 1990;323(5):301–308

11. Beck-Sague CM, Azimi P, Fonseca SN, et al. Bloodstream infections in neonatal intensive care unit patients: results of a multicenter study. *Pediatr Infect Dis J.* 1994;13(12):1110–1116

12. Liñares J, Sitges-Serra A, Garau J, Pérez JL, Martín R. Pathogenesis of catheter sepsis: a prospective study with quantitative and semiquantitative cultures of catheter hub and segments. *J Clin Microbiol.* 1985;21(3):357–360

13. Milliken J, Tait GA, Ford-Jones EL, Mindorff CM, Gold R, Mullins G. Nosocomial infections in a pediatric intensive care unit. *Crit Care Med.* 1988;16(3):233–237

14. Foglia E, Meier MD, Elward A. Ventilator-associated pneumonia in neonatal and pediatric intensive care unit patients. *Clin Microbiol Rev.* 2007;20(3):409–425

15. Huxley EJ, Viroslav J, Gray WR, Pierce AK. Pharyngeal aspiration in normal adults and patients with depressed consciousness. *Am J Med.* 1978;64(4):564–568

16. Goodwin SR, Graves SA, Haberkern CM. Aspiration in intubated premature infants. *Pediatrics.* 1985;75(1):85–88

17. Hopper AO, Kwong LK, Stevenson DK, et al. Detection of gastric contents in tracheal fluid of infants by lactose assay. *J Pediatr.* 1983;102(3):415–418

18. Farhath S, Aghai ZH, Nakhla T, et al. Pepsin, a reliable marker of gastric aspiration, is frequently detected in tracheal aspirates from premature ventilated neonates: relationship with feeding and methylxanthine therapy. *J Pediatr Gastroenterol Nutr.* 2006;43(3):336–341

19. Farhath S, He Z, Nakhla T, et al. Pepsin, a marker of gastric contents, is increased in tracheal aspirates from preterm infants who develop bronchopulmonary dysplasia. *Pediatrics.* 2008;121(2). Available at: www.pediatrics.org/cgi/content/full/121/2/e253

20. Browning DH, Graves SA. Incidence of aspiration with endotracheal tubes in children. *J Pediatr.* 1983;102(4):582–584

21. Hentschel J, Brüngger B, Stüdi K, Mühlemann K. Prospective surveillance of nosocomial infections in a Swiss NICU: low risk of pneumonia on nasal continuous positive airway pressure? *Infection.* 2005;33(5-6):350–355

22. Graham PL 3rd, Begg MD, Larson E, et al. Risk factors for late onset gram-negative sepsis in very low birth weight infants hospitalized in the neonatal intensive care unit. *Pediatr Infect Dis.* 2006;25(2):113–117

23. Stoll BJ, Hansen N, Fanaroff AA, et al. Late-onset sepsis in very low birth weight neonates: the experience of the NICHD Neonatal Research Network. *Pediatrics.* 2002;110(2 pt 1):285–291

24. Mermel LA, Allon M, Bouza E, et al. Clinical practice guidelines for the diagnosis and management of intravascular catheter-related infection: 2009 Update by the Infectious Diseases Society of America [published correction appears in *Clin Infect Dis.* 2010;50(3):457 and *Clin Infect Dis.* 2010;50(7):1079]. *Clin Infect Dis.* 2009;49(1):1–45

25. Centers for Disease Control and Prevention. Criteria for defining nosocomial pneumonia. Available at: www.cdc.gov/ncidod/hip/NNIS/members/pneumonia/final/PneuCriteriaFinal.pdf. Accessed August 1, 2011

26. Baltimore RS. The difficulty of diagnosing ventilator-associated pneumonia. *Pediatrics.* 2003;112(6 pt 1):1420–1421

27. Berger R, Arango L. Etiologic diagnosis of bacterial nosocomial pneumonia in seriously ill patients. *Crit Care Med.* 1985;13(10):833–836

28. Hill JD, Ratliff JL, Parrott JC, et al. Pulmonary pathology in acute respiratory insufficiency: lung biopsy as a diagnostic tool. *J Thorac Cardiovasc Surg.* 1976;71(1):64–71

29. Salata RA, Lederman MM, Shlaes DM, et al. Diagnosis of nosocomial pneumonia in intubated, intensive care unit patients. *Am Rev Respir Dis.* 1987;135(2):426–432

30. Griffin JJ, Meduri GU. New approaches in the diagnosis of nosocomial pneumonia. *Med Clin North Am.* 1994;78(5):1091–1122

31. Jourdain B, Novara A, Joly-Guillou ML, et al. Role of quantitative cultures of endotracheal aspirates in the diagnosis of nosocomial pneumonia. *Am J Respir Crit Care Med.* 1995;152(1):241–246

32. American Thoracic Society; Infectious Diseases Society of America. Guidelines for the management of adults with hospital-acquired, ventilator-associated, and healthcare-associated pneumonia. *Am J Respir Crit Care Med.* 2005;171(4):388–416

33. Allen RM, Dunn WF, Limper AH. Diagnosing ventilator-associated pneumonia: the role of bronchoscopy. *Mayo Clin Proc.* 1994;69(10):962–968

34. Wimberley N, Faling LJ, Bartlett JG. A fiberoptic bronchoscopy technique to obtain uncontaminated lower airway secretions for bacterial culture. *Am Rev Respir Dis.* 1979;119(3):337–343

35. Barzilay Z, Mandel M, Keren G, Davidson S. Nosocomial bacterial pneumonia in ventilated children: clinical significance of culture-positive peripheral bronchial aspirates. *J Pediatr.* 1994;112(3):421–426

36. Scheld WM, Mandell GL. Nosocomial pneumonia: pathogenesis and recent advances in diagnosis and therapy. *Rev Infect Dis.* 1991;13(suppl 9):S743–S751

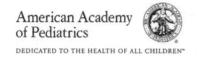

CLINICAL REPORT

Guidance on Management of Asymptomatic Neonates Born to Women With Active Genital Herpes Lesions

David W. Kimberlin, MD, Jill Baley, MD, COMMITTEE ON
INFECTIOUS DISEASES, and COMMITTEE ON FETUS AND
NEWBORN

KEY WORDS
newborn, herpes simplex virus, acyclovir, pregnancy

ABBREVIATIONS
CNS—central nervous system
CSF—cerebrospinal fluid
HSV—herpes simplex virus
HSV-1—herpes simplex virus type 1
HSV-2—herpes simplex virus type 2
IgG—immunoglobulin G
PCR—polymerase chain reaction
SEM—skin, eye, mouth

FUNDING: Funded in whole or in part with Federal funds from
the National Institute of Allergy and Infectious Diseases, National
Institutes of Health, Department of Health and Human Services,
under contract (N01-AI-30025, N01-AI-65306, N01-AI-15113, N01-AI-
62554), the General Clinical Research Unit (M01-RR00032), and
the State of Alabama. Funded by the National Institutes of Health
(NIH).

www.pediatrics.org/cgi/doi/10.1542/peds.2012-3216

doi:10.1542/peds.2012-3216

All clinical reports from the American Academy of Pediatrics
automatically expire 5 years after publication unless reaffirmed,
revised, or retired at or before that time.

PEDIATRICS (ISSN Numbers: Print, 0031-4005; Online, 1098-4275).

abstract

Herpes simplex virus (HSV) infection of the neonate is uncommon, but
genital herpes infections in adults are very common. Thus, although
treating an infant with neonatal herpes is a relatively rare occurrence,
managing infants potentially exposed to HSV at the time of delivery
occurs more frequently. The risk of transmitting HSV to an infant during delivery is determined in part by the mother's previous immunity
to HSV. Women with primary genital HSV infections who are shedding
HSV at delivery are 10 to 30 times more likely to transmit the virus to
their newborn infants than are women with recurrent HSV infection
who are shedding virus at delivery. With the availability of commercial serological tests that reliably can distinguish type-specific HSV
antibodies, it is now possible to determine the type of maternal
infection and, thus, further refine management of infants delivered
to women who have active genital HSV lesions. The management
algorithm presented herein uses both serological and virological
studies to determine the risk of HSV transmission to the neonate
who is delivered to a mother with active herpetic genital lesions and
tailors management accordingly. The algorithm does not address the
approach to asymptomatic neonates delivered to women with a history of genital herpes but no active lesions at delivery. *Pediatrics*
2013;131:e635–e646

INTRODUCTION

Herpes simplex virus (HSV) infection of the neonate is an uncommon
occurrence, with an estimated 1500 cases diagnosed annually in the
United States from a birth cohort of more than 4 000 000. In contrast,
genital herpes infections in adults are very common. Between 1 in 4
and 1 in 5 adults in the United States has genital herpes caused by
HSV type 2 (HSV-2).[1,2] In addition, HSV type 1 (HSV-1) now accounts for
at least 20% and, in some locales, more than 50% of cases of genital
herpes in the United States.[3,4] Therefore, managing infants potentially
exposed to HSV at the time of delivery is not uncommon, and prevention of the devastating outcomes of neonatal HSV disease is paramount.

Current recommendations for the management of infants after intrapartum exposure are based on expert opinion, because a randomized
controlled trial to determine whether an exposed neonate should be
treated would be unethical. However, the existing recommendations do

not take into account recent information correlating risk of transmission with type of maternal infection (primary versus recurrent) at the time of delivery.[5] The algorithm contained within this American Academy of Pediatrics (AAP) clinical report for the diagnostic and therapeutic approach to the neonate with known potential exposure to HSV during the perinatal period incorporates the most current scientific understanding of the biology, epidemiology, and pathology of HSV infection and disease.

TERMINOLOGY OF HSV INFECTION AND DISEASE

When an individual with no HSV-1 or HSV-2 antibody acquires either virus in the genital tract, a first-episode primary infection results. If a person with pre-existing HSV-1 antibody acquires HSV-2 genital infection (or vice versa), a first-episode nonprimary infection ensues. Viral reactivation from latency and subsequent antegrade translocation of virus back to skin and mucosal surfaces produces a recurrent infection.

Genital HSV infection can be either clinically apparent (eg, genital lesions) or inapparent (asymptomatic, or sub-clinical). Transmission to the neonate at the time of birth can occur with either presentation.

The distinction between neonatal HSV infection and neonatal HSV disease warrants discussion. Infection occurs when viral replication has been established, but the virus is not causing illness. Disease occurs when viral replication produces clinical signs of illness (eg, skin lesions, encephalitis, hepatitis). Once an infant is infected with HSV, progression to neonatal HSV disease is virtually certain. In an effort to prevent this progression from neonatal infection to neonatal disease, experts have recommended for many years that parenteral acyclovir be administered preemptively to HSV-infected neonates.[6]

RISK OF MATERNAL INFECTION DURING PREGNANCY

Recurrent infections are the most common form of genital HSV during pregnancy.[7] Approximately 10% of HSV-2–seronegative pregnant women have an HSV-2–seropositive sexual partner and, thus, are at risk for contracting a primary HSV-2 infection during the pregnancy[8] and transmitting the virus to their infants during delivery. Approximately one-fifth to one-third of women of childbearing age are seronegative for both HSV-1 and HSV-2,[9,10] and, among discordant couples, the chance that a woman will acquire either virus during pregnancy is estimated to be 3.7%.[11] For women who are already seropositive for HSV-1, the estimated chance of HSV-2 acquisition during the pregnancy is 1.7%.[11] Approximately two-thirds of women who acquire genital herpes during pregnancy remain asymptomatic and have no symptoms to suggest a genital HSV infection.[11] This is consistent with the finding that 60% to 80% of women who deliver an HSV-infected infant have a clinically unapparent genital HSV infection at the time of delivery and have neither a past history of genital herpes nor a sexual partner reporting a history of genital HSV.[12–14]

RISK OF NEONATAL HSV INFECTION

HSV infection of the newborn infant is acquired during 1 of 3 distinct times: intrauterine (in utero), intrapartum (perinatal), and postpartum (postnatal). The time of transmission of HSV-1 or HSV-2 for the overwhelming majority of infected infants (~85%) is in the intrapartum period. An additional 10% of infected neonates acquire HSV-1 post-natally from either a maternal or non-maternal source, and the final 5% are infected with HSV-2 or HSV-1 in utero. Five factors known to influence trans-mission of HSV from mother to neonate are:

1. Type of maternal infection (primary versus recurrent)[5,15–18];

2. Maternal HSV antibody status[5,14,19,20];

3. Duration of rupture of membranes[18];

4. Integrity of mucocutaneous barriers (eg, use of fetal scalp electrodes)[5,21,22]; and

5. Mode of delivery (cesarean versus vaginal delivery).[5]

Infants born to mothers who have a first episode of genital HSV infection near term and are shedding virus at delivery are at much greater risk of developing neonatal herpes than are infants whose mothers have recurrent genital herpes (Fig 1).[5,15–18]

The largest assessment of the influence of type of maternal infection on likelihood of neonatal transmission is a landmark study involving almost 60 000 women in labor who did not have clinical evidence of genital HSV disease, approximately 40 000 of whom had cultures performed within 48 hours of delivery (Fig 1).[5] Of these, 121 women were identified who were asymptomatically shedding HSV and who had sera available for analysis. In this large trial, 57% of infants delivered to women with first-episode primary HSV infection developed neonatal HSV disease, compared with 25% of infants delivered to women with first-episode nonprimary infection and 2% of infants delivered to women with recurrent HSV disease (Fig 1).[5]

CLINICAL MANIFESTATIONS OF NEONATAL HSV DISEASE

HSV infections acquired either intra-partum or postpartum can be classified as: (1) disease involving multiple visceral organs, including lung, liver, adrenal glands, skin, eye, and/or brain (disseminated disease); (2) central nervous system (CNS) disease, with or without skin lesions (CNS disease); and (3) disease limited to the skin, eyes, and/or mouth (skin, eye, mouth [SEM]

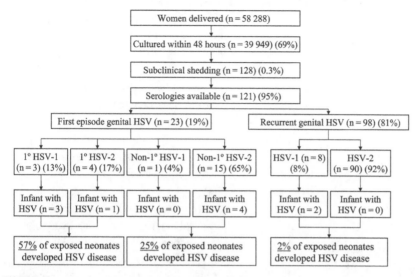

FIGURE 1
Type of maternal infection and risk of HSV transmission to the neonate.[5]

disease). This classification system is predictive of both morbidity and mortality.[23–27] Neonates with disseminated and SEM HSV disease typically present for medical attention at 10 to 12 days of age, whereas infants with CNS disease typically present at 17 to 19 days of age.[24] Overall, approximately half of all infants with neonatal HSV disease will have CNS involvement (CNS disease or disseminated disease with CNS involvement), and approximately 70% will have characteristic vesicular skin lesions (SEM disease, 83%; CNS disease, 63%; disseminated disease, 58%).[24]

DIAGNOSIS OF GENITAL HSV DISEASE

HSV can be detected from genital lesions by polymerase chain reaction (PCR) assay, viral culture, or antigen detection. Of these, PCR assay or viral culture are the testing modalities recommended by the Centers for Disease Control and Prevention for the diagnosis of genital HSV lesions.[28] The sensitivity of viral culture from genital lesions is low, especially for recurrent infection, and declines rapidly as lesions begin to heal. PCR assays for HSV DNA are more sensitive and are increasingly used for the diagnosis of genital HSV.[28,29] A

potential limitation of the PCR assay at the current time relates to its availability in all clinical settings; some smaller or more remote medical facilities have limited or no access to laboratories offering this technology. At many tertiary care centers, PCR assay results may be available within a day, whereas it takes 2 to 5 days for HSV to grow in viral culture. Typing of an HSV culture isolate or PCR assay product to determine if it is HSV-1 or HSV-2 can be accomplished by one of several techniques. The reliability of viral culture depends on the stage of the episode, with higher quantities of virus being present during the prodromal and vesicular stages than during crusting.[30] Antigen detection methods are available commercially but may not distinguish HSV-1 from HSV-2 and are not recommended by the Centers for Disease Control and Prevention for the diagnosis of genital herpes.

Before the year 2000, commercially available serological assays were unable to distinguish between HSV-1 and HSV-2 antibodies, severely limiting their utility. Over the past decade, a number of type-specific serological assays that reliably distinguish between immunoglobulin G (IgG) directed against HSV-1 and HSV-2

have been approved by the US Food and Drug Administration (Table 1). Many of these products are sold in kits that are used by clinical laboratories throughout the United States. Several additional tests that claim to distinguish between HSV-1 and HSV-2 antibody are available commercially, but high cross-reactivity rates attributable to their use of crude antigen preparations limit their utility,[31] and their use is not recommended.

DIAGNOSIS OF NEONATAL HSV DISEASE

Isolation of HSV by culture remains the definitive diagnostic method of establishing neonatal HSV disease. If skin lesions are present, a scraping of the vesicles should be transferred in appropriate viral transport media on ice to a diagnostic virology laboratory.[6] Other sites from which specimens should be obtained for culture of HSV include the conjunctivae, mouth, nasopharynx, and rectum ("surface cultures").[6] Specimens for viral culture from mucosal body sites may be combined before inoculating in cell culture to decrease costs, because the important information gathered from such cultures is the presence or absence of replicating virus rather than its precise body site. The sensitivity of PCR assay on surface specimens has not been studied; if used, surface PCR assay should be performed in addition to (and not instead of) the gold-standard surface culture. Rapid diagnostic techniques also are available, such as direct fluorescent antibody staining of vesicle scrapings or enzyme immunoassay detection of HSV antigens. These techniques are as specific but slightly less sensitive than culture.

The diagnosis of neonatal HSV CNS disease has been greatly enhanced by PCR testing of cerebrospinal fluid (CSF) specimens,[32–38] and PCR assay is now the method of choice for documenting CNS involvement in an infant

TABLE 1 Quick Reference Guide for Blood Tests to Accurately Detect Type-Specific HSV Antibodies

	Biokit HSV-2 Rapid Test (also sold as SureVue HSV-2 Rapid Test by Fisher HealthCare)	BioPlex HSV	Captia ELISA	Euroimmun Anti-HSV-1 and Anti-HSV-2 ELISA	HerpeSelect HSV-1 ELISA and HerpeSelect HSV-2 ELISA	HerpeSelect 1 and 2 Differentiation Immunoblot	Liaison HSV-2	AthenA MultiLyte
Supplier	Biokit USA	Bio-Rad Laboratories	Trinity Biotech USA	Euroimmun US LLC	Focus Diagnostics	Focus Diagnostics	DiaSorin Inc.	Inverness Medical
FDA approved	1999	2009	2004	2007	2000/2002	2000	2008	2008
Antibodies detected	HSV-2 only	HSV-1 or HSV-2 or both	HSV-1 or HSV-2 or both	HSV-1 or HSV-2	HSV-1 or HSV-2 or both	HSV-1 and/or HSV-2	HSV-1 or HSV-2	HSV-1 and/or HSV-2
Best use of test	POC test to screen or test individuals >3 mo postexposure	Screening or testing (high volume)	Screening or testing pregnant women or STD clinic patients (moderate volume)	Moderate volume	Screening or testing STD patients or pregnant women (moderate volume)	Low volume	High volume	Screening or testing (moderate to high volume)
Collection method	Finger stick, whole blood, or serum in clinic	Blood draw (sent to laboratory)	Blood draw (sent to laboratory)	Blood draw (sent to laboratory)	Blood draw (sent to laboratory)	Blood draw (sent to laboratory)	Blood draw (sent to laboratory)	Blood draw (sent to laboratory)
Test time	10 min	45 min	~2 h	~2 h	~2 h	~2 h	35 min	~2 h
FDA approved for use during pregnancy		Yes	Yes		Yes	Yes		
Test availability	Limited	Limited	Widely available		Widely available			
Web site	www.biokitusa.com	www.bio-rad.com	www.trinitybiotech.com	www.euroimmunus.com	www.herpeselect.com	www.herpeselect.com	www.diasorin.com	www.invernessmedicalpd.com
For more information	800-926-3353	800-224-6723	800-325-3424	800-913-2022			800-328-5669	877-546-8633

FDA, US Food and Drug Administration; POC, point of care; STD, sexually transmitted disease. Adapted from http://www.ashastd.org/ Accessed August 5, 2010.

suspected of having HSV disease. However, PCR assay of CSF should only be performed in conjunction with HSV surface cultures, given that up to 40% of infants with disseminated disease will not have CNS involvement, and, by definition, no infants with SEM disease will have CNS involvement. The sensitivity of CSF PCR testing in neonatal HSV disease ranges from 75% to 100%.[33,36,38] PCR analysis of CSF also should play a role in determining the duration of antiviral therapy, because available data suggest that having HSV DNA detected in CSF at or after completion of intravenous therapy is associated with poor outcomes.[36,37] All infants with a positive CSF PCR assay result for HSV DNA at the beginning of antiviral therapy should have a repeat lumbar puncture near the end of treatment to determine that HSV DNA has been cleared from the CNS.[24] Infants whose PCR assay result remains positive should continue to receive intravenous antiviral therapy until the CSF PCR assay result is negative.[24,36]

Application of PCR testing to blood specimens from infants with suspected HSV disease appears promising,[37–42] and, in the 2012 *Red Book*,[6] PCR assay of blood has been added to the laboratory evaluation for neonatal HSV disease. Data are insufficient at the current time to allow the use of serial PCR assays of blood to establish response to antiviral therapy or to guide decisions about the duration of therapy.

Serological testing is not helpful in the diagnosis of neonatal HSV infection, because transplacentally acquired maternal HSV IgG is present in most infants, given the substantial proportions of the adult American population who are HSV-1 and/or HSV-2 seropositive.

PREVENTION OF NEONATAL HSV DISEASE

Cesarean delivery in a woman with active genital lesions can reduce the infant's risk of acquiring HSV.[5,18] In

1999, the American College of Obstetricians and Gynecologists updated its management guidelines for genital herpes in pregnancy.[43] To reduce the risk of neonatal HSV disease, cesarean delivery should be performed if genital HSV lesions or prodromal symptoms are present at the time of delivery. Neonatal HSV infection has occurred despite cesarean delivery performed before the rupture of membranes.[12,44]

In women with a previous diagnosis of genital herpes, cesarean delivery to prevent neonatal HSV infection is not indicated if there are no genital lesions at the time of labor. In an effort to reduce cesarean deliveries performed for the indication of genital herpes, the use of oral acyclovir or valacyclovir near the end of pregnancy to suppress genital HSV recurrences has become increasingly common in obstetric practice. Several studies with small sample sizes suggest that suppressive acyclovir therapy during the last weeks of pregnancy decreases the occurrence of clinically apparent genital HSV disease at the time of delivery,[45–48] with an associated decrease in cesarean delivery rates for the indication of genital HSV.[45,46,49,50] However, because viral shedding still occurs (albeit with reduced frequency),[47,51] the potential for neonatal infection is not avoided completely, and cases of neonatal HSV disease in newborn infants of women who were receiving antiviral suppression recently have been reported.[52,53]

ALGORITHM FOR MANAGEMENT OF ASYMPTOMATIC NEONATES BORN VAGINALLY OR BY CESAREAN DELIVERY TO WOMEN WITH ACTIVE GENITAL HSV LESIONS (FIGS 2 AND 3)

The risk of transmitting HSV to the newborn infant during delivery is influenced directly by the mother's previous immunity to HSV; women who have primary genital HSV infections who are

shedding HSV at delivery are 10 to 30 times more likely to transmit the virus to their newborn infants than women with a recurrent infection.[5] The increased risk is attributable both to lower concentrations of transplacental HSV-specific antibodies (which also are less reactive to expressed polypeptides) in women with primary infection[19] and to the higher quantities of HSV that are shed for a longer period of time in the maternal genital tract in comparison with women who have recurrent genital HSV infection.[54] However, a substantial percentage of women with first clinical episodes of symptomatic genital herpes actually are experiencing reactivation of a previously unrecognized genital herpetic infection.[55] Thus, to tailor management of exposed neonates according to their degree of risk, one must distinguish primary versus recurrent maternal HSV infection in a manner that relies on more than just the history, or lack thereof, of genital herpes in the woman or her partner (s). Ideally, detection of HSV DNA from genital swabs obtained from women in labor would identify both symptomatic and asymptomatic HSV shedding, allowing for focused management of only those infants who are exposed; however, the technology to accomplish this on a broad scale is not readily available commercially at this time.

With the approval of commercially available serological tests that can reliably distinguish type-specific HSV antibodies (Table 1), the means to further refine management of asymptomatic neonates delivered to women with active genital HSV lesions is now possible. The algorithm detailed in Figs 2 and 3 applies only to asymptomatic neonates after vaginal or cesarean (because cesarean delivery reduces but does not eliminate the risk of neonatal HSV disease) delivery to women with active genital HSV lesions. It is intended to outline 1 approach to the management

of these infants and may not be feasible in settings with limited access to PCR assays for HSV DNA or to the newer type-specific serological tests. If, at any point during the evaluation outlined in the algorithm, an infant develops symptoms that could possibly indicate neonatal HSV disease (fever, hypothermia, lethargy, irritability, vesicular rash, seizures, etc), a full diagnostic evaluation should be undertaken, and intravenous acyclovir therapy should be initiated. In applying this algorithm, obstetric providers and pediatricians likely will need to work closely with their diagnostic laboratories to ensure that serological and virological testing is available and turnaround times are acceptable. In situations in which this is not possible, the approach detailed in the algorithm will have limited, and perhaps no, applicability.

TESTING OF WOMEN IN LABOR

Women in labor with visible genital lesions that are characteristic of HSV should have the lesions swabbed for HSV PCR and culture (AI). Any positive test result then requires further analysis to determine if the virus is HSV-1 or HSV-2. Correlation of viral type with serological status allows for determination of maternal infection classification (Table 2).

Management of Asymptomatic Neonates After Vaginal or Cesarean Delivery to Women With Lesions at Delivery and History of Genital HSV Preceding Pregnancy

For women with a history of genital herpes preceding the pregnancy, the likelihood that the current outbreak represents reactivation of latent HSV is high, and, therefore, the likelihood of transmission to the infant is low (2%). Skin and mucosal specimens (conjunctivae, mouth, nasopharynx, and rectum, and scalp electrode site, if present) should be obtained from the

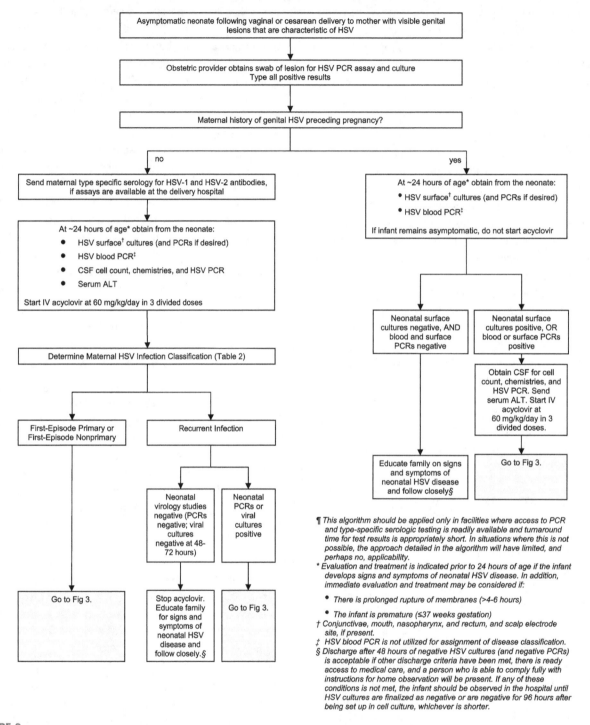

FIGURE 2

Algorithm for the evaluation of asymptomatic neonates after vaginal or cesarean delivery to women with active genital herpes lesions. ALT, alanine aminotransferase; D/C, discontinue.

neonate for culture (and PCR assay, if desired) at approximately 24 hours after delivery (BII), and blood should be sent for HSV DNA PCR assay. Acyclovir need not be started as long as the infant remains asymptomatic (BIII).

The importance of waiting until approximately 24 hours after delivery to obtain virological studies is based on the fact that a positive virological test result at that point represents actively replicating virus on the infant's mucosa,

whereas a positive test result shortly after birth could reflect only transient maternal contamination that may not lead to replication with resulting neonatal HSV disease.[56] It is permissible to discharge an asymptomatic infant after

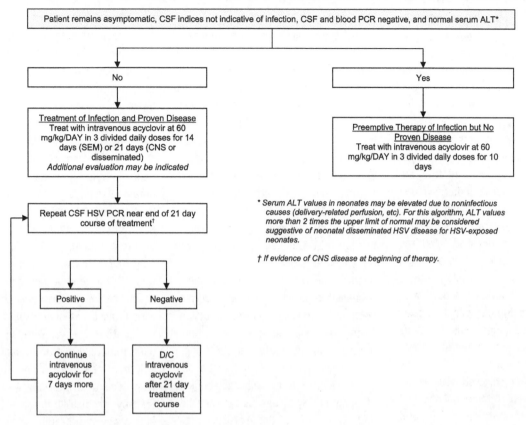

FIGURE 3

Algorithm for the treatment of asymptomatic neonates after vaginal or cesarean delivery to women with active genital herpes lesions. ALT, alanine aminotransferase; D/C, discontinue.

48 hours of negative HSV cultures (and negative PCR assay results) if other discharge criteria have been met, there is ready access to medical care, and a person who is able to comply fully with instructions for home observation will be present (BIII). If any of these conditions is not met, the infant should be observed in the hospital until HSV cultures are finalized as negative or are negative for 96 hours after being set up in cell culture, whichever is shorter.

If the surface and blood virological study results are negative at 5 days, the infant should be evaluated if signs or symptoms of neonatal HSV disease develop during the first 6 weeks of life (AII). Conversely, if the surface and blood virological study results become positive, thus confirming neonatal HSV infection, the infant should undergo a complete evaluation (lumbar puncture with CSF sent for indices and HSV DNA PCR assay, in addition to serum alanine

transaminase) to determine the extent of disease, and intravenous acyclovir should be initiated as soon as possible. If the evaluation findings are normal, indicating that the neonate has HSV infection but that it has not yet progressed to HSV disease, the infant should be treated empirically with intravenous acyclovir for 10 days to prevent progression from infection to disease (preemptive therapy) (BIII). If the evaluation findings are abnormal,

TABLE 2 Maternal Infection Classification by Genital HSV Viral Type and Maternal Serology[a]

Classification of Maternal Infection	PCR/Culture From Genital Lesion	Maternal HSV-1 and HSV-2 IgG Antibody Status
Documented first-episode primary infection	Positive, either virus	Both negative
Documented first-episode nonprimary infection	Positive for HSV-1	Positive for HSV-2 AND negative for HSV-1
	Positive for HSV-2	Positive for HSV-1 AND negative for HSV-2
Assume first-episode (primary or nonprimary) infection	Positive for HSV-1 OR HSV-2	Not available
	Negative OR not available[b]	Negative for HSV-1 and/or HSV-2 OR not available
Recurrent infection	Positive for HSV-1	Positive for HSV-1
	Positive for HSV-2	Positive for HSV-2

[a] To be used for women without a clinical history of genital herpes.

[b] When a genital lesion is strongly suspicious for HSV, clinical judgment should supersede the virological test results for the conservative purposes of this neonatal management algorithm. Conversely, if in retrospect, the genital lesion was not likely to be caused by HSV and the PCR assay result or culture is negative, departure from the evaluation and management in this conservative algorithm may be warranted.

indicating the neonate already has neonatal HSV disease, the infant should be treated for 14 to 21 days with intravenous acyclovir on the basis of the extent of neonatal HSV disease (disseminated, CNS, or SEM) (AII); if the initial CSF PCR assay result is positive for HSV DNA, a repeat lumbar puncture should be obtained near the end of therapy (eg, on day 17 or 18 of an anticipated 21-day course of therapy), and intravenous acyclovir should be discontinued at 21 days if the repeat HSV PCR assay result is negative (AII). If the "end-of-therapy" CSF PCR assay result is positive, intravenous acyclovir should be continued for another 7 days, with another repeat lumbar puncture near the end of therapy, again with decisions regarding cessation of therapy predicated on the repeat HSV CSF PCR assay result (BII). After completion of parenteral acyclovir for treatment of neonatal HSV disease, infants should receive oral acyclovir suppressive therapy for 6 months.[57]

Management of Asymptomatic Neonates After Vaginal or Cesarean Delivery to Women With Lesions at Delivery and No History of Genital HSV Preceding Pregnancy

For women without a history of genital herpes preceding pregnancy, the presence of genital lesions at delivery could represent first-episode primary infection (with a risk of transmission to the newborn infant of 57%), first-episode nonprimary infection (with a risk of transmission to the newborn infant of 25%), or recurrent infection (with a risk of transmission to the newborn infant of 2%). Thus, with the availability of type-specific serological testing, the practitioner can determine which type of infection the outbreak represents, given that the risks to the infant are so disparate. Accordingly, serological testing should be performed to determine the type of HSV infection in the mother to delineate between the 3 (Table 1).

At approximately 24 hours after delivery, neonatal skin and mucosal specimens (conjunctivae, mouth, nasopharynx, and rectum, and scalp electrode site, if present) should be obtained for culture (and PCR assay, if desired), and blood should be sent for HSV DNA PCR assay to evaluate for HSV infection. In addition, the infant should be evaluated for neonatal HSV disease (lumbar puncture with CSF sent for indices and HSV DNA PCR assay, in addition to serum alanine transaminase) at the same time, and intravenous acyclovir should be initiated pending the results of the evaluation, because the possibility is high that this could be a primary maternal infection (BIII). It is acceptable to wait to initiate therapy until approximately 24 hours after delivery in an asymptomatic neonate, because the average age at onset of neonatal HSV disease is between 1.5 and 3 weeks of age. Some practitioners advocate evaluation and treatment immediately after delivery if the infant is preterm or there has been prolonged rupture of membranes (CIII).

Laboratory correlations between virological (PCR/culture) and serological results that define maternal disease classification (first-episode primary, first-episode nonprimary, and recurrent) are presented in Table 2. The table deliberately uses a conservative estimate of first-episode infection, because the likelihood of transmission in such a situation is high. It is intended to be used to determine maternal disease classification in women without a clinical history of genital herpes.

If the mother has a documented or assumed first-episode primary or first-episode nonprimary infection (Table 2) and the neonate's evaluation results are normal, the infant should be treated empirically with intravenous acyclovir for 10 days to prevent progression from neonatal infection to disease (preemptive therapy) (BIII). If

the infant's evaluation results are abnormal, indicating the neonate already has neonatal HSV disease, the infant should be treated for 14 to 21 days with intravenous acyclovir on the basis of the extent of neonatal HSV disease (disseminated, CNS, or SEM) (AII); if the initial CSF PCR assay results are positive for HSV DNA, a repeat lumbar puncture should be obtained near the anticipated end of therapy (eg, on day 17 or 18 of therapy), and intravenous acyclovir should be discontinued at 21 days if the repeat HSV PCR assay result is negative (AII). If the end-of-therapy CSF PCR assay result is positive, the intravenous acyclovir should be continued for another 7 days, with another repeat lumbar puncture near the anticipated new end of therapy, again with decisions regarding cessation of therapy predicated on the HSV CSF PCR assay result (BII). After completion of parenteral acyclovir for treatment of neonatal HSV disease, infants should receive oral acyclovir suppressive therapy for 6 months.[57]

If the mother has recurrent genital HSV infection (that is, she has type-specific antibody to the HSV serotype detected by her genital swab) and the neonatal surface and blood virology study results are negative, acyclovir should be stopped, the parent(s) should receive education regarding signs and symptoms of neonatal HSV, and the infant may be discharged and reevaluated with any signs or symptoms of illness during the first 6 weeks of life (AII). Conversely, if virology study results are positive, confirming neonatal HSV infection, intravenous acyclovir should be continued, with the duration of treatment based on the evaluation for neonatal HSV disease. If the evaluation findings are normal, the infant should be treated empirically with intravenous acyclovir for 10 days to prevent progression from HSV infection to HSV disease (preemptive therapy) (BIII). If the evaluation findings are abnormal, the infant should be treated with intravenous acyclovir for 14 to 21 days on the basis of the extent of neonatal HSV disease (disseminated, CNS, or SEM) (AII); if the initial CSF PCR assay result is positive for HSV DNA, a repeat lumbar puncture should be obtained near the end of therapy (eg, on day 17 or 18 of an anticipated 21-day course of therapy), and intravenous acyclovir should be discontinued at 21 days if the repeat HSV PCR assay result is negative (AII). If the end-of-therapy CSF PCR assay result is positive, intravenous acyclovir should be continued for another 7 days, with another repeat lumbar puncture near the end of therapy, again with decisions regarding cessation of therapy predicated on the basis of HSV CSF PCR assay result (BII). After completion of parenteral acyclovir for treatment of neonatal HSV disease, infants should receive oral acyclovir suppressive therapy for 6 months.[57]

COMMITTEE ON INFECTIOUS DISEASES, 2012–2013

Michael T. Brady, MD, Chairperson
Carrie L. Byington, MD
H. Dele Davies, MD
Kathryn M. Edwards, MD
Mary P. Glode, MD
Mary Anne Jackson, MD
Harry L. Keyserling, MD
Yvonne A. Maldonado, MD
Dennis L. Murray, MD
Walter A. Orenstein, MD
Gordon E. Schutze, MD
Rodney E. Willoughby, MD
Theoklis E. Zaoutis, MD

LIAISONS

Marc A. Fischer, MD – *Centers for Disease Control and Prevention*
Bruce Gellin, MD – *National Vaccine Program Office*
Richard L. Gorman, MD – *National Institutes of Health*
Lucia Lee, MD – *Food and Drug Administration*
R. Douglas Pratt, MD – *Food and Drug Administration*
Jennifer S. Read, MD – *National Vaccine Program Office*
Joan Robinson, MD – *Canadian Pediatric Society*
Marco Aurelio Palazzi Safadi, MD – *Sociedad Latinoamericana de Infectologia Pediatrica (SLIPE)*
Jane Seward, MBBS, MPH – *Centers for Disease Control and Prevention*
Jeffrey R. Starke, MD – *American Thoracic Society*
Geoffrey Simon, MD – *Committee on Practice Ambulatory Medicine*
Tina Q. Tan, MD – *Pediatric Infectious Diseases Society*

EX OFFICIO

Henry H. Bernstein, DO – Red Book Online *Associate Editor*

David W. Kimberlin, MD – Red Book *Editor*
Sarah S. Long, MD – Red Book *Associate Editor*
H. Cody Meissner, MD – Visual Red Book *Associate Editor*

STAFF

Jennifer Frantz, MPH

COMMITTEE ON FETUS AND NEWBORN, 2012–2013

Lu-Ann Papile, MD, Chairperson
Jill E. Baley, MD
William Benitz, MD
Waldemar A. Carlo, MD
James Cummings, MD
Eric Eichenwald, MD
Praveen Kumar, MD
Richard A. Polin, MD
Rosemarie C. Tan, MD, PhD
Kasper S. Wang, MD

FORMER MEMBER

Kristi L. Watterberg, MD

LIAISONS

CAPT Wanda D. Barfield, MD, MPH – *Centers for Disease Control and Prevention*
George Macones, MD – *American College of Obstetricians and Gynecologists*
Ann L. Jefferies, MD – *Canadian Pediatric Society*
Erin L. Keels, APRN, MS, NNP-BC – *National Association of Neonatal Nurses*
Tonse N.K. Raju, MD, DCH – *National Institutes of Health*

STAFF

Jim Couto, MA

REFERENCES

1. Fleming DT, McQuillan GM, Johnson RE, et al. Herpes simplex virus type 2 in the United States, 1976 to 1994. *N Engl J Med.* 1997;337(16):1105–1111

2. Xu F, McQuillan GM, Kottiri BJ, et al. Trends in herpes simplex virus type 2 infection in the United States. In: 42nd Annual Meeting of the Infectious Diseases Society of America; September 30–October 3, 2004; Boston, MA. Abstract 739

3. Lafferty WE, Downey L, Celum C, Wald A. Herpes simplex virus type 1 as a cause of genital herpes: impact on surveillance and prevention. *J Infect Dis.* 2000;181(4):1454–1457

4. Kimberlin DW, Rouse DJ. Clinical practice. Genital herpes. *N Engl J Med.* 2004;350(19):1970–1977

5. Brown ZA, Wald A, Morrow RA, Selke S, Zeh J, Corey L. Effect of serologic status and cesarean delivery on transmission rates of herpes simplex virus from mother to infant. *JAMA.* 2003;289(2):203–209

6. American Academy of Pediatrics. Herpes simplex. In: Pickering LK, Baker CJ, Kimberlin DW, Long SS, eds. *Red Book: 2012 Report of the Committee on Infectious Diseases.* 29th ed. Elk Grove Village, IL: American Academy of Pediatrics; 2012:398–408

7. Whitley RJ. Herpes simplex virus infections. In: Remington JS, Klein JO, eds. *Infectious Diseases of the Fetus and Newborn Infants.* 3rd ed. Philadelphia, PA: WB Saunders Co; 1990:282–305

8. Kulhanjian JA, Soroush V, Au DS, et al. Identification of women at unsuspected risk of primary infection with herpes simplex virus type 2 during pregnancy. *N Engl J Med.* 1992;326(14):916–920

9. Xu F, Schillinger JA, Sternberg MR, et al. Seroprevalence and coinfection with herpes simplex virus type 1 and type 2 in the United States, 1988-1994. *J Infect Dis.* 2002;185(8):1019–1024

10. Xu F, Sternberg MR, Kottiri BJ, et al. Trends in herpes simplex virus type 1 and type 2 seroprevalence in the United States. *JAMA.* 2006;296(8):964–973

11. Brown ZA, Selke S, Zeh J, et al. The acquisition of herpes simplex virus during pregnancy. *N Engl J Med.* 1997;337(8):509–515

12. Whitley RJ, Corey L, Arvin A, et al. Changing presentation of herpes simplex virus

infection in neonates. *J Infect Dis.* 1988; 158(1):109–116

13. Whitley RJ, Nahmias AJ, Visintine AM, Fleming CL, Alford CA. The natural history of herpes simplex virus infection of mother and newborn. *Pediatrics.* 1980;66(4):489–494

14. Yeager AS, Arvin AM. Reasons for the absence of a history of recurrent genital infections in mothers of neonates infected with herpes simplex virus. *Pediatrics.* 1984; 73(2):188–193

15. Brown ZA, Benedetti J, Ashley R, et al. Neonatal herpes simplex virus infection in relation to asymptomatic maternal infection at the time of labor. *N Engl J Med.* 1991;324(18):1247–1252

16. Brown ZA, Vontver LA, Benedetti J, et al. Effects on infants of a first episode of genital herpes during pregnancy. *N Engl J Med.* 1987;317(20):1246–1251

17. Corey L, Wald A. Genital herpes. In: Holmes KK, Sparling PF, Mardh PA, et al, eds. *Sexually Transmitted Diseases.* 3rd ed. New York, NY: McGraw-Hill; 1999:285–312

18. Nahmias AJ, Josey WE, Naib ZM, Freeman MG, Fernandez RJ, Wheeler JH. Perinatal risk associated with maternal genital herpes simplex virus infection. *Am J Obstet Gynecol.* 1971;110(6):825–837

19. Prober CG, Sullender WM, Yasukawa LL, Au DS, Yeager AS, Arvin AM. Low risk of herpes simplex virus infections in neonates exposed to the virus at the time of vaginal delivery to mothers with recurrent genital herpes simplex virus infections. *N Engl J Med.* 1987;316(5):240–244

20. Yeager AS, Arvin AM, Urbani LJ, Kemp JA III. Relationship of antibody to outcome in neonatal herpes simplex virus infections. *Infect Immun.* 1980;29(2):532–538

21. Parvey LS, Ch'ien LT. Neonatal herpes simplex virus infection introduced by fetal-monitor scalp electrodes. *Pediatrics.* 1980; 65(6):1150–1153

22. Kaye EM, Dooling EC. Neonatal herpes simplex meningoencephalitis associated with fetal monitor scalp electrodes. *Neurology.* 1981;31(8):1045–1047

23. Kimberlin DW, Lin CY, Jacobs RF, et al; National Institute of Allergy and Infectious Diseases Collaborative Antiviral Study Group. Safety and efficacy of high-dose intravenous acyclovir in the management of neonatal herpes simplex virus infections. *Pediatrics.* 2001;108(2):230–238

24. Kimberlin DW, Lin CY, Jacobs RF, et al; National Institute of Allergy and Infectious Diseases Collaborative Antiviral Study Group. Natural history of neonatal herpes simplex virus infections in the acyclovir era. *Pediatrics.* 2001;108(2):223–229

25. Whitley R, Arvin A, Prober C, et al; Infectious Diseases Collaborative Antiviral Study Group. A controlled trial comparing vidarabine with acyclovir in neonatal herpes simplex virus infection. *N Engl J Med.* 1991;324(7):444–449

26. Whitley R, Arvin A, Prober C, et al; The National Institute of Allergy and Infectious Diseases Collaborative Antiviral Study Group. Predictors of morbidity and mortality in neonates with herpes simplex virus infections. *N Engl J Med.* 1991;324(7):450–454

27. Whitley RJ, Nahmias AJ, Soong SJ, Galasso GG, Fleming CL, Alford CA. Vidarabine therapy of neonatal herpes simplex virus infection. *Pediatrics.* 1980;66(4):495–501

28. Workowski KA, Berman S; Centers for Disease Control and Prevention (CDC). Sexually transmitted diseases treatment guidelines, 2010 [published correction appears in *MMWR Recomm Rep.* 2011;60(1):18]. *MMWR Recomm Rep.* 2010;59(RR-12):1–110

29. Wald A, Huang ML, Carrell D, Selke S, Corey L. Polymerase chain reaction for detection of herpes simplex virus (HSV) DNA on mucosal surfaces: comparison with HSV isolation in cell culture. *J Infect Dis.* 2003;188 (9):1345–1351

30. Moseley RC, Corey L, Benjamin D, Winter C, Remington ML. Comparison of viral isolation, direct immunofluorescence, and indirect immunoperoxidase techniques for detection of genital herpes simplex virus infection. *J Clin Microbiol.* 1981;13(5):913–918

31. Ashley RL. Sorting out the new HSV type specific antibody tests. *Sex Transm Infect.* 2001;77(4):232–237

32. Rowley AH, Whitley RJ, Lakeman FD, Wolinsky SM. Rapid detection of herpes-simplex-virus DNA in cerebrospinal fluid of patients with herpes simplex encephalitis. *Lancet.* 1990; 335(8687):440–441

33. Troendle-Atkins J, Demmler GJ, Buffone GJ. Rapid diagnosis of herpes simplex virus encephalitis by using the polymerase chain reaction. *J Pediatr.* 1993;123(3):376–380

34. Anderson NE, Powell KF, Croxson MC. A polymerase chain reaction assay of cerebrospinal fluid in patients with suspected herpes simplex encephalitis. *J Neurol Neurosurg Psychiatry.* 1993;56(5):520–525

35. Schlesinger Y, Storch GA. Herpes simplex meningitis in infancy. *Pediatr Infect Dis J.* 1994;13(2):141–144

36. Kimberlin DW, Lakeman FD, Arvin AM, et al; National Institute of Allergy and Infectious Diseases Collaborative Antiviral Study Group. Application of the polymerase chain reaction to the diagnosis and management of neonatal herpes simplex virus disease. *J Infect Dis.* 1996;174(6):1162–1167

37. Malm G, Forsgren M. Neonatal herpes simplex virus infections: HSV DNA in cerebrospinal fluid and serum. *Arch Dis Child Fetal Neonatal Ed.* 1999;81(1):F24–F29

38. Kimura H, Futamura M, Kito H, et al. Detection of viral DNA in neonatal herpes simplex virus infections: frequent and prolonged presence in serum and cerebrospinal fluid. *J Infect Dis.* 1991;164(2): 289–293

39. Barbi M, Binda S, Primache V, Tettamanti A, Negri C, Brambilla C. Use of Guthrie cards for the early diagnosis of neonatal herpes simplex virus disease. *Pediatr Infect Dis J.* 1998;17(3):251–252

40. Diamond C, Mohan K, Hobson A, Frenkel L, Corey L. Viremia in neonatal herpes simplex virus infections. *Pediatr Infect Dis J.* 1999;18(6):487–489

41. Lewensohn-Fuchs I, Osterwall P, Forsgren M, Malm G. Detection of herpes simplex virus DNA in dried blood spots making a retrospective diagnosis possible. *J Clin Virol.* 2003;26(1):39–48

42. Kimura H, Ito Y, Futamura M, et al. Quantitation of viral load in neonatal herpes simplex virus infection and comparison between type 1 and type 2. *J Med Virol.* 2002;67(3):349–353

43. American College of Obstetricians and Gynecologists. ACOG Practice Bulletin. Clinical management guidelines for obstetrician-gynecologists. No 82 June 2007. Management of herpes in pregnancy. *Obstet Gynecol.* 2007;109(6):1489–1498

44. Peng J, Krause PJ, Kresch M. Neonatal herpes simplex virus infection after cesarean section with intact amniotic membranes. *J Perinatol.* 1996;16(5):397–399

45. Braig S, Luton D, Sibony O, et al. Acyclovir prophylaxis in late pregnancy prevents recurrent genital herpes and viral shedding. *Eur J Obstet Gynecol Reprod Biol.* 2001;96 (1):55–58

46. Scott LL, Sanchez PJ, Jackson GL, Zeray F, Wendel GD Jr. Acyclovir suppression to prevent cesarean delivery after first-episode genital herpes. *Obstet Gynecol.* 1996;87(1): 69–73

47. Scott LL, Hollier LM, McIntire D, Sanchez PJ, Jackson GL, Wendel GD Jr. Acyclovir suppression to prevent recurrent genital herpes at delivery. *Infect Dis Obstet Gynecol.* 2002;10(2):71–77

48. Sheffield JS, Hollier LM, Hill JB, Stuart GS, Wendel GD Jr. Acyclovir prophylaxis to prevent herpes simplex virus recurrence at delivery: a systematic review. *Obstet Gynecol.* 2003;102(6):1396–1403

49. Andrews WW, Kimberlin DF, Whitley R, Cliver S, Ramsey PS, Deeter R. Valacyclovir therapy

to reduce recurrent genital herpes in pregnant women. *Am J Obstet Gynecol.* 2006;194 (3):774–781

50. Sheffield JS, Hill JB, Hollier LM, et al. Valacyclovir prophylaxis to prevent recurrent herpes at delivery: a randomized clinical trial. *Obstet Gynecol.* 2006;108(1): 141–147

51. Watts DH, Brown ZA, Money D, et al. A double-blind, randomized, placebo-controlled trial of acyclovir in late pregnancy for the reduction of herpes simplex virus shedding and cesarean delivery. *Am J Obstet Gynecol.* 2003; 188(3):836–843

52. Pinninti SG, Feja KN, Kimberlin DW, et al. Neonatal herpes disease despite maternal antenatal antiviral suppressive therapy: a multicenter case series of the first such infants reported. In: 48th Annual Meeting of the Infectious Diseases Society of America; October 22, 2010; Vancouver, British Columbia. Abstract 1841

53. Pinninti SG, Angara R, Feja KN, et al. Neonatal herpes disease following maternal antenatal antiviral suppressive therapy: a multicenter case series. *J Pediatr.* 2012; 161(1):134–138.e1–e3

54. Whitley RJ. Herpes simplex viruses. In: Fields BN, Knipe DM, Howley PM, et al, eds. *Fields Virology.* 3rd ed. Philadelphia, PA: Lippincott Raven Publishers; 1996:2297– 2342

55. Diamond C, Selke S, Ashley R, Benedetti J, Corey L. Clinical course of patients with serologic evidence of recurrent genital herpes presenting with signs and symptoms of first episode disease. *Sex Transm Dis.* 1999;26(4): 221–225

56. Turner R, Shehab Z, Osborne K, Hendley JO. Shedding and survival of herpes simplex virus from 'fever blisters'. *Pediatrics.* 1982; 70(4):547–549

57. Kimberlin DW, Whitley RJ, Wan W, et al; National Institute of Allergy and Infectious Diseases Collaborative Antiviral Study Group. Oral acyclovir suppression and neurodevelopment after neonatal herpes. *N Engl J Med.* 2011;365(14):1284–1292

APPENDIX Evidence-based Rating System Used To Determine Strength Of Recommendations

Category	Definition	Recommendation
Strength of recommendation		
A	Strong evidence for efficacy and substantial clinical benefit	Strongly recommended
B	Strong or moderate evidence for efficacy, but only limited clinical benefit	Generally recommended
C	Insufficient evidence for efficacy, or efficacy does not outweigh possible adverse consequences	Optional
D	Moderate evidence against efficacy or for adverse outcome	Generally not recommended
E	Strong evidence against efficacy or for adverse outcome	Never recommended
Quality of evidence supporting recommendation		
I	Evidence from at least 1 well-executed randomized controlled trial or 1 rigorously designed laboratory-based experimental study that has been replicated by an independent investigator	
II	Evidence from at least 1 well-designed clinical trial without randomization; cohort or case-controlled analytic studies (preferably from >1 center); multiple time-series studies; dramatic results from uncontrolled studies; or some evidence from laboratory experiments	
III	Evidence from opinions of respected authorities based on clinical or laboratory experience, descriptive studies, or reports of expert committees	

Adapted from Centers for Disease Control. 2009 guidelines for the prevention and treatment of opportunistic infections among HIV-exposed and HIV-infected children. *MMWR Recomm Rep.* 2009;58(RR-11):5.

CLINICAL REPORT   Guidance for the Clinician in Rendering Pediatric Care

American Academy
of Pediatrics

DEDICATED TO THE HEALTH OF ALL CHILDREN™

Management of Neonates Born at ≥35 0/7 Weeks' Gestation With Suspected or Proven Early-Onset Bacterial Sepsis

Karen M. Puopolo, MD, PhD, FAAP,[a,b] William E. Benitz, MD, FAAP,[c] Theoklis E. Zaoutis, MD, MSCE, FAAP,[a,d]
COMMITTEE ON FETUS AND NEWBORN, COMMITTEE ON INFECTIOUS DISEASES

abstract

The incidence of neonatal early-onset sepsis (EOS) has declined substantially over the last 2 decades, primarily because of the implementation of evidence-based intrapartum antimicrobial therapy. However, EOS remains a serious and potentially fatal illness. Laboratory tests alone are neither sensitive nor specific enough to guide EOS management decisions. Maternal and infant clinical characteristics can help identify newborn infants who are at risk and guide the administration of empirical antibiotic therapy. The incidence of EOS, the prevalence and implications of established risk factors, the predictive value of commonly used laboratory tests, and the uncertainties in the risk/benefit balance of antibiotic exposures all vary significantly with gestational age at birth. Our purpose in this clinical report is to provide a summary of the current epidemiology of neonatal sepsis among infants born at ≥35 0/7 weeks' gestation and a framework for the development of evidence-based approaches to sepsis risk assessment among these infants.

[a]Department of Pediatrics, Perelman School of Medicine, University of Pennsylvania, Philadelphia, Pennsylvania; [b]Children's Hospital of Philadelphia, and [d]Roberts Center for Pediatric Research, Philadelphia, Pennsylvania; and [c]Division of Neonatal and Developmental Medicine, Department of Pediatrics, School of Medicine, Stanford University, Palo Alto, California

Clinical reports from the American Academy of Pediatrics benefit from expertise and resources of liaisons and internal (AAP) and external reviewers. However, clinical reports from the American Academy of Pediatrics may not reflect the views of the liaisons or the organizations or government agencies that they represent.

The guidance in this report does not indicate an exclusive course of treatment or serve as a standard of medical care. Variations, taking into account individual circumstances, may be appropriate.

All clinical reports from the American Academy of Pediatrics automatically expire 5 years after publication unless reaffirmed, revised, or retired at or before that time.

DOI: https://doi.org/10.1542/peds.2018-2894

Address correspondence to Karen M. Puopolo, MD, PhD, FAAP. E-mail: puopolok@email.chop.edu

PEDIATRICS (ISSN Numbers: Print, 0031-4005; Online, 1098-4275).

To cite: Puopolo KM, Benitz WE, Zaoutis TE, AAP COMMITTEE ON FETUS AND NEWBORN, AAP COMMITTEE ON INFECTIOUS DISEASES. Management of Neonates Born at ≥35 0/7 Weeks' Gestation With Suspected or Proven Early-Onset Bacterial Sepsis. *Pediatrics.* 2018;142(6):e20182894

Early-onset sepsis (EOS) is a serious and potentially fatal complication of birth. Assessing term and late-preterm newborn infants for risk of EOS is one of the most common clinical tasks conducted by pediatric providers.[1] As the use of preventive intrapartum antibiotic therapies has increased and the incidence of EOS has decreased, physicians are challenged to identify those newborn infants who are at the highest risk of infection. Pediatric providers are particularly concerned about initially well-appearing infants with identified risk factors for EOS for fear of missing the opportunity to intervene before infants become critically ill. The need to (1) assess a newborn infant's risk of EOS, (2) determine which steps should be taken at particular levels of risk (including the administration of empirical, broad-spectrum antibiotic therapies), and (3) decide when to discontinue empirical antibiotic therapies are critically important decisions that are made daily by physicians caring for neonates.

Depending on the local structure of pediatric care, these decisions are made by community pediatricians, family physicians, emergency department physicians, newborn hospitalists, and/or neonatal intensive care specialists.

PATHOGENESIS AND CURRENT EPIDEMIOLOGY OF NEONATAL EOS

EOS is defined as a blood or cerebrospinal fluid (CSF) culture obtained within 72 hours after birth growing a pathogenic bacterial species. This microbiologic definition stands in contrast to the functional definitions of sepsis that are used in pediatric and adult patients, for whom the definition is used to specify a series of time-sensitive interventions. Before the first national guidelines were published in which researchers recommended intrapartum antibiotic prophylaxis (IAP) to prevent perinatal group B *Streptococcus* (GBS) disease,[2] the overall incidence of EOS in the United States was 3 to 4 cases per 1000 live births.[3] Currently, the incidence of EOS among infants who are born at term has declined to approximately 0.5 in 1000 live births.[4,5] The EOS incidence is higher (approximately 1 in 1000 live births) among late-preterm infants but still an order of magnitude lower than the incidence among preterm, very low birth weight infants.[4–7] Culture-confirmed meningitis among term infants is even more rare, with an incidence of 0.01 to 0.02 cases per 1000 live births.[4,8] Morbidity and mortality from EOS remain substantial; approximately 60% of term infants with EOS require neonatal intensive care for respiratory distress and/or blood pressure support.[8] Mortality is approximately 2% to 3% among infants with EOS born at ≥35 weeks' gestation.[4,5,8]

EOS primarily begins in utero and was originally described as amniotic infection syndrome.[9,10] Among term infants, the pathogenesis of EOS is most commonly that of ascending colonization and infection of the uterine compartment with maternal gastrointestinal and genitourinary flora during labor with subsequent colonization and invasive infection of the fetus and/or fetal aspiration of infected amniotic fluid. Rarely, EOS may develop at or near term before the onset of labor. Whether acquired hematogenously across the placenta or via an ascending route, bacterial infection can be a cause of stillbirth in the third trimester.[11,12] *Listeria monocytogenes*, which is usually transmitted from the mother to the fetus by the transplacental hematogenous spread of infection before the onset of labor, is an infrequent but notable cause of EOS.[13]

RISK FACTORS FOR EOS

The occurrence, severity, and duration of specific clinical risk factors can be used to assess the risk of EOS among term and late-preterm infants. Evidence has supported the predictive value of gestational age, maternal intraamniotic infection (represented either by intrapartum fever or the obstetric clinical diagnosis of chorioamnionitis), the duration of rupture of membranes (ROM), maternal GBS colonization, the administration of appropriate intrapartum antibiotic therapy, and the newborn clinical condition.[2,14–16] Surveillance studies in the United States reveal higher rates of EOS among infants who are born to mothers of African American race compared with those who are not of African American race, but race is not an independent predictor in multivariable analyses.[4,5,7] Multiple other factors associated with an increased risk of EOS (eg, twin gestation, fetal tachycardia, meconium-stained amniotic fluid) also are not independent predictors of infection.

The clinical diagnosis of chorioamnionitis has been used as a primary risk factor for identifying infants who are at risk for EOS, presenting multiple difficulties for obstetric and neonatal providers. Although most infants with EOS are born to women with this clinical diagnosis, specificity is poor; only a small proportion of infants who are born in the setting of chorioamnionitis develop EOS.[16–19] In a review of nearly 400 000 newborn infants, researchers confirmed the high rate of chorioamnionitis diagnosis among the mothers of infants with EOS but estimated that approximately 450 term infants who were exposed to chorioamnionitis would have to be treated per case of confirmed EOS.[20] These data are used to provide a strong argument against using the clinical diagnosis of chorioamnionitis as a sole indicator of risk for EOS in term infants. The identification of chorioamnionitis itself is challenging, particularly among women who are laboring at or near term. The American College of Obstetricians and Gynecologists (ACOG) has recently opted to transition away from the use of the term chorioamnionitis to the use of intraamniotic infection and has published guidance for its diagnosis and management.[21] The ACOG aligned with the recommendations of a multispecialty workshop sponsored by the *Eunice Kennedy Shriver* National Institute of Child Health and Human Development in defining a confirmed diagnosis of intraamniotic infection as 1 made by using positive amniotic fluid Gram-stain and/or culture results or by using placental histopathology.[21,22] Suspected intraamniotic infection is defined as maternal intrapartum fever (either a single maternal intrapartum temperature ≥39.0°C or a temperature of 38.0°C–38.9°C that persists for >30 minutes) and 1 or more of the following: maternal leukocytosis, purulent cervical drainage, and fetal tachycardia. The

ACOG recommends that intrapartum antibiotic therapy be administered whenever intraamniotic infection is diagnosed or suspected and when otherwise unexplained maternal fever occurs in isolation. These recommendations are based on data revealing the protective effect of intrapartum antibiotic therapy for both the mother and fetus when infection is present while acknowledging frequent uncertainty about the presence of intraamniotic infection.

ANTIBIOTIC STEWARDSHIP IN EOS MANAGEMENT

Newborn infants may be exposed to antibiotic drugs before birth in the form of GBS IAP, maternal surgical prophylaxis in cesarean deliveries, or intrapartum antibiotic therapy administered because of suspected or confirmed intraamniotic infection or other maternal infections. Combined, these indications result in an antibiotic exposure of 32% to 45% of all newborn infants.[23–25] Administered to protect mothers and newborn infants, such early antibiotic exposures may also have negative consequences for term and late-preterm infants. Researchers in retrospective studies conducted primarily among term infants have associated antibiotic administration in infancy with increased risks of later childhood health problems, such as wheezing, asthma, food allergy, inflammatory bowel disease, and childhood obesity.[26–32] Although the biologic basis of such associations is not firmly established, researchers suggest that neonatal antibiotic administration alters the developing gut microbiome.[33–35] Intrapartum antibiotic administration has been associated with changes in stool bacterial composition at 1 week, 3 months, and 12 months of age.[34,35] The impact of breastfeeding on gut dysbiosis may be important given that mother-infant separation for EOS evaluation can delay the initiation of

breastfeeding and increase formula supplementation.[36] Although the relationship between early neonatal antibiotic exposure and subsequent childhood health remains to be defined, current evidence reveals that such exposures do affect newborn infants in the short-term; therefore, physicians should consider the risk/benefit balance of initiating antibiotic therapy for the risk of EOS as well as for continuing empirical antibiotic therapy in the absence of a culture-confirmed infection.

RISK STRATIFICATION FOR TERM AND LATE-PRETERM INFANTS

Three approaches currently exist for the use of risk factors to identify infants who are at increased risk of EOS, as detailed in the following sections. Each approach has merits and limitations, and each is a reasonable approach to risk assessment among infants who are born at ≥35 weeks' gestation. No strategy can be used to immediately identify all infants who will develop EOS or avoid the treatment of a substantial number of infants who are uninfected. Therefore, each strategy must include measures to monitor infants who are not initially identified and to minimize the duration of antibiotic administration to infants who are uninfected. Those at birth centers should develop institutional approaches that are best suited to their local resources and structures. Optimally, the effect of the chosen approach should be measured to identify low-frequency adverse events and to affirm efficacy.

Categorical Risk Factor Assessment

A categorical risk factor assessment includes risk factor threshold values to identify infants who are at increased risk for EOS. Algorithms for the management of GBS-specific EOS have been used as a general framework for the prevention of all EOS.[3,37,38] Risk factors used in such algorithms included (1) any

newborn infant who is ill appearing; (2) a mother with a clinical diagnosis of chorioamnionitis; (3) a mother who is colonized with GBS and who received inadequate IAP, with a duration of ROM being >18 hours or birth before 37 weeks' gestation; or (4) a mother who is colonized with GBS who received inadequate IAP but with no additional risk factors. Recommendations in these algorithms include the following: laboratory testing and empirical antibiotic therapy for infants in categories 1 and 2, laboratory testing for category 3, and observation in the hospital for ≥48 hours for category 4.

Different versions of this approach have been published since 1996 and have been incorporated by physicians into local algorithms. An advantage of using categorical risk factors is that substantial data have been reported that are used to address the effects on GBS-specific disease and on the frequency of neonatal EOS evaluation.[3,39–45] Limitations of this approach include a lack of clear definitions for newborn clinical illness, difficulties in establishing the clinical diagnosis of maternal chorioamnionitis, an inconsistent consideration of intrapartum antibiotics, and the absence of guidance on what is used to define abnormal laboratory test results in the newborn infant.

Multivariate Risk Assessment

A multivariate risk assessment includes an individualized synthesis of established risk factors and the newborn clinical condition to estimate each infant's risk of EOS. A cohort of 608 000 newborn infants was used to develop predictive models for culture-confirmed EOS based on objective data that are known at the moment of birth[7] and the evolving newborn condition during the first 6 to 12 hours after birth.[46] The objective data include gestational age, the highest maternal intrapartum temperature, the maternal GBS colonization status, the duration of ROM, and the type and duration of intrapartum antibiotic therapies. The predictive models were used to develop a Web-based Neonatal Early-Onset Sepsis Risk Calculator with recommended clinical algorithms that are based on the final risk estimate.[47] Blood culture and enhanced clinical observation are recommended for infants with an EOS risk estimated at ≥1 per 1000 live births, and blood culture and empirical antibiotic therapy are recommended for infants with an EOS risk estimated at ≥3 per 1000 live births. A prospective validation in 204 685 infants revealed that blood culture testing declined by 66%, and empirical antibiotic administration declined by 48% with this approach compared with the previous use of a categorical risk algorithm based on recommendations by the Centers for Disease Control and Prevention (CDC).[44] No adverse effects of the multivariate risk approach were noted during birth hospitalization. Readmissions for culture-confirmed infection during the week after discharge from the birth hospital were rare (approximately 5 in 100 000 births) and did not differ by the approach (sepsis risk calculator versus CDC risk algorithm) used at birth.

The advantages of the multivariate approach are that it (1) is used to provide differential information on an individual infant's risk rather than place infants in categories with a wide range of risk, (2) includes only objective data and not a clinical diagnosis of maternal chorioamnionitis, and (3) results in relatively few well-appearing newborn infants being treated empirically with antibiotic agents. Potential concerns are derived from the anticipated effect on birth hospitals because this multivariate approach necessitates increased clinical surveillance for some

infants in the well nursery and/ or postpartum care unit. The classification of infants as clinically ill, equivocal, or well appearing requires ongoing clinical assessment over the first 12 hours after birth.[44,46,48] Workflow changes could be needed to accommodate changes in the frequency of vital signs and other clinical assessments for infants who are identified as being at moderate risk of EOS. Those at institutions opting for this approach may set different risk thresholds for specific actions other than those that are validated[44,48] but should also consider quantifying the effect of the chosen risk thresholds to affirm safety and efficacy.

Risk Assessment Primarily Based on Newborn Clinical Condition

A third strategy consists of the reliance on clinical signs of illness to identify infants with EOS. Under this approach, regardless of any estimation of neonatal or maternal risk factors for EOS, infants who appear ill at birth and those who develop signs of illness over the first 48 hours after birth are either treated empirically with antibiotic agents or further evaluated by laboratory screening. Among term and late-preterm infants, good clinical condition at birth is associated with a reduction in risk for EOS of approximately 60% to 70%.[44,46] A multidisciplinary panel sponsored by the *Eunice Kennedy Shriver* National Institute of Child Health and Human Development advocated that infants be flagged for risk of EOS on the basis of the obstetric diagnosis of suspected intraamniotic infection but that those conducting newborn evaluation primarily rely on clinical observation alone for well-appearing term and late-preterm infants.[22] Those at several centers have reported experience with strategies based on the identification of at-risk newborn infants using categorical or multivariate approaches to risk accompanied by laboratory tests

and serial examinations of at-risk newborn infants.[42,49–53] Researchers at 1 center in Italy reported a cohort of 7628 term infants who were managed with a categorical approach to risk identification and compared the outcomes with a cohort of 7611 infants who were managed with serial physical examinations every 4 to 6 hours through 48 hours of age. Significant decreases in the use of laboratory tests, blood cultures, and empirical antibiotic agents were observed in the second cohort. Two infants who developed EOS in the second cohort were identified as they developed signs of illness.[42]

The primary advantage of this approach is a significant reduction in the rate of antibiotic use. Those at institutions adopting such an approach will need to decide whether to adopt a categorical or multivariate approach for the identification of infants who are at risk. Alternatively, providers can decide to conduct serial clinical evaluations on all newborn infants without regard to risk of EOS. The latter approach would provide a means of identifying infants who develop EOS despite a low estimate of risk and initially reassuring clinical condition. Such cases occur at rate of approximately 1 in 10 000 live births among term and late-preterm infants.[46] Potential disadvantages of this approach are that it can require significant changes to newborn care at birth hospitals, including the establishment of processes to ensure universal serial, structured, documented examinations and the development of clear criteria for additional evaluation and empirical antibiotic administration. Frequent medical examinations of all newborn infants may be variably acceptable to families and may add significantly to the cost of well nursery care. Importantly, physicians and families must understand that the identification of initially well-appearing infants who develop clinical illness is not a failure of care but rather an anticipated outcome of this approach to EOS risk management.

LABORATORY TESTING

Blood Culture

In the absence of validated, clinically available molecular diagnostics, blood culture remains the diagnostic standard for EOS. Newborn surface cultures and gastric aspirate analysis cannot be used to diagnose EOS, and urine culture is not indicated in sepsis evaluations performed at <72 hours of age. In modern blood culture systems, optimized enriched culture media with antimicrobial neutralization properties, continuous-read detection systems, and specialized pediatric culture bottles are used. Concerns have been raised about the incomplete detection of low-level bacteremia and the effect of intrapartum antibiotic administration.[22,54] However, these systems are used to reliably detect bacteremia at a level of 1 to 10 colony-forming units per mL if a minimum blood volume of 1 mL is inoculated. Furthermore, researchers in several studies have reported no effect of intrapartum antibiotic therapy on time to positivity.[55–59] Culture media containing antimicrobial neutralization elements efficiently neutralize β-lactam antibiotic agents and gentamicin.[55] A median blood culture time to positivity of <24 hours is reported among term infants when using contemporary blood culture techniques.[60–63] Despite the performance characteristics of modern blood cultures, a prolonged empirical antibiotic treatment of term newborn infants who are critically ill may occasionally be appropriate despite negative culture results.

Pediatric blood culture bottles generally require a minimum inoculum of 1 mL of blood for optimal recovery of organisms.[64,65] The use of 2 separate culture bottles may provide the opportunity to determine if commensal species are true infections by comparing growth in the 2 cultures.[66,67] The use of 1 aerobic and 1 anaerobic culture bottle may be done to optimize the organism recovery of rare strict anaerobic species,[68] and most neonatal pathogens, including GBS, *Escherichia coli*, and *Staphylococcus aureus*, will grow under anaerobic conditions. Anaerobic blood culture is routinely performed as part of sepsis evaluation among obstetric and other adult patients. Those at individual centers may benefit from collaborative discussion with those at the laboratory where cultures are processed to optimize local processes.

CSF Culture

CSF culture should ideally be performed along with blood culture and before the initiation of empirical antibiotic therapy for infants who are at the highest risk of EOS. Among infants born at ≥35 weeks' gestation, those at the highest risk include those with critical illness. CSF cell counts obtained after the initiation of empirical antibiotic therapy may be difficult to interpret.[69,70] However, physicians must balance the challenges of CSF interpretation with the realities of care: lumbar puncture should not be performed if the newborn infant's clinical condition would be compromised or antibiotic initiation would be delayed by the procedure. Meningitis was diagnosed clinically in 4% of EOS cases in CDC surveillance, but only half of the diagnoses were made by using CSF culture, reflecting the practical difficulties in performing lumbar puncture.[4] CSF culture and analysis should be performed if blood cultures grow a pathogen to optimize the type and duration of antibiotic therapy. CSF culture and analysis do not need to be performed in the vast majority of term infants for whom blood cultures are sterile. The incidence of culture-confirmed meningitis in the absence of culture-confirmed bacteremia is approximately 1 to 2 cases per 100 000 live births.[4,8] Physicians may, therefore, use their best judgment to determine when CSF analysis should be performed in the absence of documented bacteremia.

White Blood Cell Count

The white blood cell (WBC) count, immature/total neutrophil ratio (I/T), and absolute neutrophil count (ANC) are commonly used to assess the risk of EOS. Multiple clinical factors can affect the WBC count and differential, including gestational age at birth, sex, and mode of delivery.[71–74] Fetal bone marrow depression attributable to maternal preeclampsia or placental insufficiency and prolonged exposure to inflammatory signals, such as those associated with the premature ROM, frequently result in abnormal values in the absence of infection. As the incidence of EOS declines, the clinical utility of the WBC count also declines. Researchers in 2 large, multicenter studies applied the likelihood ratio, a test characteristic that is independent of disease incidence, to assess the relationship between WBC count and culture-confirmed EOS among term and late-preterm infants and found that none of the components (WBC count, I/T, nor ANC) performed well. Extreme values (total WBC count <5000/μL [I/T >0.3; ANC <2000/μL] in one study[73] and WBC count <1000/μL [ANC <100/μL; and I/T >0.5] in the other[75]) were associated with the highest likelihood ratios but very low sensitivities. WBC count >20 000/μL and platelet counts were not associated with EOS in either study. The I/T squared (I/T divided by the ANC) performed better than any of the more traditional tests and was independent of age in hours but also had modest sensitivity and specificity.[76]

Other Inflammatory Markers

Researchers in multiple studies address other markers of inflammation, including C-reactive protein (CRP), procalcitonin, interleukins (ILs) (soluble IL-2 receptor, IL-6, and IL-8), tumor necrosis factor α, and CD64.[77–80] Both CRP and procalcitonin concentrations increase in newborn infants in response to a variety of inflammatory stimuli, including infection, asphyxia, and pneumothorax. Procalcitonin concentrations also increase naturally over the first 24 to 36 hours after birth.[79] Single values of CRP or procalcitonin obtained after birth to assess the risk of EOS are neither sensitive nor specific to guide EOS care decisions. Consistently normal values of CRP and procalcitonin over the first 48 hours of age are associated with the absence of EOS, but serial abnormal values alone should not be used to decide whether to administer antibiotics in the absence of culture-confirmed infection. Additionally, at this time, a serial evaluation of inflammatory markers should not be used to assess well-appearing term newborn infants for risk of EOS.

TREATMENT OF EOS

The microbial causes of EOS in the United States have been unchanged over the past 10 years. Researchers in national surveillance studies continue to identify GBS as the most common bacteria isolated in EOS cases among term and late-preterm infants, accounting for approximately 40% to 45% of all cases,[4,5] followed by E coli in approximately 10% to 15% of cases. The remaining cases are caused primarily by other Gram-positive organisms (predominantly viridans group streptococci and enterococci), and approximately 5% are caused by other Gram-negative

organisms. S aureus (approximately 3%–4%) and L monocytogenes (approximately 1%–2%) are less common causes of EOS among term infants.[4,5]

Ampicillin and gentamicin, in combination, is the first choice for empirical therapy for EOS. This combination will be effective against GBS, most other streptococcal and enterococcal species, and L monocytogenes. Although two-thirds of E coli EOS isolates and most other Gram-negative EOS isolates are resistant to ampicillin, the majority remain sensitive to gentamicin.[4] Extended-spectrum β-lactamase–producing organisms are rarely reported among EOS cases in the United States. Therefore, the routine empirical use of broader-spectrum antibiotic agents is typically not justified and may be harmful.[81] Nonetheless, approximately 7% of E coli cases (1.7% of all EOS cases) were resistant to both ampicillin and gentamicin in recent CDC surveillance studies.[4] Among term newborn infants who are critically ill, the empirical addition of broader-spectrum therapy should be considered until culture results are available.

When EOS is confirmed by using blood culture, lumbar puncture should be performed if not previously done. Serial daily blood cultures should be performed until microbiological sterility is documented. In definitive antibiotic therapy, providers should use the narrowest spectrum of appropriate antibiotics. The duration of therapy should be guided by expert references (eg, the American Academy of Pediatrics Red Book: Report of the Committee on Infectious Diseases) and informed by using CSF analysis results and the achievement of sterile cultures. Consultation with infectious disease specialists can be considered for cases that are complicated by meningitis or other site-specific infections and for

cases that are caused by resistant or atypical organisms. Among term infants with unexplained critical cardiorespiratory illness, an empirical course of antibiotic therapy may be justified even in the absence of culture-confirmed infection. Most often, however, antibiotic therapy should be discontinued when blood cultures are sterile at 36 to 48 hours of incubation unless there is evidence of site-specific infection. Continuing empirical antibiotic therapy in response to laboratory test abnormalities alone is rarely justified, particularly among well-appearing term infants.

PREVENTION STRATEGIES

The only proven preventive strategy for EOS is the appropriate administration of maternal IAP. Recommendations from national professional organizations should be followed for the administration of GBS intrapartum prophylaxis as well as for the administration of intrapartum antibiotic therapy when there is suspected or confirmed intraamniotic infection. Neonatal practices are focused on the identification and empirical antibiotic treatment of newborn infants who are at risk for EOS; these practices cannot prevent EOS. The empirical administration of intramuscular penicillin to all newborn infants to prevent neonatal GBS-specific EOS is not justified and is not endorsed by the American Academy of Pediatrics. Neither GBS IAP nor any neonatal EOS practice will prevent late-onset GBS infection[3,82,83] or any other form of late-onset bacterial infection.

SUMMARY POINTS

We include the following summary points:

1. The epidemiology of EOS differs substantially between term and/or late-preterm infants and very preterm infants.

2. Infants born at ≥35 0/7 weeks' gestation can be stratified by the level of risk for EOS. Acceptable approaches to risk stratification include the following:

o categorical algorithms in which threshold values for intrapartum risk factors are used;

o multivariate risk assessment based on both intrapartum risk factors and infant examinations. The Neonatal Early-Onset Sepsis Risk Calculator[47] is an example of this approach; and

o serial physical examination to detect the presence of clinical signs of illness after birth. This approach may begin with a categorical or multivariate assessment to identify newborn infants who are at risk and will be subjected to serial monitoring, or this may be applied to all newborn infants.

3. Birth centers should consider the development of locally tailored, documented guidelines for EOS risk assessment and clinical management. Ongoing surveillance once guidelines are implemented is recommended.

4. The diagnosis of EOS is made by using blood or CSF cultures. EOS cannot be diagnosed by using laboratory tests, such as a complete blood cell count or CRP or by using surface cultures, gastric aspirate analysis, or urine culture.

5. The combination of ampicillin and gentamicin is the appropriate empirical antibiotic regimen for most infants who are at risk for EOS. The empirical administration of additional broad-spectrum agents may be indicated in term infants who are critically ill until appropriate culture results are known.

6. When blood cultures are sterile, antibiotic therapy should be discontinued by 36 to 48 hours of incubation unless there is clear evidence of site-specific infection.

LEAD AUTHORS

Karen M. Puopolo, MD, PhD, FAAP
William E. Benitz, MD, FAAP
Theoklis E. Zaoutis, MD, MSCE, FAAP

COMMITTEE ON FETUS AND NEWBORN, 2017–2018

James Cummings, MD, Chairperson
Sandra Juul, MD
Ivan Hand, MD
Eric Eichenwald, MD
Brenda Poindexter, MD
Dan L. Stewart, MD
Susan W. Aucott, MD
Karen M. Puopolo, MD
Jay P. Goldsmith, MD
Kristi Watterberg, MD, Immediate Past Chairperson

LIAISONS

Kasper S. Wang, MD – *American Academy of Pediatrics Section on Surgery*
Thierry Lacaze, MD – *Canadian Paediatric Society*
Joseph Wax, MD – *American College of Obstetricians and Gynecologists*
Tonse N.K. Raju, MD, DCH – *National Institutes of Health*
Wanda Barfield, MD, MPH, CAPT USPHS – *Centers for Disease Control and Prevention*
Erin Keels, MS, APRN, NNP-BC – *National Association of Neonatal Nurses*

STAFF

Jim Couto, MA

COMMITTEE ON INFECTIOUS DISEASES, 2017–2018

Carrie L. Byington, MD, FAAP, Chairperson
Yvonne A. Maldonado, MD, FAAP, Vice Chairperson
Ritu Banerjee, MD, PhD, FAAP
Elizabeth D. Barnett, MD, FAAP
James D. Campbell, MD, MS, FAAP
Jeffrey S. Gerber, MD, PhD, FAAP
Ruth Lynfield, MD, FAAP
Flor M. Munoz, MD, MSc, FAAP
Dawn Nolt, MD, MPH, FAAP
Ann-Christine Nyquist, MD, MSPH, FAAP
Sean T. O'Leary, MD, MPH, FAAP
Mobeen H. Rathore, MD, FAAP
Mark H. Sawyer, MD, FAAP
William J. Steinbach, MD, FAAP
Tina Q. Tan, MD, FAAP
Theoklis E. Zaoutis, MD, MSCE, FAAP

EX OFFICIO

David W. Kimberlin, MD, FAAP – *Red Book* Editor

Michael T. Brady, MD, FAAP – *Red Book* Associate Editor
Mary Anne Jackson, MD, FAAP – *Red Book* Associate Editor
Sarah S. Long, MD, FAAP – *Red Book* Associate Editor
Henry H. Bernstein, DO, MHCM, FAAP – *Red Book* Online Associate Editor
H. Cody Meissner, MD, FAAP – Visual *Red Book* Associate Editor

LIAISONS

Amanda C. Cohn, MD, FAAP – *Centers for Disease Control and Prevention*
Jamie Deseda-Tous, MD – *Sociedad Latinoamericana de Infectologia Pediatrica*
Karen M. Farizo, MD – *United States Food and Drug Administration*
Marc Fischer, MD, FAAP – *Centers for Disease Control and Prevention*
Natasha Halasa, MD, MPH, FAAP – *Pediatric Infectious Diseases Society*
Nicole Le Saux, MD – *Canadian Paediatric Society*
Scot Moore, MD, FAAP – *Committee on Practice Ambulatory Medicine*
Angela K. Shen, ScD, MPH – *National Vaccine Program Office*
Neil S. Silverman, MD – *American College of Obstetricians and Gynecologists*
James J. Stevermer, MD, MSPH, FAAFP – *American Academy of Family Physicians*
Jeffrey R. Starke, MD, FAAP – *American Thoracic Society*
Kay M. Tomashek, MD, MPH, DTM – *National Institutes of Health*

STAFF

Jennifer M. Frantz, MPH

ABBREVIATIONS

ACOG: American College of Obstetricians and Gynecologists
ANC: absolute neutrophil count
CDC: Centers for Disease Control and Prevention
CRP: C-reactive protein
CSF: cerebrospinal fluid
EOS: early-onset sepsis
GBS: group B *Streptococcus*
IAP: intrapartum antibiotic prophylaxis
IL: interleukin
I/T: immature/total neutrophil ratio
ROM: rupture of membranes
WBC: white blood cell

FINANCIAL DISCLOSURE: The authors have indicated they have no financial relationships relevant to this article to disclose.

FUNDING: No external funding.

POTENTIAL CONFLICT OF INTEREST: The authors have indicated they have no potential conflicts of interest to disclose.

COMPANION PAPER: A companion to this article can be found online at www.pediatrics.org/cgi/doi/10.1542/peds.2018-2896.

REFERENCES

1. Mukhopadhyay S, Taylor JA, Von Kohorn I, et al. Variation in sepsis evaluation across a national network of nurseries. *Pediatrics.* 2017;139(3):e20162845

2. Verani JR, McGee L, Schrag SJ; Division of Bacterial Diseases, National Center for Immunization and Respiratory Diseases, Centers for Disease Control and Prevention (CDC). Prevention of perinatal group B streptococcal disease–revised guidelines from CDC, 2010. *MMWR Recomm Rep.* 2010;59(RR-10):1–36

3. Schuchat A, Zywicki SS, Dinsmoor MJ, et al. Risk factors and opportunities for prevention of early-onset neonatal sepsis: a multicenter case-control study. *Pediatrics.* 2000;105(1, pt 1):21–26

4. Schrag SJ, Farley MM, Petit S, et al. Epidemiology of invasive early-onset neonatal sepsis, 2005 to 2014. *Pediatrics.* 2016;138(6):e20162013

5. Weston EJ, Pondo T, Lewis MM, et al. The burden of invasive early-onset neonatal sepsis in the United States, 2005-2008. *Pediatr Infect Dis J.* 2011;30(11):937–941

6. Stoll BJ, Hansen NI, Bell EF, et al; Eunice Kennedy Shriver National Institute of Child Health and Human Development Neonatal Research Network. Trends in care practices, morbidity, and mortality of extremely preterm neonates, 1993-2012. *JAMA.* 2015;314(10):1039–1051

7. Puopolo KM, Draper D, Wi S, et al. Estimating the probability of neonatal early-onset infection on the basis of maternal risk factors. *Pediatrics.* 2011;128(5). Available at: www.pediatrics.org/cgi/content/full/128/5/e1155

8. Stoll BJ, Hansen NI, Sánchez PJ, et al; Eunice Kennedy Shriver National Institute of Child Health and Human Development Neonatal Research Network. Early onset neonatal sepsis: the burden of group B Streptococcal and *E. coli* disease continues. *Pediatrics.* 2011;127(5):817–826

9. Benirschke K. Routes and types of infection in the fetus and the newborn. *AMA J Dis Child.* 1960;99(6):714–721

10. Blanc WA. Pathways of fetal and early neonatal infection. Viral placentitis, bacterial and fungal chorioamnionitis. *J Pediatr.* 1961;59(4):473–496

11. Goldenberg RL, McClure EM, Saleem S, Reddy UM. Infection-related stillbirths. *Lancet.* 2010;375(9724):1482–1490

12. Gibbs RS, Roberts DJ. Case records of the Massachusetts General Hospital. Case 27-2007. A 30-year-old pregnant woman with intrauterine fetal death. *N Engl J Med.* 2007;357(9):918–925

13. Lamont RF, Sobel J, Mazaki-Tovi S, et al. Listeriosis in human pregnancy: a systematic review. *J Perinat Med.* 2011;39(3):227–236

14. Escobar GJ, Li DK, Armstrong MA, et al. Neonatal sepsis workups in infants >/=2000 grams at birth: a population-based study. *Pediatrics.* 2000;106(2, pt 1):256–263

15. Benitz WE, Gould JB, Druzin ML. Risk factors for early-onset group B streptococcal sepsis: estimation of odds ratios by critical literature review. *Pediatrics.* 1999;103(6). Available at: www.pediatrics.org/cgi/content/full/103/6/e77

16. Mukhopadhyay S, Puopolo KM. Risk assessment in neonatal early onset sepsis. *Semin Perinatol.* 2012;36(6):408–415

17. Jackson GL, Engle WD, Sendelbach DM, et al. Are complete blood cell counts useful in the evaluation of asymptomatic neonates exposed to suspected chorioamnionitis? *Pediatrics.* 2004;113(5):1173–1180

18. Jackson GL, Rawiki P, Sendelbach D, Manning MD, Engle WD. Hospital course and short-term outcomes of term and late preterm neonates following exposure to prolonged rupture of membranes and/or chorioamnionitis. *Pediatr Infect Dis J.* 2012;31(1):89–90

19. Kiser C, Nawab U, McKenna K, Aghai ZH. Role of guidelines on length of therapy in chorioamnionitis and neonatal sepsis. *Pediatrics.* 2014;133(6):992–998

20. Wortham JM, Hansen NI, Schrag SJ, et al; Eunice Kennedy Shriver NICHD Neonatal Research Network. Chorioamnionitis and culture-confirmed, early-onset neonatal infections. *Pediatrics.* 2016;137(1):e20152316

21. Heine RP, Puopolo KM, Beigi R, Silverman NS, El-Sayed YY; Committee on Obstetric Practice. Committee opinion no. 712: intrapartum management of intraamniotic infection. *Obstet Gynecol.* 2017;130(2):e95–e101

22. Higgins RD, Saade G, Polin RA, et al; Chorioamnionitis Workshop Participants. Evaluation and management of women and newborns with a maternal diagnosis of chorioamnionitis: summary of a workshop. *Obstet Gynecol.* 2016;127(3):426–436

23. Van Dyke MK, Phares CR, Lynfield R, et al. Evaluation of universal antenatal screening for group B *streptococcus.* *N Engl J Med.* 2009;360(25):2626–2636

24. Persaud RR, Azad MB, Chari RS, Sears MR, Becker AB, Kozyrskyj AL; CHILD Study Investigators. Perinatal antibiotic exposure of neonates in Canada and associated risk factors: a population-based study. *J Matern Fetal Neonatal Med.* 2015;28(10):1190–1195

25. Stokholm J, Schjørring S, Pedersen L, et al. Prevalence and predictors of antibiotic administration during

pregnancy and birth. *PLoS One.* 2013;8(12):e82932

26. Ajslev TA, Andersen CS, Gamborg M, Sørensen TI, Jess T. Childhood overweight after establishment of the gut microbiota: the role of delivery mode, pre-pregnancy weight and early administration of antibiotics. *Int J Obes.* 2011;35(4):522–529

27. Alm B, Erdes L, Möllborg P, et al. Neonatal antibiotic treatment is a risk factor for early wheezing. *Pediatrics.* 2008;121(4):697–702

28. Alm B, Goksör E, Pettersson R, et al. Antibiotics in the first week of life is a risk factor for allergic rhinitis at school age. *Pediatr Allergy Immunol.* 2014;25(5):468–472

29. Risnes KR, Belanger K, Murk W, Bracken MB. Antibiotic exposure by 6 months and asthma and allergy at 6 years: findings in a cohort of 1, 401 US children. *Am J Epidemiol.* 2011;173(3):310–318

30. Russell SL, Gold MJ, Hartmann M, et al. Early life antibiotic-driven changes in microbiota enhance susceptibility to allergic asthma. *EMBO Rep.* 2012;13(5):440–447

31. Saari A, Virta LJ, Sankilampi U, Dunkel L, Saxen H. Antibiotic exposure in infancy and risk of being overweight in the first 24 months of life. *Pediatrics.* 2015;135(4):617–626

32. Trasande L, Blustein J, Liu M, Corwin E, Cox LM, Blaser MJ. Infant antibiotic exposures and early-life body mass. *Int J Obes.* 2013;37(1):16–23

33. Greenwood C, Morrow AL, Lagomarcino AJ, et al. Early empiric antibiotic use in preterm infants is associated with lower bacterial diversity and higher relative abundance of *Enterobacter.* *J Pediatr.* 2014;165(1):23–29

34. Corvaglia L, Tonti G, Martini S, et al. Influence of intrapartum antibiotic prophylaxis for group B *Streptococcus* on gut microbiota in the first month of life. *J Pediatr Gastroenterol Nutr.* 2016;62(2):304–308

35. Azad MB, Konya T, Persaud RR, et al; CHILD Study Investigators. Impact of maternal intrapartum antibiotics, method of birth and breastfeeding on gut microbiota during the first year of life: a prospective cohort study. *BJOG.* 2016;123(6):983–993

36. Mukhopadhyay S, Lieberman ES, Puopolo KM, Riley LE, Johnson LC. Effect of early-onset sepsis evaluations on in-hospital breastfeeding practices among asymptomatic term neonates. *Hosp Pediatr.* 2015;5(4):203–210

37. Centers for Disease Control and Prevention. Prevention of perinatal group B streptococcal disease: a public health perspective. Centers for Disease Control and Prevention [published correction appears in *MMWR Morb Mortal Wkly Rep.* 1996;45(31):679]. *MMWR Recomm Rep.* 1996;45(RR-7):1–24

38. Schrag S, Gorwitz R, Fultz-Butts K, Schuchat A. Prevention of perinatal group B streptococcal disease. Revised guidelines from CDC. *MMWR Recomm Rep.* 2002;51(RR-11):1–22

39. Schrag SJ, Zywicki S, Farley MM, et al. Group B streptococcal disease in the era of intrapartum antibiotic prophylaxis. *N Engl J Med.* 2000;342(1):15–20

40. Schrag SJ, Zell ER, Lynfield R, et al; Active Bacterial Core Surveillance Team. A population-based comparison of strategies to prevent early-onset group B streptococcal disease in neonates. *N Engl J Med.* 2002;347(4):233–239

41. Puopolo KM, Escobar GJ. Early-onset sepsis: a predictive model based on maternal risk factors. *Curr Opin Pediatr.* 2013;25(2):161–166

42. Cantoni L, Ronfani L, Da Riol R, Demarini S; Perinatal Study Group of the Region Friuli-Venezia Giulia. Physical examination instead of laboratory tests for most infants born to mothers colonized with group B *Streptococcus*: support for the Centers for Disease Control and Prevention's 2010 recommendations. *J Pediatr.* 2013;163(2):568–573

43. Mukhopadhyay S, Dukhovny D, Mao W, Eichenwald EC, Puopolo KM. 2010 perinatal GBS prevention guideline and resource utilization. *Pediatrics.* 2014;133(2):196–203

44. Kuzniewicz MW, Puopolo KM, Fischer A, et al. A quantitative, risk-based approach to the management of neonatal early-onset sepsis. *JAMA Pediatr.* 2017;171(4):365–371

45. Mukhopadhyay S, Eichenwald EC, Puopolo KM. Neonatal early-onset sepsis evaluations among well-appearing infants: projected impact of changes in CDC GBS guidelines. *J Perinatol.* 2013;33(3):198–205

46. Escobar GJ, Puopolo KM, Wi S, et al. Stratification of risk of early-onset sepsis in newborns ≥ 34 weeks' gestation. *Pediatrics.* 2014;133(1):30–36

47. Northern California Kaiser-Permanente. Neonatal Early-Onset Sepsis Calculator. Available at: https://neonatalsepsiscal culator.kaiserpermanente.org. Accessed April 5, 2018

48. Dhudasia MB, Mukhopadhyay S, Puopolo KM. Implementation of the sepsis risk calculator at an academic birth hospital. *Hosp Pediatr.* 2018;8(5):243–250

49. Ottolini MC, Lundgren K, Mirkinson LJ, Cason S, Ottolini MG. Utility of complete blood count and blood culture screening to diagnose neonatal sepsis in the asymptomatic at risk newborn. *Pediatr Infect Dis J.* 2003;22(5):430–434

50. Flidel-Rimon O, Galstyan S, Juster-Reicher A, Rozin I, Shinwell ES. Limitations of the risk factor based approach in early neonatal sepsis evaluations. *Acta Paediatr.* 2012;101(12):e540–e544

51. Hashavya S, Benenson S, Ergaz-Shaltiel Z, Bar-Oz B, Averbuch D, Eventov-Friedman S. The use of blood counts and blood cultures to screen neonates born to partially treated group B *Streptococcus*-carrier mothers for early-onset sepsis: is it justified? *Pediatr Infect Dis J.* 2011;30(10):840–843

52. Berardi A, Fornaciari S, Rossi C, et al. Safety of physical examination alone for managing well-appearing neonates ≥ 35 weeks' gestation at risk for early-onset sepsis. *J Matern Fetal Neonatal Med.* 2015;28(10):1123–1127

53. Joshi NS, Gupta A, Allan JM, et al. Clinical monitoring of well-appearing infants born to mothers with chorioamnionitis. *Pediatrics.* 2018;141(4):e20172056

54. Wynn JL, Wong HR, Shanley TP, Bizzarro MJ, Saiman L, Polin RA. Time for a neonatal-specific consensus definition

for sepsis. *Pediatr Crit Care Med.* 2014;15(6):523–528

55. Dunne WM Jr, Case LK, Isgriggs L, Lublin DM. In-house validation of the BACTEC 9240 blood culture system for detection of bacterial contamination in platelet concentrates. *Transfusion.* 2005;45(7):1138–1142

56. Flayhart D, Borek AP, Wakefield T, Dick J, Carroll KC. Comparison of BACTEC PLUS blood culture media to BacT/Alert FA blood culture media for detection of bacterial pathogens in samples containing therapeutic levels of antibiotics. *J Clin Microbiol.* 2007;45(3):816–821

57. Jorgensen JH, Mirrett S, McDonald LC, et al. Controlled clinical laboratory comparison of BACTEC plus aerobic/F resin medium with BacT/Alert aerobic FAN medium for detection of bacteremia and fungemia. *J Clin Microbiol.* 1997;35(1):53–58

58. Krisher KK, Gibb P, Corbett S, Church D. Comparison of the BacT/Alert PF pediatric FAN blood culture bottle with the standard pediatric blood culture bottle, the Pedi-BacT. *J Clin Microbiol.* 2001;39(8):2880–2883

59. Nanua S, Weber C, Isgriggs L, Dunne WM Jr. Performance evaluation of the VersaTREK blood culture system for quality control testing of platelet units. *J Clin Microbiol.* 2009;47(3):817–818

60. Garcia-Prats JA, Cooper TR, Schneider VF, Stager CE, Hansen TN. Rapid detection of microorganisms in blood cultures of newborn infants utilizing an automated blood culture system. *Pediatrics.* 2000;105(3, pt 1):523–527

61. Sarkar SS, Bhagat I, Bhatt-Mehta V, Sarkar S. Does maternal intrapartum antibiotic treatment prolong the incubation time required for blood cultures to become positive for infants with early-onset sepsis? *Am J Perinatol.* 2015;32(4):357–362

62. Guerti K, Devos H, Ieven MM, Mahieu LM. Time to positivity of neonatal blood cultures: fast and furious? *J Med Microbiol.* 2011;60(pt 4):446–453

63. Jardine L, Davies MW, Faoagali J. Incubation time required for neonatal blood cultures to become positive. *J Paediatr Child Health.* 2006;42(12):797–802

64. Schelonka RL, Chai MK, Yoder BA, Hensley D, Brockett RM, Ascher DP. Volume of blood required to detect common neonatal pathogens. *J Pediatr.* 1996;129(2):275–278

65. Yaacobi N, Bar-Meir M, Shchors I, Bromiker R. A prospective controlled trial of the optimal volume for neonatal blood cultures. *Pediatr Infect Dis J.* 2015;34(4):351–354

66. Sarkar S, Bhagat I, DeCristofaro JD, Wiswell TE, Spitzer AR. A study of the role of multiple site blood cultures in the evaluation of neonatal sepsis. *J Perinatol.* 2006;26(1):18–22

67. Struthers S, Underhill H, Albersheim S, Greenberg D, Dobson S. A comparison of two versus one blood culture in the diagnosis and treatment of coagulase-negative *staphylococcus* in the neonatal intensive care unit. *J Perinatol.* 2002;22(7):547–549

68. Mukhopadhyay S, Puopolo KM. Clinical and microbiologic characteristics of early-onset sepsis among very low birth weight infants: opportunities for antibiotic stewardship. *Pediatr Infect Dis J.* 2017;36(5):477–481

69. Garges HP, Moody MA, Cotten CM, et al. Neonatal meningitis: what is the correlation among cerebrospinal fluid cultures, blood cultures, and cerebrospinal fluid parameters? *Pediatrics.* 2006;117(4):1094–1100

70. Greenberg RG, Smith PB, Cotten CM, Moody MA, Clark RH, Benjamin DK Jr. Traumatic lumbar punctures in neonates: test performance of the cerebrospinal fluid white blood cell count. *Pediatr Infect Dis J.* 2008;27(12):1047–1051

71. Christensen RD, Henry E, Jopling J, Wiedmeier SE. The CBC: reference ranges for neonates. *Semin Perinatol.* 2009;33(1):3–11

72. Manroe BL, Weinberg AG, Rosenfeld CR, Browne R. The neonatal blood count in health and disease. I. Reference values for neutrophilic cells. *J Pediatr.* 1979;95(1):89–98

73. Newman TB, Puopolo KM, Wi S, Draper D, Escobar GJ. Interpreting complete blood counts soon after birth in newborns at risk for sepsis. *Pediatrics.* 2010;126(5):903–909

74. Schmutz N, Henry E, Jopling J, Christensen RD. Expected ranges for blood neutrophil concentrations of neonates: the Manroe and Mouzinho charts revisited. *J Perinatol.* 2008;28(4):275–281

75. Hornik CP, Benjamin DK, Becker KC, et al. Use of the complete blood cell count in early-onset neonatal sepsis. *Pediatr Infect Dis J.* 2012;31(8):799–802

76. Newman TB, Draper D, Puopolo KM, Wi S, Escobar GJ. Combining immature and total neutrophil counts to predict early onset sepsis in term and late preterm newborns: use of the I/T². *Pediatr Infect Dis J.* 2014;33(8):798–802

77. Benitz WE. Adjunct laboratory tests in the diagnosis of early-onset neonatal sepsis. *Clin Perinatol.* 2010;37(2):421–438

78. Lynema S, Marmer D, Hall ES, Meinzen-Derr J, Kingma PS. Neutrophil CD64 as a diagnostic marker of sepsis: impact on neonatal care. *Am J Perinatol.* 2015;32(4):331–336

79. Su H, Chang SS, Han CM, et al. Inflammatory markers in cord blood or maternal serum for early detection of neonatal sepsis-a systemic review and meta-analysis. *J Perinatol.* 2014;34(4):268–274

80. Chiesa C, Panero A, Rossi N, et al. Reliability of procalcitonin concentrations for the diagnosis of sepsis in critically ill neonates. *Clin Infect Dis.* 1998;26(3):664–672

81. Clark RH, Bloom BT, Spitzer AR, Gerstmann DR. Empiric use of ampicillin and cefotaxime, compared with ampicillin and gentamicin, for neonates at risk for sepsis is associated with an increased risk of neonatal death. *Pediatrics.* 2006;117(1):67–74

82. Jordan HT, Farley MM, Craig A, et al; Active Bacterial Core Surveillance (ABCs), Emerging Infections Program Network, CDC. Revisiting the need for vaccine prevention of late-onset neonatal group B streptococcal disease: a multistate, population-based analysis. *Pediatr Infect Dis J.* 2008;27(12):1057–1064

83. Phares CR, Lynfield R, Farley MM, et al; Active Bacterial Core Surveillance/ Emerging Infections Program Network. Epidemiology of invasive group B streptococcal disease in the United States, 1999-2005. *JAMA.* 2008;299(17):2056–2065

CLINICAL REPORT Guidance for the Clinician in Rendering Pediatric Care

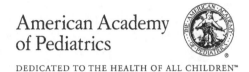

DEDICATED TO THE HEALTH OF ALL CHILDREN™

Management of Neonates Born at ≤34 6/7 Weeks' Gestation With Suspected or Proven Early-Onset Bacterial Sepsis

Karen M. Puopolo, MD, PhD, FAAP,[a,b] William E. Benitz, MD, FAAP,[c] Theoklis E. Zaoutis, MD, MSCE, FAAP,[a,d]
COMMITTEE ON FETUS AND NEWBORN, COMMITTEE ON INFECTIOUS DISEASES

abstract

Early-onset sepsis (EOS) remains a serious and often fatal illness among infants born preterm, particularly among newborn infants of the lowest gestational age. Currently, most preterm infants with very low birth weight are treated empirically with antibiotics for risk of EOS, often for prolonged periods, in the absence of a culture-confirmed infection. Retrospective studies have revealed that antibiotic exposures after birth are associated with multiple subsequent poor outcomes among preterm infants, making the risk/benefit balance of these antibiotic treatments uncertain. Gestational age is the strongest single predictor of EOS, and the majority of preterm births occur in the setting of other factors associated with risk of EOS, making it difficult to apply risk stratification strategies to preterm infants. Laboratory tests alone have a poor predictive value in preterm EOS. Delivery characteristics of extremely preterm infants present an opportunity to identify those with a lower risk of EOS and may inform decisions to initiate or extend antibiotic therapies. Our purpose for this clinical report is to provide a summary of the current epidemiology of preterm neonatal sepsis and provide guidance for the development of evidence-based approaches to sepsis risk assessment among preterm newborn infants.

[a]Department of Pediatrics, Perelman School of Medicine, University of Pennsylvania, Philadelphia, Pennsylvania; [b]Children's Hospital of Philadelphia, and [d]Roberts Center for Pediatric Research, Philadelphia, Pennsylvania; and [c]Division of Neonatal and Developmental Medicine, Department of Pediatrics, School of Medicine, Stanford University, Palo Alto, California

DOI: https://doi.org/10.1542/peds.2018-2896

Address correspondence to Karen M. Puopolo, MD, PhD, FAAP. E-mail: puopolok@email.chop.edu

PEDIATRICS (ISSN Numbers: Print, 0031-4005; Online, 1098-4275).

To cite: Puopolo KM, Benitz WE, Zaoutis TE, AAP COMMITTEE ON FETUS AND NEWBORN, AAP COMMITTEE ON INFECTIOUS DISEASES. Management of Neonates Born at ≤34 6/7 Weeks' Gestation With Suspected or Proven Early-Onset Bacterial Sepsis. *Pediatrics.* 2018;142(6):e20182896

Antibiotics are administered shortly after birth to nearly all preterm infants with very low birth weight (VLBW) (birth weight <1500 g) because of the risk of early-onset sepsis (EOS).[1–4] Physicians are often reluctant to discontinue antibiotics once initiated for many reasons, including the relatively high risk of EOS among preterm infants and the relatively high rate of mortality attributable to infection. Particularly among infants with VLBW, neonatal clinicians must determine which infants are most likely to have EOS when nearly all have some degree of respiratory or systemic instability. Poor predictive performance of common laboratory tests and concerns regarding the unreliability of blood cultures add to the difficulty in discriminating at-risk infants. Because gestational age is the strongest predictor of EOS and approximately two-thirds of preterm births are associated with preterm labor, premature rupture of membranes (PROM), or clinical chorioamnionitis,[5] risk stratification strategies cannot be applied to preterm newborn infants in the same manner as for term neonates.

PATHOGENESIS AND CURRENT EPIDEMIOLOGY OF PRETERM NEONATAL EOS

Preterm EOS is defined as a blood or cerebrospinal fluid (CSF) culture obtained within 72 hours after birth that is growing a pathogenic bacterial species. This microbiological definition stands in contrast to the functional definitions of sepsis used in pediatric and adult patients, for whom the definition is used to specify a series of time-sensitive interventions. The current overall incidence of EOS in the United States is approximately 0.8 cases per 1000 live births.[6] A disproportionate number of cases occur among infants born preterm in a manner that is inversely proportional to gestational age at birth. The incidence of EOS is approximately 0.5 cases per 1000 infants born at ≥37 weeks' gestation, compared with approximately 1 case per 1000 infants born at 34 to 36 weeks' gestation, 6 cases per 1000 infants born at <34 weeks' gestation, 20 cases per 1000 infants born at <29 weeks' gestation, and 32 cases per 1000 infants born at 22 to 24 weeks' gestation.[6–10] The incidence of EOS has declined among term infants over the past 25 years, a change attributed to the implementation of evidence-based intrapartum antimicrobial therapy. The impact of such therapies on preterm infants is less clear. Authors of the most recent studies report an EOS incidence among infants with VLBW ranging from 9 to 11 cases per 1000 infants with VLBW,

whereas studies from the early 1990s revealed rates of 19 to 32 per 1000 infants.[10,11] Improvements among VLBW incidence may be limited to those born at older gestational ages. No significant change over time was observed in a study of 34 636 infants born from 1993 to 2012 at 22 to 28 weeks' gestation, with the reported incidence ranging from 20.5 to 24.4 per 1000 infants.[8] Morbidity and mortality from EOS remain substantial: 95% of preterm infants with EOS require neonatal intensive care for respiratory distress and/or blood pressure support, and 75% of deaths from EOS occur among infants with VLBW.[6,10] The mortality rate among those with EOS is an order of magnitude higher among preterm compared with term infants, whether measured by gestational age (1.6% at ≥37 weeks, 30% at 25–28 weeks, and approximately 50% at 22–24 weeks)[7,8,10] or birth weight (3.5% among those born at ≥1500 g vs 35% for those born at <1500 g).[6]

The pathogenesis of preterm EOS is complex. EOS primarily begins in utero and was originally described as the "amniotic infection syndrome."[12,13] Among term infants, EOS pathogenesis most commonly develops during labor and involves ascending colonization and infection of the uterine compartment with maternal gastrointestinal and genitourinary flora, with subsequent colonization and invasive infection of the fetus and/or fetal aspiration of infected amniotic fluid. This intrapartum sequence may be responsible for EOS that develops after PROM or during preterm labor that is induced for maternal indications. However, the pathogenesis of preterm EOS likely begins before the onset of labor in many cases of preterm labor and/or PROM. Intraamniotic infection (IAI) may cause stillbirth in the second and third trimesters.[14] In approximately 25% of cases, IAI is the cause of preterm labor and PROM, particularly

when these occur at the lowest gestational ages; evidence suggests that microbial-induced maternal inflammation can initiate parturition and elicit fetal inflammatory responses.[5,15–18] Organisms isolated from the intrauterine compartment of women with preterm labor, PROM, or both are primarily vaginal in origin and include low-virulence species, such as *Ureaplasma*, as well as anaerobic species and well-recognized neonatal pathogens, such as *Escherichia coli* and group B *Streptococcus* (GBS).[16–18] The isolation of maternal oral flora and, more rarely, *Listeria monocytogenes*, suggests a transplacental pathway for some IAIs.[16,18–20] Inflammation inciting parturition may not, however, always be attributable to IAI. Inflammation resulting from immune-mediated rejection of the fetal or placental compartment (from maternal extrauterine infection), as well as that incited by reproductive or nonreproductive microbiota, may all contribute to the pathogenesis of preterm labor and PROM, complicating the interpretation of placental pathology.[15,20]

RISK FACTORS FOR PRETERM EOS

Multiple clinical risk factors have been used to assess the risk of EOS among infants born at ≤34 6/7 weeks' gestation. Univariate analyses of risk factors for EOS among preterm infants have been used to identify gestational age, birth weight, PROM and prolonged rupture of membranes (ROM), preterm onset of labor, maternal age and race, maternal intrapartum fever, mode of delivery, and administration of intrapartum antibiotics to be associated with risk of EOS; however, the independent contribution of any specific factor other than gestational age has been difficult to quantify. For example, among term infants, there is a linear relationship between the duration of ROM and the risk of EOS.[9]

In contrast, the relationship between PROM and the risk of EOS is not simply described by its occurrence or duration but modified by gestational age as well as by the additional presence of clinical chorioamnionitis and the administration of latency and intrapartum antibiotics.[17,21–24] These observations are likely related to uncertainty regarding the role of intrauterine infection and cervical structural defects in the pathogenesis of spontaneous PROM.[24,25]

The clinical diagnosis of chorioamnionitis has been used as a primary risk factor for identifying infants at risk for EOS. Most preterm infants with EOS are born to women with this clinical diagnosis.[4,26–29] The American College of Obstetricians and Gynecologists (ACOG) recently advocated for using the term "intraamniotic infection" rather than chorioamnionitis (which is primarily a histologic diagnosis) and published guidance for its diagnosis and management.[30] A confirmed diagnosis of IAI is made by a positive result on an amniotic fluid Gram-stain, culture, or placental histopathology. Suspected IAI is diagnosed by maternal intrapartum fever (either a single documented maternal intrapartum temperature of ≥39.0°C or a temperature of 38.0–38.9°C that persists for >30 minutes) and 1 or more of the following: (1) maternal leukocytosis, (2) purulent cervical drainage, and (3) fetal tachycardia. The ACOG recommends that intrapartum antibiotics be administered whenever IAI is diagnosed or suspected and when otherwise unexplained maternal fever occurs during labor. Chorioamnionitis or IAI is strongly associated with EOS in preterm infants, with a number needed to treat of only 6 to 40 infants per case of confirmed EOS.[4,26–29] Conversely, the absence of clinical and histologic chorioamnionitis may be used to identify a group of preterm infants who are at a lower

risk for EOS. In a study of 15 318 infants born at 22 to 28 weeks' gestation, those born by cesarean delivery with membrane rupture at delivery and without clinical chorioamnionitis were significantly less likely to have EOS or die before 12 hours of age.[4] The number needed to treat for infants born in these circumstances was approximately 200; with the additional absence of histologic chorioamnionitis, the number needed to treat is approximately 380.[4] Another study of 109 cases of EOS occurring among 5313 infants with VLBW over a 25-year period revealed that 97% of cases occurred in infants born with some combination of PROM, preterm labor, or concern for IAI.[29] In that report, 2 cases of listeriosis occurred in the context of unexplained fetal distress in otherwise uncomplicated pregnancies.

ANTIBIOTIC STEWARDSHIP IN PRETERM EOS MANAGEMENT

Currently, most premature infants with VLBW are treated empirically with antibiotics for risk of EOS, often for prolonged periods, even in the absence of a culture-confirmed infection. Prolonged empirical antibiotics are administered to approximately 35% to 50% of infants with a low gestational age, with significant center-specific variation.[1–4] Antibiotic drugs are administered for many reasons, including the relatively high incidence of EOS among preterm infants, the relatively high rate of mortality attributable to infection, and the frequency of clinical instability after birth. Empirical antibiotics administered to very preterm infants in the first days after birth have been associated with an increased risk of subsequent poor outcomes.[1,4,31–33] One multicenter study of 4039 infants born from 1998 to 2001 with a birth weight of <1000 g revealed that those infants who died or had a diagnosis of necrotizing

enterocolitis (NEC) before hospital discharge were significantly more likely to have received prolonged empirical antibiotic therapy in the first week after birth.[1] The authors of the study estimated that the risk of NEC increased by 7% for each additional day of antibiotics administered in the absence of culture-confirmed EOS. Authors of a single-center study of infants with VLBW estimated that the risk of NEC increased by 20% for each additional day of antibiotics administered in the absence of a culture-confirmed infection.[31] Authors of another study of 11 669 infants with VLBW assessed the overall rate of antibiotic use and found that higher rates during the first week after birth or during the entire hospitalization were both associated with increased mortality, even when adjusted for multiple predictors of neonatal morbidity and mortality.[33] One concern in each of these studies is that some infants categorized as uninfected may in fact have suffered from EOS. Yet, even among 5640 infants born at 22 to 28 weeks' gestation at a lower risk for EOS, those who received prolonged empirical antibiotic therapy during the first week after birth had higher rates of death and bronchopulmonary dysplasia.[4] Several explanations are possible for all of these findings, including simply that physicians administer the most antibiotics to the sickest infants. Other potential mechanisms include the role of antibiotics in promoting dysbiosis of the gut, skin, and respiratory tract, affecting the interactions between colonizing flora in maintaining health and promoting immunity; it is also possible that antibiotics and dysbiosis function as modulators of vascular development.[34,35] Although the full relationship between early neonatal antibiotic exposures and subsequent childhood health remains to be defined, current evidence suggests that such exposures do affect preterm infants. Physicians should consider the risk/benefit balance of initiating antibiotic therapy for risk of EOS as well as for continuing empirical antibiotic therapy in the absence of a culture-confirmed infection.

RISK CATEGORIZATION FOR PRETERM INFANTS

Perhaps the greatest contributor to the nearly universal practice of empirical antibiotic administration to preterm infants is the uncertainty in EOS risk assessment. Because gestational age is the strongest predictor of EOS, and two-thirds of preterm births are associated with preterm labor, PROM, or clinical concern for intrauterine infection,[5] risk stratification strategies cannot be applied to preterm infants in the same manner as for term neonates. In particular, the Neonatal Early-Onset Sepsis Risk Calculator does not apply to infants born before 34 0/7 weeks' gestation.[36] The objective of EOS risk assessment among preterm infants is, therefore, to determine which infants are at the lowest risk for infection and who, despite clinical instability, may be spared administration of empirical antibiotics. The circumstances of preterm birth may provide the best current approach to EOS management for preterm infants.

Preterm Infants at Lower Risk for EOS

Criteria for preterm infants to be considered at a lower risk for EOS include the following: (1) obstetric indications for preterm birth (such as maternal preeclampsia or other noninfectious medical illness or placental insufficiency), (2) birth by cesarean delivery, and (3) absence of labor, attempts to induce labor, or any ROM before delivery. Acceptable initial approaches to these infants might include (1) no laboratory evaluation and no empirical antibiotic therapy, or (2) a blood culture and clinical monitoring. For infants who do not improve after initial stabilization and/or those

who have severe systemic instability, the administration of empirical antibiotics may be reasonable but is not mandatory.

Infants in this category who are born by vaginal or cesarean delivery after efforts to induce labor and/or ROM before delivery are subject to factors associated with the pathogenesis of EOS during delivery. If any concern for infection arises during the process of delivery, the infant should be managed as recommended below for preterm infants at a higher risk for EOS. Otherwise, an acceptable approach to these infants is to obtain a blood culture and to initiate antibiotic therapy for infants with respiratory and/or cardiovascular instability after birth.

Preterm Infants at Higher Risk for EOS

Infants born preterm because of cervical incompetence, preterm labor, PROM, chorioamnionitis or IAI, and/or acute and otherwise unexplained onset of nonreassuring fetal status are at the highest risk for EOS. In these cases, IAI may be the cause of preterm birth or a secondary complication of PROM and cervical dilatation. IAI may also be the cause of unexplained fetal distress. The most reasonable approach to these infants is to perform a blood culture and start empirical antibiotic treatment. Obtaining CSF for culture before the administration of antibiotics should be considered if the infant will tolerate the procedure and if it will not delay the initiation of antibiotic therapy.

LABORATORY TESTING

Blood Culture

In the absence of validated, clinically available molecular diagnostic tests, a blood culture remains the diagnostic standard for EOS. Newborn surface cultures and gastric aspirate analysis cannot be used to diagnose EOS, and a urine culture is not indicated in

sepsis evaluations performed at <72 hours of age. Modern blood culture systems use optimized enriched culture media with antimicrobial neutralization properties, continuous-read detection systems, and specialized pediatric culture bottles. Although concerns have been raised regarding incomplete detection of low-level bacteremia and the effects of intrapartum antibiotic administration,[27,37] these systems reliably detect bacteremia at a level of 1 to 10 colony-forming units if a minimum of 1 mL of blood is inoculated; authors of several studies report no effect of intrapartum antibiotics on time to positivity.[38–42] Culture media containing antimicrobial neutralization elements efficiently neutralize β-lactam antibiotics and gentamicin.[39] A median blood culture time to positivity <24 hours is reported among VLBW infants when using contemporary blood culture techniques.[29,43–46] Pediatric blood culture bottles generally require a minimum of 1 mL of blood for optimal recovery of organisms.[47,48] The use of 2 separate bottles may provide the opportunity to determine if commensal species are true infections by comparing growth in the two.[49,50] Use of 1 aerobic and 1 anaerobic culture bottle may optimize organism recovery. Most neonatal pathogens, including GBS, *E coli*, coagulase-negative *Staphylococcus*, and *Staphylococcus aureus*, will grow in anaerobic conditions. One study revealed that with routine use of both pediatric aerobic and adult anaerobic blood cultures, strict anaerobic species (primarily *Bacteroides fragilis*) were isolated in 16% of EOS cases in preterm infants with VLBW.[29] An anaerobic blood culture is routinely performed among adult patients at risk for infection and can be used for neonatal blood cultures. Individual centers may benefit from collaborative discussion with the laboratory where cultures are processed to optimize local processes.

CSF Culture

The incidence of meningitis is higher among preterm infants (approximately 0.7 cases per 1000 live births at 22–28 weeks' gestation)[4] compared with the incidence in the overall birth population (approximately 0.02–0.04 cases per 1000 live births).[6, 10] In the study of differential EOS risk among very preterm infants, meningitis did not occur at all among lower-risk preterm infants.[4] The true incidence of meningitis among preterm infants may be underestimated because of the common practice of performing a lumbar puncture after the initiation of empirical antibiotic therapy. Although most preterm infants with culture-confirmed early-onset meningitis grow the same organism from blood cultures, the concordance is not 100%, and CSF cell count parameters may not always identify meningitis.[51] If a CSF culture has not been obtained before the initiation of empirical antibiotics, physicians should balance the physiologic stability of the infant, the risk of EOS, and the potential harms associated with prolonged antibiotic therapy when making the decision to perform a lumbar puncture in preterm infants who are critically ill.

White Blood Cell Count

The white blood cell (WBC) count, differential (immature-to-total neutrophil ratio), and absolute neutrophil count are commonly used to assess risk of EOS. Multiple clinical factors can affect the WBC count and differential, including gestational age at birth, sex, and mode of delivery.[52–55] Fetal bone marrow depression attributable to maternal preeclampsia or placental insufficiency, as well as prolonged exposure to inflammatory signals (such as PROM), frequently result in abnormal values in the absence

of infection. Most studies in which the performance characteristics of the complete blood cell (CBC) count in predicting infection is addressed have been focused on term infants. In 1 large multicenter study, the authors assessed the relationship between the WBC count and culture-confirmed EOS and analyzed data separately for infants born at <34 weeks' gestation.[56] They found that all components of the CBC count lacked sensitivity for predicting EOS. The highest likelihood ratios (LRs) for EOS were associated with extreme values. A positive LR of >3 (ie, a likelihood of infection at least 3 times higher than the entire group of infants born at <34 weeks' gestation) was associated with a WBC count of <1000 cells per μL, an absolute neutrophil count of <1000, and an immature-to-total neutrophil ratio of >0.25. A total WBC count of >50 000 cells per μL (LR, 2.3) and a platelet count of <50 000 (LR, 2.2) had a modest relationship to EOS.

Other Inflammatory Markers

Other markers of inflammation, including C-reactive protein (CRP), procalcitonin, interleukins (soluble interleukin 2 receptor, interleukin 6, and interleukin 8), tumor necrosis factor α, and CD64 are addressed in multiple studies.[57–60] Both CRP and procalcitonin concentrations increase in newborn infants in response to a variety of inflammatory stimuli, including infection, asphyxia, and pneumothorax. Procalcitonin concentrations also increase naturally over the first 24 to 36 hours after birth.[60] Single values of CRP or procalcitonin obtained after birth to assess the risk of EOS are neither sufficiently sensitive nor specific to guide EOS care decisions. Consistently normal values of CRP and procalcitonin over the first 48 hours of age are associated with the absence of EOS, but serial abnormal values alone should not be used to extend antibiotic therapy in the

absence of a culture-confirmed infection.

TREATMENT OF PRETERM EOS

The microbiology of EOS in the United States is largely unchanged over the past 10 years. Authors of national surveillance studies continue to identify *E coli* as the most common bacteria isolated in EOS cases that occur among preterm infants, whether defined by a gestational age of <34 weeks or by a birth weight of <1500 g. Overall, *E coli* is isolated in approximately 50%, and GBS is isolated in approximately 20% of all EOS cases occurring among infants born at <34 weeks' gestation.[6] Fungal organisms are isolated in <1% of cases. Approximately 10% of cases are caused by other Gram-positive organisms (predominantly viridans group streptococci and enterococci), and approximately 20% of cases are caused by other Gram-negative organisms. *S aureus* (approximately 1%–2%) and *L monocytogenes* (approximately 1%) are uncommon causes of preterm EOS.[4,6,11] If an anaerobic culture is routinely performed, strict anaerobic bacteria are isolated in up to 15% of EOS cases among preterm infants with VLBW, with *B fragilis* being the predominant anaerobic species isolated.[29]

Ampicillin and gentamicin are the first choice for empirical therapy for EOS. This combination will be effective against GBS, most other streptococcal and enterococcal species, and *L monocytogenes*. Although two-thirds of *E coli* EOS isolates and most other Gram-negative EOS isolates are resistant to ampicillin, the majority remain sensitive to gentamicin.[6] Extended-spectrum, β-lactamase-producing organisms are only rarely reported among EOS cases in the United States. Therefore, the routine empirical use of broader-spectrum antibiotics is not warranted and may be harmful.[61]

Nonetheless, 1% to 2% of *E coli* cases were resistant to both ampicillin and gentamicin in recent surveillance studies by the Centers for Disease Control and Prevention, and *B fragilis* is not uniformly sensitive to these medications.[6,62] Therefore, among preterm infants who are severely ill and at the highest risk for Gram-negative EOS (such as infants with VLBW born after prolonged PROM and infants exposed to prolonged courses of antepartum antibiotic therapy[63–65]), the empirical addition of broader-spectrum antibiotic therapy may be considered until culture results are available. The choice of additional therapy should be guided by local antibiotic resistance data.

When EOS is confirmed by a blood culture, a lumbar puncture should be performed if not previously done. Antibiotic therapy should use the narrowest spectrum of appropriate agents once antimicrobial sensitivities are known. The duration of therapy should be guided by expert references (eg, the American Academy of Pediatrics [AAP] *Red Book: Report of the Committee on Infectious Diseases*) and informed by the results of a CSF analysis and the achievement of sterile blood and CSF cultures. Consultation with infectious disease specialists should be considered for cases complicated by meningitis or other site-specific infections and for cases with complex antibiotic resistance patterns.

When initial blood culture results are negative, antibiotic therapy should be discontinued by 36 to 48 hours of incubation, unless there is evidence of site-specific infection. Persistent cardiorespiratory instability is common among infants with VLBW and is not alone an indication for prolonged empirical antibiotic administration. Continuing empirical antibiotic administration in response to laboratory test abnormalities alone is rarely justified, particularly among preterm infants born in the setting of

maternal obstetric conditions known to affect fetal hematopoiesis.

PREVENTION STRATEGIES

The only proven preventive strategy for EOS is the appropriate administration of maternal intrapartum antibiotic prophylaxis. The most current recommendations from national organizations, such as the AAP, ACOG, and Centers for Disease Control and Prevention, should be followed for the administration of GBS intrapartum prophylaxis as well as for the administration of intrapartum antibiotic therapy when there is suspected or confirmed IAI. Neonatal practices are focused on the identification and empirical antibiotic treatment of preterm neonates at risk for EOS; these practices cannot prevent EOS. The empirical administration of intramuscular penicillin to all newborn infants to prevent neonatal, GBS-specific EOS is not justified and is not endorsed by the AAP. Neither GBS intrapartum antibiotic prophylaxis nor any neonatal EOS practice will prevent late-onset GBS infection or any other form of late-onset bacterial infection. Preterm infants are particularly susceptible to late-onset GBS infection, with approximately 40% of late-onset GBS cases occurring among infants born at ≤34 6/7 weeks' gestation.[66,67]

SUMMARY POINTS

1. The epidemiology, microbiology, and pathogenesis of EOS differ substantially between term infants and preterm infants with VLBW.

2. Infants born at ≤34 6/7 weeks' gestation can be categorized by level of risk for EOS by the circumstances of their preterm birth.

   o Infants born preterm by cesarean delivery because of maternal noninfectious illness

or placental insufficiency in the absence of labor, attempts to induce labor, or ROM before delivery are at a relatively low risk for EOS. Depending on the clinical condition of the neonate, physicians should consider the risk/benefit balance of an EOS evaluation and empirical antibiotic therapy.

   o Infants born preterm because of maternal cervical incompetence, preterm labor, PROM, clinical concern for IAI, or acute onset of unexplained nonreassuring fetal status are at the highest risk for EOS. Such neonates should undergo EOS evaluation with a blood culture and empirical antibiotic treatment.

   o Obstetric and neonatal care providers should communicate and document the circumstances of preterm birth to facilitate EOS risk assessment among preterm infants.

3. Clinical centers should consider the development of locally appropriate written guidelines for preterm EOS risk assessment and clinical management. After guidelines are implemented, ongoing surveillance, designed to identify low-frequency adverse events and affirm efficacy, is recommended.

4. The diagnosis of EOS is made by a blood or CSF culture. EOS cannot be diagnosed by laboratory tests alone, such as CBC count or CRP levels.

5. The combination of ampicillin and gentamicin is the most appropriate empirical antibiotic regimen for infants at risk for EOS. Empirical administration of additional broad-spectrum antibiotics may be indicated in preterm infants who are severely ill and at a high risk for EOS, particularly after prolonged antepartum maternal antibiotic treatment.

6. When blood cultures are sterile, antibiotic therapy should be discontinued by 36 to 48 hours of incubation, unless there is clear evidence of site-specific infection. Persistent cardiorespiratory instability is common among preterm infants with VLBW and is not alone an indication for prolonged empirical antibiotic administration. Laboratory test abnormalities alone rarely justify prolonged empirical antibiotic administration, particularly among preterm infants at a lower risk for EOS.

LEAD AUTHORS

Karen M. Puopolo, MD, PhD, FAAP
William E. Benitz, MD, FAAP
Theoklis E. Zaoutis, MD, MSCE, FAAP

COMMITTEE ON FETUS AND NEWBORN, 2017–2018

James Cummings, MD, Chairperson
Sandra Juul, MD
Ivan Hand, MD
Eric Eichenwald, MD
Brenda Poindexter, MD
Dan L. Stewart, MD
Susan W. Aucott, MD
Karen M. Puopolo, MD, PhD, FAAP
Jay P. Goldsmith, MD
Kristi Watterberg, MD, Immediate Past Chairperson

LIAISONS

Kasper S. Wang, MD – *American Academy of Pediatrics Section on Surgery*
Thierry Lacaze, MD – *Canadian Paediatric Society*
Joseph Wax, MD – *American College of Obstetricians and Gynecologists*
Tonse N.K. Raju, MD, DCH – *National Institutes of Health*

Wanda Barfield, MD, MPH, CAPT USPHS – *Centers for Disease Control and Prevention*
Erin Keels, MS, APRN, NNP-BC – *National Association of Neonatal Nurses*

STAFF

Jim Couto, MA

COMMITTEE ON INFECTIOUS DISEASES, 2017–2018

Carrie L. Byington, MD, FAAP, Chairperson
Yvonne A. Maldonado, MD, FAAP, Vice Chairperson
Ritu Banerjee, MD, PhD, FAAP
Elizabeth D. Barnett, MD, FAAP
James D. Campbell, MD, MS, FAAP
Jeffrey S. Gerber, MD, PhD, FAAP
Ruth Lynfield, MD, FAAP
Flor M. Munoz, MD, MSc, FAAP
Dawn Nolt, MD, MPH, FAAP
Ann-Christine Nyquist, MD, MSPH, FAAP
Sean T. O'Leary, MD, MPH, FAAP
Mobeen H. Rathore, MD, FAAP
Mark H. Sawyer, MD, FAAP
William J. Steinbach, MD, FAAP
Tina Q. Tan, MD, FAAP
Theoklis E. Zaoutis, MD, MSCE, FAAP

EX OFFICIO

David W. Kimberlin, MD, FAAP – *Red Book* Editor
Michael T. Brady, MD, FAAP – *Red Book* Associate Editor
Mary Anne Jackson, MD, FAAP – *Red Book* Associate Editor
Sarah S. Long, MD, FAAP – *Red Book* Associate Editor
Henry H. Bernstein, DO, MHCM, FAAP – *Red Book* Online Associate Editor
H. Cody Meissner, MD, FAAP – Visual *Red Book* Associate Editor

LIAISONS

Amanda C. Cohn, MD, FAAP – *Centers for Disease Control and Prevention*
Jamie Deseda-Tous, MD – *Sociedad Latinoamericana de Infectología Pediátrica*

Karen M. Farizo, MD – *US Food and Drug Administration*
Marc Fischer, MD, FAAP – *Centers for Disease Control and Prevention*
Natasha Halasa, MD, MPH, FAAP – *Pediatric Infectious Diseases Society*
Nicole Le Saux, MD – *Canadian Pediatric Society*
Scot Moore, MD, FAAP – *Committee on Practice Ambulatory Medicine*
Angela K. Shen, ScD, MPH – *National Vaccine Program Office*
Neil S. Silverman, MD – *American College of Obstetricians and Gynecologists*
James J. Stevermer, MD, MSPH, FAAFP – *American Academy of Family Physicians*
Jeffrey R. Starke, MD, FAAP – *American Thoracic Society*
Kay M. Tomashek, MD, MPH, DTM – *National Institutes of Health*

STAFF

Jennifer M. Frantz, MPH

ABBREVIATIONS

AAP: American Academy of Pediatrics
ACOG: American College of Obstetricians and Gynecologists
CBC: complete blood cell
CRP: C-reactive protein
CSF: cerebrospinal fluid
EOS: early-onset sepsis
GBS: group B *Streptococcus*
IAI: intraamniotic infection
LR: likelihood ratio
NEC: necrotizing enterocolitis
PROM: premature rupture of membranes
ROM: rupture of membranes
VLBW: very low birth weight
WBC: white blood cell

FINANCIAL DISCLOSURE: The authors have indicated they have no financial relationships relevant to this article to disclose.

FUNDING: No external funding.

POTENTIAL CONFLICT OF INTEREST: The authors have indicated they have no potential conflicts of interest to disclose.

COMPANION PAPER: A companion to this article can be found online at www.pediatrics.org/cgi/doi/10.1542/peds.2018-2894.

REFERENCES

1. Cotten CM, Taylor S, Stoll B, et al; NICHD Neonatal Research Network. Prolonged duration of initial empirical antibiotic treatment is associated with increased rates of necrotizing enterocolitis and death for extremely low birth weight infants. *Pediatrics.* 2009;123(1):58–66

2. Cordero L, Ayers LW. Duration of empiric antibiotics for suspected early-onset sepsis in extremely low birth weight infants. *Infect Control Hosp Epidemiol.* 2003;24(9):662–666

3. Oliver EA, Reagan PB, Slaughter JL, Buhimschi CS, Buhimschi IA. Patterns of empiric antibiotic administration

for presumed early-onset neonatal sepsis in neonatal intensive care units in the United States. *Am J Perinatol.* 2017;34(7):640–647

4. Puopolo KM, Mukhopadhyay S, Hansen NI, et al; NICHD Neonatal Research Network. Identification of extremely premature infants at low risk for early-onset sepsis. *Pediatrics.* 2017;140(5):e20170925

5. Goldenberg RL, Culhane JF, Iams JD, Romero R. Epidemiology and causes of preterm birth. *Lancet.* 2008;371(9606):75–84

6. Schrag SJ, Farley MM, Petit S, et al. Epidemiology of invasive early-onset neonatal sepsis, 2005 to 2014. *Pediatrics.* 2016;138(6):e20162013

7. Weston EJ, Pondo T, Lewis MM, et al. The burden of invasive early-onset neonatal sepsis in the United States, 2005-2008. *Pediatr Infect Dis J.* 2011;30(11):937–941

8. Stoll BJ, Hansen NI, Bell EF, et al; Eunice Kennedy Shriver National Institute of Child Health and Human Development Neonatal Research Network. Trends in care practices, morbidity, and mortality of extremely preterm neonates, 1993-2012. *JAMA.* 2015;314(10):1039–1051

9. Puopolo KM, Draper D, Wi S, et al. Estimating the probability of neonatal early-onset infection on the basis of maternal risk factors. *Pediatrics.* 2011;128(5). Available at: www.pediatrics. org/cgi/content/full/128/5/e1155

10. Stoll BJ, Hansen NI, Sánchez PJ, et al; Eunice Kennedy Shriver National Institute of Child Health and Human Development Neonatal Research Network. Early onset neonatal sepsis: the burden of group B streptococcal and *E. coli* disease continues. *Pediatrics.* 2011;127(5):817–826

11. Stoll BJ, Hansen NI, Higgins RD, et al; National Institute of Child Health and Human Development. Very low birth weight preterm infants with early onset neonatal sepsis: the predominance of gram-negative infections continues in the National Institute of Child Health and Human Development Neonatal Research Network, 2002-2003. *Pediatr Infect Dis J.* 2005;24(7):635–639

12. Benirschke K. Routes and types of infection in the fetus and the newborn. *AMA J Dis Child.* 1960;99(6):714–721

13. Blanc WA. Pathways of fetal and early neonatal infection. Viral placentitis, bacterial and fungal chorioamnionitis. *J Pediatr.* 1961;59:473–496

14. Goldenberg RL, McClure EM, Saleem S, Reddy UM. Infection-related stillbirths. *Lancet.* 2010;375(9724):1482–1490

15. Romero R, Dey SK, Fisher SJ. Preterm labor: one syndrome, many causes. *Science.* 2014;345(6198):760–765

16. Goldenberg RL, Hauth JC, Andrews WW. Intrauterine infection and preterm delivery. *N Engl J Med.* 2000;342(20):1500–1507

17. Carroll SG, Ville Y, Greenough A, et al. Preterm prelabour amniorrhexis: intrauterine infection and interval between membrane rupture and delivery. *Arch Dis Child Fetal Neonatal Ed.* 1995;72(1):F43–F46

18. Muglia LJ, Katz M. The enigma of spontaneous preterm birth. *N Engl J Med.* 2010;362(6):529–535

19. Lamont RF, Sobel J, Mazaki-Tovi S, et al. Listeriosis in human pregnancy: a systematic review. *J Perinat Med.* 2011;39(3):227–236

20. Vinturache AE, Gyamfi-Bannerman C, Hwang J, Mysorekar IU, Jacobsson B; Preterm Birth International Collaborative (PREBIC). Maternal microbiome - a pathway to preterm birth. *Semin Fetal Neonatal Med.* 2016;21(2):94–99

21. Hanke K, Hartz A, Manz M, et al; German Neonatal Network (GNN). Preterm prelabor rupture of membranes and outcome of very-low-birth-weight infants in the German Neonatal Network. *PLoS One.* 2015;10(4):e0122564

22. Ofman G, Vasco N, Cantey JB. Risk of early-onset sepsis following preterm, prolonged rupture of membranes with or without chorioamnionitis. *Am J Perinatol.* 2016;33(4):339–342

23. Dutta S, Reddy R, Sheikh S, Kalra J, Ray P, Narang A. Intrapartum antibiotics and risk factors for early onset sepsis. *Arch Dis Child Fetal Neonatal Ed.* 2010;95(2):F99–F103

24. Parry S, Strauss JF III. Premature rupture of the fetal membranes. *N Engl J Med.* 1998;338(10):663–670

25. American College of Obstetricians and Gynecologists' Committee on Practice Bulletins—Obstetrics. Practice bulletin no. 172: premature rupture of membranes. *Obstet Gynecol.* 2016;128(4):e165–e177

26. Benitz WE, Gould JB, Druzin ML. Risk factors for early-onset group B streptococcal sepsis: estimation of odds ratios by critical literature review. *Pediatrics.* 1999;103(6). Available at: www.pediatrics.org/cgi/content/full/103/6/e77

27. Higgins RD, Saade G, Polin RA, et al; Chorioamnionitis Workshop Participants. Evaluation and management of women and newborns with a maternal diagnosis of chorioamnionitis: summary of a workshop. *Obstet Gynecol.* 2016;127(3):426–436

28. Wortham JM, Hansen NI, Schrag SJ, et al; Eunice Kennedy Shriver NICHD Neonatal Research Network. Chorioamnionitis and culture-confirmed, early-onset neonatal infections. *Pediatrics.* 2016;137(1):e20152323

29. Mukhopadhyay S, Puopolo KM. Clinical and microbiologic characteristics of early-onset sepsis among very low birth weight infants: opportunities for antibiotic stewardship. *Pediatr Infect Dis J.* 2017;36(5):477–481

30. Committee on Obstetric Practice. Committee opinion no. 712: intrapartum management of intraamniotic infection. *Obstet Gynecol.* 2017;130(2):e95–e101

31. Alexander VN, Northrup V, Bizzarro MJ. Antibiotic exposure in the newborn intensive care unit and the risk of necrotizing enterocolitis. *J Pediatr.* 2011;159(3):392–397

32. Kuppala VS, Meinzen-Derr J, Morrow AL, Schibler KR. Prolonged initial empirical antibiotic treatment is associated with adverse outcomes in premature infants. *J Pediatr.* 2011;159(5):720–725

33. Ting JY, Synnes A, Roberts A, et al; Canadian Neonatal Network Investigators. Association between

antibiotic use and neonatal mortality and morbidities in very low-birth-weight infants without culture-proven sepsis or necrotizing enterocolitis. *JAMA Pediatr.* 2016;170(12):1181–1187

34. Vangay P, Ward T, Gerber JS, Knights D. Antibiotics, pediatric dysbiosis, and disease. *Cell Host Microbe.* 2015;17(5):553–564

35. Kinlay S, Michel T, Leopold JA. The future of vascular biology and medicine. *Circulation.* 2016;133(25):2603–2609

36. Kaiser Permanente Division of Research. Neonatal early-onset sepsis calculator. Available at: https://neonatalsepsiscalculator. kaiserpermanente.org. Accessed April 5, 2018

37. Wynn JL, Wong HR, Shanley TP, Bizzarro MJ, Saiman L, Polin RA. Time for a neonatal-specific consensus definition for sepsis. *Pediatr Crit Care Med.* 2014;15(6):523–528

38. Dunne WM Jr, Case LK, Isgriggs L, Lublin DM. In-house validation of the BACTEC 9240 blood culture system for detection of bacterial contamination in platelet concentrates. *Transfusion.* 2005;45(7):1138–1142

39. Flayhart D, Borek AP, Wakefield T, Dick J, Carroll KC. Comparison of BACTEC PLUS blood culture media to BacT/Alert FA blood culture media for detection of bacterial pathogens in samples containing therapeutic levels of antibiotics. *J Clin Microbiol.* 2007;45(3):816–821

40. Jorgensen JH, Mirrett S, McDonald LC, et al. Controlled clinical laboratory comparison of BACTEC plus aerobic/F resin medium with BacT/Alert aerobic FAN medium for detection of bacteremia and fungemia. *J Clin Microbiol.* 1997;35(1):53–58

41. Krisher KK, Gibb P, Corbett S, Church D. Comparison of the BacT/Alert PF pediatric FAN blood culture bottle with the standard pediatric blood culture bottle, the Pedi-BacT. *J Clin Microbiol.* 2001;39(8):2880–2883

42. Nanua S, Weber C, Isgriggs L, Dunne WM Jr. Performance evaluation of the VersaTREK blood culture system for quality control testing of platelet units. *J Clin Microbiol.* 2009;47(3):817–818

43. Garcia-Prats JA, Cooper TR, Schneider VF, Stager CE, Hansen TN. Rapid detection of microorganisms in blood cultures of newborn infants utilizing an automated blood culture system. *Pediatrics.* 2000;105(3 pt 1):523–527

44. Sarkar SS, Bhagat I, Bhatt-Mehta V, Sarkar S. Does maternal intrapartum antibiotic treatment prolong the incubation time required for blood cultures to become positive for infants with early-onset sepsis? *Am J Perinatol.* 2015;32(4):357–362

45. Guerti K, Devos H, Ieven MM, Mahieu LM. Time to positivity of neonatal blood cultures: fast and furious? *J Med Microbiol.* 2011;60(pt 4):446–453

46. Jardine L, Davies MW, Faoagali J. Incubation time required for neonatal blood cultures to become positive. *J Paediatr Child Health.* 2006;42(12):797–802

47. Schelonka RL, Chai MK, Yoder BA, Hensley D, Brockett RM, Ascher DP. Volume of blood required to detect common neonatal pathogens. *J Pediatr.* 1996;129(2):275–278

48. Yaacobi N, Bar-Meir M, Shchors I, Bromiker R. A prospective controlled trial of the optimal volume for neonatal blood cultures. *Pediatr Infect Dis J.* 2015;34(4):351–354

49. Sarkar S, Bhagat I, DeCristofaro JD, Wiswell TE, Spitzer AR. A study of the role of multiple site blood cultures in the evaluation of neonatal sepsis. *J Perinatol.* 2006;26(1):18–22

50. Struthers S, Underhill H, Albersheim S, Greenberg D, Dobson S. A comparison of two versus one blood culture in the diagnosis and treatment of coagulase-negative *staphylococcus* in the neonatal intensive care unit. *J Perinatol.* 2002;22(7):547–549

51. Garges HP, Moody MA, Cotten CM, et al. Neonatal meningitis: what is the correlation among cerebrospinal fluid cultures, blood cultures, and cerebrospinal fluid parameters? *Pediatrics.* 2006;117(4):1094–1100

52. Manroe BL, Weinberg AG, Rosenfeld CR, Browne R. The neonatal blood count in health and disease. I. Reference values for neutrophilic cells. *J Pediatr.* 1979;95(1):89–98

53. Schmutz N, Henry E, Jopling J, Christensen RD. Expected ranges for blood neutrophil concentrations of neonates: the Manroe and Mouzinho charts revisited. *J Perinatol.* 2008;28(4):275–281

54. Christensen RD, Henry E, Jopling J, Wiedmeier SE. The CBC: reference ranges for neonates. *Semin Perinatol.* 2009;33(1):3–11

55. Newman TB, Puopolo KM, Wi S, Draper D, Escobar GJ. Interpreting complete blood counts soon after birth in newborns at risk for sepsis. *Pediatrics.* 2010;126(5):903–909

56. Hornik CP, Benjamin DK, Becker KC, et al. Use of the complete blood cell count in early-onset neonatal sepsis. *Pediatr Infect Dis J.* 2012;31(8): 799–802

57. Benitz WE. Adjunct laboratory tests in the diagnosis of early-onset neonatal sepsis. *Clin Perinatol.* 2010;37(2):421–438

58. Lynema S, Marmer D, Hall ES, Meinzen-Derr J, Kingma PS. Neutrophil CD64 as a diagnostic marker of sepsis: impact on neonatal care. *Am J Perinatol.* 2015;32(4):331–336

59. Su H, Chang SS, Han CM, et al. Inflammatory markers in cord blood or maternal serum for early detection of neonatal sepsis-a systemic review and meta-analysis. *J Perinatol.* 2014;34(4):268–274

60. Chiesa C, Panero A, Rossi N, et al. Reliability of procalcitonin concentrations for the diagnosis of sepsis in critically ill neonates. *Clin Infect Dis.* 1998;26(3):664–672

61. Clark RH, Bloom BT, Spitzer AR, Gerstmann DR. Empiric use of ampicillin and cefotaxime, compared with ampicillin and gentamicin, for neonates at risk for sepsis is associated with an increased risk of neonatal death. *Pediatrics.* 2006;117(1):67–74

62. Snydman DR, Jacobus NV, McDermott LA, et al. Lessons learned from the anaerobe survey: historical perspective and review of the most recent data (2005-2007). *Clin Infect Dis.* 2010;50(suppl 1):S26–S33

63. Stoll BJ, Hansen N, Fanaroff AA, et al. Changes in pathogens causing early-onset sepsis in very-low-birth-weight infants. *N Engl J Med.* 2002;347(4):240–247

64. Schrag SJ, Hadler JL, Arnold KE, Martell-Cleary P, Reingold A, Schuchat A. Risk factors for invasive, early-onset *Escherichia coli* infections in the era of widespread intrapartum antibiotic use. *Pediatrics.* 2006;118(2):570–576

65. Puopolo KM, Eichenwald EC. No change in the incidence of ampicillin-resistant, neonatal, early-onset sepsis over 18 years. *Pediatrics.* 2010;125(5). Available at: www.pediatrics.org/cgi/content/full/125/5/e1031

66. Jordan HT, Farley MM, Craig A, et al; Active Bacterial Core Surveillance (ABCs)/Emerging Infections Program Network, CDC. Revisiting the need for vaccine prevention of late-onset neonatal group B streptococcal disease: a multistate, population-based analysis. *Pediatr Infect Dis J.* 2008;27(12):1057–1064

67. Phares CR, Lynfield R, Farley MM, et al; Active Bacterial Core Surveillance/Emerging Infections Program Network. Epidemiology of invasive group B streptococcal disease in the United States, 1999-2005. *JAMA.* 2008;299(17):2056–2065

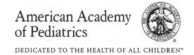

American Academy
of Pediatrics
DEDICATED TO THE HEALTH OF ALL CHILDREN™

Guidance for the Clinician in
Rendering Pediatric Care

CLINICAL REPORT

Strategies for Prevention of Health Care–Associated Infections in the NICU

Richard A. Polin, MD, Susan Denson, MD, Michael T. Brady, MD, THE COMMITTEE ON FETUS AND NEWBORN and COMMITTEE ON INFECTIOUS DISEASES

KEY WORDS
health care–associated infection, nosocomial infection, neonatal ICU, NICU, antibiotics, neonate, newborn

ABBREVIATIONS
CDC—Centers for Disease Control and Prevention
CI—confidence interval
ESBL—extended-spectrum β-lactamase
RR—relative risk

www.pediatrics.org/cgi/doi/10.1542/peds.2012-0145

doi:10.1542/peds-2012-0145

All clinical reports from the American Academy of Pediatrics automatically expire 5 years after publication unless reaffirmed, revised, or retired at or before that time.

PEDIATRICS (ISSN Numbers: Print, 0031-4005; Online, 1098-4275).

abstract

Health care–associated infections in the NICU result in increased morbidity and mortality, prolonged lengths of stay, and increased medical costs. Neonates are at high risk of acquiring health care–associated infections because of impaired host-defense mechanisms, limited amounts of protective endogenous flora on skin and mucosal surfaces at time of birth, reduced barrier function of their skin, use of invasive procedures and devices, and frequent exposure to broad-spectrum antibiotic agents. This clinical report reviews management and prevention of health care–associated infections in newborn infants. *Pediatrics* 2012;129:e1085–e1093

INTRODUCTION

Health care–associated infections in the NICU are infections acquired in the hospital while receiving treatment of other conditions. Although they are less likely to cause mortality than early-onset infections, they have considerable health and economic consequences. Most health care–associated infections in the NICU result from the instrumentation and procedures required to preserve an infant's life. Thus, it is not possible to lower the rate of health care–associated infections merely by limiting the use of procedures. Furthermore, it is no longer acceptable to consider health care–associated infections as a consequence of neonatal intensive care. Rather, it is incumbent on clinicians to minimize risks of infection by performing invasive procedures only when needed and in the safest manner possible. There is evidence to support the concept that proactive strategies to prevent health care–associated infections in the NICU are possible,[1–5] although data supporting specific infection-control interventions in neonates are lacking. Although neonates clearly have unique vulnerabilities, there is no reason to believe that interventions shown to be effective in the pediatric ICU or adult ICU would not be equally effective in the NICU. Because of unique issues confronting the vulnerable neonate, however, these interventions may require some accommodations and further study.

STRATEGIES FOR THE PREVENTION OF HEALTH CARE–ASSOCIATED INFECTIONS

Hand Hygiene

Hand hygiene remains the most effective method for reducing health care–associated infections.[6] Hospitals with higher rates of hand hygiene compliance have lower rates of central line bloodstream infection; however, compliance with hand hygiene practices is less than optimal.[7] A recent meta-analysis concluded that educational programs and multidisciplinary quality-improvement teams can be effective in increasing compliance with hand hygiene procedures[8]; however, each of the 33 studies included more than 1 intervention, and it was difficult to determine which was most efficacious. The Centers for Disease Control and Prevention (CDC) published guidelines for hand hygiene in health care settings in 2002.[9] Although the guidelines were widely accepted and disseminated by members of the National Nosocomial Infection Surveillance System, a recent analysis demonstrated that implementation of these guidelines had no effect on hand hygiene compliance rates (mean, 56.6%).[10]

The sixth edition of the *Guidelines for Perinatal Care*[11] recommends use of an antiseptic soap or an alcohol-based gel or foam for routine hand sanitizing if hands are not visibly soiled. When hands are visibly contaminated, they should first be washed with soap and water. Larson et al[12] compared the effectiveness of a traditional antiseptic hand wash with an alcohol hand sanitizer in reducing bacterial colonization. There were no differences in mean microbial counts on nurses' hands or infection rates among patients in the NICU; however, nurses' skin condition improved during the alcohol phase. Other studies have demonstrated the effectiveness of alcohol-based products, but there are no data to suggest they are superior. Compliance with hand hygiene may be enhanced if alcohol-based products are available at each infant's bedside.

In May 2009, the World Health Organization published new consensus recommendations for hand hygiene.[13] The guidelines provide a comprehensive overview of hand hygiene in health care and evidence- and consensus-based recommendations for successful implementation. Consensus recommendations were categorized according to the CDC/Healthcare Infection Control Practice Advisory Committee grading system (Tables 1 and 2). A partial list of recommendations relevant to the NICU is shown in Table 3.

Prevention of Central Line–Associated Bloodstream Infections

Catheter-related bloodstream infections are the most common hospital-acquired infections in the NICU. Central line–related infections are in large part a result of poor technique at the time of placement and ongoing care of the catheter site. Attempts to reduce the incidence of central line–associated bloodstream infections primarily fall into 1 of 5 categories: (1) clinical practice guidelines for the insertion and maintenance of indwelling lines[14]; (2) prophylactic administration of antibiotic agents (including antibiotic lock therapy); (3) topical emollients to reduce skin penetrance of bacteria; (4) promotion of breastfeeding; and (5) gowning for visitors and attendants. The goal of all infection-control programs should be to reduce the rate of central line–associated bloodstream infections to zero.

Both chlorhexidine (2%) and povidone-iodine are recommended for skin antisepsis in infants 2 months or older[15,16]; however, chlorhexidine is not approved by the US Food and Drug Administration for infants younger than 2 months. In a randomized trial, use of a chlorhexidine-impregnated gauze dressing (0.5% chlorhexidine gluconate in a 70% alcohol solution) in infants of very low birth weight reduced central venous catheter colonization when compared with use of a 10% povidone-iodine scrub but did not reduce the incidence of central line–associated bloodstream infections.[17] Notably, in the chlorhexidine group, contact dermatitis occurred in

TABLE 1 Evidence Grading System

Ranking System for Evidence According to the CDC/Healthcare Infection Control Practice Advisory Committee System
Category IA: Strongly recommended for implementation and strongly supported by well-designed experimental, clinical, or epidemiologic studies.
Category IB: Strongly recommended for implementation and supported by some experimental, clinical, or epidemiologic studies and a strong theoretical rational.
Category IC: Required for implementation, as mandated by federal and/or state regulation or standard.
Category II: Suggested for implementation and supported by suggestive clinical or epidemiologic studies or a theoretical rationale or a consensus by a panel of experts.

TABLE 2 Infectious Diseases Society of America/US Public Health Service Grading System for Ranking Recommendations for Clinical Guidelines

Category, Grade	Definition
Strength of recommendation	
A	Good evidence to support a recommendation for use
B	Moderate evidence to support a recommendation for use
C	Poor evidence to support a recommendation for use
Quality of evidence	
I	Evidence from ≥1 properly randomized controlled trial
II	Evidence from ≥1 well-designed clinical trial, without randomization; from cohort or case-controlled analytic studies (preferably from >1 center); from multiple time series; or from dramatic results from uncontrolled experiments
III	Evidence from opinions of respected authorities, based on clinical experience, descriptive studies, or reports from expert committees

TABLE 3 World Health Organization Recommendations for Hand Hygiene

- Wash hands with soap and water when visibly dirty or soiled with blood or other body fluids (IB) or after using the toilet (II).
- Use of an alcohol-based hand rub for all routine antisepsis is recommended for all clinical settings if the hands are not soiled (IA). If an alcohol-based hand rub is not obtainable, wash hands with soap and water (IB). Brushes are no longer recommended (even for surgical scrubs) (IB).
- Perform hand hygiene:
  - Before and after touching the patient (IB).
  - Before handling an invasive device for patient care, regardless of whether gloves are worn (IB).
  - After contact with body fluids or excretions, mucous membranes, nonintact skin, or wound dressings (IA).
  - If moving from a contaminated body site to another body site during care of the same patient (IB).
  - After contact with inanimate surfaces and objects (including medical equipment) in the immediate vicinity of the patient (IB).
  - After removing sterile (II) or nonsterile gloves (IB).
- Selection and handling of hand hygiene agents:
  - Provide products with a low irritancy potential (IB).
  - To maximize acceptance of hand hygiene products by health care workers, solicit input regarding the skin tolerance, feel, and fragrance of any products under consideration (IB).
  - Determine any known interaction between products used to clean hands, skin care products, and the types of gloves used in the institution (II).
  - Ensure that dispensers are accessible at point of care (IB).
  - Provide alternative hand hygiene products for health care workers with confirmed allergies or adverse reactions to standard products (II).
  - When alcohol-based hand rub is available in the health care facility, use of antimicrobial soap is not recommended (II).
  - Soap and alcohol-based hand rub should not be used concomitantly (II).
- Use of gloves:
  - The use of gloves does not replace the need for hand hygiene (IB).
  - Wear gloves when it can be reasonably anticipated that contact with blood or other potentially infectious materials, mucous membranes, or nonintact skin will occur (IC).
  - Remove gloves after caring for a patient. Do not wear the same pair of gloves for more than 1 patient (IB).
  - Change or remove gloves during patient care if moving from a contaminated body site to either another body site (including nonintact skin, mucous membrane, or medical device) within the same patient or the environment (II).
- Other aspects of hand hygiene:
  - Do not wear artificial fingernails or extenders when having direct contact with the patient (IA).
  - Keep natural nails short.
- Hand hygiene promotion programs:
  - In hand hygiene–promotion programs for health care workers, focus specifically on factors currently found to have a significant influence on behavior and not solely on the type of hand hygiene product. The strategy should be multifaceted and multimodal and include education and senior executive support for implementation (IA).
  - Educate health care workers about the type of patient-care activities that can result in hand contamination and about the advantages and disadvantages of various methods used to clean their hands (II).
  - Monitor health care workers' adherence to recommended hand hygiene practices and provide them with performance feedback (IA).
  - Encourage partnerships between patients, their families, and health care workers to promote hand hygiene in the health care setting (II).

15% of neonates weighing less than 1000 g. In a meta-analysis of studies comparing chlorhexidine gluconate solution with a povidone-iodine solution, the overall risk reduction (for central line–associated bloodstream infections) with chlorhexidine gluconate compared with a povidone-iodine solution was approximately 50%.[18]

Extraluminal contamination of the intracutaneous tract is believed to be responsible for catheter-related infections that happen in the week after placement.[19] Catheters are more mobile during the first week after insertion and can slide in and out of the insertion site, drawing organisms down into the catheter tract. Techniques to reduce the likelihood of extraluminal contamination include proper hand hygiene, aseptic catheter insertion (including use of a maximal sterile barrier for catheter insertion and care [IA]), use of a topical antiseptic (IA), and use of sterile dressing (IA). Although transparent dressings permit easier inspection of the catheter site, they have no proven benefit in reducing infection.[20] Catheter sites must be monitored visually or by palpation on a daily basis (IB) and should be redressed and cleaned on a weekly basis (IA). In neonates, there are no data indicating that tunneled catheters have a lower risk of infection than nontunneled catheters.[21]

After the first week of placement, intraluminal colonization after hub manipulation and contamination is responsible for most central line–associated bloodstream infections.[19] Mahieu et al[22] demonstrated that the frequency of catheter manipulations was directly related to the frequency of central line–associated bloodstream infections. Tubing used to administer blood products or lipid emulsions should be changed daily (IB). Tubing used to infuse dextrose and amino acids should be replaced every 4 to 7 days. It is important to remove all central venous catheters when they are no longer essential (1A). Many NICUs remove central catheters when the volume of enteral feedings reaches 80 to 100 mL/kg per day. Topical antibiotic agents or creams should not be used at the insertion site for catheters (1B).

Guidelines for the prevention of intravascular catheter-related infections have been published.[23] These guidelines make specific recommendations for umbilical catheters. Levels of evidence are indicated in parentheses (Table 4).

Recently, there has been a focus on implementing "NICU care bundles" to reduce the incidence of hospital-acquired infections. Care bundles are groups of interventions (extrapolated from studies in adults or recommendations from professional organizations) that are likely to be effective. This multifaceted approach has reduced the incidence of health care–associated sepsis in each center or groups of centers where it has been implemented.[24–27]

Coagulase-negative staphylococci are the most common cause of central line–associated bloodstream infections in the United States. Therefore, the use of low-dose vancomycin in parenteral alimentation solutions (at concentrations above the minimal inhibitory concentration) has been suggested as a way to decrease the incidence of bacteremia attributable to coagulase-negative staphylococci. Five randomized clinical trials of low-dose vancomycin in preterm neonates have been conducted, all of which date from the late 1990s. In 4 of the studies, there was a statistically significant reduction in the incidence of coagulase-negative staphylococcal sepsis (relative risk [RR], 0.11; 95% confidence interval [CI], 0.05–0.24)[28];

however, there were no significant differences in mortality or length of stay. The use of antibiotic lock therapy has also been investigated. Lock solutions containing vancomycin are instilled into the catheter lumen to reduce intraluminal colonization. Most randomized clinical trials of antibiotic lock therapy have been completed in adults and older children.[29] A meta-analysis of these trials demonstrated a significant reduction in bloodstream infections (RR, 0.49; 95% CI, 0.26–0.95). Use of vancomycin as a true lock solution (instilling it for a defined period rather than flushing it through the catheter) conferred greater benefit. The single study of antibiotic lock therapy in the neonatal population[30] demonstrated a statistically significant reduction in central line–associated bloodstream infections (RR, 0.13; 95% CI, 0.01–0.57). No increase in vancomycin resistance occurred in this study; however, the study was not sufficiently powered to address that question. Because of the concern for development of vancomycin-resistant organisms and the lack of long-term efficacy data, neither continuous infusions of vancomycin nor antibiotic lock therapy can be recommended.

Invasive fungal infections are responsible for 9% to 12% of health care–associated infections in infants weighing less than 1500 g.[31] In a prospective study from the National Institute for

Child Health and Human Development research network, 9% of infants weighing less than 1000 g developed candidiasis.[32] Death or neurodevelopment impairment occurred in 73% of these infants. Prophylactic fluconazole has been suggested as a way to decrease the incidence of invasive fungal disease. The rationale is that prevention of fungal colonization in high-risk infants will lower the risk of invasive disease. A meta-analysis of 5 trials comparing systemic fluconazole with placebo, demonstrated a statistically significant reduction in the incidence of invasive fungal infections (RR, 0.48; 95% CI, 0.31–0.73)[33]; however, there was no significant difference in the incidence of death before discharge from the hospital and insufficient data to assess neurodevelopmental outcomes. There is a concern that the use of azoles to prevent fungal infections will lead to an increase in fluconazole resistance or will result in toxicity, especially among the most immature infants for whom there are limited pharmacokinetic data.

In many NICUs, it is policy that care providers and visitors wear gowns on entering the nursery. Eight trials have evaluated the benefit of gowning.[34] A meta-analysis demonstrated that there was no significant effect of a gowning policy on reducing the incidence of systemic nosocomial infection (RR, 1.24; 95% CI, 0.90–1.71). For that reason,

TABLE 4 Guidelines for the Prevention of Intravascular Catheter-related Infections

1. Remove and do not replace umbilical artery catheters if any signs of central line–associated bloodstream infection, vascular insufficiency in the lower extremities, or thrombosis are present (Category II).
2. Remove and do not replace umbilical venous catheters if any signs of central line–associated bloodstream infection or thrombosis are present (Category II).
3. Cleanse the umbilical insertion site with an antiseptic before catheter insertion. Avoid tincture of iodine because of the potential effect on the neonatal thyroid. Other iodine-containing products (eg, povidone-iodine) can be used (Category IB).
4. Do not use topical antibiotic ointment or creams on catheter insertion sites because of the potential to promote fungal infections and antimicrobial resistance (Category IA).
5. Add low doses of heparin (0.25–1.0 U/mL) to the fluid infused through umbilical arterial catheter (Category IB).
6. Remove umbilical catheters as soon as possible when no longer needed or when any sign of vascular insufficiency to the lower extremities is observed. Optimally, umbilical artery catheters should not be left in place for more than 5 d (Category II).
7. Umbilical venous catheters should be removed as soon as possible when no longer needed but can be used up to 14 d if managed aseptically (Category II).
8. An umbilical catheter may be replaced if it is malfunctioning and there is no other indication for catheter removal and the total duration of catheterization has not exceeded 5 d for an umbilical artery catheter or 14 d for an umbilical vein catheter (Category II).

gowns should not be required for routine admission to the NICU by health care workers or visitors. Despite the lack of overall benefit, gowns and gloves should be worn when an infant is colonized with a resistant or invasive pathogen, consistent with appropriate isolation requirements. Additional personal protective equipment may be required on the basis of isolation requirements of the specific pathogen or clinical condition and the activity or procedure to be performed.

Prevention of Health Care–Associated Pneumonia

The CDC published guidelines for preventing health care–associated pneumonia in 2003.[35] These guidelines were not specifically designed to address the unique issues facing the mechanically ventilated patient in the NICU; however, many of the recommendations are relevant to all patient populations.

General concepts discussed in the CDC document include the following:

1. Staff Education and Involvement in Infection Prevention. All providers should receive appropriate information relating to the epidemiology of and infection control procedures for preventing health care–associated pneumonia. There should be procedures in place to ensure worker competency, including performance of appropriate infection-control activities. Staff should be involved with implementation of interventions to prevent health care–associated pneumonia using performance-improvement tools and techniques (IA).

2. Infection and Microbiologic Surveillance. Surveillance for health care–associated pneumonia in patients in the NICU should be performed to determine trends and help identify outbreaks or other problems (IB). Routine surveillance cultures of

patients or equipment should not be performed (II).

3. Prevention of Transmission of Microorganisms. Within the NICU, risks for acquisition of microorganisms that could result in health care–associated pneumonia can be reduced by (1) proper sterilization or disinfection and maintenance of equipment and devices (IA), and (2) prevention of person-to-person transmission of bacteria by use of Standard Precautions as well as other isolation practices when appropriate (IA).

4. Modifying Host Risk for Infection. Aspiration is a major risk for the development of health care–associated pneumonia. Devices such as endotracheal tubes, tracheostomy tubes, or enteral tubes should be removed from patients as soon as appropriate and clinically indicated (IB). In the absence of medical contraindication(s), the head of the bed should be elevated at an angle of 30 to 45 degrees for mechanically ventilated patients (II). A comprehensive oral-hygiene program should be followed for the infant (II).

Suctioning practices and position of the infant in the bed may influence tracheal colonization. The use of closed-suctioning systems allows endotracheal suctioning without disconnecting patients from the ventilator. Closed-suctioning methods reduce physiologic disruptions (hypoxia and decrease in heart rate), and NICU nurses judged them to be easier to use than an open system.[36,37] Closed-suctioning systems provide an opportunity for bacterial contamination when pooled secretions in the lumen are reintroduced into the lower respiratory tract with repeat suctioning. On the other hand, closed-suctioning systems could potentially reduce environmental contamination of the endotracheal tube. In studies evaluating mechanically ventilated adults, airway colonization was more common when

closed-suctioning systems were used,[38,39] but ventilator-associated pneumonia rates were equal to or slightly less than the rates among patients managed with open systems.[38–40] CDC recommendations[35] do not endorse one system over the other, and there is no recommendation addressing the frequency at which closed-suctioning systems should be changed.

Tracheal colonization from oropharyngeal contamination is less common among neonates on mechanical ventilation when the neonates are placed in a lateral position on the bed as compared with the supine position (30% for lateral versus 87% for supine; $P < .01$).[41] Keeping the endotracheal tube and the ventilator circuit in a horizontal position might reduce tracking of oropharyngeal sections down into the lower respiratory tract.[42] The lateral position also is associated with reduced aspiration of gastric secretions into the trachea.[41] Using a nonsupine position may reduce the risk of ventilator-associated pneumonia.[43]

Other Strategies to Reduce Health Care–Associated Infections in the NICU

The skin of the preterm newborn infant has compromised barrier and immune function. In addition, the skin of the extremely preterm infant can be easily damaged and serve as a portal for the entry of organisms into the bloodstream. Topical emollients have been used to decrease transepidermal water losses and have been suggested as a method to decrease health care–associated infections. In a meta-analysis of 4 trials completed in industrialized countries, a significantly increased risk of coagulase-negative staphylococcal infection was found in infants treated with prophylactic topical ointment.[44] In contrast, infants born at <33 weeks' gestation in Bangladesh treated topically with sunflower oil were 41% less likely to develop health care–associated infections than were control infants.[45] The lack of effectiveness of topical emollients in industrialized countries may be attributable to different mechanisms of transcutaneous sepsis. In industrialized countries, instrumentation is used more commonly, and sites of insertion can serve as a portal for bacterial invasion. In developing countries, environmental contamination and malnutrition play a greater role, and invasive devices are used less frequently. Therefore, bacterial invasion is likely attributable to microscopic sites of skin barrier compromise, which might be protected by the use of an emollient.

The use of human milk feedings has been associated with a lower risk of sepsis and necrotizing enterocolitis in preterm infants.[46] Human milk contains a large number of immunoprotective substances, prebiotics, and probiotics and has been shown to decrease the incidence of gastrointestinal and respiratory infections in infancy.[47] Although a number of randomized clinical trials and cohort studies have concluded that human milk feedings had a protective effect on infection in preterm infants, a meta-analysis of 9 studies (6 cohort and 3 randomized clinical trials from India) failed to show an advantage of human milk feedings.[48] The authors believed there were serious methodologic flaws in all of the cohort studies, "including poor study design, inadequate sample sizes, neglecting to account for some confounders, failure to eliminate the effects associated with maternal choice of feeding method and other sociodemographic variables." In addition, the definition of human milk feedings was not consistent among studies. It is important to note that necrotizing enterocolitis was excluded from this systematic review.

A number of other practices may provide opportunities to reduce colonization of the critically ill neonate with health care–associated pathogens or to modify the risk of developing disease if colonized. Specific practices that may provide benefit include (1) appropriate vaccination of health care workers (eg, influenza vaccine and tetanus toxoid, reduced diphtheria toxoid, and acellular pertussis, adsorbed); (2) cohorting in selected outbreak situations; and (3) visitation guidelines to identify ill/infected visitors.

Antibiotic Use and Misuse

The use and misuse of antibiotics can be associated with alteration in neonates' microflora and the development of antibiotic resistance. This is a particular concern within the confines of a NICU, where there is a population of vulnerable children who have medical conditions that may require frequent and/or prolonged antibiotic use, long hospitalizations, crowded conditions, and frequent contact and interventions.

Antimicrobial resistance can be intrinsic (ie, present without exposure to antimicrobial agents) or acquired. An example of intrinsic resistance is the resistance of Gram-negative organisms to vancomycin. Acquired antimicrobial resistance is driven by antimicrobial exposure, as is seen in methicillin-resistant *Staphylococcus aureus* and the extended-spectrum β-lactamase (ESBL)-producing organisms. These patterns of resistance represent adaptations of bacteria to antibiotic exposure.

Judicious use of antibiotic agents is commonly recommended as appropriate in the NICU, but it is not commonly practiced. The critically ill nature of patients in the NICU prompts frequent and prolonged use of antimicrobial agents. Judicious use of antibiotic agents in the NICU would include limiting use to only those situations in which a bacterial infection is likely, discontinuing empirical treatment when a bacterial infection has not been identified,

changing the antibiotic agents administered to those with the narrowest spectrum on the basis of susceptibility testing, and treating for the appropriate duration. Although clinical situations will vary, these principles remain consistent. It is also relevant to consider the potential for different antibiotic agents to drive the development of resistance. ESBL-producing organisms (primarily Gram-negative enteric agents) are present in many NICUs because of the frequent use of third-generation cephalosporins and other broad-spectrum β-lactam antibiotic agents. Curtailing the use of third-generation cephalosporins and using other antibiotic agents, such as aminoglycosides for empirical therapy, has been associated with less antibiotic resistance, including ESBL-producing organisms. Good infection-control practices also play a significant role in reducing horizontal transmission of antibiotic-resistant bacteria.

The Infectious Diseases Society of America and the Society for Healthcare Epidemiology of America have developed guidelines for "Antimicrobial Stewardship" to reduce antimicrobial resistance.[49] These guidelines are designed to address programmatic changes that improve control of antibiotic resistance (see Table 1 for levels of evidence). Strategies that might be helpful in the NICU setting include the following: (1) auditing antimicrobial use of practitioners and providing feedback (IA); (2) formulary restriction and preauthorization requirements for selected antimicrobial agents (IB); (3) education of prescribers and nurses concerning the role of antimicrobial use and the development of resistance (IB); (4) development of clinical guidelines/pathways for selected conditions (IA); (5) antimicrobial order forms (IB); (6) specific plans for streamlining (broad- to narrow-spectrum antibiotic agents) or deescalating (elimination of redundant or unnecessary) antimicrobial agents (IB); (7) dose optimization on the basis of individual characteristics (eg, weight, renal status, drug-drug interactions) (IB); and (8) switching from parenteral to oral antibiotic agents when appropriate and feasible (IB). Data are not sufficient to recommend antimicrobial cycling or routine use of combination therapy merely to prevent the development of resistance; however, antimicrobial combinations may be valuable for preventing development of resistance in specific circumstances.

CONCLUSIONS

Health care–associated infections are an important medical morbidity facing an already vulnerable group of infants. The epidemiology and strategies that can reduce these infections are well known; however, implementation of strategies that can influence the occurrence of health care–associated infections within the NICU requires a concerted team effort by all individuals who participate in the care of these infants. Each care provider must understand his or her role in preventing health care–associated infections and have a willingness to modify behaviors such that they comply with recognized infection-control practices. All too frequently, the health of a tiny infant whose life is being saved through the use of the best in 21st-century technology is jeopardized by the smallest of acts—such as a care provider neglecting to wash his or her hands. Recognition of the importance of even the most basic care practices can result in behavior modification within the NICU and improve compliance with established infection-control practices.

LEAD AUTHORS
Richard A. Polin, MD
Susan Denson, MD
Michael T. Brady, MD

COMMITTEE ON FETUS AND NEWBORN, 2011–2012
Lu-Ann Papile, MD, Chairperson
Jill E. Baley, MD
Waldemar A. Carlo, MD
James J. Cummings, MD
Praveen Kumar, MD
Richard A. Polin, MD
Rosemarie C. Tan, MD, PhD
Kristi L. Watterberg, MD

LIAISONS
CAPT Wanda D. Barfield, MD, MPH – *Centers for Disease Control and Prevention*
Ann L. Jefferies, MD – *Canadian Pediatric Society*
George A. Macones, MD – *American College of Obstetricians and Gynecologists*
Rosalie O. Mainous, PhD, APRN, NNP-BC – *National Association of Neonatal Nurses*
Tonse N. K. Raju, MD, DCH – *National Institutes of Health*
Kasper S .Wang, MD – *AAP Section on Surgery*

STAFF
Jim Couto, MA

COMMITTEE ON INFECTIOUS DISEASES, 2011–2012
Michael T. Brady, MD, Chairperson
Carrie L. Byington, MD
H. Dele Davies, MD
Kathryn M. Edwards, MD
Mary P. Glode, MD
Mary Anne Jackson, MD
Harry L. Keyserling, MD
Yvonne A. Maldonado, MD
Dennis L. Murray, MD
Walter A. Orenstein, MD
Gordon E. Schutze, MD
Rodney E. Willoughby, MD
Theoklis E. Zaoutis, MD

LIAISONS
Marc A. Fischer, MD – *Centers for Disease Control and Prevention*
Bruce Gellin, MD – *National Vaccine Program Office*
Richard L. Gorman, MD – *National Institutes of Health*
Lucia Lee, MD – *Food and Drug Administration*
R. Douglas Pratt, MD – *Food and Drug Administration*
Jennifer S. Read, MD – *National Vaccine Program Office*
Joan Robinson, MD – *Canadian Pediatric Society*
Marco Aurelio Palazzi Safadi, MD – *Sociedad Latinoamericana de Infectologia Pediatrica (SLIPE)*
Jane Seward, MBBS, MPH – *Centers for Disease Control and Prevention*
Jeffrey R. Starke, MD – *American Thoracic Society*
Geoffrey Simon, MD – *Committee on Practice Ambulatory Medicine*
Tina Q. Tan, MD – *Pediatric Infectious Diseases Society*

EX OFFICIO
Carol J. Baker, MD – Red Book *Associate Editor*
Henry H. Bernstein, DO – Red Book *Associate Editor*
David W. Kimberlin, MD – Red Book *Associate Editor*
Sarah S. Long, MD – Red Book *Online Associate Editor*
H. Cody Meissner, MD – Visual Red Book *Associate Editor*
Larry K. Pickering, MD – Red Book *Editor*

CONSULTANT
Lorry G. Rubin, MD

STAFF
Jennifer Frantz, MPH

REFERENCES

1. Bizzarro MJ, Sabo B, Noonan M, Bonfiglio MP, Northrup V, Diefenbach K; Central Venous Catheter Initiative Committee. A quality improvement initiative to reduce central line-associated bloodstream infections in a neonatal intensive care unit. *Infect Control Hosp Epidemiol*. 2010;31(3):241–248

2. Cimiotti JP, Haas J, Saiman L, Larson EL. Impact of staffing on bloodstream infections in the neonatal intensive care unit. *Arch Pediatr Adolesc Med*. 2006;160(8):832–836

3. Garland JS, Uhing MR. Strategies to prevent bacterial and fungal infection in the neonatal intensive care unit. *Clin Perinatol*. 2009;36(1):1–13

4. Garland JS. Strategies to prevent ventilator-associated pneumonia in neonates. *Clin Perinatol*. 2010;37(3):629–643

5. Payne NR, Finkelstein MJ, Liu M, Kaempf JW, Sharek PJ, Olsen S. NICU practices and outcomes associated with 9 years of quality improvement collaboratives. *Pediatrics*. 2010; 125(3):437–446

6. Larson E. Skin hygiene and infection prevention: more of the same or different approaches? *Clin Infect Dis.* 1999;29(5):1287–1294

7. Harbarth S, Pittet D, Grady L, et al. Interventional study to evaluate the impact of an alcohol-based hand gel in improving hand hygiene compliance. *Pediatr Infect Dis J.* 2002;21(6):489–495

8. Aboelela SW, Stone PW, Larson EL. Effectiveness of bundled behavioural interventions to control healthcare-associated infections: a systematic review of the literature. *J Hosp Infect.* 2007;66(2):101–108

9. Boyce JM, Pittet D; Healthcare Infection Control Practices Advisory Committee; HICPAC/SHEA/APIC/IDSA Hand Hygiene Task Force; Society for Healthcare Epidemiology of America/Association for Professionals in Infection Control/Infectious Diseases Society of America. Guideline for Hand Hygiene in Health-Care Settings. Recommendations of the Healthcare Infection Control Practices Advisory Committee and the HICPAC/SHEA/APIC/IDSA Hand Hygiene Task Force. *MMWR Recomm Rep.* 2002;51(RR-16):1–45, quiz CE1–CE4

10. Larson EL, Quiros D, Lin SX. Dissemination of the CDC's Hand Hygiene Guideline and impact on infection rates. *Am J Infect Control.* 2007;35(10):666–675

11. American Academy of Pediatrics, American College of Obstetricians and Gynecologists. *Guidelines for Perinatal Care.* Infection control. In: Lockwood CJ, Lemons JA, eds. 6th ed. Elk Grove Village, IL: American Academy of Pediatrics; 2007:349–370

12. Larson EL, Cimiotti J, Haas J, et al. Effect of antiseptic handwashing vs alcohol sanitizer on health care-associated infections in neonatal intensive care units. *Arch Pediatr Adolesc Med.* 2005;159(4):377–383

13. Pittet D, Allegranzi B, Boyce J; World Health Organization World Alliance for Patient Safety First Global Patient Safety Challenge Core Group of Experts. The World Health Organization Guidelines on Hand Hygiene in Health Care and their consensus recommendations. *Infect Control Hosp Epidemiol.* 2009;30(7):611–622

14. O'Grady NP, Alexander M, Dellinger EP, et al; Healthcare Infection Control Practices Advisory Committee. Guidelines for the prevention of intravascular catheter-related infections. *Am J Infect Control.* 2002;30(8 suppl 1):476–489

15. Garland JS, Alex CP, Uhing MR, Peterside IE, Rentz A, Harris MC. Pilot trial to compare tolerance of chlorhexidine gluconate to povidone-iodine antisepsis for central venous catheter placement in neonates. *J Perinatol.* 2009;29(12):808–813

16. Datta MK, Clarke P. Current practices of skin antisepsis for central venous catheter insertion in UK tertiary-level neonatal units. *Arch Dis Child Fetal Neonatal Ed.* 2008;93(4):F328

17. Garland JS, Alex CP, Mueller CD, et al. A randomized trial comparing povidone-iodine to a chlorhexidine gluconate-impregnated dressing for prevention of central venous catheter infections in neonates. *Pediatrics.* 2001;107(6):1431–1436

18. Chaiyakunapruk N, Veenstra DL, Lipsky BA, Saint S. Chlorhexidine compared with povidone-iodine solution for vascular catheter-site care: a meta-analysis. *Ann Intern Med.* 2002;136(11):792–801

19. Garland JS, Alex CP, Sevallius JM, et al. Cohort study of the pathogenesis and molecular epidemiology of catheter-related bloodstream infection in neonates with peripherally inserted central venous catheters. *Infect Control Hosp Epidemiol.* 2008;29(3):243–249

20. Hoffmann KK, Weber DJ, Samsa GP, Rutala WA. Transparent polyurethane film as an intravenous catheter dressing. A meta-analysis of the infection risks. *JAMA.* 1992;267(15):2072–2076

21. Chien LY, Macnab Y, Aziz K, Andrews W, McMillan DD, Lee SK; Canadian Neonatal Network. Variations in central venous catheter-related infection risks among Canadian neonatal intensive care units. *Pediatr Infect Dis J.* 2002;21(6):505–511

22. Mahieu LM, De Muynck AO, Ieven MM, De Dooy JJ, Goossens HJ, Van Reempts PJ. Risk factors for central vascular catheter-associated bloodstream infections among patients in a neonatal intensive care unit. *J Hosp Infect.* 2001;48(2):108–116

23. O'Grady NP, Alexander M, Burns LA, et al; Healthcare Infection Control Practices Advisory Committee (HICPAC). Guidelines for the prevention of intravascular catheter-related infections. *Clin Infect Dis.* 2011;52(9):e162–e193

24. Kilbride HW, Wirtschafter DD, Powers RJ, Sheehan MB. Implementation of evidence-based potentially better practices to decrease nosocomial infections. *Pediatrics.* 2003;111(4 pt 2). Available at: www.pediatrics.org/cgi/content/full/111/supplement_E1/e519

25. Bloom BT, Craddock A, Delmore PM, et al. Reducing acquired infections in the NICU: observing and implementing meaningful differences in process between high and low acquired infection rate centers. *J Perinatol.* 2003;23(6):489–492

26. Andersen C, Hart J, Vemgal P, Harrison C. Prospective evaluation of a multi-factorial prevention strategy on the impact of nosocomial infection in very-low-birth weight infants. *J Hosp Infect.* 2005;61(2):162–167

27. Aly H, Herson V, Duncan A, et al. Is bloodstream infection preventable among premature infants? A tale of two cities. *Pediatrics.* 2005;115(6):1513–1518

28. Craft AP, Finer NN, Barrington KJ. Vancomycin for prophylaxis against sepsis in preterm neonates. *Cochrane Database Syst Rev.* 2000;(2):CD001971

29. Safdar N, Maki DG. Use of vancomycin-containing lock or flush solutions for prevention of bloodstream infection associated with central venous access devices: a meta-analysis of prospective, randomized trials. *Clin Infect Dis.* 2006;43(4):474–484

30. Garland JS, Alex CP, Henrickson KJ, McAuliffe TL, Maki DG. A vancomycin-heparin lock solution for prevention of nosocomial bloodstream infection in critically ill neonates with peripherally inserted central venous catheters: a prospective, randomized trial. *Pediatrics.* 2005;116(2). Available at: www.pediatrics.org/cgi/content/full/116/2/e198

31. Stoll BJ, Hansen N, Fanaroff AA, et al. Late-onset sepsis in very low birth weight neonates: the experience of the NICHD Neonatal Research Network. *Pediatrics.* 2002;110(2 pt 1):285–291

32. Benjamin DK Jr, Stoll BJ, Gantz MG, et al. Neonatal candidiasis: epidemiology, risk factors, and clinical judgment. *Pediatrics.* 2010;126(4). Available at: www.pediatrics.org/cgi/content/full/126/4/e865

33. Clerihew L, Austin N, McGuire W. Prophylactic systemic antifungal agents to prevent mortality and morbidity in very low birth weight infants. *Cochrane Database Syst Rev.* 2007;(4):CD003850

34. Webster J, Pritchard MA. Gowning by attendants and visitors in newborn nurseries for prevention of neonatal morbidity and mortality. *Cochrane Database Syst Rev.* 2003;(3):CD003670

35. Tablan OC, Anderson LJ, Besser R, Bridges C, Hajjeh R; CDC; ; Healthcare Infection Control Practices Advisory Committee. Guidelines for preventing health-care—associated pneumonia, 2003: recommendations of CDC and the Healthcare Infection Control Practices Advisory Committee. *MMWR Recomm Rep.* 2004;53(RR-3):1–36

36. Cordero L, Sananes M, Ayers LW. Comparison of a closed (Trach Care MAC) with an open endotracheal suction system in small premature infants. *J Perinatol.* 2000;20(3):151–156

37. Woodgate PG, Flenady V. Tracheal suctioning without disconnection in intubated ventilated neonates. *Cochrane Database Syst Rev.* 2001;(2):CD003065

38. Deppe SA, Kelly JW, Thoi LL, et al. Incidence of colonization, nosocomial pneumonia, and

mortality in critically ill patients using a Trach Care closed-suction system versus an open-suction system: prospective, randomized study. *Crit Care Med.* 1990;18(12):1389–1393

39. Johnson KL, Kearney PA, Johnson SB, Niblett JB, MacMillan NL, McClain RE. Closed versus open endotracheal suctioning: costs and physiologic consequences. *Crit Care Med.* 1994;22(4):658–666

40. Combes P, Fauvage B, Oleyer C. Nosocomial pneumonia in mechanically ventilated patients, a prospective randomised evaluation of the Stericath closed suctioning system. *Intensive Care Med.* 2000;26(7):878–882

41. Torres A, Serra-Batlles J, Ros E, et al. Pulmonary aspiration of gastric contents in patients receiving mechanical ventilation: the effect of body position. *Ann Intern Med.* 1992;116(7):540–543

42. Aly H, Badawy M, El-Kholy A, Nabil R, Mohamed A. Randomized, controlled trial on tracheal colonization of ventilated infants: can gravity prevent ventilator-associated pneumonia? *Pediatrics.* 2008;122(4):770–774

43. Drakulovic MB, Torres A, Bauer TT, Nicolas JM, Nogué S, Ferrer M. Supine body position as a risk factor for nosocomial pneumonia in mechanically ventilated patients: a randomised trial. *Lancet.* 1999;354(9193):1851–1858

44. Soll RF, Edwards WH. Emollient ointment for preventing infection in preterm infants. *Cochrane Database Syst Rev.* 2000;(2):CD001150

45. Darmstadt GL, Saha SK, Ahmed AS, et al. Effect of topical treatment with skin barrier-enhancing emollients on nosocomial infections in preterm infants in Bangladesh: a randomised controlled trial. *Lancet.* 2005;365(9464):1039–1045

46. Schanler RJ. Evaluation of the evidence to support current recommendations to meet the needs of premature infants: the role of human milk. *Am J Clin Nutr.* 2007;85(2):625S–628S

47. Goldman AS. The immune system in human milk and the developing infant. *Breastfeed Med.* 2007;2(4):195–204

48. de Silva A, Jones PW, Spencer SA. Does human milk reduce infection rates in preterm infants? A systematic review. *Arch Dis Child Fetal Neonatal Ed.* 2004;89(6):F509–F513

49. Dellit TH, Owens RC, McGowan JE Jr, et al Infectious Diseases Society of America; Society for Healthcare Epidemiology of America. Infectious Diseases Society of America and the Society for Healthcare Epidemiology of America guidelines for developing an institutional program to enhance antimicrobial stewardship. *Clin Infect Dis.* 2007;44(2):159–177

SECTION 6

Complications/ Issues

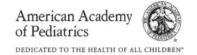

American Academy
of Pediatrics
DEDICATED TO THE HEALTH OF ALL CHILDREN™

Guidance for the Clinician in
Rendering Pediatric Care

CLINICAL REPORT

Assessment and Management of Inguinal Hernia in Infants

abstract

Inguinal hernia repair in infants is a routine surgical procedure. However, numerous issues, including timing of the repair, the need to explore the contralateral groin, use of laparoscopy, and anesthetic approach, remain unsettled. Given the lack of compelling data, consideration should be given to large, prospective, randomized controlled trials to determine best practices for the management of inguinal hernias in infants. *Pediatrics* 2012;130:768–773

INTRODUCTION

Inguinal hernia is a common condition requiring surgical repair in the pediatric age group. The incidence of inguinal hernias is approximately 3% to 5% in term infants and 13% in infants born at less than 33 weeks of gestational age.[1] Inguinal hernias in both term and preterm infants are commonly repaired shortly after diagnosis to avoid incarceration of the hernia. Given the lack of definitive data, optimal timing for repair of inguinal hernias in infants remains debatable. This report reviews the embryology and natural history of inguinal hernias as well as published data regarding the timing and approach to inguinal hernia repair in infants.

EMBRYOLOGY AND NATURAL HISTORY OF THE PATENT PROCESSUS VAGINALIS

Complete understanding of the issues related to surgical repair of an inguinal hernia requires an understanding of the embryology of descent of the testes and the formation of the processus vaginalis.

Testicular descent involves 2 phases: intra-abdominal and extra-abdominal.[2] During the intra-abdominal phase, the testis, which derives from the bipotential gonad originating at the urogenital ridge, is attached to the diaphragm by the craniosuspensory ligament. In the male fetus, regression of the craniosuspensory ligament results in transabdominal migration of the testis between 8 and 15 weeks postconception. Simultaneously, there is thickening of the gubernaculum, which attaches the testis to the scrotum through the external and internal rings of the inguinal canal. As the male fetus grows and the abdomen elongates, the testis is essentially anchored by the thickened gubernaculum.[3] In the female fetus, the craniosuspensory ligament is maintained; hence, the ovary retains its dorsal (retrocoelomic or retroperitoneal)

Kasper S. Wang, MD, and the COMMITTEE ON FETUS AND NEWBORN AND SECTION ON SURGERY

KEY WORDS
inguinal hernia, infants, surgery, anesthesia, laparoscopy

ABBREVIATION
PPV—patent processus vaginalis

This document is copyrighted and is property of the American Academy of Pediatrics and its Board of Directors. All authors have filed conflict of interest statements with the American Academy of Pediatrics. Any conflicts have been resolved through a process approved by the Board of Directors. The American Academy of Pediatrics has neither solicited nor accepted any commercial involvement in the development of the content of this publication.

The guidance in this report does not indicate an exclusive course of treatment or serve as a standard of medical care. Variations, taking into account individual circumstances, may be appropriate.

www.pediatrics.org/cgi/doi/10.1542/peds.2012-2008

doi:10.1542/peds.2012-2008

All clinical reports from the American Academy of Pediatrics automatically expire 5 years after publication unless reaffirmed, revised, or retired at or before that time.

PEDIATRICS (ISSN Numbers: Print, 0031-4005; Online, 1098-4275).

intra-abdominal location. In addition, the gubernaculum does not thicken but persists as the ovarian round ligament.

The second phase occurs between 25 and 35 weeks of gestation.[4] The testis descends from its retroperitoneal, intra-abdominal location through the inguinal canal, drawing with it an extension of the peritoneal lining, which defines the processus vaginalis. Normally, the processus vaginalis obliterates and involutes, leaving no communication between the intra-abdominal peritoneal cavity and the extra-abdominal inguinal canal and scrotum. This enveloping involuted layer is the tunica vaginalis. Both human in vitro tissue culture and rodent model studies implicate genito-femoral nerve innervation as critical for regulation of gubernacular length as well as obliteration of the processus vaginalis.[5–7] Incomplete involution results in a patent processus vaginalis (PPV), through which fluid can travel and accumulate extra-abdominally as a hydrocele. If the communication is large, intra-abdominal structures such as bowel may herniate, resulting in an indirect inguinal hernia. The relation of the processus vaginalis with testicular descent is thought to explain why more than 90% of pediatric inguinal hernias are diagnosed in boys.[1] Involution of the left processus vaginalis precedes that of right, which is consistent with the observation that 60% of indirect inguinal hernias occur on the right side.[8]

The prevalence of PPV is highest during infancy and declines with age. Congenital hydroceles, which are essentially clinically apparent PPV, usually resolve spontaneously within 18 to 24 months.[9,10] The reported prevalence of PPV is as high as 80% in term male infants.[11] However, this prevalence is generally extrapolated from findings at time of exploration of the contralateral internal ring during time of inguinal hernia repair. Thus, most reported rates of bilateral PPV are derived from observations in patients with symptomatic unilateral inguinal hernias and likely overestimate the true prevalence of PPV in the general population. Rowe et al reported a 64% rate of contralateral PPV identified at the time of inguinal hernia repair in infants younger than 2 months. Reported rates of contralateral PPV decrease to between 33% and 50% in children younger than 1 year of age and are as low as 15% by 5 years of age.[12–16] Not all cases of PPV result in inguinal hernias. The estimated childhood risk of developing an inguinal hernia if there is a PPV is between 25% and 50%.[17,18] Even though the true prevalence of a PPV in the general pediatric population is likely lower than contralateral PPV reported at the time of hernia repair, it is clearly greatest at birth and declines with increasing age.

RATIONALE AND TIMING FOR ELECTIVE INGUINAL HERNIA REPAIR IN INFANTS

All inguinal hernias in infants are repaired to avoid the risk of incarceration of bowel and gonadal infarction and atrophy.[19–22] However, these risks must be balanced against the risk of potential operative and anesthetic complications. Unfortunately, data regarding these risks are not definitive.

Many investigators have sought to define the risk of inguinal hernia incarceration in young children. However, the physical features of hernia, such as the size of the abdominal wall defect, the amount of the herniating intestine, and the ease with which it can be reduced, do not consistently predict the risk of incarceration. Attempts have been made to correlate the age at diagnosis, the duration between diagnosis and hernia repair, and infants' gestational age with risk of inguinal hernia incarceration. Notably, in an analysis of a Canadian administrative database containing more than 1000 children with inguinal hernia, Zamakshary et al showed that children younger than 1 year had a twofold greater risk of inguinal hernia incarceration when repair was performed ≥14 days after diagnosis compared with children who had repair performed between 1 and 2 years of age.[23] Vaos et al reported a retrospective analysis of preterm infants undergoing inguinal hernia repair at 1 of 2 institutions.[24] They noted that infants undergoing repair later than 1 week after diagnosis were at significantly greater risk of inguinal hernia incarceration, postoperative hernia recurrence, and testicular atrophy, compared with infants undergoing earlier repair. Lautz et al analyzed the risk of inguinal hernia incarceration in approximately 49 000 preterm infants using the 2003 and 2006 Kids' Inpatient Databases.[25] They determined that the overall rate of inguinal hernia incarceration was approximately 16% and that the risk was greatest in infants in whom surgery was delayed beyond 40 weeks' corrected gestational age (21%) compared with those repaired between 36 and 39 weeks (9%) corrected age or less than 36 weeks corrected gestational age (11%). Furthermore, 28% of former preterm infants undergoing repair during a subsequent hospitalization were noted to have inguinal hernia incarceration, suggesting an even greater risk with further delay. Although fraught with limitations inherent to administrative databases, the conclusions of this study are compelling.

Conversely, other data indicate that delay in inguinal hernia repair is associated with low rates of inguinal hernia incarceration. Lee et al reported a 4.6% rate of hernia incarceration in 172 former preterm infants within a single Kaiser system hospital. Of the 127 infants who were discharged from the hospital with known inguinal hernias and scheduled for a planned elective outpatient repair, there were no episodes of inguinal hernia incarceration while awaiting repair.[26] Uemura et al reported comparable inguinal hernia incarceration rates in 19 preterm infants (birth weight range 492–2401 g) who underwent repair at more than 2 weeks after diagnosis, compared with 21 preterm infants who underwent more urgent repair.[27] Although these studies suggest that inguinal hernia repair can be delayed, the data are not as compelling as those suggesting repair on a more urgent basis.

Inguinal hernia repair is associated with operative complications, including hernia recurrence, vas deferens injury, and testicular atrophy, the rates of which vary from 1% to 8%.[28–31] Long-term complications include chronic pain and infertility in adulthood.[32] In a single-institution, retrospective analysis, Moss et al observed low recurrence and complication rates up to 5 years after surgical repair in infants younger than 2 months of age.[33] Conversely, a retrospective analysis by Baird et al revealed a higher rate of complications in infants who were 43 weeks' corrected gestational age or younger, compared with those who underwent repair at an older age.[34] They speculated that the greater friability of the hernia sac in former preterm infants predisposes to repair failure.

Early repair of inguinal hernias in preterm infants must be further balanced against the risk of postoperative apnea after general anesthesia. Historically, the rate of postoperative apnea in preterm infants has been reported to be as high as 49%.[35,36] The risk of postoperative apnea is associated with perioperative anemia and a history of preoperative apnea as well as associated comorbidities.[35,37] Vaos et al noted that preterm infants

undergoing inguinal hernia repair within 1 week of diagnosis experienced a significantly greater rate of apnea compared with those undergoing repair later.[24] Melone et al reported on a cohort of 127 former preterm infants (mean gestational age, 32.7 weeks) who underwent outpatient inguinal hernia repair at a mean corrected gestational age of 45.3 weeks. The authors identified only 2 infants who experienced episodes of apnea: 1 in the operating room, the other postdischarge. They concluded that because the apnea rate is so low, elective outpatient inguinal hernia repair is a feasible option for preterm infants. Lee et al reported no episodes of apnea in a cohort of preterm infants (30.7 weeks' gestation at birth) undergoing outpatient elective hernia repair.[26] However, the authors noted that 13 of 45 former preterm infants who underwent elective inguinal hernia repair before discharge from the NICU remained intubated for longer than 2 days postoperatively.

Younger corrected gestational age is associated with a greater risk of apnea.[38] Allen et al noted a nearly 9% rate of postoperative apnea in their cohort of 57 preterm infants undergoing inguinal hernia repair.[39] In a subset analysis, infants who experienced apnea episodes tended to be younger (41 weeks' corrected gestational age compared with 47 weeks' corrected gestational age); had significantly higher perioperative risk, as measured by American Society of Anesthesia scores (2.6 compared with 1.8); and were more likely to have received intraoperative narcotic and muscle relaxation compared with infants who were not apneic. A recent meta-analysis concluded that former preterm infants undergoing general anesthesia who are less than 46 weeks' corrected gestational age should be observed for at least 12 hours postoperatively and that those who are between 46 and 60

weeks' corrected gestational age should receive more individualized care on the basis of the presence or absence of associated comorbidities.[40]

To reduce the incidence of postoperative apnea, spinal, rather than general, anesthesia has been used for inguinal hernia repair in preterm infants.[41–43] Although some studies have been encouraging, none have been adequately powered. Indeed, Craven et al published a Cochrane Collaboration analysis in which only 108 patients from 4 small randomized or quasi-randomized studies comparing spinal and general anesthesia were identified.[44] The authors concluded that there was no evidence that spinal anesthesia was associated with a reduction in postoperative apnea, bradycardia, or oxygen desaturation. Furthermore, the authors concluded that a large, randomized controlled trial was necessary to determine whether spinal anesthesia reduces postoperative cardiorespiratory complications; to date, no such study has been reported.

Over the past decade, studies performed in rodents and nonhuman primates have shown a dose-dependent association of neuronal apoptosis with general anesthetic agents, including ketamine, propofol, and isoflurane.[45–47] Importantly, there is emerging evidence that the use of general anesthesia in infancy may be associated with long-term neurocognitive and developmental problems, specifically after multiple exposures to general anesthesia before 3 years of age.[48] DiMaggio et al, using a New York State Medicaid database, showed that children younger than 3 years who were given general anesthesia for inguinal hernia repair had a greater than twofold risk of developmental or behavioral disorders than did age-matched control children.[49] A potential bias of this study is that children undergoing surgery at a young age may also be predisposed to learning or cognitive disorders. Bartels et al attempted to address this issue by using the Netherlands Twin Registry to evaluate monozygotic concordant-discordant twins. In a study of 1143 monozygotic twin pairs, exposure to anesthesia before 3 years of age was associated with reduced educational achievement.[50] However, there was no difference in outcome between twin pairs when one twin had undergone anesthesia and the other had not. The authors concluded that there is no causal relationship between anesthesia exposure and learning disabilities. Hansen et al recently compared ninth-grade test scores of nearly 2700 Swedish children who had undergone inguinal hernia repair as infants with those of randomly selected age-matched controls and found no difference in test performance.[51] Clearly, the issue of whether anesthetic exposure as an infant affects long-term neurodevelopment is unsettled. Two large clinical studies are under way to address this issue.[52]

Ultimately, the timing of preterm infant inguinal hernia repair varies widely in practice. In a 2005 survey of members of the American Academy of Pediatrics Section on Surgery, 63% reported routinely performing hernia repairs just before discharge from the NICU, 18% performed repairs at a specific corrected gestational age, and 5% performed repairs when it was convenient.[53] If a hernia was discovered after discharge, 53% of respondents would repair the hernia when it was convenient, and 27% of respondents would wait to repair until the infant was between 38 and 60 weeks' corrected gestational age (mean, 53.1 weeks' corrected gestational age). In a previous survey performed in 1993, surgeons were more likely to repair an inguinal hernia when convenient.[54]

Timing of inguinal hernia repair in preterm and term infants represents a balance of the risks of inguinal hernia incarceration and of postoperative respiratory complications. At present, the literature does not clearly define what these risks are and how they should be balanced.

CONTRALATERAL INGUINAL EXPLORATION

The utility of contralateral inguinal exploration in children is an area of active debate. The rationale for attempting to diagnose a contralateral PPV is that repair can be performed to prevent any potential contralateral incarceration with no additive anesthetic risk. Historically, surgeons performed routine open contralateral inguinal explorations to identify PPV in either all children or in selected populations (ie, former preterm infants or children younger than 2 years). Marulaiah et al suggested that routine contralateral exploration is not indicated, given the risks associated with such exploration, such as spermatic cord injury.[55] Alternatively, given the high incidence of subsequent hernias if a contralateral PPV is encountered, others support routine exploration.[13,56,57] Lee et al indicated that it is cost-effective to perform routine contralateral groin explorations.[58] Results from the aforementioned 2005 survey of American Academy of Pediatrics Section on Surgery members revealed a variety of practices; 15% of respondents indicated that they never explore the contralateral side in a male patient, 12% responded that they always do, and 73% responded that they had an age cutoff beyond which they would not explore.[53] Respondents also had a wide variation of practices when caring for a girl with a unilateral hernia. For both male and female patients with hernias, however, results of the survey revealed that there were significant reductions in the routine explorations of the contralateral side compared with results from the same survey performed in 1996.[54] Various diagnostic modalities, such as the physical examination, herniography, or ultrasonographic examination are not particularly sensitive or specific, thus making these efforts unreliable.[56,59] With the advent of laparoscopic techniques, inspection of the contralateral internal ring has become increasingly popular as the method of choice for evaluating for a PPV. According to survey responses, use of laparoscopy as the modality with which to explore the contralateral ring has increased from 6% in 1996 to 37% in 2005.[53,54] Use of laparoscopy to explore the contralateral groin has likely increased since then.

LAPAROSCOPIC APPROACH TO INGUINAL HERNIA REPAIR IN INFANTS

Laparoscopic repair has been used effectively in preterm infants. Various techniques have been described, but all routinely use a port placed in the umbilicus to visualize the internal ring. Reported hernia recurrence rates are comparable to those associated with open repair.[60,61] However, data regarding the risk of testicular atrophy are not available.[62,63] A prospective, randomized, single-blinded trial comparing laparoscopic to open repair of inguinal hernias showed that children who were older than 3 months of age when laparoscopic repair was performed required significantly fewer doses of pain medication.[64] The utility of laparoscopic repair of inguinal hernias in younger infants remains undetermined to date.

CONCLUSIONS

- Inguinal hernias are common in the infant population. The risk of hernia incarceration drives the preference to pursue surgical repair.
- Data regarding optimal timing of repair are conflicting and inadequate.

- There is no consensus on when or if contralateral inguinal exploration is necessary.

- Data regarding a laparoscopic approach to inguinal hernia repairs suggest that it is comparable to the standard open technique.

- Given the lack of data supporting evidence-based approaches to inguinal hernias in infants, consideration should be given to large, prospective, randomized, controlled trials to answer these important questions.

LEAD AUTHOR

Kasper S. Wang, MD

COMMITTEE ON FETUS AND NEWBORN, 2011–2012

Lu-Ann Papile, MD, Chairperson
Jill E. Baley, MD
William Benitz, MD
James Cummings, MD
Waldemar A. Carlo, MD
Praveen Kumar, MD
Richard A. Polin, MD
Rosemarie C. Tan, MD, PhD
Kristi L. Watterberg, MD

LIAISONS

CAPT Wanda Denise Barfield, MD, MPH—*Centers for Disease Control and Prevention*
George Macones, MD—*American College of Obstetricians and Gynecologists*
Ann L. Jefferies, MD—*Canadian Pediatric Society*
Rosalie O. Mainous, PhD, RNC, NNP—*National Association of Neonatal Nurses*

Tonse N. K. Raju, MD, DCH—*National Institutes of Health*

STAFF

Jim Couto, MA

SECTION ON SURGERY EXECUTIVE COMMITTEE, 2011–2012

Mary L. Brandt, MD, Chairperson
Robert C. Shamberger MD, Immediate Past Chairperson
Michael G. Caty, MD
Kurt F. Heiss, MD
George W. Holcomb, III, MD
Rebecka L. Meyers, MD
R. Lawrence Moss, MD
Frederick J. Rescorla, MD

STAFF

Vivan Thorne

REFERENCES

1. Grosfeld JL. Current concepts in inguinal hernia in infants and children. *World J Surg.* 1989;13(5):506–515

2. Hughes IA, Acerini CL. Factors controlling testis descent. *Eur J Endocrinol.* 2008;159 (suppl 1):S75–S82

3. Beasley SW, Hutson JM. The role of the gubernaculum in testicular descent. *J Urol.* 1988;140(5 pt 2):1191–1193

4. Skandalakis JE, Colborn GL, Androulakis JA, Skandalakis LJ, Pemberton LB. Embryologic and anatomic basis of inguinal herniorrhaphy. *Surg Clin North Am.* 1993;73(4):799–836

5. Al Shareef Y, Sourial M, Hutson JM. Exogenous calcitonin gene-related peptide perturbs the direction and length of gubernaculum in capsaicin-treated rats. *Pediatr Surg Int.* 2007; 23(4):305–308

6. Ting AY, Huynh J, Farmer P, et al. The role of hepatocyte growth factor in the humoral regulation of inguinal hernia closure. *J Pediatr Surg.* 2005;40(12):1865–1868

7. Hutson JM, Temelcos C. Could inguinal hernia be treated medically? *Med Hypotheses.* 2005;64(1):37–40

8. Brandt ML. Pediatric hernias. *Surg Clin North Am.* 2008;88(1):27–43, vii–viii

9. Osifo OD, Osaigbovo EO. Congenital hydrocele: prevalence and outcome among male children who underwent neonatal circumcision in Benin City, Nigeria. *J Pediatr Urol.* 2008;4(3):178–182

10. O'Neill J, Rowe M, Grosfeld J, Fonkalsrud E, Coran A, eds. *Inguinal Hernia and Hydrocele.*

Pediatric Surgery. Vol 2. 5th ed. St Louis, MO: Mosby; 1998:1071–1086

11. Snyder WH, Greany FM. Inguinal hernia. In: Mustard WT, Ravitch MM, Snyder WH, eds. *Pediatric Surgery.* 2nd ed. Chicago, IL: Year Book Medical; 1969: 692–704

12. Rowe MI, Copelson LW, Clatworthy HW. The patent processus vaginalis and the inguinal hernia. *J Pediatr Surg.* 1969;4(1):102–107

13. Holcomb GW, III, Morgan WM, III, Brock JW III. Laparoscopic evaluation for contralateral patent processus vaginalis: Part II. *J Pediatr Surg.* 1996;31(8):1170–1173

14. Wolf SA, Hopkins JW. Laparoscopic incidence of contralateral patent processus vaginalis in boys with clinical unilateral inguinal hernias. *J Pediatr Surg.* 1994;29 (8):1118–1120, discussion 1120–1121

15. Geisler DP, Jegathesan S, Parmley MC, McGee JM, Nolen MG, Broughan TA. Laparoscopic exploration for the clinically undetected hernia in infancy and childhood. *Am J Surg.* 2001;182(6):693–696

16. Saad S, Mansson J, Saad A, Goldfarb MA. Ten-year review of groin laparoscopy in 1001 pediatric patients with clinical unilateral inguinal hernia: an improved technique with transhernia multiple-channel scope. *J Pediatr Surg.* 2011;46(5):1011–1014

17. Snyder WH. *Pediatric Surgery.* Vol 1. Chicago, IL: Year Book Medical Publishers; 1962

18. McGregor DB, Halverson K, McVay CB. The unilateral pediatric inguinal hernia: Should the contralateral side by explored? *J Pediatr Surg.* 1980;15(3):313–317

19. Krieger NR, Shochat SJ, McGowan V, Hartman GE. Early hernia repair in the premature infant: long-term follow-up. *J Pediatr Surg.* 1994;29(8):978–981, discussion 981–982

20. Misra D, Hewitt G, Potts SR, Brown S, Boston VE. Inguinal herniotomy in young infants, with emphasis on premature neonates. *J Pediatr Surg.* 1994;29(11):1496–1498

21. Puri P, Guiney EJ, O'Donnell B. Inguinal hernia in infants: the fate of the testis following incarceration. *J Pediatr Surg.* 1984; 19(1):44–46

22. Rescorla FJ, Grosfeld JL. Inguinal hernia repair in the perinatal period and early infancy: clinical considerations. *J Pediatr Surg.* 1984;19(6):832–837

23. Zamakhshary M, To T, Guan J, Langer JC. Risk of incarceration of inguinal hernia among infants and young children awaiting elective surgery. *CMAJ.* 2008;179(10):1001–1005

24. Vaos G, Gardikis S, Kambouri K, Sigalas I, Kourakis G, Petoussis G. Optimal timing for repair of an inguinal hernia in premature infants. *Pediatr Surg Int.* 2010;26(4):379–385

25. Lautz TB, Raval MV, Reynolds M. Does timing matter? A national perspective on the risk of incarceration in premature neonates with inguinal hernia. *J Pediatr.* 2011;158(4):573–577

26. Lee SL, Gleason JM, Sydorak RM. A critical review of premature infants with inguinal hernias: optimal timing of repair, incarceration risk, and postoperative apnea. *J Pediatr Surg.* 2011;46(1):217–220

27. Uemura S, Woodward AA, Amerena R, Drew J. Early repair of inguinal hernia in premature babies. *Pediatr Surg Int.* 1999;15(1): 36–39

28. Ein SH, Njere I, Ein A. Six thousand three hundred sixty-one pediatric inguinal hernias: a 35-year review. *J Pediatr Surg.* 2006; 41(5):980–986

29. Skinner MA, Grosfeld JL. Inguinal and umbilical hernia repair in infants and children. *Surg Clin North Am.* 1993;73(3):439–449

30. Harvey MH, Johnstone MJ, Fossard DP. Inguinal herniotomy in children: a five year survey. *Br J Surg.* 1985;72(6):485–487

31. Hecker WC, Ring-Mrozik E. Results of follow-up of operations in pediatric patients with indirect inguinal hernia [in German]. *Langenbecks Arch Chir.* 1987;371(2):115–121

32. Zendejas B, Zarroug AE, Erben YM, Holley CT, Farley DR. Impact of childhood inguinal hernia repair in adulthood: 50 years of follow-up. *J Am Coll Surg.* 2010;211(6):762–768

33. Moss RL, Hatch EI Jr;. Inguinal hernia repair in early infancy. *Am J Surg.* 1991;161 (5):596–599

34. Baird R, Gholoum S, Laberge JM, Puligandla P. Prematurity, not age at operation or incarceration, impacts complication rates of inguinal hernia repair. *J Pediatr Surg.* 2011;46(5):908–911

35. Welborn LG, Hannallah RS, Luban NL, Fink R, Ruttimann UE. Anemia and postoperative apnea in former preterm infants. *Anesthesiology.* 1991;74(6):1003–1006

36. Malviya S, Swartz J, Lerman J. Are all preterm infants younger than 60 weeks postconceptual age at risk for post-anesthetic apnea? *Anesthesiology.* 1993;78 (6):1076–1081

37. Liu LM, Coté CJ, Goudsouzian NG, et al. Life-threatening apnea in infants recovering from anesthesia. *Anesthesiology.* 1983;59 (6):506–510

38. Coté CJ, Zaslavsky A, Downes JJ, et al. Postoperative apnea in former preterm infants after inguinal herniorrhaphy. A combined analysis. *Anesthesiology.* 1995;82 (4):809–822

39. Allen GS, Cox CS, Jr;White N, Khalil S, Rabb M, Lally KP. Postoperative respiratory complications in ex-premature infants after inguinal herniorrhaphy. *J Pediatr Surg.* 1998;33(7):1095–1098

40. Walther-Larsen S, Rasmussen LS. The former preterm infant and risk of postoperative apnoea: recommendations for management. *Acta Anaesthesiol Scand.* 2006;50(7):888–893

41. Gallagher TM, Crean PM. Spinal anaesthesia in infants born prematurely. *Anaesthesia.* 1989;44(5):434–436

42. Schwartz N, Eisenkraft JB, Dolgin S. Spinal anesthesia for the high-risk infant. *Mt Sinai J Med.* 1988;55(5):399–403

43. Welborn LG, Rice LJ, Hannallah RS, Broadman LM, Ruttimann UE, Fink R. Postoperative apnea in former preterm infants: prospective comparison of spinal and general anesthesia. *Anesthesiology.* 1990;72(5):838–842

44. Craven PD, Badawi N, Henderson-Smart DJ, O'Brien M. Regional (spinal, epidural, caudal) versus general anaesthesia in preterm infants undergoing inguinal herniorrhaphy in early infancy. *Cochrane Database Syst Rev.* 2003;(3):CD003669

45. Jevtovic-Todorovic V, Hartman RE, Izumi Y, et al. Early exposure to common anesthetic agents causes widespread neurodegeneration in the developing rat brain and persistent learning deficits. *J Neurosci.* 2003;23(3):876–882

46. Slikker W, Jr;Zou X, Hotchkiss CE, et al. Ketamine-induced neuronal cell death in the perinatal rhesus monkey. *Toxicol Sci.* 2007;98(1):145–158

47. Fredriksson A, Pontén E, Gordh T, Eriksson P. Neonatal exposure to a combination of N-methyl-D-aspartate and gamma-aminobutyric acid type A receptor anesthetic agents potentiates apoptotic neurodegeneration and persistent behavioral deficits. *Anesthesiology.* 2007;107(3):427–436

48. Wilder RT, Flick RP, Sprung J, et al. Early exposure to anesthesia and learning disabilities in a population-based birth cohort. *Anesthesiology.* 2009;110(4):796–804

49. DiMaggio C, Sun LS, Kakavouli A, Byrne MW, Li G. A retrospective cohort study of the association of anesthesia and hernia repair surgery with behavioral and developmental disorders in young children. *J Neurosurg Anesthesiol.* 2009;21(4):286–291

50. Bartels M, Althoff RR, Boomsma DI. Anesthesia and cognitive performance in children: no evidence for a causal relationship. *Twin Res Hum Genet.* 2009;12 (3):246–253

51. Hansen TG, Pedersen JK, Henneberg SW, et al. Academic performance in adolescence after inguinal hernia repair in infancy: a nationwide cohort study. *Anesthesiology.* 2011;114(5):1076–1085

52. Sun L. Early childhood general anaesthesia exposure and neurocognitive development. *Br J Anaesth.* 2010;105(suppl 1):i61–i68

53. Antonoff MB, Kreykes NS, Saltzman DA, Acton RD. American Academy of Pediatrics Section on Surgery hernia survey revisited. *J Pediatr Surg.* 2005;40(6):1009–1014

54. Wiener ES, Touloukian RJ, Rodgers BM, et al. Hernia survey of the Section on Surgery of the American Academy of Pediatrics. *J Pediatr Surg.* 1996;31(8):1166–1169

55. Marulaiah M, Atkinson J, Kukkady A, Brown S, Samarakkody U. Is contralateral exploration necessary in preterm infants with unilateral inguinal hernia? *J Pediatr Surg.* 2006;41(12):2004–2007

56. Valusek PA, Spilde TL, Ostlie DJ, et al. Laparoscopic evaluation for contralateral patent processus vaginalis in children with unilateral inguinal hernia. *J Laparoendosc Adv Surg Tech A.* 2006;16(6):650–653

57. Ron O, Eaton S, Pierro A. Systematic review of the risk of developing a metachronous contralateral inguinal hernia in children. *Br J Surg.* 2007;94(7):804–811

58. Lee SL, Sydorak RM, Lau ST. Laparoscopic contralateral groin exploration: is it cost effective? *J Pediatr Surg.* 2010;45(4):793–795

59. Miltenburg DM, Nuchtern JG, Jaksic T, Kozinetiz C, Brandt ML. Laparoscopic evaluation of the pediatric inguinal hernia—a meta-analysis. *J Pediatr Surg.* 1998;33(6): 874–879

60. Schier F, Montupet P, Esposito C. Laparoscopic inguinal herniorrhaphy in children: a three-center experience with 933 repairs. *J Pediatr Surg.* 2002;37(3):395–397

61. Dutta S, Albanese C. Transcutaneous laparoscopic hernia repair in children: a prospective review of 275 hernia repairs with minimum 2-year follow-up. *Surg Endosc.* 2009;23(1):103–107

62. Schier F. Laparoscopic inguinal hernia repair-a prospective personal series of 542 children. *J Pediatr Surg.* 2006;41(6):1081–1084

63. Takehara H, Yakabe S, Kameoka K. Laparoscopic percutaneous extraperitoneal closure for inguinal hernia in children: clinical outcome of 972 repairs done in 3 pediatric surgical institutions. *J Pediatr Surg.* 2006; 41(12):1999–2003

64. Chan KL, Hui WC, Tam PK. Prospective randomized single-center, single-blind comparison of laparoscopic vs open repair of pediatric inguinal hernia. *Surg Endosc.* 2005;19(7):927–932

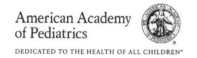

American Academy
of Pediatrics
DEDICATED TO THE HEALTH OF ALL CHILDREN™

Guidance for the Clinician in
Rendering Pediatric Care

CLINICAL REPORT

Hypothermia and Neonatal Encephalopathy

abstract

Data from large randomized clinical trials indicate that therapeutic hypothermia, using either selective head cooling or systemic cooling, is an effective therapy for neonatal encephalopathy. Infants selected for cooling must meet the criteria outlined in published clinical trials. The implementation of cooling needs to be performed at centers that have the capability to manage medically complex infants. Because the majority of infants who have neonatal encephalopathy are born at community hospitals, centers that perform cooling should work with their referring hospitals to implement education programs focused on increasing the awareness and identification of infants at risk for encephalopathy, and the initial clinical management of affected infants. *Pediatrics* 2014;133:1146–1150

COMMITTEE ON FETUS AND NEWBORN

KEY WORDS
hypothermia, hyperthermia, neonatal encephalopathy, infant, head cooling

ABBREVIATIONS
aEEG—amplitude-integrated electroencephalography
EEG—electroencephalography
CI—confidence interval
NICHD—National Institute of Child Health and Human Development
RR—relative risk

BACKGROUND

In 2005, the National Institute of Child Health and Human Development (NICHD) convened a workshop to evaluate the status of knowledge regarding the safety and efficacy of hypothermia as a neuroprotective therapy for neonatal hypoxic-ischemic encephalopathy.[1] Shortly thereafter, the Committee on Fetus and Newborn of the American Academy of Pediatrics published a commentary supporting the recommendation of the workshop that the widespread implementation of hypothermia outside the limits of controlled trials was premature.[2] In 2010, the *Eunice Kennedy Shriver* NICHD organized a follow-up to the 2005 workshop to review available evidence.[3] The purpose of this clinical report is to review briefly the current knowledge regarding the efficacy and safety of therapeutic hypothermia, to point out major gaps in knowledge that were identified at the 2010 workshop, and to suggest a framework for the implementation of hypothermia. The intended audience is neonatal/perinatal medicine practitioners.

PRELIMINARY STUDIES

Neuronal rescue of encephalopathic newborn infants using induced hypothermia is one of the few therapeutic modalities in neonatology that was studied extensively in animal models before clinical application in humans. From animal studies, it was noted that cooling the brain to approximately 32°C to 34°C starting within 5.5 hours after a hypoxic/ischemic insult and continuing to cool for 12 to 72 hours resulted in improved neuropathologic and functional outcomes.[4] After showing consistent benefit in animal models, the safety, feasibility, and practicality of using induced hypothermia in infants who have neonatal encephalopathy were investigated in

www.pediatrics.org/cgi/doi/10.1542/peds.2014-0899

doi:10.1542/peds.2014-0899

PEDIATRICS (ISSN Numbers: Print, 0031-4005; Online, 1098-4275).

several small studies. Data from these preliminary clinical studies indicated that reducing body temperature by 2°C to 3°C for a prolonged period of time was possible and that the changes in blood pressure, heart rate, and cardiac output noted were of little clinical significance.[5–7]

Large Randomized Clinical Trials of Hypothermic Neural Rescue (Table 1)

Six large randomized clinical trials of induced hypothermia for neonatal encephalopathy were published from 2005 to 2011.[8–13] Although there were some differences in the method of cooling and selection of subjects, in all trials infants were at least 35 weeks' gestation at birth; randomization was completed within 6 hours of birth; the target temperature was 33.5°C to 34.5°C; the intervention period was 72 hours, followed by slow rewarming (0.5°C/hour); and the primary outcome measure was the combined rate of death or disability, assessed at 18 to 22 months of age. Some trials used preferential head cooling with mild body cooling,[8,11] and others used whole-body cooling[9,10,12,13]; however, all trials continuously monitored both the degree of cooling and core body temperature. In addition, 3 trials used either amplitude-integrated electroencephalography (aEEG) or electroencephalography (EEG) for the assessment of severity of encephalopathy and enrollment of infants.[8,10,12]

Each of the 6 published trials was powered to detect a difference in the primary composite outcome of death or disability at 18 to 24 months of age, and all showed a benefit with cooling; in 4 of the 6 studies, this reached statistical significance. Rates of death or disability were similar in the control groups for 4 of the 6 studies, suggesting that patient selection and treatment were likely similar in these trials.[8–10,13] A published meta-analysis that included a small pilot study[5] as well as the 6 large published clinical trials demonstrated a reduction in the relative risk (RR) of the composite outcome of death or major neurodevelopmental disability at 18 to 24 months of age by 24% (RR, 0.76; 95% confidence interval [CI], 0.69–0.84).[14] A beneficial effect was noted both in infants who had moderate encephalopathy (RR, 0.67; 95% CI, 0.56–0.81) and those who had severe encephalopathy (RR 0.83; 95% CI, 0.74–0.92). The number of infants who need to be treated to prevent 1 infant from dying or becoming disabled is 6 for infants who have moderate encephalopathy and 7 for those who have severe encephalopathy. A review by the Cochrane collaboration that included 11 randomized controlled trials comprising 1505 term and late preterm infants who had moderate/severe encephalopathy demonstrated similar results.[15] The reduction in death or major neurodevelopmental disability to 18 months of age for treated infants was 25% overall; 32% for infants who had moderate encephalopathy and

TABLE 1 Therapeutic Hypothermia Clinical Trials

Clinical Trial	Entry Criteria
CoolCap	Gestational age ≥36 weeks and ≤6 hours of age AND Apgar score ≤5 at 10 minutes after birth OR Continued need for resuscitation at 10 minutes after birth OR pH <7.00 or base deficit ≥16 mmol/L or more on an umbilical cord blood sample or an arterial or venous blood sample obtained within 60 minutes of birth AND Moderate or severe encephalopathy on clinical examination AND Moderately or severely abnormal background of at least 20 minutes' duration or seizure activity on amplitude integrated electroencephalogram (aEEG) after one hour of age
Whole Body Cooling	Gestational age ≥36 weeks and ≤6 hours of age AND pH ≤7.00 or base deficit ≥16 mmol/L in an umbilical cord blood sample or any blood sample obtained within the first hour after birth[a] AND Moderate or severe encephalopathy on clinical examination
TOBY	Gestational age ≥36 weeks and ≤6 hours of age AND Apgar score ≤5 at 10 minutes after birth OR Continued need for resuscitation 10 minutes after birth OR pH <7.00 or base deficit ≥16 mmol/L on umbilical cord or arterial or capillary blood sample obtained within 60 minutes after birth AND Moderate or severe encephalopathy on clinical examination AND Abnormal background activity of at least 30 minutes' duration or seizures on amplitude integrated electroencephalogram (aEEG)

[a] If blood gas is not available or pH is between 7.01 and 7.15 or base deficit is between 10 and 15.9 mmol/L on blood sample obtained within the first hour of birth, two additional criteria are needed: a history of an acute perinatal event (eg, cord prolapse, fetal heart rate decelerations) and either the need for assisted ventilation initiated at birth and continued for 10 minutes or an Apgar score ≤5 at 10 minutes after birth.

18% for those who had severe encephalopathy.

Follow-up beyond infancy has been reported for subjects enrolled in the CoolCap trial and the NICHD Whole-Body Cooling trial.[16,17] Because the follow-up rate at 7 to 8 years of age was only 50% in the CoolCap trial, there were insufficient data to ascertain the long-term risk or benefits of selective head cooling. In the NICHD follow-up study, there was no statistical difference in the composite primary outcome of death or IQ <70 at 6 to 7 years of age between the treated and usual care cohorts ($P = .06$). Hypothermia treatment was associated with a reduction in the secondary outcomes of death (RR, 0.66; 95% CI, 0.45–0.97) and death or cerebral palsy (RR, 0.71; 95% CI, 0.54–0.95).

Observations From Large Clinical Trials

Adverse effects observed with hypothermia were infrequent in the target temperature ranges used in published clinical trials. The most common adverse effects were sinus bradycardia and prolongation of the QT interval on electrocardiogram, both of which are physiologic responses to hypothermia. Reddening or hardening of the skin (systemic hypothermia) and on the scalp (selective head cooling) and subcutaneous fat necrosis occurred rarely. The reported rates of coagulopathy, sepsis, and pneumonia were essentially the same in treated and control infants. When published studies were aggregated in a meta-analysis, the adverse effects of hypothermia included an increase in sinus bradycardia and a significant increase in thrombocytopenia (platelet count <150 000/mm^3).[15]

Both the TOBY and NICHD trial noted an adverse effect of pyrexia on neurologic outcome among infants allocated to standard care.[18,19] In both

trials, approximately 30% of the control group had a rectal or esophageal temperature greater than 38°C recorded on at least 1 occasion. The risk for death or disability among infants who had an elevated rectal temperature was increased by threefold in the TOBY trial, whereas in the NICHD trial, the risk for adverse outcome was increased threefold to fourfold, with each degree Celsius increase in the highest quartile of esophageal temperature. It is not known whether the elevated temperatures observed in the 2 trials caused additional brain injury or whether the elevated temperatures were the manifestation of existing hypoxic-ischemic brain injury.

Knowledge Gained From Large Clinical Trials

Approximately 1200 infants were enrolled in the 6 large clinical trials of therapeutic hypothermia. Analyses of aggregate data, as well as data from registries, indicate that moderate hypothermia initiated within 6 hours of birth and continued for 72 hours is a safe and modestly effective neural rescue strategy for infants born at greater than 35 weeks of gestational age who have clinical evidence of moderate or severe neonatal encephalopathy.

Areas of Uncertainty

Because there was little variability among published clinical trials, questions remain regarding the optimal timing for the initiation of cooling and the depth and duration of therapy. There are several ongoing randomized clinical trials that are designed to assess the efficacy of initiating cooling between 6 and 12 hours of age, using a deeper depth of cooling (32°C), or cooling for a longer duration (120 hours) (NCT 01192776, NCT 00614744). In addition, information regarding the safety and efficacy of cooling treatment of encephalopathic infants born

at less than 35 weeks of gestational age is lacking, but preliminary information may be available in the near future (NCT 1793129).

There is also uncertainty regarding the safety and efficacy of initiating cooling before transfer to a center offering therapeutic hypothermia. However, data from the Vermont Oxford Encephalopathic Registry indicate that as many as a third of encephalopathic infants, many of whom were born in other facilities, were not admitted to a neonatal ICU until after 6 hours of age.[20] In a study in which active cooling with cool packs was started on arrival of the transport team at the referring center, approximately one-third of the 35 infants had a rectal temperature below 32°C on arrival at the cooling center.[21] A similar rate of excessive cooling on arrival was noted when passive cooling was used (3 of 18 infants).[22] Using a carefully designed protocol for passive cooling at the referral hospital and on transport, Kendall et al noted that 67% of the 39 infants were within target temperature range (33°C–34°C) on arrival at the cooling center, and 11% had a rectal temperature below 32°C.[23] There have been 2 observational studies from the United Kingdom of servo-controlled cooling in the field.[24,25] Application of this mode of cooling led to significantly less overcooling and greater success in maintaining rectal temperature in the target range when compared with passive cooling.

Clinical Trials of Adjuvant Therapies for Neonatal Encephalopathy

Because the incidence of death and disability remains high after treatment with cooling (approximately 40%), there is an urgent need for additional therapies to further improve outcomes of infants who have acute encephalopathy. Promising neuroprotective agents include antiepileptic drugs, erythropoietin, melatonin, and xenon. Phase I and II trials of xenon (NCT 00934700, NCT 01545271) and topiramate (NCT 01241019, NCT 01765218) as adjuvant therapy to hypothermia are underway. A phase II study of erythropoietin using doses of 1000 U/kg intravenously in infants undergoing cooling is planned (NCT 01913340) and a phase I and II study of darbepoetin as concurrent therapy with cooling is in progress.[26] There is also a phase I–II study assessing the safety and efficacy of clonidine therapy during cooling for neonatal encephalopathy (NCT 01862250).

CONCLUSIONS

1. Medical centers offering hypothermia should be capable of providing comprehensive clinical care, including mechanical ventilation; physiologic (vital signs, temperature) and biochemical (blood gas) monitoring; neuroimaging, including MRI; seizure detection and monitoring with aEEG or EEG; neurologic consultation; and a system in place for monitoring longitudinal neurodevelopmental outcome.

2. Infants offered hypothermia should meet inclusion criteria outlined in published clinical trials (see Table 1). Eligibility criteria include a pH of ≤7.0 or a base deficit of ≥16 mmol/L in a sample of umbilical cord blood or blood obtained during the first hour after birth,

history of an acute perinatal event, a 10-minute Apgar score of <5, or assisted ventilation initiated at birth and continued for at least 10 minutes. In addition, a neurologic examination demonstrating moderate to severe encephalopathy is essential. If preferential head cooling is used, an abnormal background activity on either EEG or aEEG also is required.

3. Training programs and infrastructure need to be established and maintained in a highly organized and reproducible manner to ensure patient safety. Each center offering hypothermia therapy needs to develop a written protocol and monitor management and outcomes. Training needs to include awareness and timely identification of infants at risk for encephalopathy and an appropriate assessment of infants who have encephalopathy. Educational endeavors need to involve obstetric care providers; labor, delivery, nursery, and postpartum personnel; and pediatric care providers.

4. Outreach education to community hospitals needs to be implemented. Specific issues include the awareness and timely identification of infants at risk for encephalopathy and prevention of extreme hypothermia and hyperthermia.

5. Cooling infants who are born at less than 35 weeks' gestation or those who have mild encephalopathy, cooling for longer than 72 hours, cooling at a temperature lower than that used in published clinical trials, and the use of adjuvant therapies should only be performed in a research setting and with informed parental consent.

LEAD AUTHOR

Lu-Ann Papile, MD, FAAP

COMMITTEE ON FETUS AND NEWBORN, 2012–2013

Lu-Ann Papile, MD, FAAP, Chairperson
Jill E. Baley, MD, FAAP
William Benitz, MD, FAAP
James Cummings, MD, FAAP
Waldemar A. Carlo, MD, FAAP
Eric Eichenwald, MD, FAAP
Praveen Kumar, MD, FAAP
Richard A. Polin, MD, FAAP
Rosemarie C. Tan, MD, PhD, FAAP
Kasper S. Wang, MD, FAAP

LIAISONS

CAPT Wanda Denise Barfield, MD, MPH, FAAP – *Centers for Disease Control and Prevention*
George Macones, MD – *American College of Obstetricians and Gynecologists*
Ann L. Jefferies, MD – *Canadian Paediatric Society*
Erin L. Keels APRN, MS, NNP-BC – *National Association of Neonatal Nurses*
Tonse N. K. Raju, MD, DCH, FAAP – *National Institutes of Health*

STAFF

Jim Couto, MA

REFERENCES

1. Higgins RD, Raju TNK, Perlman J, et al. Hypothermia and perinatal asphyxia: executive summary of the National Institute of Child Health and Human Development workshop. *J Pediatr.* 2006;148(2):170–175

2. Blackmon LR, Stark AR; American Academy of Pediatrics Committee on Fetus and Newborn. Hypothermia: a neuroprotective therapy for neonatal hypoxic-ischemic encephalopathy. *Pediatrics.* 2006;117(3):942–948

3. Higgins RD, Raju T, Edwards D, et al. Hypothermia and other treatment options for neonatal encephalopathy: an executive summary of the Eunice Kennedy Shriver NICHD Workshop. *J Pediatr.* 2011:159(5).e1–858.e1

4. Gunn AJ, Gunn TR. The 'pharmacology' of neuronal rescue with cerebral hypothermia. *Early Hum Dev.* 1998;53(1):19–35

5. Gunn AJ, Gluckman PD, Gunn TR. Selective head cooling in newborn infants after

perinatal asphyxia: a safety study. *Pediatrics.* 1998;102(4 pt 1):885–892

6. Azzopardi D, Robertson NJ, Cowan FM, Rutherford MA, Rampling M, Edwards AD. Pilot study of treatment with whole body hypothermia for neonatal encephalopathy. *Pediatrics.* 2000;106(4):684–694

7. Gebauer CM, Knuepfer M, Robel-Tillig E, Pulzer F, Vogtmann C. Hemodynamics among neonates with hypoxic-ischemic encephalopathy during whole-body hypothermia and

passive rewarming. *Pediatrics*. 2006;117(3): 843–850

8. Gluckman PD, Wyatt JS, Azzopardi D, et al. Selective head cooling with mild systemic hypothermia after neonatal encephalopathy: multicentre randomised trial. *Lancet*. 2005;365(9460):663–670

9. Shankaran S, Laptook AR, Ehrenkranz RA, et al; National Institute of Child Health and Human Development Neonatal Research Network. Whole-body hypothermia for neonates with hypoxic-ischemic encephalopathy. *N Engl J Med*. 2005;353(15):1574–1584

10. Azzopardi DV, Strohm B, Edwards AD, et al; TOBY Study Group. Moderate hypothermia to treat perinatal asphyxial encephalopathy. *N Engl J Med*. 2009;361(14):1349–1358

11. Zhou WH, Cheng GQ, Shao XM, et al; China Study Group. Selective head cooling with mild systemic hypothermia after neonatal hypoxic-ischemic encephalopathy: a multicenter randomized controlled trial in China. *J Pediatr*. 2010;157(3):367–372, e1–e3

12. Simbruner G, Mittal RA, Rohlmann F, Muche R; neo.nEURO.network Trial Participants. Systemic hypothermia after neonatal encephalopathy: outcomes of neo.nEURO.network RCT. *Pediatrics*. 2010;126(4). Available at: www.pediatrics.org/cgi/content/full/126/4/e771

13. Jacobs SE, Morley CJ, Inder TE, et al; Infant Cooling Evaluation Collaboration. Whole-body hypothermia for term and near-term newborns with hypoxic-ischemic encepha-lopathy: a randomized controlled trial. *Arch Pediatr Adolesc Med*. 2011;165(8):692–700

14. Tagin MA, Woolcott CG, Vincer MJ, Whyte RK, Stinson DA. Hypothermia for neonatal hypoxic ischemic encephalopathy: an updated systematic review and meta-analysis. *Arch Pediatr Adolesc Med*. 2012;166(6):558–566

15. Jacobs SE, Berg M, Hunt R, et al. Cooling for newborns with hypoxic ischaemic encephalopathy. *Cochrane Database Syst Rev* 2013;(1):CD003311. doi: 10. 1002/14651858. CD003311.pub3. Review

16. Shankaran S, Pappas A, McDonald SA, et al; Eunice Kennedy Shriver NICHD Neonatal Research Network. Childhood outcomes after hypothermia for neonatal encephalopathy. *N Engl J Med*. 2012;366(22):2085–2092

17. Guillet R, Edwards AD, Thorenson M, et al. CoolCap Trial Group. Seven-to eight year follow-up of the CoolCap trial of head cooling for neonatal encephalopathy. *Pediatr Res*. 2012;71(2):205–209

18. Wyatt JS, Gluckman PD, Liu PY, et al. Cool-Cap Study Group. Determination of outcomes after head cooling for neonatal encephalopathy. *Pediatrics*. 2007;119(5): 912–921

19. Laptook A, Tyson J, Shankaran S, et al; National Institute of Child Health and Human Development Neonatal Research Network. Elevated temperature after hypoxic-ischemic encephalopathy: risk factor for adverse outcomes. *Pediatrics*. 2008;122(3):491–499

20. Pfister RH, Bingham P, Edwards EM, et al. The Vermont Oxford Neonatal Encephalopathy Registry: rationale, methods, and initial results. *BMC Pediatr*. 2012;12:84

21. Fairchild K, Sokora D, Scott J, Zanelli S. Therapeutic hypothermia on neonatal transport: 4-year experience in a single NICU. *J Perinatol*. 2010;30(5):324–329

22. Hallberg B, Olson L, Bartocci M, Edqvist I, Blennow M. Passive induction of hypothermia during transport of asphyxiated infants: a risk of excessive cooling. *Acta Paediatr*. 2009;98(6):942–946

23. Kendall GS, Kapetanakis A, Ratnavel N, Azzopardi D, Robertson NJ; Cooling on Retrieval Study Group. Passive cooling for initiation of therapeutic hypothermia in neonatal encephalopathy. *Arch Dis Child Fetal Neonatal Ed*. 2010;95(6):F408–F412

24. Johnston ED, Becher J-C, Mitchell AP, Stenson BJ. Provision of servo-controlled cooling during neonatal transport. *Arch Dis Child Fetal Neonatal Ed*. 2012;97(5): F365–F367

25. Chaudhary R, Farrer K, Broster S, McRitchie L, Austin T. Active versus passive cooling during neonatal transport. *Pediatrics*. 2013;132(5):841–846

26. Wu YW, Bauer LA, Ballard RA, et al. Erythropoietin for neuroprotection in neonatal encephalopathy: safety and pharmacokinetics. *Pediatrics*. 2012;130(4):683–691

AMERICAN ACADEMY OF PEDIATRICS

CLINICAL PRACTICE GUIDELINE

Subcommittee on Hyperbilirubinemia

Management of Hyperbilirubinemia in the Newborn Infant 35 or More Weeks of Gestation

ABSTRACT. Jaundice occurs in most newborn infants. Most jaundice is benign, but because of the potential toxicity of bilirubin, newborn infants must be monitored to identify those who might develop severe hyperbilirubinemia and, in rare cases, acute bilirubin encephalopathy or kernicterus. The focus of this guideline is to reduce the incidence of severe hyperbilirubinemia and bilirubin encephalopathy while minimizing the risks of unintended harm such as maternal anxiety, decreased breastfeeding, and unnecessary costs or treatment. Although kernicterus should almost always be preventable, cases continue to occur. These guidelines provide a framework for the prevention and management of hyperbilirubinemia in newborn infants of 35 or more weeks of gestation. In every infant, we recommend that clinicians 1) promote and support successful breastfeeding; 2) perform a systematic assessment before discharge for the risk of severe hyperbilirubinemia; 3) provide early and focused follow-up based on the risk assessment; and 4) when indicated, treat newborns with phototherapy or exchange transfusion to prevent the development of severe hyperbilirubinemia and, possibly, bilirubin encephalopathy (kernicterus). *Pediatrics* 2004; 114:297–316; *hyperbilirubinemia, newborn, kernicterus, bilirubin encephalopathy, phototherapy.*

ABBREVIATIONS. AAP, American Academy of Pediatrics; TSB, total serum bilirubin; TcB, transcutaneous bilirubin; G6PD, glucose-6-phosphate dehydrogenase; $ETCO_c$, end-tidal carbon monoxide corrected for ambient carbon monoxide; B/A, bilirubin/albumin; UB, unbound bilirubin.

BACKGROUND

In October 1994, the Provisional Committee for Quality Improvement and Subcommittee on Hyperbilirubinemia of the American Academy of Pediatrics (AAP) produced a practice parameter dealing with the management of hyperbilirubinemia in the healthy term newborn.[1] The current guideline represents a consensus of the committee charged by the AAP with reviewing and updating the existing guideline and is based on a careful review of the evidence, including a comprehensive literature review by the New England Medical Center Evidence-Based Practice Center.[2] (See "An Evidence-Based Review of Important Issues Concerning Neonatal Hyperbilirubinemia"[3] for a description of the methodology, questions addressed, and conclusions of this report.) This guideline is intended for use by hospitals and pediatricians, neonatologists, family physicians, physician assistants, and advanced practice nurses who treat newborn infants in the hospital and as outpatients. A list of frequently asked questions and answers for parents is available in English and Spanish at www.aap.org/family/jaundicefaq. htm.

DEFINITION OF RECOMMENDATIONS

The evidence-based approach to guideline development requires that the evidence in support of a policy be identified, appraised, and summarized and that an explicit link between evidence and recommendations be defined. Evidence-based recommendations are based on the quality of evidence and the balance of benefits and harms that is anticipated when the recommendation is followed. This guideline uses the definitions for quality of evidence and balance of benefits and harms established by the AAP Steering Committee on Quality Improvement Management.[4] See Appendix 1 for these definitions.

The draft practice guideline underwent extensive peer review by committees and sections within the AAP, outside organizations, and other individuals identified by the subcommittee as experts in the field. Liaison representatives to the subcommittee were invited to distribute the draft to other representatives and committees within their specialty organizations. The resulting comments were reviewed by the subcommittee and, when appropriate, incorporated into the guideline.

BILIRUBIN ENCEPHALOPATHY AND KERNICTERUS

Although originally a pathologic diagnosis characterized by bilirubin staining of the brainstem nuclei and cerebellum, the term "kernicterus" has come to be used interchangeably with both the acute and chronic findings of bilirubin encephalopathy. Bilirubin encephalopathy describes the clinical central nervous system findings caused by bilirubin toxicity to the basal ganglia and various brainstem nuclei. To avoid confusion and encourage greater consistency in the literature, the committee recommends that in infants the term "acute bilirubin encephalopathy" be used to describe the acute manifestations of bilirubin

PEDIATRICS (ISSN 0031 4005). Copyright © 2004 by the American Academy of Pediatrics.

toxicity seen in the first weeks after birth and that the term "kernicterus" be reserved for the chronic and permanent clinical sequelae of bilirubin toxicity.

See Appendix 1 for the clinical manifestations of acute bilirubin encephalopathy and kernicterus.

FOCUS OF GUIDELINE

The overall aim of this guideline is to promote an approach that will reduce the frequency of severe neonatal hyperbilirubinemia and bilirubin encephalopathy and minimize the risk of unintended harm such as increased anxiety, decreased breastfeeding, or unnecessary treatment for the general population and excessive cost and waste. Recent reports of kernicterus indicate that this condition, although rare, is still occurring.[2,5–10]

Analysis of these reported cases of kernicterus suggests that if health care personnel follow the recommendations listed in this guideline, kernicterus would be largely preventable.

These guidelines emphasize the importance of universal systematic assessment for the risk of severe hyperbilirubinemia, close follow-up, and prompt intervention when indicated. The recommendations apply to the care of infants at 35 or more weeks of gestation. These recommendations seek to further the aims defined by the Institute of Medicine as appropriate for health care:[11] safety, effectiveness, efficiency, timeliness, patient-centeredness, and equity. They specifically emphasize the principles of patient safety and the key role of timeliness of interventions to prevent adverse outcomes resulting from neonatal hyperbilirubinemia.

The following are the key elements of the recommendations provided by this guideline. Clinicians should:

1. Promote and support successful breastfeeding.
2. Establish nursery protocols for the identification and evaluation of hyperbilirubinemia.
3. Measure the total serum bilirubin (TSB) or transcutaneous bilirubin (TcB) level on infants jaundiced in the first 24 hours.
4. Recognize that visual estimation of the degree of jaundice can lead to errors, particularly in darkly pigmented infants.
5. Interpret all bilirubin levels according to the infant's age in hours.
6. Recognize that infants at less than 38 weeks' gestation, particularly those who are breastfed, are at higher risk of developing hyperbilirubinemia and require closer surveillance and monitoring.
7. Perform a systematic assessment on all infants before discharge for the risk of severe hyperbilirubinemia.
8. Provide parents with written and verbal information about newborn jaundice.
9. Provide appropriate follow-up based on the time of discharge and the risk assessment.
10. Treat newborns, when indicated, with phototherapy or exchange transfusion.

PRIMARY PREVENTION

In numerous policy statements, the AAP recommends breastfeeding for all healthy term and near-term newborns. This guideline strongly supports this general recommendation.

RECOMMENDATION 1.0: Clinicians should advise mothers to nurse their infants at least 8 to 12 times per day for the first several days[12] (evidence quality C: benefits exceed harms).

Poor caloric intake and/or dehydration associated with inadequate breastfeeding may contribute to the development of hyperbilirubinemia.[6,13,14] Increasing the frequency of nursing decreases the likelihood of subsequent significant hyperbilirubinemia in breast-fed infants.[15–17] Providing appropriate support and advice to breastfeeding mothers increases the likelihood that breastfeeding will be successful.

Additional information on how to assess the adequacy of intake in a breastfed newborn is provided in Appendix 1.

RECOMMENDATION 1.1: The AAP recommends against routine supplementation of nondehydrated breastfed infants with water or dextrose water (evidence quality B and C: harms exceed benefits).

Supplementation with water or dextrose water will not prevent hyperbilirubinemia or decrease TSB levels.[18,19]

SECONDARY PREVENTION

RECOMMENDATION 2.0: Clinicians should perform ongoing systematic assessments during the neonatal period for the risk of an infant developing severe hyperbilirubinemia.

Blood Typing

RECOMMENDATION 2.1: All pregnant women should be tested for ABO and Rh (D) blood types and have a serum screen for unusual isoimmune antibodies (evidence quality B: benefits exceed harms).

RECOMMENDATION 2.1.1: If a mother has not had prenatal blood grouping or is Rh-negative, a direct antibody test (or Coombs' test), blood type, and an Rh (D) type on the infant's (cord) blood are strongly recommended (evidence quality B: benefits exceed harms).

RECOMMENDATION 2.1.2: If the maternal blood is group O, Rh-positive, it is an option to test the cord blood for the infant's blood type and direct antibody test, but it is not required provided that there is appropriate surveillance, risk assessment before discharge, and follow-up[20] (evidence quality C: benefits exceed harms).

Clinical Assessment

RECOMMENDATION 2.2: Clinicians should ensure that all infants are routinely monitored for the development of jaundice, and nurseries should have established protocols for the assessment of jaundice. Jaundice should be assessed whenever the infant's vital signs are measured but no less than every 8 to 12 hours (evidence quality D: benefits versus harms exceptional).

In newborn infants, jaundice can be detected by blanching the skin with digital pressure, revealing the underlying color of the skin and subcutaneous tissue. The assessment of jaundice must be per-

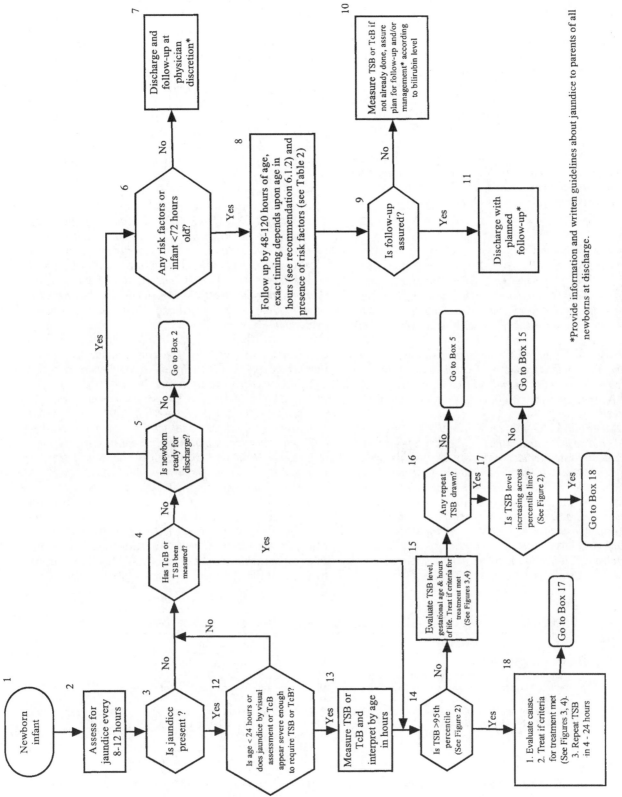

Fig 1. Algorithm for the management of jaundice in the newborn nursery.

*Provide information and written guidelines about jaundice to parents of all newborns at discharge.

formed in a well-lit room or, preferably, in daylight at a window. Jaundice is usually seen first in the face and progresses caudally to the trunk and extremities,[21] but visual estimation of bilirubin levels from the degree of jaundice can lead to errors.[22–24] In most infants with TSB levels of less than 15 mg/dL (257 μmol/L), noninvasive TcB-measurement devices can provide a valid estimate of the TSB level.[2,25–29] See Appendix 1 for additional information on the clinical evaluation of jaundice and the use of TcB measurements.

RECOMMENDATION 2.2.1: Protocols for the assessment of jaundice should include the circumstances in which nursing staff can obtain a TcB level or order a TSB measurement (evidence quality D: benefits versus harms exceptional).

Laboratory Evaluation

RECOMMENDATION 3.0: A TcB and/or TSB measurement should be performed on every infant who is jaundiced in the first 24 hours after birth (Fig 1 and Table 1)[30] (evidence quality C: benefits exceed harms). The need for and timing of a repeat TcB or TSB measurement will depend on the zone in which the TSB falls (Fig 2),[25,31] the age of the infant, and the evolution of the hyperbilirubinemia. Recommendations for TSB measurements after the age of 24 hours are provided in Fig 1 and Table 1.

See Appendix 1 for capillary versus venous bilirubin levels.

RECOMMENDATION 3.1: A TcB and/or TSB measurement should be performed if the jaundice appears excessive for the infant's age (evidence quality D: benefits versus harms exceptional). If there is any doubt about the degree of jaundice, the TSB or TcB should be measured. Visual estimation of bilirubin levels from the degree of jaundice can lead to errors, particularly in darkly pigmented infants (evidence quality C: benefits exceed harms).

RECOMMENDATION 3.2: All bilirubin levels should be interpreted according to the infant's age in hours (Fig 2) (evidence quality C: benefits exceed harms).

Cause of Jaundice

RECOMMENDATION 4.1: The possible cause of jaundice should be sought in an infant receiving phototherapy or whose TSB level is rising rapidly (ie, crossing percentiles [Fig 2]) and is not explained by the history and physical examination (evidence quality D: benefits versus harms exceptional).

RECOMMENDATION 4.1.1: Infants who have an elevation of direct-reacting or conjugated bilirubin should have a urinalysis and urine culture.[32] Additional laboratory evaluation for sepsis should be performed if indicated by history and physical examination (evidence quality C: benefits exceed harms).

See Appendix 1 for definitions of abnormal levels of direct-reacting and conjugated bilirubin.

RECOMMENDATION 4.1.2: Sick infants and those who are jaundiced at or beyond 3 weeks should have a measurement of total and direct or conjugated bilirubin to identify cholestasis (Table 1) (evidence quality D: benefit versus harms exceptional). The results of the newborn thyroid and galactosemia screen should also be checked in these infants (evidence quality D: benefits versus harms exceptional).

RECOMMENDATION 4.1.3: *If the direct-reacting or conjugated bilirubin level is elevated, additional evaluation for the causes of cholestasis is recommended (evidence quality C: benefits exceed harms).*

RECOMMENDATION 4.1.4: *Measurement of the glucose-6-phosphate dehydrogenase (G6PD) level is recommended for a jaundiced infant who is receiving phototherapy and whose family history or ethnic or geographic origin suggest the likelihood of G6PD deficiency or for an infant in whom the response to phototherapy is poor (Fig 3) (evidence quality C: benefits exceed harms).*

G6PD deficiency is widespread and frequently unrecognized, and although it is more common in the populations around the Mediterranean and in the Middle East, Arabian peninsula, Southeast Asia, and Africa, immigration and intermarriage have transformed G6PD deficiency into a global problem.[33,34]

TABLE 1. Laboratory Evaluation of the Jaundiced Infant of 35 or More Weeks' Gestation	
Indications	Assessments
Jaundice in first 24 h	Measure TcB and/or TSB
Jaundice appears excessive for infant's age	Measure TcB and/or TSB
Infant receiving phototherapy or TSB rising rapidly (ie, crossing percentiles [Fig 2]) and unexplained by history and physical examination	Blood type and Coombs' test, if not obtained with cord blood
	Complete blood count and smear
	Measure direct or conjugated bilirubin
	It is an option to perform reticulocyte count, G6PD, and ETCO$_c$, if available
	Repeat TSB in 4–24 h depending on infant's age and TSB level
TSB concentration approaching exchange levels or not responding to phototherapy	Perform reticulocyte count, G6PD, albumin, ETCO$_c$, if available
Elevated direct (or conjugated) bilirubin level	Do urinalysis and urine culture. Evaluate for sepsis if indicated by history and physical examination
Jaundice present at or beyond age 3 wk, or sick infant	Total and direct (or conjugated) bilirubin level
	If direct bilirubin elevated, evaluate for causes of cholestasis
	Check results of newborn thyroid and galactosemia screen, and evaluate infant for signs or symptoms of hypothyroidism

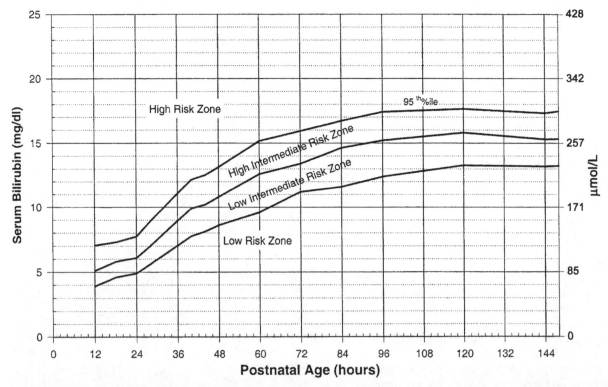

Fig 2. Nomogram for designation of risk in 2840 well newborns at 36 or more weeks' gestational age with birth weight of 2000 g or more or 35 or more weeks' gestational age and birth weight of 2500 g or more based on the hour-specific serum bilirubin values. The serum bilirubin level was obtained before discharge, and the zone in which the value fell predicted the likelihood of a subsequent bilirubin level exceeding the 95th percentile (high-risk zone) as shown in Appendix 1, Table 4. Used with permission from Bhutani et al.[31] See Appendix 1 for additional information about this nomogram, which should not be used to represent the natural history of neonatal hyperbilirubinemia.

Furthermore, G6PD deficiency occurs in 11% to 13% of African Americans, and kernicterus has occurred in some of these infants.[5,33] In a recent report, G6PD deficiency was considered to be the cause of hyperbilirubinemia in 19 of 61 (31.5%) infants who developed kernicterus.[5] (See Appendix 1 for additional information on G6PD deficiency.)

Risk Assessment Before Discharge

RECOMMENDATION 5.1: Before discharge, every newborn should be assessed for the risk of developing severe hyperbilirubinemia, and all nurseries should establish protocols for assessing this risk. Such assessment is particularly important in infants who are discharged before the age of 72 hours (evidence quality C: benefits exceed harms).

RECOMMENDATION 5.1.1: The AAP recommends 2 clinical options used individually or in combination for the systematic assessment of risk: predischarge measurement of the bilirubin level using TSB or TcB and/or assessment of clinical risk factors. Whether either or both options are used, appropriate follow-up after discharge is essential (evidence quality C: benefits exceed harms).

The best documented method for assessing the risk of subsequent hyperbilirubinemia is to measure the TSB or TcB level[25,31,35–38] and plot the results on a nomogram (Fig 2). A TSB level can be obtained at the time of the routine metabolic screen, thus obviating the need for an additional blood sample. Some authors have suggested that a TSB measurement should be part of the routine screening of all newborns.[5,31] An infant whose predischarge TSB is in the

low-risk zone (Fig 2) is at very low risk of developing severe hyperbilirubinemia.[5,38]

Table 2 lists those factors that are clinically signif-

TABLE 2. Risk Factors for Development of Severe Hyperbilirubinemia in Infants of 35 or More Weeks' Gestation (in Approximate Order of Importance)

Major risk factors
 Predischarge TSB or TcB level in the high-risk zone (Fig 2)[25,31]
 Jaundice observed in the first 24 h[30]
 Blood group incompatibility with positive direct antiglobulin test, other known hemolytic disease (eg, G6PD deficiency), elevated ETCO$_c$
 Gestational age 35–36 wk[39,40]
 Previous sibling received phototherapy[40,41]
 Cephalohematoma or significant bruising[39]
 Exclusive breastfeeding, particularly if nursing is not going well and weight loss is excessive[39,40]
 East Asian race[39]*
Minor risk factors
 Predischarge TSB or TcB level in the high intermediate-risk zone[25,31]
 Gestational age 37–38 wk[39,40]
 Jaundice observed before discharge[40]
 Previous sibling with jaundice[40,41]
 Macrosomic infant of a diabetic mother[42,43]
 Maternal age ≥25 y[39]
 Male gender[39,40]
Decreased risk (these factors are associated with decreased risk of significant jaundice, listed in order of decreasing importance)
 TSB or TcB level in the low-risk zone (Fig 2)[25,31]
 Gestational age ≥41 wk[39]
 Exclusive bottle feeding[39,40]
 Black race[38]*
 Discharge from hospital after 72 h[40,44]

* Race as defined by mother's description.

icant and most frequently associated with an increase in the risk of severe hyperbilirubinemia. But, because these risk factors are common and the risk of hyperbilirubinemia is small, individually the factors are of limited use as predictors of significant hyperbilirubinemia.[39] Nevertheless, if no risk factors are present, the risk of severe hyperbilirubinemia is extremely low, and the more risk factors present, the greater the risk of severe hyperbilirubinemia.[39] The important risk factors most frequently associated with severe hyperbilirubinemia are breastfeeding, gestation below 38 weeks, significant jaundice in a previous sibling, and jaundice noted before discharge.[39,40] A formula-fed infant of 40 or more weeks' gestation is at very low risk of developing severe hyperbilirubinemia.[39]

Hospital Policies and Procedures

RECOMMENDATION 6.1: *All hospitals should provide written and verbal information for parents at the time of discharge, which should include an explanation of jaundice, the need to monitor infants for jaundice, and advice on how monitoring should be done (evidence quality D: benefits versus harms exceptional).*

An example of a parent-information handout is available in English and Spanish at www.aap.org/family/jaundicefaq.htm.

Follow-up

RECOMMENDATION 6.1.1: *All infants should be examined by a qualified health care professional in the first few days after discharge to assess infant well-being and the presence or absence of jaundice. The timing and location of this assessment will be determined by the length of stay in the nursery, presence or absence of risk factors for hyperbilirubinemia (Table 2 and Fig 2), and risk of other neonatal problems (evidence quality C: benefits exceed harms).*

Timing of Follow-up

RECOMMENDATION 6.1.2: *Follow-up should be provided as follows:*

Infant Discharged	Should Be Seen by Age
Before age 24 h	72 h
Between 24 and 47.9 h	96 h
Between 48 and 72 h	120 h

For some newborns discharged before 48 hours, 2 follow-up visits may be required, the first visit between 24 and 72 hours and the second between 72 and 120 hours. Clinical judgment should be used in determining follow-up. Earlier or more frequent follow-up should be provided for those who have risk factors for hyperbilirubinemia (Table 2), whereas those discharged with few or no risk factors can be seen after longer intervals (evidence quality C: benefits exceed harms).

RECOMMENDATION 6.1.3: *If appropriate follow-up cannot be ensured in the presence of elevated risk for developing severe hyperbilirubinemia, it may be necessary to delay discharge either until appropriate follow-up can be ensured or the period of greatest risk has passed (72-96 hours) (evidence quality D: benefits versus harms exceptional).*

Follow-up Assessment

RECOMMENDATION 6.1.4: *The follow-up assessment should include the infant's weight and percent change from birth weight, adequacy of intake, the pattern of voiding and stooling, and the presence or absence of jaundice (evidence quality C: benefits exceed harms). Clinical judgment should be used to determine the need for a bilirubin measurement. If there is any doubt about the degree of jaundice, the TSB or TcB level should be measured. Visual estimation of bilirubin levels can lead to errors, particularly in darkly pigmented infants (evidence quality C: benefits exceed harms).*

See Appendix 1 for assessment of the adequacy of intake in breastfeeding infants.

TREATMENT

Phototherapy and Exchange Transfusion

RECOMMENDATION 7.1: *Recommendations for treatment are given in Table 3 and Figs 3 and 4 (evidence quality C: benefits exceed harms). If the TSB does not fall or continues to rise despite intensive phototherapy, it is very likely that hemolysis is occurring. The committee's recommendations for discontinuing phototherapy can be found in Appendix 2.*

RECOMMENDATION 7.1.1: *In using the guidelines for phototherapy and exchange transfusion (Figs 3 and 4), the direct-reacting (or conjugated) bilirubin level should not be subtracted from the total (evidence quality D: benefits versus harms exceptional).*

In unusual situations in which the direct bilirubin level is 50% or more of the total bilirubin, there are no good data to provide guidance for therapy, and consultation with an expert in the field is recommended.

RECOMMENDATION 7.1.2: *If the TSB is at a level at which exchange transfusion is recommended (Fig 4) or if the TSB level is 25 mg/dL (428 μmol/L) or higher at any time, it is a medical emergency and the infant should be admitted immediately and directly to a hospital pediatric service for intensive phototherapy. These infants should not be referred to the emergency department, because it delays the initiation of treatment[54] (evidence quality C: benefits exceed harms).*

RECOMMENDATION 7.1.3: *Exchange transfusions should be performed only by trained personnel in a neonatal intensive care unit with full monitoring and resuscitation capabilities (evidence quality D: benefits versus harms exceptional).*

RECOMMENDATION 7.1.4: *In isoimmune hemolytic disease, administration of intravenous γ-globulin (0.5-1 g/kg over 2 hours) is recommended if the TSB is rising despite intensive phototherapy or the TSB level is within 2 to 3 mg/dL (34-51 μmol/L) of the exchange level (Fig 4).[55] If necessary, this dose can be repeated in 12 hours (evidence quality B: benefits exceed harms).*

Intravenous γ-globulin has been shown to reduce the need for exchange transfusions in Rh and ABO hemolytic disease.[55–58] Although data are limited, it is reasonable to assume that intravenous γ-globulin will also be helpful in the other types of Rh hemolytic disease such as anti-C and anti-E.

TABLE 3. Example of a Clinical Pathway for Management of the Newborn Infant Readmitted for Phototherapy or Exchange Transfusion

Treatment
  Use intensive phototherapy and/or exchange transfusion as indicated in Figs 3 and 4 (see Appendix 2 for details of phototherapy use)
Laboratory tests
  TSB and direct bilirubin levels
  Blood type (ABO, Rh)
  Direct antibody test (Coombs')
  Serum albumin
  Complete blood cell count with differential and smear for red cell morphology
  Reticulocyte count
  $ETCO_c$ (if available)
  G6PD if suggested by ethnic or geographic origin or if poor response to phototherapy
  Urine for reducing substances
  If history and/or presentation suggest sepsis, perform blood culture, urine culture, and cerebrospinal fluid for protein, glucose, cell count, and culture
Interventions
  If TSB ≥25 mg/dL (428 μmol/L) or ≥20 mg/dL (342 μmol/L) in a sick infant or infant <38 wk gestation, obtain a type and crossmatch, and request blood in case an exchange transfusion is necessary
  In infants with isoimmune hemolytic disease and TSB level rising in spite of intensive phototherapy or within 2–3 mg/dL (34–51 μmol/L) of exchange level (Fig 4), administer intravenous immunoglobulin 0.5–1 g/kg over 2 h and repeat in 12 h if necessary
  If infant's weight loss from birth is >12% or there is clinical or biochemical evidence of dehydration, recommend formula or expressed breast milk. If oral intake is in question, give intravenous fluids.
For infants receiving intensive phototherapy
  Breastfeed or bottle-feed (formula or expressed breast milk) every 2–3 h
  If TSB ≥25 mg/dL (428 μmol/L), repeat TSB within 2–3 h
  If TSB 20–25 mg/dL (342–428 μmol/L), repeat within 3–4 h. If TSB <20 mg/dL (342 μmol/L), repeat in 4–6 h. If TSB continues to fall, repeat in 8–12 h
  If TSB is not decreasing or is moving closer to level for exchange transfusion or the TSB/albumin ratio exceeds levels shown in Fig 4, consider exchange transfusion (see Fig 4 for exchange transfusion recommendations)
  When TSB is <13–14 mg/dL (239 μmol/L), discontinue phototherapy
  Depending on the cause of the hyperbilirubinemia, it is an option to measure TSB 24 h after discharge to check for rebound

Serum Albumin Levels and the Bilirubin/Albumin Ratio

RECOMMENDATION 7.1.5: It is an option to measure the serum albumin level and consider an albumin level of less than 3.0 g/dL as one risk factor for lowering the threshold for phototherapy use (see Fig 3) (evidence quality D: benefits versus risks exceptional.).

RECOMMENDATION 7.1.6: If an exchange transfusion is being considered, the serum albumin level should be measured and the bilirubin/albumin (B/A) ratio used in conjunction with the TSB level and other factors in determining the need for exchange transfusion (see Fig 4) (evidence quality D: benefits versus harms exceptional).

The recommendations shown above for treating hyperbilirubinemia are based primarily on TSB levels and other factors that affect the risk of bilirubin encephalopathy. This risk might be increased by a prolonged (rather than a brief) exposure to a certain TSB level.[59,60] Because the published data that address this issue are limited, however, it is not possible to provide specific recommendations for intervention based on the duration of hyperbilirubinemia.

See Appendix 1 for the basis for recommendations 7.1 through 7.1.6 and for the recommendations provided in Figs 3 and 4. Appendix 1 also contains a discussion of the risks of exchange transfusion and the use of B/A binding.

Acute Bilirubin Encephalopathy

RECOMMENDATION 7.1.7: Immediate exchange transfusion is recommended in any infant who is jaun-diced and manifests the signs of the intermediate to advanced stages of acute bilirubin encephalopathy[61,62] (hypertonia, arching, retrocollis, opisthotonos, fever, high-pitched cry) even if the TSB is falling (evidence quality D: benefits versus risks exceptional).

Phototherapy

RECOMMENDATION 7.2: All nurseries and services treating infants should have the necessary equipment to provide intensive phototherapy (see Appendix 2) (evidence quality D: benefits exceed risks).

Outpatient Management of the Jaundiced Breastfed Infant

RECOMMENDATION 7.3: In breastfed infants who require phototherapy (Fig 3), the AAP recommends that, if possible, breastfeeding should be continued (evidence quality C: benefits exceed harms). It is also an option to interrupt temporarily breastfeeding and substitute formula. This can reduce bilirubin levels and/or enhance the efficacy of phototherapy[63–65] (evidence quality B: benefits exceed harms). In breastfed infants receiving phototherapy, supplementation with expressed breast milk or formula is appropriate if the infant's intake seems inadequate, weight loss is excessive, or the infant seems dehydrated.

IMPLEMENTATION STRATEGIES

The Institute of Medicine[11] recommends a dramatic change in the way the US health care system

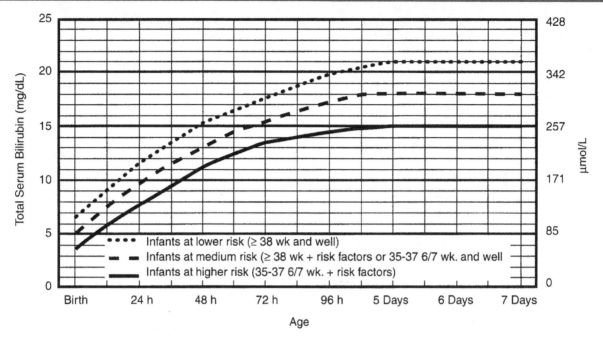

- Use total bilirubin. Do not subtract direct reacting or conjugated bilirubin.
- Risk factors = isoimmune hemolytic disease, G6PD deficiency, asphyxia, significant lethargy, temperature instability, sepsis, acidosis, or albumin < 3.0g/dL (if measured)
- For well infants 35-37 6/7 wk can adjust TSB levels for intervention around the medium risk line. It is an option to intervene at lower TSB levels for infants closer to 35 wks and at higher TSB levels for those closer to 37 6/7 wk.
- It is an option to provide conventional phototherapy in hospital or at home at TSB levels 2-3 mg/dL (35-50mmol/L) below those shown but home phototherapy should not be used in any infant with risk factors.

Fig 3. Guidelines for phototherapy in hospitalized infants of 35 or more weeks' gestation.

Note: These guidelines are based on limited evidence and the levels shown are approximations. The guidelines refer to the use of intensive phototherapy which should be used when the TSB exceeds the line indicated for each category. Infants are designated as "higher risk" because of the potential negative effects of the conditions listed on albumin binding of bilirubin,[45–47] the blood-brain barrier,[48] and the susceptibility of the brain cells to damage by bilirubin.[48]

"Intensive phototherapy" implies irradiance in the blue-green spectrum (wavelengths of approximately 430–490 nm) of at least 30 μW/cm^2 per nm (measured at the infant's skin directly below the center of the phototherapy unit) and delivered to as much of the infant's surface area as possible. Note that irradiance measured below the center of the light source is much greater than that measured at the periphery. Measurements should be made with a radiometer specified by the manufacturer of the phototherapy system.

See Appendix 2 for additional information on measuring the dose of phototherapy, a description of intensive phototherapy, and of light sources used. If total serum bilirubin levels approach or exceed the exchange transfusion line (Fig 4), the sides of the bassinet, incubator, or warmer should be lined with aluminum foil or white material.[50] This will increase the surface area of the infant exposed and increase the efficacy of phototherapy.[51]

If the total serum bilirubin does not decrease or continues to rise in an infant who is receiving intensive phototherapy, this strongly suggests the presence of hemolysis.

Infants who receive phototherapy and have an elevated direct-reacting or conjugated bilirubin level (cholestatic jaundice) may develop the bronze-baby syndrome. See Appendix 2 for the use of phototherapy in these infants.

ensures the safety of patients. The perspective of safety as a purely individual responsibility must be replaced by the concept of safety as a property of systems. Safe systems are characterized by a shared knowledge of the goal, a culture emphasizing safety, the ability of each person within the system to act in a manner that promotes safety, minimizing the use of memory, and emphasizing the use of standard procedures (such as checklists), and the involvement of patients/families as partners in the process of care.

These principles can be applied to the challenge of preventing severe hyperbilirubinemia and kernicterus. A systematic approach to the implementation of these guidelines should result in greater safety. Such approaches might include

- The establishment of standing protocols for nursing assessment of jaundice, including testing TcB and TSB levels, without requiring physician orders.

- Checklists or reminders associated with risk factors, age at discharge, and laboratory test results that provide guidance for appropriate follow-up.
- Explicit educational materials for parents (a key component of all AAP guidelines) concerning the identification of newborns with jaundice.

FUTURE RESEARCH

Epidemiology of Bilirubin-Induced Central Nervous System Damage

There is a need for appropriate epidemiologic data to document the incidence of kernicterus in the newborn population, the incidence of other adverse effects attributable to hyperbilirubinemia and its management, and the number of infants whose TSB levels exceed 25 or 30 mg/dL (428-513 μmol/L). Organizations such as the Centers for Disease Control and Prevention should implement strategies for appropriate data gathering to identify the number of

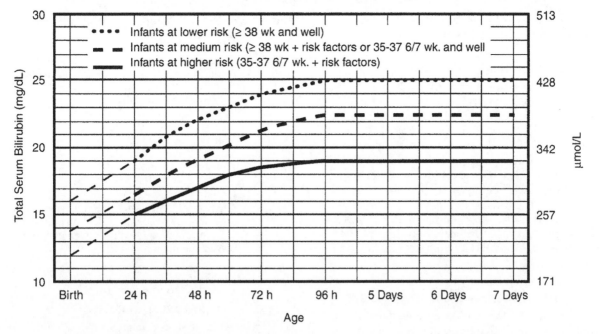

- The dashed lines for the first 24 hours indicate uncertainty due to a wide range of clinical circumstances and a range of responses to phototherapy.
- Immediate exchange transfusion is recommended if infant shows signs of acute bilirubin encephalopathy (hypertonia, arching, retrocollis, opisthotonos, fever, high pitched cry) or if TSB is ≥5 mg/dL (85 μmol/L) above these lines.
- Risk factors - isoimmune hemolytic disease, G6PD deficiency, asphyxia, significant lethargy, temperature instability, sepsis, acidosis.
- Measure serum albumin and calculate B/A ratio (See legend)
- Use total bilirubin. Do not subtract direct reacting or conjugated bilirubin
- If infant is well and 35-37 6/7 wk (median risk) can individualize TSB levels for exchange based on actual gestational age.

Fig 4. Guidelines for exchange transfusion in infants 35 or more weeks' gestation.

Note that these suggested levels represent a consensus of most of the committee but are based on limited evidence, and the levels shown are approximations. See ref. 3 for risks and complications of exchange transfusion. During birth hospitalization, exchange transfusion is recommended if the TSB rises to these levels despite intensive phototherapy. For readmitted infants, if the TSB level is above the exchange level, repeat TSB measurement every 2 to 3 hours and consider exchange if the TSB remains above the levels indicated after intensive phototherapy for 6 hours.

The following B/A ratios can be used together with but in not in lieu of the TSB level as an additional factor in determining the need for exchange transfusion[52]:

Risk Category	B/A Ratio at Which Exchange Transfusion Should be Considered	
	TSB mg/dL/Alb, g/dL	TSB μmol/L/Alb, μmol/L
Infants ≥38 0/7 wk	8.0	0.94
Infants 35 0/7–36 6/7 wk and well or ≥38 0/7 wk if higher risk or isoimmune hemolytic disease or G6PD deficiency	7.2	0.84
Infants 35 0/7–37 6/7 wk if higher risk or isoimmune hemolytic disease or G6PD deficiency	6.8	0.80

If the TSB is at or approaching the exchange level, send blood for immediate type and crossmatch. Blood for exchange transfusion is modified whole blood (red cells and plasma) crossmatched against the mother and compatible with the infant.[53]

infants who develop serum bilirubin levels above 25 or 30 mg/dL (428-513 μmol/L) and those who develop acute and chronic bilirubin encephalopathy. This information will help to identify the magnitude of the problem; the number of infants who need to be screened and treated to prevent 1 case of kernicterus; and the risks, costs, and benefits of different strategies for prevention and treatment of hyperbilirubinemia. In the absence of these data, recommendations for intervention cannot be considered definitive.

Effect of Bilirubin on the Central Nervous System

The serum bilirubin level by itself, except when it is extremely high and associated with bilirubin encephalopathy, is an imprecise indicator of long-term neurodevelopmental outcome.[2] Additional studies are needed on the relationship between central nervous system damage and the duration of hyperbilirubinemia, the binding of bilirubin to albumin, and changes seen in the brainstem auditory evoked response. These studies could help to better identify risk, clarify the effect of bilirubin on the central nervous system, and guide intervention.

Identification of Hemolysis

Because of their poor specificity and sensitivity, the standard laboratory tests for hemolysis (Table 1) are frequently unhelpful.[66,67] However, end-tidal carbon monoxide, corrected for ambient carbon monoxide (ETCO$_c$), levels can confirm the presence or absence of hemolysis, and measurement of ETCO$_c$ is the only clinical test that provides a direct measurement of the rate of heme catabolism and the rate of bilirubin production.[68,69] Thus, ETCO$_c$ may be helpful in determining the degree of surveillance needed and the timing of intervention. It is not yet known, however, how ETCO$_c$ measurements will affect management.

Nomograms and the Measurement of Serum and TcB

It would be useful to develop an age-specific (by hour) nomogram for TSB in populations of newborns that differ with regard to risk factors for hyperbilirubinemia. There is also an urgent need to improve the precision and accuracy of the measurement of TSB in the clinical laboratory.[70,71] Additional studies are also needed to develop and validate noninvasive (transcutaneous) measurements of serum bilirubin and to understand the factors that affect these measurements. These studies should also assess the cost-effectiveness and reproducibility of TcB measurements in clinical practice.[2]

Pharmacologic Therapy

There is now evidence that hyperbilirubinemia can be effectively prevented or treated with tin-mesoporphyrin,[72–75] a drug that inhibits the production of heme oxygenase. Tin-mesoporphyrin is not approved by the US Food and Drug Administration. If approved, tin-mesoporphyrin could find immediate application in preventing the need for exchange transfusion in infants who are not responding to phototherapy.[75]

Dissemination and Monitoring

Research should be directed toward methods for disseminating the information contained in this guideline to increase awareness on the part of physicians, residents, nurses, and parents concerning the issues of neonatal hyperbilirubinemia and strategies for its management. In addition, monitoring systems should be established to identify the impact of these guidelines on the incidence of acute bilirubin encephalopathy and kernicterus and the use of phototherapy and exchange transfusions.

CONCLUSIONS

Kernicterus is still occurring but should be largely preventable if health care personnel follow the recommendations listed in this guideline. These recommendations emphasize the importance of universal, systematic assessment for the risk of severe hyperbilirubinemia, close follow-up, and prompt intervention, when necessary.

SUBCOMMITTEE ON HYPERBILIRUBINEMIA
M. Jeffrey Maisels, MB, BCh, Chairperson
Richard D. Baltz, MD
Vinod K. Bhutani, MD
Thomas B. Newman, MD, MPH
Heather Palmer, MB, BCh
Warren Rosenfeld, MD
David K. Stevenson, MD
Howard B. Weinblatt, MD

CONSULTANT
Charles J. Homer, MD, MPH, Chairperson
   American Academy of Pediatrics Steering
   Committee on Quality Improvement and
   Management

STAFF
Carla T. Herrerias, MPH

ACKNOWLEDGMENTS

M.J.M. received grant support from Natus Medical, Inc, for multinational study of ambient carbon monoxide; WellSpring Pharmaceutical Corporation for study of Stannsoporfin (tin-mesoporphyrin); and Minolta, Inc, for study of the Minolta/Hill-Rom Air-Shields transcutaneous jaundice meter model JM-103. V.K.B. received grant support from WellSpring Pharmaceutical Corporation for study of Stannsoporfin (tin-mesoporphyrin) and Natus Medical, Inc, for multinational study of ambient carbon monoxide and is a consultant (volunteer) to SpectrX (BiliChek transcutaneous bilirubinometer). D.K.S. is a consultant to and holds stock options through Natus Medical, Inc.

The American Academy of Pediatrics Subcommittee on Hyperbilirubinemia gratefully acknowledges the help of the following organizations, committees, and individuals who reviewed drafts of this guideline and provided valuable criticisms and commentary: American Academy of Pediatrics Committee on Nutrition; American Academy of Pediatrics Committee on Practice and Ambulatory Medicine; American Academy of Pediatrics Committee on Child Health Financing; American Academy of Pediatrics Committee on Medical Liability; American Academy of Pediatrics Committee on Fetus and Newborn; American Academy of Pediatrics Section on Perinatal Pediatrics; Centers for Disease Control and Prevention; Parents of Infants and Children With Kernicterus (PICK); Charles Ahlfors, MD; Daniel Batton, MD; Thomas Bojko, MD; Sarah Clune, MD; Sudhakar Ezhuthachan, MD; Lawrence Gartner, MD; Cathy Hammerman, MD; Thor Hansen, MD; Lois Johnson, MD; Michael Kaplan, MB, ChB; Tony McDonagh, PhD; Gerald Merenstein, MD; Mary O'Shea, MD; Max Perlman, MD; Ronald Poland, MD; Alex Robertson, MD; Firmino Rubaltelli, MD; Steven Shapiro, MD; Stanford Singer, MD; Ann Stark, MD; Gautham Suresh, MD; Margot VandeBor, MD; Hank Vreman, PhD; Philip Walson, MD; Jon Watchko, MD; Richard Wennberg, MD; and Chap-Yung Yeung, MD.

REFERENCES

1. American Academy of Pediatrics, Provisional Committee for Quality Improvement and Subcommittee on Hyperbilirubinemia. Practice parameter: management of hyperbilirubinemia in the healthy term newborn. *Pediatrics.* 1994;94:558–562
2. Ip S, Glicken S, Kulig J, Obrien R, Sege R, Lau J. *Management of Neonatal Hyperbilirubinemia.* Rockville, MD: US Department of Health and Human Services, Agency for Healthcare Research and Quality; 2003. AHRQ Publication 03-E011
3. Ip S, Chung M, Kulig J. et al. An evidence-based review of important issues concerning neonatal hyperbilirubinemia. *Pediatrics.* 2004;113(6). Available at: www.pediatrics.org/cgi/content/full/113/6/e644
4. American Academy of Pediatrics, Steering Committee on Quality Improvement and Management. A taxonomy of recommendations. *Pediatrics.* 2004; In press
5. Johnson LH, Bhutani VK, Brown AK. System-based approach to management of neonatal jaundice and prevention of kernicterus. *J Pediatr.* 2002;140:396–403

6. Maisels MJ, Newman TB. Kernicterus in otherwise healthy, breast-fed term newborns. *Pediatrics.* 1995;96:730–733

7. MacDonald M. Hidden risks: early discharge and bilirubin toxicity due to glucose-6-phosphate dehydrogenase deficiency. *Pediatrics.* 1995;96: 734–738

8. Penn AA, Enzman DR, Hahn JS, Stevenson DK. Kernicterus in a full term infant. *Pediatrics.* 1994;93:1003–1006

9. Washington EC, Ector W, Abboud M, Ohning B, Holden K. Hemolytic jaundice due to G6PD deficiency causing kernicterus in a female newborn. *South Med J.* 1995;88:776–779

10. Ebbesen F. Recurrence of kernicterus in term and near-term infants in Denmark. *Acta Paediatr.* 2000;89:1213–1217

11. Institue of Medicine. *Crossing the Quality Chasm: A New Health System for the 21st Century.* Washington, DC: National Academy Press; 2001

12. American Academy of Pediatrics, American College of Obstetricians and Gynecologists. *Guidelines for Perinatal Care.* 5th ed. Elk Grove Village, IL: American Academy of Pediatrics; 2002:220–224

13. Bertini G, Dani C, Trochin M, Rubaltelli F. Is breastfeeding really favoring early neonatal jaundice? *Pediatrics.* 2001;107(3). Available at: www.pediatrics.org/cgi/content/full/107/3/e41

14. Maisels MJ, Gifford K. Normal serum bilirubin levels in the newborn and the effect of breast-feeding. *Pediatrics.* 1986;78:837–843

15. Yamauchi Y, Yamanouchi I. Breast-feeding frequency during the first 24 hours after birth in full-term neonates. *Pediatrics.* 1990;86:171–175

16. De Carvalho M, Klaus MH, Merkatz RB. Frequency of breastfeeding and serum bilirubin concentration. *Am J Dis Child.* 1982;136:737–738

17. Varimo P, Similä S, Wendt L, Kolvisto M. Frequency of breast feeding and hyperbilirubinemia [letter]. *Clin Pediatr (Phila).* 1986;25:112

18. De Carvalho M, Holl M, Harvey D. Effects of water supplementation on physiological jaundice in breast-fed babies. *Arch Dis Child.* 1981;56: 568–569

19. Nicoll A, Ginsburg R, Tripp JH. Supplementary feeding and jaundice in newborns. *Acta Paediatr Scand.* 1982;71:759–761

20. Madlon-Kay DJ. Identifying ABO incompatibility in newborns: selective vs automatic testing. *J Fam Pract.* 1992;35:278–280

21. Kramer LI. Advancement of dermal icterus in the jaundiced newborn. *Am J Dis Child.* 1969;118:454–458

22. Moyer VA, Ahn C, Sneed S. Accuracy of clinical judgment in neonatal jaundice. *Arch Pediatr Adolesc Med.* 2000;154:391–394

23. Davidson LT, Merritt KK, Weech AA. Hyperbilirubinemia in the newborn. *Am J Dis Child.* 1941;61:958–980

24. Tayaba R, Gribetz D, Gribetz I, Holzman IR. Noninvasive estimation of serum bilirubin. *Pediatrics.* 1998;102(3). Available at: www.pediatrics. org/cgi/content/full/102/3/e28

25. Bhutani V, Gourley GR, Adler S, Kreamer B, Dalman C, Johnson LH. Noninvasive measurement of total serum bilirubin in a multiracial predischarge newborn population to assess the risk of severe hyperbilirubinemia. *Pediatrics.* 2000;106(2). Available at: www.pediatrics.org/cgi/content/full/106/2/e17

26. Yasuda S, Itoh S, Isobe K, et al. New transcutaneous jaundice device with two optical paths. *J Perinat Med.* 2003;31:81–88

27. Maisels MJ, Ostrea EJ Jr, Touch S, et al. Evaluation of a new transcutaneous bilirubinometer. *Pediatrics.* 2004;113:1638–1645

28. Ebbesen F, Rasmussen LM, Wimberley PD. A new transcutaneous bilirubinometer, bilicheck, used in the neonatal intensive care unit and the maternity ward. *Acta Paediatr.* 2002;91:203–211

29. Rubaltelli FF, Gourley GR, Loskamp N, et al. Transcutaneous bilirubin measurement: a multicenter evaluation of a new device. *Pediatrics.* 2001;107:1264–1271

30. Newman TB, Liljestrand P, Escobar GJ. Jaundice noted in the first 24 hours after birth in a managed care organization. *Arch Pediatr Adolesc Med.* 2002;156:1244–1250

31. Bhutani VK, Johnson L, Sivieri EM. Predictive ability of a predischarge hour-specific serum bilirubin for subsequent significant hyperbilirubinemia in healthy term and near-term newborns. *Pediatrics.* 1999;103: 6–14

32. Garcia FJ, Nager AL. Jaundice as an early diagnostic sign of urinary tract infection in infancy. *Pediatrics.* 2002;109:846–851

33. Kaplan M, Hammerman C. Severe neonatal hyperbilirubinemia: a potential complication of glucose-6-phosphate dehydrogenase deficiency. *Clin Perinatol.* 1998;25:575–590

34. Valaes T. Severe neonatal jaundice associated with glucose-6-phosphate dehydrogenase deficiency: pathogenesis and global epidemiology. *Acta Paediatr Suppl.* 1994;394:58–76

35. Alpay F, Sarici S, Tosuncuk HD, Serdar MA, Inanç N, Gökçay E. The value of first-day bilirubin measurement in predicting the development of significant hyperbilirubinemia in healthy term newborns. *Pediatrics.*

2000;106(2). Available at: www.pediatrics.org/cgi/content/full/106/2/e16

36. Carbonell X, Botet F, Figueras J, Riu-Godo A. Prediction of hyperbilirubinaemia in the healthy term newborn. *Acta Paediatr.* 2001;90:166–170

37. Kaplan M, Hammerman C, Feldman R, Brisk R. Predischarge bilirubin screening in glucose-6-phosphate dehydrogenase-deficient neonates. *Pediatrics.* 2000;105:533–537

38. Stevenson DK, Fanaroff AA, Maisels MJ, et al. Prediction of hyperbilirubinemia in near-term and term infants. *Pediatrics.* 2001;108:31–39

39. Newman TB, Xiong B, Gonzales VM, Escobar GJ. Prediction and prevention of extreme neonatal hyperbilirubinemia in a mature health maintenance organization. *Arch Pediatr Adolesc Med.* 2000;154:1140–1147

40. Maisels MJ, Kring EA. Length of stay, jaundice, and hospital readmission. *Pediatrics.* 1998;101:995–998

41. Gale R, Seidman DS, Dollberg S, Stevenson DK. Epidemiology of neonatal jaundice in the Jerusalem population. *J Pediatr Gastroenterol Nutr.* 1990;10:82–86

42. Berk MA, Mimouni F, Miodovnik M, Hertzberg V, Valuck J. Macrosomia in infants of insulin-dependent diabetic mothers. *Pediatrics.* 1989; 83:1029–1034

43. Peevy KJ, Landaw SA, Gross SJ. Hyperbilirubinemia in infants of diabetic mothers. *Pediatrics.* 1980;66:417–419

44. Soskolne El, Schumacher R, Fyock C, Young ML, Schork A. The effect of early discharge and other factors on readmission rates of newborns. *Arch Pediatr Adolesc Med.* 1996;150:373–379

45. Ebbesen F, Brodersen R. Risk of bilirubin acid precipitation in preterm infants with respiratory distress syndrome: considerations of blood/brain bilirubin transfer equilibrium. *Early Hum Dev.* 1982;6:341–355

46. Cashore WJ, Oh W, Brodersen R. Reserve albumin and bilirubin toxicity index in infant serum. *Acta Paediatr Scand.* 1983;72:415–419

47. Cashore WJ. Free bilirubin concentrations and bilirubin-binding affinity in term and preterm infants. *J Pediatr.* 1980;96:521–527

48. Bratlid D. How bilirubin gets into the brain. *Clin Perinatol.* 1990;17: 449–465

49. Wennberg RP. Cellular basis of bilirubin toxicity. *N Y State J Med.* 1991;91:493–496

50. Eggert P, Stick C, Schroder H. On the distribution of irradiation intensity in phototherapy. Measurements of effective irradiance in an incubator. *Eur J Pediatr.* 1984;142:58–61

51. Maisels MJ. Why use homeopathic doses of phototherapy? *Pediatrics.* 1996;98:283–287

52. Ahlfors CE. Criteria for exchange transfusion in jaundiced newborns. *Pediatrics.* 1994;93:488–494

53. American Association of Blood Banks Technical Manual Committee. Perinatal issues in transfusion practice. In: Brecher M, ed. *Technical Manual.* Bethesda, MD: American Association of Blood Banks; 2002: 497–515

54. Garland JS, Alex C, Deacon JS, Raab K. Treatment of infants with indirect hyperbilirubinemia. Readmission to birth hospital vs nonbirth hospital. *Arch Pediatr Adolesc Med.* 1994;148:1317–1321

55. Gottstein R, Cooke R. Systematic review of intravenous immunoglobulin in haemolytic disease of the newborn. *Arch Dis Child Fetal Neonatal Ed.* 2003;88:F6–F10

56. Sato K, Hara T, Kondo T, Iwao H, Honda S, Ueda K. High-dose intravenous gammaglobulin therapy for neonatal immune haemolytic jaundice due to blood group incompatibility. *Acta Paediatr Scand.* 1991; 80:163–166

57. Rubo J, Albrecht K, Lasch P, et al. High-dose intravenous immune globulin therapy for hyperbilirubinemia caused by Rh hemolytic disease. *J Pediatr.* 1992;121:93–97

58. Hammerman C, Kaplan M, Vreman HJ, Stevenson DK. Intravenous immune globulin in neonatal ABO isoimmunization: factors associated with clinical efficacy. *Biol Neonate.* 1996;70:69–74

59. Johnson L, Boggs TR. Bilirubin-dependent brain damage: incidence and indications for treatment. In: Odell GB, Schaffer R, Simopoulos AP, eds. *Phototherapy in the Newborn: An Overview.* Washington, DC: National Academy of Sciences; 1974:122–149

60. Ozmert E, Erdem G, Topcu M. Long-term follow-up of indirect hyperbilirubinemia in full-term Turkish infants. *Acta Paediatr.* 1996;85: 1440–1444

61. Volpe JJ. *Neurology of the Newborn.* 4th ed. Philadelphia, PA: W. B. Saunders; 2001

62. Harris M, Bernbaum J, Polin J, Zimmerman R, Polin RA. Developmental follow-up of breastfed term and near-term infants with marked hyperbilirubinemia. *Pediatrics.* 2001;107:1075–1080

63. Osborn LM, Bolus R. Breast feeding and jaundice in the first week of life. *J Fam Pract.* 1985;20:475–480

64. Martinez JC, Maisels MJ, Otheguy L, et al. Hyperbilirubinemia in the breast-fed newborn: a controlled trial of four interventions. *Pediatrics.* 1993;91:470–473

65. Amato M, Howald H, von Muralt G. Interruption of breast-feeding versus phototherapy as treatment of hyperbilirubinemia in full-term infants. *Helv Paediatr Acta.* 1985;40:127–131

66. Maisels MJ, Gifford K, Antle CE, Leib GR. Jaundice in the healthy newborn infant: a new approach to an old problem. *Pediatrics.* 1988;81:505–511

67. Newman TB, Easterling MJ. Yield of reticulocyte counts and blood smears in term infants. *Clin Pediatr (Phila).* 1994;33:71–76

68. Herschel M, Karrison T, Wen M, Caldarelli L, Baron B. Evaluation of the direct antiglobulin (Coombs') test for identifying newborns at risk for hemolysis as determined by end-tidal carbon monoxide concentration (ETCOc); and comparison of the Coombs' test with ETCOc for detecting significant jaundice. *J Perinatol.* 2002;22:341–347

69. Stevenson DK, Vreman HJ. Carbon monoxide and bilirubin production in neonates. *Pediatrics.* 1997;100:252–254

70. Vreman HJ, Verter J, Oh W, et al. Interlaboratory variability of bilirubin measurements. *Clin Chem.* 1996;42:869–873

71. Lo S, Doumas BT, Ashwood E. Performance of bilirubin determinations in US laboratories—revisited. *Clin Chem.* 2004;50:190–194

72. Kappas A, Drummond GS, Henschke C, Valaes T. Direct comparison of Sn-mesoporphyrin, an inhibitor of bilirubin production, and phototherapy in controlling hyperbilirubinemia in term and near-term newborns. *Pediatrics.* 1995;95:468–474

73. Martinez JC, Garcia HO, Otheguy L, Drummond GS, Kappas A. Control of severe hyperbilirubinemia in full-term newborns with the inhibitor of bilirubin production Sn-mesoporphyrin. *Pediatrics.* 1999;103:1–5

74. Suresh G, Martin CL, Soll R. Metalloporphyrins for treatment of unconjugated hyperbilirubinemia in neonates. *Cochrane Database Syst Rev.* 2003;2:CD004207

75. Kappas A, Drummond GS, Munson DP, Marshall JR. Sn-mesoporphyrin interdiction of severe hyperbilirubinemia in Jehovah's Witness newborns as an alternative to exchange transfusion. *Pediatrics.* 2001;108:1374–1377

APPENDIX 1: Additional Notes

Definitions of Quality of Evidence and Balance of Benefits and Harms

The Steering Committee on Quality Improvement and Management categorizes evidence quality in 4 levels:

1. Well-designed, randomized, controlled trials or diagnostic studies on relevant populations
2. Randomized, controlled trials or diagnostic studies with minor limitations; overwhelming, consistent evidence from observational studies
3. Observational studies (case-control and cohort design)
4. Expert opinion, case reports, reasoning from first principles

The AAP defines evidence-based recommendations as follows:[1]

- Strong recommendation: the committee believes that the benefits of the recommended approach clearly exceed the harms of that approach and that the quality of the supporting evidence is either excellent or impossible to obtain. Clinicians should follow these recommendations unless a clear and compelling rationale for an alternative approach is present.
- Recommendation: the committee believes that the benefits exceed the harms, but the quality of evidence on which this recommendation is based is not as strong. Clinicians should also generally follow these recommendations but should be alert to new information and sensitive to patient prefer-

ences. In this guideline, the term "should" implies a recommendation by the committee.

- Option: either the quality of the evidence that exists is suspect or well-performed studies have shown little clear advantage to one approach over another. Patient preference should have a substantial role in influencing clinical decision-making when a policy is described as an option.
- No recommendation: there is a lack of pertinent evidence and the anticipated balance of benefits and harms is unclear.

Anticipated Balance Between Benefits and Harms

The presence of clear benefits or harms supports stronger statements for or against a course of action. In some cases, however, recommendations are made when analysis of the balance of benefits and harms provides an exceptional dysequilibrium and it would be unethical or impossible to perform clinical trials to "prove" the point. In these cases the balance of benefit and harm is termed "exceptional."

Clinical Manifestations of Acute Bilirubin Encephalopathy and Kernicterus

Acute Bilirubin Encephalopathy

In the early phase of acute bilirubin encephalopathy, severely jaundiced infants become lethargic and hypotonic and suck poorly.[2,3] The intermediate phase is characterized by moderate stupor, irritability, and hypertonia. The infant may develop a fever and high-pitched cry, which may alternate with drowsiness and hypotonia. The hypertonia is manifested by backward arching of the neck (retrocollis) and trunk (opisthotonos). There is anecdotal evidence that an emergent exchange transfusion at this stage, in some cases, might reverse the central nervous system changes.[4] The advanced phase, in which central nervous system damage is probably irreversible, is characterized by pronounced retrocollis-opisthotonos, shrill cry, no feeding, apnea, fever, deep stupor to coma, sometimes seizures, and death.[2,3,5]

Kernicterus

In the chronic form of bilirubin encephalopathy, surviving infants may develop a severe form of athetoid cerebral palsy, auditory dysfunction, dental-enamel dysplasia, paralysis of upward gaze, and, less often, intellectual and other handicaps. Most infants who develop kernicterus have manifested some or all of the signs listed above in the acute phase of bilirubin encephalopathy. However, occasionally there are infants who have developed very high bilirubin levels and, subsequently, the signs of kernicterus but have exhibited few, if any, antecedent clinical signs of acute bilirubin encephalopathy.[3,5,6]

Clinical Evaluation of Jaundice and TcB Measurements

Jaundice is usually seen in the face first and progresses caudally to the trunk and extremities,[7] but because visual estimation of bilirubin levels from the degree of jaundice can lead to errors,[8–10] a low threshold should be used for measuring the TSB.

Devices that provide a noninvasive TcB measurement have proven very useful as screening tools,[11] and newer instruments give measurements that provide a valid estimate of the TSB level.[12–17] Studies using the new TcB-measurement instruments are limited, but the data published thus far suggest that in most newborn populations, these instruments generally provide measurements within 2 to 3 mg/dL (34–51 μmol/L) of the TSB and can replace a measurement of serum bilirubin in many circumstances, particularly for TSB levels less than 15 mg/dL (257 μmol/L).[12–17] Because phototherapy "bleaches" the skin, both visual assessment of jaundice and TcB measurements in infants undergoing phototherapy are not reliable. In addition, the ability of transcutaneous instruments to provide accurate measurements in different racial groups requires additional study.[18,19] The limitations of the accuracy and reproducibility of TSB measurements in the clinical laboratory[20–22] must also be recognized and are discussed in the technical report.[23]

Capillary Versus Venous Serum Bilirubin Measurement

Almost all published data regarding the relationship of TSB levels to kernicterus or developmental outcome are based on capillary blood TSB levels. Data regarding the differences between capillary and venous TSB levels are conflicting.[24,25] In 1 study the capillary TSB levels were higher, but in another they were lower than venous TSB levels.[24,25] Thus, obtaining a venous sample to "confirm" an elevated capillary TSB level is not recommended, because it will delay the initiation of treatment.

Direct-Reacting and Conjugated Bilirubin

Although commonly used interchangeably, direct-reacting bilirubin is not the same as conjugated bilirubin. Direct-reacting bilirubin is the bilirubin that reacts directly (without the addition of an accelerating agent) with diazotized sulfanilic acid. Conjugated bilirubin is bilirubin made water soluble by binding with glucuronic acid in the liver. Depending on the technique used, the clinical laboratory will report total and direct-reacting or unconjugated and conjugated bilirubin levels. In this guideline and for clinical purposes, the terms may be used interchangeably.

Abnormal Direct and Conjugated Bilirubin Levels

Laboratory measurement of direct bilirubin is not precise,[26] and values between laboratories can vary widely. If the TSB is at or below 5 mg/dL (85 μmol/L), a direct or conjugated bilirubin of more than 1.0 mg/dL (17.1 μmol/L) is generally considered abnormal. For TSB values higher than 5 mg/dL (85 μmol/L), a direct bilirubin of more than 20% of the TSB is considered abnormal. If the hospital laboratory measures conjugated bilirubin using the Vitros (formerly Ektachem) system (Ortho-Clinical Diagnostics, Raritan, NJ), any value higher than 1 mg/dL is considered abnormal.

Assessment of Adequacy of Intake in Breastfeeding Infants

The data from a number of studies[27–34] indicate that unsupplemented, breastfed infants experience their maximum weight loss by day 3 and, on average, lose 6.1% ± 2.5% (SD) of their birth weight. Thus, ~5% to 10% of fully breastfed infants lose 10% or more of their birth weight by day 3, suggesting that adequacy of intake should be evaluated and the infant monitored if weight loss is more than 10%.[35] Evidence of adequate intake in breastfed infants also includes 4 to 6 thoroughly wet diapers in 24 hours and the passage of 3 to 4 stools per day by the fourth day. By the third to fourth day, the stools in adequately breastfed infants should have changed from meconium to a mustard yellow, mushy stool.[36] The above assessment will also help to identify breastfed infants who are at risk for dehydration because of inadequate intake.

Nomogram for Designation of Risk

Note that this nomogram (Fig 2) does not describe the natural history of neonatal hyperbilirubinemia, particularly after 48 to 72 hours, for which, because of sampling bias, the lower zones are spuriously elevated.[37] This bias, however, will have much less effect on the high-risk zone (95th percentile in the study).[38]

G6PD Dehydrogenase Deficiency

It is important to look for G6PD deficiency in infants with significant hyperbilirubinemia, because some may develop a sudden increase in the TSB. In addition, G6PD-deficient infants require intervention at lower TSB levels (Figs 3 and 4). It should be noted also that in the presence of hemolysis, G6PD levels can be elevated, which may obscure the diagnosis in the newborn period so that a normal level in a hemolyzing neonate does not rule out G6PD deficiency.[39] If G6PD deficiency is strongly suspected, a repeat level should be measured when the infant is 3 months old. It is also recognized that immediate laboratory determination of G6PD is generally not available in most US hospitals, and thus translating the above information into clinical practice is cur-

TABLE 4. Risk Zone as a Predictor of Hyperbilirubinemia[39]

TSB Before Discharge	Newborns (Total = 2840), n (%)	Newborns Who Subsequently Developed a TSB Level >95th Percentile, n (%)
High-risk zone (>95th percentile)	172 (6.0)	68 (39.5)
High intermediate-risk zone	356 (12.5)	46 (12.9)
Low intermediate-risk zone	556 (19.6)	12 (2.26)
Low-risk zone	1756 (61.8)	0

rently difficult. Nevertheless, practitioners are reminded to consider the diagnosis of G6PD deficiency in infants with severe hyperbilirubinemia, particularly if they belong to the population groups in which this condition is prevalent. This is important in the African American population, because these infants, as a group, have much lower TSB levels than white or Asian infants.[40,41] Thus, severe hyperbilirubinemia in an African American infant should always raise the possibility of G6PD deficiency.

Basis for the Recommendations 7.1.1 Through 7.1.6 and Provided in Figs 3 and 4

Ideally, recommendations for when to implement phototherapy and exchange transfusions should be based on estimates of when the benefits of these interventions exceed their risks and cost. The evidence for these estimates should come from randomized trials or systematic observational studies. Unfortunately, there is little such evidence on which to base these recommendations. As a result, treatment guidelines must necessarily rely on more uncertain estimates and extrapolations. For a detailed discussion of this question, please see "An Evidence-Based Review of Important Issues Concerning Neonatal Hyperbilirubinemia."[23]

The recommendations for phototherapy and exchange transfusion are based on the following principles:

- The main demonstrated value of phototherapy is that it reduces the risk that TSB levels will reach a level at which exchange transfusion is recommended.[42–44] Approximately 5 to 10 infants with TSB levels between 15 and 20 mg/dL (257–342 μmol/L) will receive phototherapy to prevent the TSB in 1 infant from reaching 20 mg/dL (the number needed to treat).[12] Thus, 8 to 9 of every 10 infants with these TSB levels will not reach 20 mg/dL (342 μmol/L) even if they are not treated. Phototherapy has proven to be a generally safe procedure, although rare complications can occur (see Appendix 2).
- Recommended TSB levels for exchange transfusion (Fig 4) are based largely on the goal of keeping TSB levels below those at which kernicterus has been reported.[12,45–48] In almost all cases, exchange transfusion is recommended only after phototherapy has failed to keep the TSB level below the exchange transfusion level (Fig 4).
- The recommendations to use phototherapy and exchange transfusion at lower TSB levels for infants of lower gestation and those who are sick are based on limited observations suggesting that sick infants (particularly those with the risk factors listed in Figs 3 and 4)[49–51] and those of lower gestation[51–54] are at greater risk for developing kernicterus at lower bilirubin levels than are well infants of more than 38 6/7 weeks' gestation. Nevertheless, other studies have not confirmed all of these associations.[52,55,56] There is no doubt, however, that infants at 35 to 37 6/7 weeks' gestation are at a much greater risk of developing very high

TSB levels.[57,58] Intervention for these infants is based on this risk as well as extrapolations from more premature, lower birth-weight infants who do have a higher risk of bilirubin toxicity.[52,53]
- For all newborns, treatment is recommended at lower TSB levels at younger ages because one of the primary goals of treatment is to prevent additional increases in the TSB level.

Subtle Neurologic Abnormalities Associated With Hyperbilirubinemia

There are several studies demonstrating measurable transient changes in brainstem-evoked potentials, behavioral patterns, and the infant's cry[59–63] associated with TSB levels of 15 to 25 mg/dL (257–428 μmol/L). In these studies, the abnormalities identified were transient and disappeared when the serum bilirubin levels returned to normal with or without treatment.[59,60,62,63]

A few cohort studies have found an association between hyperbilirubinemia and long-term adverse neurodevelopmental effects that are more subtle than kernicterus.[64–67] Current studies, however, suggest that although phototherapy lowers the TSB levels, it has no effect on these long-term neurodevelopmental outcomes.[68–70]

Risks of Exchange Transfusion

Because exchange transfusions are now rarely performed, the risks of morbidity and mortality associated with the procedure are difficult to quantify. In addition, the complication rates listed below may not be generalizable to the current era if, like most procedures, frequency of performance is an important determinant of risk. Death associated with exchange transfusion has been reported in approximately 3 in 1000 procedures,[71,72] although in otherwise well infants of 35 or more weeks' gestation, the risk is probably much lower.[71–73] Significant morbidity (apnea, bradycardia, cyanosis, vasospasm, thrombosis, necrotizing enterocolitis) occurs in as many as 5% of exchange transfusions,[71] and the risks associated with the use of blood products must always be considered.[74] Hypoxic-ischemic encephalopathy and acquired immunodeficiency syndrome have occurred in otherwise healthy infants receiving exchange transfusions.[73,75]

Serum Albumin Levels and the B/A Ratio

The legends to Figs 3 and 4 and recommendations 7.1.5 and 7.1.6 contain references to the serum albumin level and the B/A ratio as factors that can be considered in the decision to initiate phototherapy (Fig 3) or perform an exchange transfusion (Fig 4). Bilirubin is transported in the plasma tightly bound to albumin, and the portion that is unbound or loosely bound can more readily leave the intravascular space and cross the intact blood-brain barrier.[76] Elevations of unbound bilirubin (UB) have been associated with kernicterus in sick preterm newborns.[77,78] In addition, elevated UB concentrations are more closely associated than TSB levels with transient abnormalities in the audiometric brainstem response in term[79] and preterm[80] infants. Long-term studies relating B/A binding in infants to developmental outcome are limited and conflicting.[69,81,82] In addition, clinical laboratory measurement of UB is not currently available in the United States.

The ratio of bilirubin (mg/dL) to albumin (g/dL) does correlate with measured UB in newborns[83] and can be used as an approximate surrogate for the measurement of UB. It must be recognized, however, that both albumin levels and the ability of albumin to bind bilirubin vary significantly between newborns.[83,84] Albumin binding of bilirubin is impaired in sick infants,[84–86] and some studies show an increase in binding with increasing gestational[86,87] and postnatal[87,88] age, but others have not found a significant effect of gestational age on binding.[89] Furthermore, the risk of bilirubin encephalopathy is unlikely to be a simple function of the TSB level or the concentration of UB but is more likely a combination of both (ie, the total amount of bilirubin available [the miscible pool of bilirubin] as well as the tendency of bilirubin to enter the tissues [the UB concentration]).[83] An additional factor is the possible susceptibility of the cells of the central nervous system to damage by bilirubin.[90] It is therefore a clinical option to use the B/A ratio together with, but not in lieu of, the TSB level as an additional factor in determining the need for exchange transfusion[83] (Fig 4).

REFERENCES

1. American Academy of Pediatrics, Steering Committee on Quality Improvement and Management. Classification of recommendations for clinical practice guidelines. *Pediatrics*. 2004; In press
2. Johnson LH, Bhutani VK, Brown AK. System-based approach to management of neonatal jaundice and prevention of kernicterus. *J Pediatr*. 2002;140:396–403
3. Volpe JJ. *Neurology of the Newborn*. 4th ed. Philadelphia, PA: W. B. Saunders; 2001
4. Harris M, Bernbaum J, Polin J, Zimmerman R, Polin RA. Developmental follow-up of breastfed term and near-term infants with marked hyperbilirubinemia. *Pediatrics*. 2001;107:1075–1080
5. Van Praagh R. Diagnosis of kernicterus in the neonatal period. *Pediatrics*. 1961;28:870–876
6. Jones MH, Sands R, Hyman CB, Sturgeon P, Koch FP. Longitudinal study of incidence of central nervous system damage following erythroblastosis fetalis. *Pediatrics*. 1954;14:346–350
7. Kramer LI. Advancement of dermal icterus in the jaundiced newborn. *Am J Dis Child*. 1969;118:454–458
8. Moyer VA, Ahn C, Sneed S. Accuracy of clinical judgment in neonatal jaundice. *Arch Pediatr Adolesc Med*. 2000;154:391–394
9. Davidson LT, Merritt KK, Weech AA. Hyperbilirubinemia in the newborn. *Am J Dis Child*. 1941;61:958–980
10. Tayaba R, Gribetz D, Gribetz I, Holzman IR. Noninvasive estimation of serum bilirubin. *Pediatrics*. 1998;102(3). Available at: www.pediatrics.org/cgi/content/full/102/3/e28
11. Maisels MJ, Kring E. Transcutaneous bilirubinometry decreases the need for serum bilirubin measurements and saves money. *Pediatrics*. 1997;99:599–601
12. Ip S, Glicken S, Kulig J, Obrien R, Sege R, Lau J. *Management of Neonatal Hyperbilirubinemia*. Rockville, MD: US Department of Health and Human Services, Agency for Healthcare Research and Quality; 2003. AHRQ Publication 03-E011
13. Bhutani V, Gourley GR, Adler S, Kreamer B, Dalman C, Johnson LH. Noninvasive measurement of total serum bilirubin in a multiracial predischarge newborn population to assess the risk of severe hyperbilirubinemia. *Pediatrics*. 2000;106(2). Available at: www.pediatrics.org/cgi/content/full/106/2/e17
14. Yasuda S, Itoh S, Isobe K, et al. New transcutaneous jaundice device with two optical paths. *J Perinat Med*. 2003;31:81–88
15. Maisels MJ, Ostrea EJ Jr, Touch S, et al. Evaluation of a new transcutaneous bilirubinometer. *Pediatrics*. 2004;113:1638–1645
16. Ebbesen F, Rasmussen LM, Wimberley PD. A new transcutaneous bilirubinometer, bilicheck, used in the neonatal intensive care unit and the maternity ward. *Acta Paediatr*. 2002;91:203–211
17. Rubaltelli FF, Gourley GR, Loskamp N, et al. Transcutaneous bilirubin measurement: a multicenter evaluation of a new device. *Pediatrics*. 2001;107:1264–1271
18. Engle WD, Jackson GL, Sendelbach D, Manning D, Frawley W. Assessment of a transcutaneous device in the evaluation of neonatal hyperbilirubinemia in a primarily Hispanic population. *Pediatrics*. 2002;110:61–67
19. Schumacher R. Transcutaneous bilirubinometry and diagnostic tests: "the right job for the tool." *Pediatrics*. 2002;110:407–408
20. Vreman HJ, Verter J, Oh W, et al. Interlaboratory variability of bilirubin measurements. *Clin Chem*. 1996;42:869–873
21. Doumas BT, Eckfeldt JH. Errors in measurement of total bilirubin: a perennial problem. *Clin Chem*. 1996;42:845–848
22. Lo S, Doumas BT, Ashwood E. Performance of bilirubin determinations in US laboratories—revisited. *Clin Chem*. 2004;50:190–194
23. Ip S, Chung M, Kulig J. et al. An evidence-based review of important issues concerning neonatal hyperbilirubinemia. *Pediatrics*. 2004;113(6). Available at: www.pediatrics.org/cgi/content/full/113/6/e644
24. Leslie GI, Philips JB, Cassady G. Capillary and venous bilirubin values: are they really different? *Am J Dis Child*. 1987;141:1199–1200
25. Eidelman AI, Schimmel MS, Algur N, Eylath U. Capillary and venous bilirubin values: they are different—and how [letter]! *Am J Dis Child*. 1989;143:642
26. Watkinson LR, St John A, Penberthy LA. Investigation into paediatric bilirubin analyses in Australia and New Zealand. *J Clin Pathol*. 1982;35:52–58
27. Bertini G, Dani C, Trochin M, Rubaltelli F. Is breastfeeding really favoring early neonatal jaundice? *Pediatrics*. 2001;107(3). Available at: www.pediatrics.org/cgi/content/full/107/3/e41
28. De Carvalho M, Klaus MH, Merkatz RB. Frequency of breastfeeding and serum bilirubin concentration. *Am J Dis Child*. 1982;136:737–738
29. De Carvalho M, Holl M, Harvey D. Effects of water supplementation on physiological jaundice in breast-fed babies. *Arch Dis Child*. 1981;56:568–569
30. Nicoll A, Ginsburg R, Tripp JH. Supplementary feeding and jaundice in newborns. *Acta Paediatr Scand*. 1982;71:759–761
31. Butler DA, MacMillan JP. Relationship of breast feeding and weight loss to jaundice in the newborn period: review of the literature and results of a study. *Cleve Clin Q*. 1983;50:263–268
32. De Carvalho M, Robertson S, Klaus M. Fecal bilirubin excretion and serum bilirubin concentration in breast-fed and bottle-fed infants. *J Pediatr*. 1985;107:786–790
33. Gourley GR, Kreamer B, Arend R. The effect of diet on feces and jaundice during the first three weeks of life. *Gastroenterology*. 1992;103:660–667
34. Maisels MJ, Gifford K. Breast-feeding, weight loss, and jaundice. *J Pediatr*. 1983;102:117–118
35. Laing IA, Wong CM. Hypernatraemia in the first few days: is the incidence rising? *Arch Dis Child Fetal Neonatal Ed*. 2002;87:F158–F162
36. Lawrence RA. Management of the mother-infant nursing couple. In: *A Breastfeeding Guide for the Medical Profession*. 4th ed. St Louis, MO: Mosby-Year Book, Inc; 1994:215-277
37. Maisels MJ, Newman TB. Predicting hyperbilirubinemia in newborns: the importance of timing. *Pediatrics*. 1999;103:493–495
38. Bhutani VK, Johnson L, Sivieri EM. Predictive ability of a predischarge hour-specific serum bilirubin for subsequent significant hyperbilirubinemia in healthy term and near-term newborns. *Pediatrics*. 1999;103:6–14
39. Beutler E. Glucose-6-phosphate dehydrogenase deficiency. *Blood*. 1994;84:3613–3636
40. Linn S, Schoenbaum SC, Monson RR, Rosner B, Stubblefield PG, Ryan KJ. Epidemiology of neonatal hyperbilirubinemia. *Pediatrics*. 1985;75:770–774
41. Newman TB, Easterling MJ, Goldman ES, Stevenson DK. Laboratory evaluation of jaundiced newborns: frequency, cost and yield. *Am J Dis Child*. 1990;144:364–368
42. Martinez JC, Maisels MJ, Otheguy L, et al. Hyperbilirubinemia in the breast-fed newborn: a controlled trial of four interventions. *Pediatrics*. 1993;91:470–473
43. Maisels MJ. Phototherapy—traditional and nontraditional. *J Perinatol*. 2001;21(suppl 1):S93–S97
44. Brown AK, Kim MH, Wu PY, Bryla DA. Efficacy of phototherapy in prevention and management of neonatal hyperbilirubinemia. *Pediatrics*. 1985;75:393–400

45. Armitage P, Mollison PL. Further analysis of controlled trials of treatment of hemolytic disease of the newborn. *J Obstet Gynaecol Br Emp*. 1953;60:602–605

46. Mollison PL, Walker W. Controlled trials of the treatment of haemolytic disease of the newborn. *Lancet*. 1952;1:429–433

47. Hsia DYY, Allen FH, Gellis SS, Diamond LK. Erythroblastosis fetalis. VIII. Studies of serum bilirubin in relation to kernicterus. *N Engl J Med*. 1952;247:668–671

48. Newman TB, Maisels MJ. Does hyperbilirubinemia damage the brain of healthy full-term infants? *Clin Perinatol*. 1990;17:331–358

49. Ozmert E, Erdem G, Topcu M. Long-term follow-up of indirect hyperbilirubinemia in full-term Turkish infants. *Acta Paediatr*. 1996;85: 1440–1444

50. Perlman JM, Rogers B, Burns D. Kernicterus findings at autopsy in 2 sick near-term infants. *Pediatrics*. 1997;99:612–615

51. Gartner LM, Snyder RN, Chabon RS, Bernstein J. Kernicterus: high incidence in premature infants with low serum bilirubin concentration. *Pediatrics*. 1970;45:906–917

52. Watchko JF, Oski FA. Kernicterus in preterm newborns: past, present, and future. *Pediatrics*. 1992;90:707–715

53. Watchko J, Claassen D. Kernicterus in premature infants: current prevalence and relationship to NICHD Phototherapy Study exchange criteria. *Pediatrics*. 1994;93(6 Pt 1):996–999

54. Stern L, Denton RL. Kernicterus in small, premature infants. *Pediatrics*. 1965;35:486–485

55. Turkel SB, Guttenberg ME, Moynes DR, Hodgman JE. Lack of identifiable risk factors for kernicterus. *Pediatrics*. 1980;66:502–506

56. Kim MH, Yoon JJ, Sher J, Brown AK. Lack of predictive indices in kernicterus. A comparison of clinical and pathologic factors in infants with or without kernicterus. *Pediatrics*. 1980;66:852–858

57. Newman TB, Xiong B, Gonzales VM, Escobar GJ. Prediction and prevention of extreme neonatal hyperbilirubinemia in a mature health maintenance organization. *Arch Pediatr Adolesc Med*. 2000;154:1140–1147

58. Newman TB, Escobar GJ, Gonzales VM, Armstrong MA, Gardner MN, Folck BF. Frequency of neonatal bilirubin testing and hyperbilirubinemia in a large health maintenance organization. *Pediatrics*. 1999;104: 1198–1203

59. Vohr BR. New approaches to assessing the risks of hyperbilirubinemia. *Clin Perinatol*. 1990;17:293–306

60. Perlman M, Fainmesser P, Sohmer H, Tamari H, Wax Y, Pevsmer B. Auditory nerve-brainstem evoked responses in hyperbilirubinemic neonates. *Pediatrics*. 1983;72:658–664

61. Nakamura H, Takada S, Shimabuku R, Matsuo M, Matsuo T, Negishi H. Auditory and brainstem responses in newborn infants with hyperbilirubinemia. *Pediatrics*. 1985;75:703–708

62. Nwaesei CG, Van Aerde J, Boyden M, Perlman M. Changes in auditory brainstem responses in hyperbilirubinemic infants before and after exchange transfusion. *Pediatrics*. 1984;74:800–803

63. Wennberg RP, Ahlfors CE, Bickers R, McMurtry CA, Shetter JL. Abnormal auditory brainstem response in a newborn infant with hyperbilirubinemia: improvement with exchange transfusion. *J Pediatr*. 1982;100:624–626

64. Soorani-Lunsing I, Woltil H, Hadders-Algra M. Are moderate degrees of hyperbilirubinemia in healthy term neonates really safe for the brain? *Pediatr Res*. 2001;50:701–705

65. Grimmer I, Berger-Jones K, Buhrer C, Brandl U, Obladen M. Late neurological sequelae of non-hemolytic hyperbilirubinemia of healthy term neonates. *Acta Paediatr*. 1999;88:661–663

66. Seidman DS, Paz I, Stevenson DK, Laor A, Danon YL, Gale R. Neonatal hyperbilirubinemia and physical and cognitive performance at 17 years of age. *Pediatrics*. 1991;88:828–833

67. Newman TB, Klebanoff MA. Neonatal hyperbilirubinemia and long-term outcome: another look at the collaborative perinatal project. *Pediatrics*. 1993;92:651–657

68. Scheidt PC, Bryla DA, Nelson KB, Hirtz DG, Hoffman HJ. Phototherapy for neonatal hyperbilirubinemia: six-year follow-up of the National Institute of Child Health and Human Development clinical trial. *Pediatrics*. 1990;85:455–463

69. Scheidt PC, Graubard BI, Nelson KB, et al. Intelligence at six years in relation to neonatal bilirubin levels: follow-up of the National Institute of Child Health and Human Development Clinical Trial of Phototherapy. *Pediatrics*. 1991;87:797–805

70. Seidman DS, Paz I, Stevenson DK, Laor A, Danon YL, Gale R. Effect of phototherapy for neonatal jaundice on cognitive performance. *J Perinatol*. 1994;14:23–28

71. Keenan WJ, Novak KK, Sutherland JM, Bryla DA, Fetterly KL. Morbidity and mortality associated with exchange transfusion. *Pediatrics*. 1985; 75:417–421

72. Hovi L, Siimes MA. Exchange transfusion with fresh heparinized blood is a safe procedure: Experiences from 1069 newborns. *Acta Paediatr Scand*. 1985;74:360–365

73. Jackson JC. Adverse events associated with exchange transfusion in healthy and ill newborns. *Pediatrics*. 1997;99(5):e7. Available at: www.pediatrics.org/cgi/content/full/99/5/e7

74. Schreiber GB, Busch MP, Kleinman SH, Korelitz JJ. The risk of transfusion-transmitted viral infections. *N Engl J Med*. 1996;334:1685–1690

75. Maisels MJ, Newman TB. Kernicterus in otherwise healthy, breast-fed term newborns. *Pediatrics*. 1995;96:730–733

76. Bratlid D. How bilirubin gets into the brain. *Clin Perinatol*. 1990;17: 449–465

77. Cashore WJ, Oh W. Unbound bilirubin and kernicterus in low-birth-weight infants. *Pediatrics*. 1982;69:481–485

78. Nakamura H, Yonetani M, Uetani Y, Funato M, Lee Y. Determination of serum unbound bilirubin for prediction of kernicterus in low birth-weight infants. *Acta Paediatr Jpn*. 1992;34:642–647

79. Funato M, Tamai H, Shimada S, Nakamura H. Vigintiphobia, unbound bilirubin, and auditory brainstem responses. *Pediatrics*. 1994;93:50–53

80. Amin SB, Ahlfors CE, Orlando MS, Dalzell LE, Merle KS, Guillet R. Bilirubin and serial auditory brainstem responses in premature infants. *Pediatrics*. 2001;107:664–670

81. Johnson L, Boggs TR. Bilirubin-dependent brain damage: incidence and indications for treatment. In: Odell GB, Schaffer R, Simopoulos AP, eds. *Phototherapy in the Newborn: An Overview*. Washington, DC: National Academy of Sciences; 1974:122–149

82. Odell GB, Storey GNB, Rosenberg LA. Studies in kernicterus. 3. The saturation of serum proteins with bilirubin during neonatal life and its relationship to brain damage at five years. *J Pediatr*. 1970;76:12–21

83. Ahlfors CE. Criteria for exchange transfusion in jaundiced newborns. *Pediatrics*. 1994;93:488–494

84. Cashore WJ. Free bilirubin concentrations and bilirubin-binding affinity in term and preterm infants. *J Pediatr*. 1980;96:521–527

85. Ebbesen F, Brodersen R. Risk of bilirubin acid precipitation in preterm infants with respiratory distress syndrome: considerations of blood/brain bilirubin transfer equilibrium. *Early Hum Dev*. 1982;6:341–355

86. Cashore WJ, Oh W, Brodersen R. Reserve albumin and bilirubin toxicity index in infant serum. *Acta Paediatr Scand*. 1983;72:415–419

87. Ebbesen F, Nyboe J. Postnatal changes in the ability of plasma albumin to bind bilirubin. *Acta Paediatr Scand*. 1983;72:665–670

88. Esbjorner E. Albumin binding properties in relation to bilirubin and albumin concentrations during the first week of life. *Acta Paediatr Scand*. 1991;80:400–405

89. Robertson A, Sharp C, Karp W. The relationship of gestational age to reserve albumin concentration for binding of bilirubin. *J Perinatol*. 1988; 8:17–18

90. Wennberg RP. Cellular basis of bilirubin toxicity. *N Y State J Med*. 1991;91:493–496

APPENDIX 2: Phototherapy

There is no standardized method for delivering phototherapy. Phototherapy units vary widely, as do the types of lamps used in the units. The efficacy of phototherapy depends on the dose of phototherapy administered as well as a number of clinical factors (Table 5).[1]

Measuring the Dose of Phototherapy

Table 5 shows the radiometric quantities used in measuring the phototherapy dose. The quantity most commonly reported in the literature is the spectral irradiance. In the nursery, spectral irradiance can be measured by using commercially available radiometers. These instruments take a single measurement across a band of wavelengths, typically 425 to 475 or 400 to 480 nm. Unfortunately, there is no standardized method for reporting phototherapy dosages in the clinical literature, so it is difficult to compare published studies on the efficacy of phototherapy and manufacturers' data for the irradiance produced by different systems.[2] Measurements of irradiance from the same system, using different radiometers,

TABLE 5. Factors That Affect the Dose and Efficacy of Phototherapy

Factor	Mechanism/Clinical Relevance	Implementation and Rationale	Clinical Application
Spectrum of light emitted	Blue-green spectrum is most effective. At these wavelengths, light penetrates skin well and is absorbed maximally by bilirubin.	Special blue fluorescent tubes or other light sources that have most output in the blue-green spectrum and are most effective in lowering TSB.	Use special blue tubes or LED light source with output in blue-green spectrum for intensive PT.
Spectral irradiance (irradiance in certain wavelength band) delivered to surface of infant	$\uparrow$ irradiance $\rightarrow$ $\uparrow$ rate of decline in TSB	Irradiance is measured with a radiometer as $\mu W/cm^2$ per nm. Standard PT units deliver 8–10 $\mu W/cm^2$ per nm (Fig 6). Intensive PT requires >30 $\mu W/cm^2$ per nm.	If special blue fluorescent tubes are used, bring tubes as close to infant as possible to increase irradiance (Fig 6). Note: This cannot be done with halogen lamps because of the danger of burn. Special blue tubes 10–15 cm above the infant will produce an irradiance of at least 35 $\mu W/cm^2$ per nm.
Spectral power (average spectral irradiance across surface area)	$\uparrow$ surface area exposed $\rightarrow$ $\uparrow$ rate of decline in TSB	For intensive PT, expose maximum surface area of infant to PT.	Place lights above and fiber-optic pad or special blue fluorescent tubes* below the infant. For maximum exposure, line sides of bassinet, warmer bed, or incubator with aluminum foil.
Cause of jaundice	PT is likely to be less effective if jaundice is due to hemolysis or if cholestasis is present. ($\uparrow$ direct bilirubin)		When hemolysis is present, start PT at lower TSB levels. Use intensive PT. Failure of PT suggests that hemolysis is the cause of jaundice. If $\uparrow$ direct bilirubin, watch for bronze baby syndrome or blistering.
TSB level at start of PT	The higher the TSB, the more rapid the decline in TSB with PT.		Use intensive PT for higher TSB levels. Anticipate a more rapid decrease in TSB when TSB >20 mg/dL (342 $\mu mol/L$).

PT indicates phototherapy; LED, light-emitting diode.
* Available in the Olympic BiliBassinet (Olympic Medical, Seattle, WA).

can also produce significantly different results. The width of the phototherapy lamp's emissions spectrum (narrow versus broad) will affect the measured irradiance. Measurements under lights with a very focused emission spectrum (eg, blue light-emitting diode) will vary significantly from one radiometer to another, because the response spectra of the radiometers vary from manufacturer to manufacturer. Broader-spectrum lights (fluorescent and halogen) have fewer variations among radiometers. Manufacturers of phototherapy systems generally recommend the specific radiometer to be used in measuring the dose of phototherapy when their system is used.

It is important also to recognize that the measured irradiance will vary widely depending on where the measurement is taken. Irradiance measured below the center of the light source can be more than double that measured at the periphery, and this dropoff at the periphery will vary with different phototherapy units. Ideally, irradiance should be measured at multiple sites under the area illuminated by the unit and the measurements averaged. The International Electrotechnical Commission[3] defines the "effective surface area" as the intended treatment surface that is illuminated by the phototherapy light. The commission uses 60 × 30 cm as the standard-sized surface.

Is It Necessary to Measure Phototherapy Doses Routinely?

Although it is not necessary to measure spectral irradiance before each use of phototherapy, it is important to perform periodic checks of phototherapy units to make sure that an adequate irradiance is being delivered.

The Dose-Response Relationship of Phototherapy

Figure 5 shows that there is a direct relationship between the irradiance used and the rate at which the serum bilirubin declines under phototherapy.[4] The data in Fig 5 suggest that there is a saturation point beyond which an increase in the irradiance produces no added efficacy. We do not know, however, that a saturation point exists. Because the conversion of bilirubin to excretable photoproducts is partly irreversible and follows first-order kinetics, there may not be a saturation point, so we do not know the maximum effective dose of phototherapy.

Effect on Irradiance of the Light Spectrum and the Distance Between the Infant and the Light Source

Figure 6 shows that as the distance between the light source and the infant decreases, there is a corresponding increase in the spectral irradiance.[5] Fig 6 also demonstrates the dramatic difference in irradi-

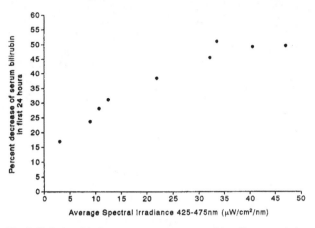

Fig 5. Relationship between average spectral irradiance and decrease in serum bilirubin concentration. Term infants with nonhemolytic hyperbilirubinemia were exposed to special blue lights (Phillips TL 52/20W) of different intensities. Spectral irradiance was measured as the average of readings at the head, trunk, and knees. Drawn from the data of Tan.[4] Source: *Pediatrics*. 1996;98: 283-287.

ance produced within the important 425- to 475-nm band by different types of fluorescent tubes.

What is Intensive Phototherapy?

Intensive phototherapy implies the use of high levels of irradiance in the 430- to 490-nm band (usually 30 $\mu W/cm^2$ per nm or higher) delivered to as much of the infant's surface area as possible. How this can be achieved is described below.

Using Phototherapy Effectively

Light Source

The spectrum of light delivered by a phototherapy unit is determined by the type of light source and

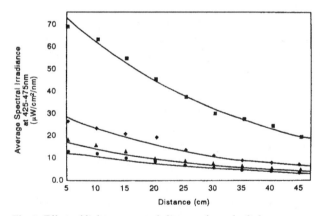

Fig 6. Effect of light source and distance from the light source to the infant on average spectral irradiance. Measurements were made across the 425- to 475-nm band by using a commercial radiometer (Olympic Bilimeter Mark II) and are the average of measurements taken at different locations at each distance (irradiance at the center of the light is much higher than at the periphery). The phototherapy unit was fitted with eight 24-in fluorescent tubes. ■ indicates special blue, General Electric 20-W F20T12/BB tube; ◆, blue, General Electric 20-W F20T12/B tube; ▲, daylight blue, 4 General Electric 20-W F20T12/B blue tubes and 4 Sylvania 20-W F20T12/D daylight tubes; •, daylight, Sylvania 20-W F20T12/D daylight tube. Curves were plotted by using linear curve fitting (True Epistat, Epistat Services, Richardson, TX). The best fit is described by the equation $y = Ae^{Bx}$. Source: *Pediatrics*. 1996;98:283-287.

any filters used. Commonly used phototherapy units contain daylight, cool white, blue, or "special blue" fluorescent tubes. Other units use tungsten-halogen lamps in different configurations, either free-standing or as part of a radiant warming device. Recently, a system using high-intensity gallium nitride light-emitting diodes has been introduced.[6] Fiber-optic systems deliver light from a high-intensity lamp to a fiber-optic blanket. Most of these devices deliver enough output in the blue-green region of the visible spectrum to be effective for standard phototherapy use. However, when bilirubin levels approach the range at which intensive phototherapy is recommended, maximal efficiency must be sought. The most effective light sources currently commercially available for phototherapy are those that use special blue fluorescent tubes[7] or a specially designed light-emitting diode light (Natus Inc, San Carlos, CA).[6] The special blue fluorescent tubes are labeled F20T12/BB (General Electric, Westinghouse, Sylvania) or TL52/20W (Phillips, Eindhoven, The Netherlands). It is important to note that special blue tubes provide much greater irradiance than regular blue tubes (labeled F20T12/B) (Fig 6). Special blue tubes are most effective because they provide light predominantly in the blue-green spectrum. At these wavelengths, light penetrates skin well and is absorbed maximally by bilirubin.[7]

There is a common misconception that ultraviolet light is used for phototherapy. The light systems used do not emit significant ultraviolet radiation, and the small amount of ultraviolet light that is emitted by fluorescent tubes and halogen bulbs is in longer wavelengths than those that cause erythema. In addition, almost all ultraviolet light is absorbed by the glass wall of the fluorescent tube and the Plexiglas cover of the phototherapy unit.

Distance From the Light

As can be seen in Fig 6, the distance of the light source from the infant has a dramatic effect on the spectral irradiance, and this effect is most significant when special blue tubes are used. To take advantage of this effect, the fluorescent tubes should be placed as close to the infant as possible. To do this, the infant should be in a bassinet, not an incubator, because the top of the incubator prevents the light from being brought sufficiently close to the infant. In a bassinet, it is possible to bring the fluorescent tubes within approximately 10 cm of the infant. Naked term infants do not become overheated under these lights. It is important to note, however, that the halogen spot phototherapy lamps cannot be positioned closer to the infant than recommended by the manufacturers without incurring the risk of a burn. When halogen lamps are used, manufacturers recommendations should be followed. The reflectors, light source, and transparent light filters (if any) should be kept clean.

Surface Area

A number of systems have been developed to provide phototherapy above and below the infant.[8,9] One commercially available system that does this is the BiliBassinet (Olympic Medical, Seattle, WA). This unit provides special blue fluorescent tubes above and below the infant. An alternative is to place fiberoptic pads below an infant with phototherapy lamps above. One disadvantage of fiber-optic pads is that they cover a relatively small surface area so that 2 or 3 pads may be needed.[5] When bilirubin levels are extremely high and must be lowered as rapidly as possible, it is essential to expose as much of the infant's surface area to phototherapy as possible. In these situations, additional surface-area exposure can be achieved by lining the sides of the bassinet with aluminum foil or a white cloth.[10]

In most circumstances, it is not necessary to remove the infant's diaper, but when bilirubin levels approach the exchange transfusion range, the diaper should be removed until there is clear evidence of a significant decline in the bilirubin level.

What Decline in the Serum Bilirubin Can You Expect?

The rate at which the bilirubin declines depends on the factors listed in Table 5, and different responses can be expected depending on the clinical circumstances. When bilirubin levels are extremely high (more than 30 mg/dL [513 μmol/L]), and intensive phototherapy is used, a decline of as much as 10 mg/dL (171 μmol/L) can occur within a few hours,[11] and a decrease of at least 0.5 to 1 mg/dL per hour can be expected in the first 4 to 8 hours.[12] On average, for infants of more than 35 weeks' gestation readmitted for phototherapy, intensive phototherapy can produce a decrement of 30% to 40% in the initial bilirubin level by 24 hours after initiation of phototherapy.[13] The most significant decline will occur in the first 4 to 6 hours. With standard phototherapy systems, a decrease of 6% to 20% of the initial bilirubin level can be expected in the first 24 hours.[8,14]

Intermittent Versus Continuous Phototherapy

Clinical studies comparing intermittent with continuous phototherapy have produced conflicting results.[15–17] Because all light exposure increases bilirubin excretion (compared with darkness), no plausible scientific rationale exists for using intermittent phototherapy. In most circumstances, however, phototherapy does not need to be continuous. Phototherapy may be interrupted during feeding or brief parental visits. Individual judgment should be exercised. If the infant's bilirubin level is approaching the exchange transfusion zone (Fig 4), phototherapy should be administered continuously until a satisfactory decline in the serum bilirubin level occurs or exchange transfusion is initiated.

Hydration

There is no evidence that excessive fluid administration affects the serum bilirubin concentration. Some infants who are admitted with high bilirubin levels are also mildly dehydrated and may need supplemental fluid intake to correct their dehydration. Because these infants are almost always breastfed, the best fluid to use in these circumstances is a milk-based formula, because it inhibits the enterohepatic circulation of bilirubin and should help to lower the serum bilirubin level. Because the photo-

products responsible for the decline in serum bilirubin are excreted in urine and bile,[18] maintaining adequate hydration and good urine output should help to improve the efficacy of phototherapy. Unless there is evidence of dehydration, however, routine intravenous fluid or other supplementation (eg, with dextrose water) of term and near-term infants receiving phototherapy is not necessary.

When Should Phototherapy Be Stopped?

There is no standard for discontinuing phototherapy. The TSB level for discontinuing phototherapy depends on the age at which phototherapy is initiated and the cause of the hyperbilirubinemia.[13] For infants who are readmitted after their birth hospitalization (usually for TSB levels of 18 mg/dL [308 μmol/L] or higher), phototherapy may be discontinued when the serum bilirubin level falls below 13 to 14 mg/dL (239-239 μmol/L). Discharge from the hospital need not be delayed to observe the infant for rebound.[13,19,20] If phototherapy is used for infants with hemolytic diseases or is initiated early and discontinued before the infant is 3 to 4 days old, a follow-up bilirubin measurement within 24 hours after discharge is recommended.[13] For infants who are readmitted with hyperbilirubinemia and then discharged, significant rebound is rare, but a repeat TSB measurement or clinical follow-up 24 hours after discharge is a clinical option.[13]

Home Phototherapy

Because the devices available for home phototherapy may not provide the same degree of irradiance or surface-area exposure as those available in the hospital, home phototherapy should be used only in infants whose bilirubin levels are in the "optional phototherapy" range (Fig 3); it is not appropriate for infants with higher bilirubin concentrations. As with hospitalized infants, it is essential that serum bilirubin levels be monitored regularly.

Sunlight Exposure

In their original description of phototherapy, Cremer et al[21] demonstrated that exposure of newborns to sunlight would lower the serum bilirubin level. Although sunlight provides sufficient irradiance in the 425- to 475-nm band to provide phototherapy, the practical difficulties involved in safely exposing a naked newborn to the sun either inside or outside (and avoiding sunburn) preclude the use of sunlight as a reliable therapeutic tool, and it therefore is not recommended.

Complications

Phototherapy has been used in millions of infants for more than 30 years, and reports of significant toxicity are exceptionally rare. Nevertheless, phototherapy in hospital separates mother and infant, and eye patching is disturbing to parents. The most important, but uncommon, clinical complication occurs in infants with cholestatic jaundice. When these infants are exposed to phototherapy, they may develop a dark, grayish-brown discoloration of the skin, serum, and urine (the bronze infant syndrome).[22] The pathogenesis of this syndrome is unknown, but it may be related to an accumulation of porphyrins and other metabolites in the plasma of infants who develop cholestasis.[22,23] Although it occurs exclusively in infants with cholestasis, not all infants with cholestatic jaundice develop the syndrome.

This syndrome generally has had few deleterious consequences, and if there is a need for phototherapy, the presence of direct hyperbilirubinemia should not be considered a contraindication to its use. This is particularly important in sick neonates. Because the products of phototherapy are excreted in the bile, the presence of cholestasis will decrease the efficacy of phototherapy. Nevertheless, infants with direct hyperbilirubinemia often show some response to phototherapy. In infants receiving phototherapy who develop the bronze infant syndrome, exchange transfusion should be considered if the TSB is in the intensive phototherapy range and phototherapy does not promptly lower the TSB. Because of the paucity of data, firm recommendations cannot be made. Note, however, that the direct serum bilirubin should not be subtracted from the TSB concentration in making decisions about exchange transfusions (see Fig 4).

Rarely, purpura and bullous eruptions have been described in infants with severe cholestatic jaundice receiving phototherapy,[24,25] and severe blistering and photosensitivity during phototherapy have occurred in infants with congenital erythropoietic porphyria.[26,27] Congenital porphyria or a family history of porphyria is an absolute contraindication to the use of phototherapy, as is the concomitant use of drugs or agents that are photosensitizers.[28]

REFERENCES

1. Maisels MJ. Phototherapy—traditional and nontraditional. *J Perinatol.* 2001;21(suppl 1):S93–S97
2. Fiberoptic phototherapy systems. *Health Devices.* 1995;24:132–153
3. International Electrotechnical Commission. Medical electrical equipment—part 2-50: particular requirements for the safety of infant phototherapy equipment. 2000. IEC 60601-2-50. Available at www.iec.ch. Accessed June 7, 2004
4. Tan KL. The pattern of bilirubin response to phototherapy for neonatal hyperbilirubinemia. *Pediatr Res.* 1982;16:670–674
5. Maisels MJ. Why use homeopathic doses of phototherapy? *Pediatrics.* 1996;98:283–287
6. Seidman DS, Moise J, Ergaz Z, et al. A new blue light-emitting phototherapy device: a prospective randomized controlled study. *J Pediatr.* 2000;136:771–774
7. Ennever JF. Blue light, green light, white light, more light: treatment of neonatal jaundice. *Clin Perinatol.* 1990;17:467–481
8. Garg AK, Prasad RS, Hifzi IA. A controlled trial of high-intensity double-surface phototherapy on a fluid bed versus conventional phototherapy in neonatal jaundice. *Pediatrics.* 1995;95:914–916
9. Tan KL. Phototherapy for neonatal jaundice. *Clin Perinatol.* 1991;18:423–439
10. Eggert P, Stick C, Schroder H. On the distribution of irradiation intensity in phototherapy. Measurements of effective irradiance in an incubator. *Eur J Pediatr.* 1984;142:58–61
11. Hansen TW. Acute management of extreme neonatal jaundice—the potential benefits of intensified phototherapy and interruption of enterohepatic bilirubin circulation. *Acta Paediatr.* 1997;86:843–846
12. Newman TB, Liljestrand P, Escobar GJ. Infants with bilirubin levels of 30 mg/dL or more in a large managed care organization. *Pediatrics.* 2003;111(6 Pt 1):1303–1311
13. Maisels MJ, Kring E. Bilirubin rebound following intensive phototherapy. *Arch Pediatr Adolesc Med.* 2002;156:669–672
14. Tan KL. Comparison of the efficacy of fiberoptic and conventional phototherapy for neonatal hyperbilirubinemia. *J Pediatr.* 1994;125:607–612
15. Rubaltelli FF, Zanardo V, Granati B. Effect of various phototherapy regimens on bilirubin decrement. *Pediatrics.* 1978;61:838–841
16. Maurer HM, Shumway CN, Draper DA, Hossaini AA. Controlled trial comparing agar, intermittent phototherapy, and continuous phototherapy for reducing neonatal hyperbilirubinemia. *J Pediatr.* 1973;82:73–76
17. Lau SP, Fung KP. Serum bilirubin kinetics in intermittent phototherapy of physiological jaundice. *Arch Dis Child.* 1984;59:892–894
18. McDonagh AF, Lightner DA. 'Like a shrivelled blood orange'—bilirubin, jaundice, and phototherapy. *Pediatrics.* 1985;75:443–455
19. Yetman RJ, Parks DK, Huseby V, Mistry K, Garcia J. Rebound bilirubin levels in infants receiving phototherapy. *J Pediatr.* 1998;133:705–707
20. Lazar L, Litwin A, Merlob P. Phototherapy for neonatal nonhemolytic hyperbilirubinemia. Analysis of rebound and indications for discontinuing therapy. *Clin Pediatr (Phila).* 1993;32:264–267
21. Cremer RJ, Perryman PW, Richards DH. Influence of light on the hyperbilirubinemia of infants. *Lancet.* 1958;1(7030):1094–1097
22. Rubaltelli FF, Jori G, Reddi E. Bronze baby syndrome: a new porphyrin-related disorder. *Pediatr Res.* 1983;17:327–330
23. Meisel P, Jahrig D, Theel L, Ordt A, Jahrig K. The bronze baby syndrome: consequence of impaired excretion of photobilirubin? *Photobiochem Photobiophys.* 1982;3:345–352
24. Mallon E, Wojnarowska F, Hope P, Elder G. Neonatal bullous eruption as a result of transient porphyrinemia in a premature infant with hemolytic disease of the newborn. *J Am Acad Dermatol.* 1995;33:333–336
25. Paller AS, Eramo LR, Farrell EE, Millard DD, Honig PJ, Cunningham BB. Purpuric phototherapy-induced eruption in transfused neonates: relation to transient porphyrinemia. *Pediatrics.* 1997;100:360–364
26. Tonz O, Vogt J, Filippini L, Simmler F, Wachsmuth ED, Winterhalter KH. Severe light dermatosis following phototherapy in a newborn infant with congenital erythropoietic urophyria [in German]. *Helv Paediatr Acta.* 1975;30:47–56
27. Soylu A, Kavukcu S, Turkmen M. Phototherapy sequela in a child with congenital erythropoietic porphyria. *Eur J Pediatr.* 1999;158:526–527
28. Kearns GL, Williams BJ, Timmons OD. Fluorescein phototoxicity in a premature infant. *J Pediatr.* 1985;107:796–798

All clinical practice guidelines from the American Academy of Pediatrics automatically expire 5 years after publication unless reaffirmed, revised, or retired at or before that time.

ERRATUM

Two errors appeared in the American Academy of Pediatrics clinical practice guideline, titled "Management of Hyperbilirubinemia in the Newborn Infant 35 or More Weeks of Gestation," that was published in the July 2004 issue of *Pediatrics* (2004;114:297–316). On page 297, Background section, first paragraph, the second sentence should read: "The current guideline represents a consensus of the committee charged by the AAP with reviewing and updating the existing guideline and is based on a careful review of the evidence, including a comprehensive literature review by the Agency for Healthcare Research and Quality and the New England Medical Center Evidence-Based Practice Center.[2]" On page 308, Appendix 1, first paragraph, the 4 levels of evidence quality should have been labeled A, B, C, and D rather than 1, 2, 3, and 4, respectively. The American Academy of Pediatrics regrets these errors.

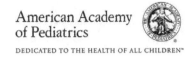

American Academy
of Pediatrics
DEDICATED TO THE HEALTH OF ALL CHILDREN™

Guidance for the Clinician in
Rendering Pediatric Care

CLINICAL REPORT

Neonatal Drug Withdrawal

abstract

Maternal use of certain drugs during pregnancy can result in transient neonatal signs consistent with withdrawal or acute toxicity or cause sustained signs consistent with a lasting drug effect. In addition, hospitalized infants who are treated with opioids or benzodiazepines to provide analgesia or sedation may be at risk for manifesting signs of withdrawal. This statement updates information about the clinical presentation of infants exposed to intrauterine drugs and the therapeutic options for treatment of withdrawal and is expanded to include evidence-based approaches to the management of the hospitalized infant who requires weaning from analgesics or sedatives. *Pediatrics* 2012;129:e540–e560

INTRODUCTION

Use and abuse of drugs, alcohol, and tobacco contribute significantly to the health burden of society. The 2009 National Survey on Drug Use and Health reported that recent (within the past month) use of illicit drugs, binge or heavy alcohol ingestion, and use of tobacco products occurred in 8.7%, 23.7%, and 27.7%, respectively, of the population 12 years or older.[1] Numerous case reports have documented the use of a variety of drugs by women of childbearing age (Table 1). Intrauterine exposure to certain drugs may cause congenital anomalies and/or fetal growth restriction, increase the risk of preterm birth, produce signs of withdrawal or toxicity in the neonate, or impair normal neurodevelopment.[2] Fetal exposure to marijuana, the illicit drug most commonly used by pregnant women, does not cause clinically important neonatal withdrawal signs but may have subtle effects on long-term neurobehavioral outcomes.[3] With the use of computer-assisted interviewing techniques that preserved confidentiality, the 2009 National Survey on Drug Use and Health noted that 4.5% of pregnant women 15 to 44 years of age reported recent use of illicit drugs (eg, marijuana, cocaine, hallucinogens, heroin, methamphetamines, and nonmedical use of prescription drugs). Binge or heavy drinking in the first trimester was reported by 11.9%, and recent tobacco use was reported by 15.3%. Rates of recent illicit drug use and smoking were lower among pregnant compared with non-pregnant women across all age groups, except for those 15 to 17 years of age. In the latter age group, the rates of illicit drug use and smoking were higher among those who were pregnant compared with those who were not pregnant (15.8% vs 13.0% and 20.6% vs 13.9%, respectively). The reported rates of illicit drug use most likely underestimate true rates, because the percentage of pregnant women who report the recent use of illicit drugs on screening interviews can

Mark L. Hudak, MD, Rosemarie C. Tan, MD,, PhD, THE COMMITTEE ON DRUGS, and THE COMMITTEE ON FETUS AND NEWBORN

KEY WORDS
opioid, methadone, heroin, fentanyl, benzodiazepine, cocaine, methamphetamine, SSRI, drug withdrawal, neonate, abstinence syndrome

ABBREVIATIONS
CNS—central nervous system
DTO—diluted tincture of opium
ECMO—extracorporeal membrane oxygenation
FDA—Food and Drug Administration
5-HIAA—5-hydroxyindoleacetic acid
ICD-9—International Classification of Diseases, Ninth Revision
NAS—neonatal abstinence syndrome
SSRI—selective serotonin reuptake inhibitor

www.pediatrics.org/cgi/doi/10.1542/peds.2011-3212

doi:10.1542/peds.2011-3212

All clinical reports from the American Academy of Pediatrics automatically expire 5 years after publication unless reaffirmed, revised, or retired at or before that time.

PEDIATRICS (ISSN Numbers: Print, 0031-4005; Online, 1098-4275).

TABLE 1 Major Drugs of Abuse[a]

Opioids	CNS Stimulants	CNS Depressants	Hallucinogens
Agonists	Amphetamines	Alcohol	Indolealkylamines (LSD, psilocin, psilocybin, DMT, DET)
Morphine	Dextroamphetamine (Dexedrine)	Barbiturates	Phenylethylamines (mescaline, peyote)
Codeine	Methamphetamine	Benzodiazepines	Phenylisopropylamines (MDA, MMDA, MDMA, MDEA)
Methadone	Amphetamine sulfate	Other sedative-hypnotics	Inhalants
Meperidine (Demerol)	Amphetamine congeners	Methaqualone (Quaalude)	Solvents and aerosols (glues, gasoline, paint thinner, cleaning solutions, nail polish remover, Freon)
Oxycodone (Percodan, OxyIR, Percolone, Roxicodone, Percocet, OxyContin)	Benzphetamine (Didrex)	Glutethimide (Doriden)	Nitrites
Propoxyphene (Darvon)	Diethylpropion (Tenuate)	Chloral hydrate	Nitrous oxide
Hydromorphone (Dilaudid)	Fenfluramine	Cannabinoids	
Hydrocodone (Lortab, Vicodin)	Phendimetrazine (Adipost, Bontril, Prelu-2)	Marijuana	
Fentanyl (Sublimaze)	Phentermine (Adipex-P, Zantryl)	Hashish	
Tramadol (Ultram, Ultracet)	Cocaine		
Heroin	Methylphenidate (Ritalin, Concerta)		
Antagonists	Pemoline (Cylert)		
Naloxone (Narcan)	Phenylpropanolamine		
Naltrexone (ReVia)	Phencyclidines		
Mixed Agonist-Antagonists	Nicotine		
Pentazocine (Talwin)			
Buprenorphine (Buprenex)			

DET, diethyltryptamine; DMT, dimethyltryptamine; LSD, lysergic acid diethylamide; MDA, methylenedioxyamphetamine; MDEA, 3,4-methylenedioxyethamphetamine; MDMA, 3,4-methylene-dioxymethamphetamine (ecstasy); and MMDA, 3-methoxy-4,5-methylenedioxyamphetamine.
[a] Adapted from Milhorn.[160]

be substantially lower than that determined by drug screening using biological samples. For infants, the use of *International Classification of Diseases, Ninth Revision* (*ICD-9*)-based hospital discharge databases to determine the incidence of neonatal drug withdrawal secondary to intrauterine exposure has in the past underestimated the incidence of this condition.[4] Data compiled by the Agency for Healthcare Research and Quality and by the Florida Department of Health attest to an increased incidence and/or recognition of neonatal withdrawal syndrome (ICD-9 code 779.5). Nationally, the number of infants coded at discharge with neonatal withdrawal increased from 7653 in 1995 to 11 937 in 2008. In Florida, the number of newborns discharged with ICD-9 code 779.5 climbed by more than 10-fold, from 0.4 to 4.4 discharges per 1000 live births, from 1995 to 2009. An indeterminate part of these observed increases has resulted from more liberal use of prescription opiates in pregnant women to palliate a wide variety of etiologies of acute or chronic pain. In a recent report, chronic use of narcotic prescriptions (use for ≥1 intrapartum month) among pregnant women cared for at a single clinic increased fivefold from 1998 to 2008, and 5.6% of infants delivered to these women manifested signs of neonatal withdrawal.[5]

Signs characteristic of neonatal withdrawal have been attributed to intrauterine exposure to a variety of drugs (Table 2). Other drugs cause signs in neonates because of acute toxicity. Chronic in utero exposure to a drug (eg, alcohol) can lead to permanent phenotypical and/or neurodevelopmental-behavioral abnormalities consistent with drug effect. Signs and symptoms of withdrawal worsen as drug levels decrease, whereas signs and symptoms of acute toxicity abate with drug elimination. Clinically important neonatal withdrawal most commonly results from intrauterine opioid exposure. The constellation of clinical findings associated with opioid withdrawal has been termed the neonatal abstinence syndrome (NAS). Among neonates exposed to opioids in utero, withdrawal signs will develop in 55% to 94%.[6–9] Neonatal withdrawal signs have also been described in infants exposed antenatally to benzodiazepines,[10,11] barbiturates,[12,13] and alcohol.[14,15]

COCAINE AND OTHER STIMULANTS

An abstinence syndrome after intrauterine exposure to central nervous system (CNS) stimulants such as cocaine and amphetamine has not been clearly defined. Many studies that have assessed behavior and neurologic signs in cocaine-exposed infants have used scoring systems that were designed to evaluate opioid withdrawal. Neurobehavioral abnormalities[16,17] frequently occur in neonates with intrauterine cocaine exposure, most frequently on the second or third postnatal days.[18] These abnormalities may include irritability, hyperactivity, tremors, high-pitched cry, and excessive sucking. Because cocaine or its metabolites may be detected in neonatal urine

TABLE 2 Maternal Nonnarcotic Drugs That Cause Neonatal Psychomotor Behavior Consistent With Withdrawal

Drug	Signs	Onset of Signs	Duration of Signs[a]	Ref. No.
Alcohol	Hyperactivity, crying, irritability, poor suck, tremors, seizures; onset of signs at birth, poor sleeping pattern, hyperphagia, diaphoresis	3–12 h	18 mo	14,15
Barbiturates	Irritability, severe tremors, hyperacusis, excessive crying, vasomotor instability, diarrhea, restlessness, increased tone, hyperphagia, vomiting, disturbed sleep; onset first 24 h of life or as late as 10–14 d of age	1–14 d	4-6 mo with prescription	12,13
Caffeine	Jitteriness, vomiting, bradycardia, tachypnea	At birth	1-7 d	161
Chlordiazepoxide	Irritability, tremors; signs may start at 21 d	Days–weeks	9 mo; 11/2 mo with prescription	11
Clomipramine	Hypothermia, cyanosis, tremors; onset 12 h of age		4 d with prescription	162
Diazepam	Hypotonia, poor suck, hypothermia, apnea, hypertonia, hyperreflexia, tremors, vomiting, hyperactivity, tachypnea (mother receiving multiple drug therapy)	Hours–weeks	8 mo; 10–66 d with prescription	10
Ethchlorvynol	Lethargy, jitteriness, hyperphagia, irritability, poor suck, hypotonia (mother receiving multiple drug therapy)		Possibly 10 d with prescription	163
Glutethimide	Increased tone, tremors, opisthotonos, high-pitched cry, hyperactivity, irritability, colic		6 mo	164
Hydroxyzine	Tremors, irritability, hyperactivity, jitteriness, shrill cry, myoclonic jerks, hypotonia, increased respiratory and heart rates, feeding problems, clonic movements (mother receiving multiple drug therapy)		5 wk with prescription	58
Meprobamate	Irritability, tremors, poor sleep patterns, abdominal pain		9 mo; 3 mo with prescription	165
SSRIs	Crying, irritability, tremors, poor suck, feeding difficulty, hypertonia, tachypnea, sleep disturbance, hypoglycemia, seizures	Hours–days	1–4 wk	31–33,35

[a] Prescription indicates the infant was treated with pharmacologic agents, and the natural course of the signs may have been shortened.

for as long as 7 days after delivery,[18] observed abnormalities in exposed infants may reflect drug effect rather than withdrawal. In an unmasked study, 6%, 14%, and 35% of infants exposed to cocaine only, heroin only, or cocaine plus heroin, respectively, qualified for treatment on the basis of scoring.[19] Several studies that used masked evaluators found that cocaine-exposed infants had either no[20,21] or minimal[22] withdrawal signs compared with cocaine-naïve infants (ie, those never exposed). Eyler et al[16] conducted a prospective controlled study of 3 groups of infants: 1 group had no documented exposure to cocaine by history or by maternal and infant urine testing; a second group was cocaine exposed but had negative urine screening at birth; and a third group had cocaine metabolites detected in neonatal urine. Observers masked to infant status performed assessments using the Brazelton Neonatal Behavioral Assessment Scale.[23] Infants who were positive for cocaine metabolites did not differ significantly

from metabolite-negative infants with a history of exposure nor from cocaine-naïve infants. These findings supported neither a withdrawal nor a drug toxicity syndrome. Cocaine-exposed infants have been described as having a higher incidence of abnormal auditory brainstem responses and EEGs, compared with nonexposed infants.[24,25] In another study, infants with heavy exposure to cocaine had similar Brazelton findings at 2 to 3 days of age as did infants with light or no exposure; however, by 17 days of age, heavily exposed infants were more excitable and demonstrated poorer state regulation.[26] No published studies have carefully evaluated pharmacologic treatment of infants with signs attributable to prenatal cocaine exposure.

Methamphetamine abuse has been reported among pregnant women,[27] although overall rates are low compared with cocaine and appear to have decreased in the general population between 2006 and 2008.[1] Methamphetamine is an extremely potent

sympathomimetic agent that induces euphoria and increases alertness and self-confidence, because it produces a massive efflux of dopamine in the CNS. Pregnant women who abuse methamphetamine are at increased risk of preterm birth, placental abruption, fetal distress, and intrauterine growth restriction at rates similar to those for pregnant women who use cocaine. In 1 study, only 4% of infants exposed to methamphetamine were treated for drug withdrawal, but it was not possible to exclude concomitant abuse of other drugs as contributory in all cases.[27] There are reports of long-term adverse neurotoxic effects of in utero methamphetamine exposure on behavior, cognitive skills, and physical dexterity.[28,29]

SELECTIVE SEROTONIN REUPTAKE INHIBITORS

Selective serotonin reuptake inhibitors (SSRIs) are a class of antidepressant medications that became available for widespread clinical use in 1988. SSRIs (eg, fluoxetine [Prozac], paroxetine [Paxil], sertraline [Zoloft], citalopram [Celexa], escitalopram [Lexapro], and fluvoxamine [Luvox]) are now the most frequently used drugs to treat depression both in the general population and in pregnant women.[30] Case reports,[31] adverse drug reaction reports,[32] and prospective studies[33,34] linked third-trimester use of SSRIs in pregnant women to a constellation of neonatal signs that include continuous crying, irritability, jitteriness, and/or restlessness; shivering; fever; tremors; hypertonia or rigidity; tachypnea or respiratory distress; feeding difficulty; sleep disturbance; hypoglycemia; and seizures.[35] The onset of these signs ranged from several hours to several days after birth and usually resolved within 1 to 2 weeks. In 1 infant exposed to paroxetine, signs persisted through 4 weeks of age.[36] In severely affected infants, a short-term course of chlorpromazine provided measurable relief of symptoms.[36]

Several authors have discussed whether these signs are better explained by serotonin syndrome (attributable to increased serotonin concentration in the intersynaptic cleft) or by SSRI withdrawal (attributable to a relative hyposerotonergic state).[30,32,35,37–40] In adults, treatment with a single SSRI may cause mild to moderate serotonin syndrome, but severe signs are more likely to occur when 2 or more drugs that increase serotonin concentration by different mechanisms are prescribed.[35] In adults, serotonin syndrome is characterized by the following triad of clinical signs: changes in mental status (agitation, confusion); autonomic hyperactivity (fever, tachycardia, tachypnea, diaphoresis, mydriasis); and neuromuscular abnormalities (tremor, clonus, hyperreflexia, hypertonia). On the other hand, serotonin withdrawal in adults manifests with subjective symptoms that include anxiety, headache,

nausea, fatigue, low mood, and, rarely, extrapyramidal signs such as dystonia. Hence, in most cases, the clinical syndrome reported among neonates born to mothers on SSRI treatment is consistent with a gradual resolution of a hyperserotonergic condition rather than with the evolution of a hyposerotonergic state. Still, in a few cases, drug withdrawal may be a better explanation.[35]

Biochemical studies that correlate serial serum SSRI (or active metabolite) concentrations and markers of CNS serotonin activity (eg, 5-hydroxyindoleacetic acid [5-HIAA], a metabolite of serotonin) with changes in clinical signs could be helpful in differentiating toxicity from withdrawal. In adults, cerebrospinal fluid concentrations of 5-HIAA (but not serum concentrations of serotonin) correlate inversely with increased CNS serotonin activity that results from SSRI treatment. One prospective study compared concentrations of SSRI and active metabolites at birth, 2 days of life, and 2 weeks of life; cord blood monoamine and metabolite; and serial serotonergic scores in infants born to mothers on treatment with SSRIs and those of SSRI-naïve control infants.[39] The infants born to mothers on SSRIs had an average serotonergic score fourfold greater than SSRI-naïve infants. Cord blood 5-HIAA concentrations were inversely related to the initial serotonergic score, and the resolution of neonatal signs correlated with rapid declines in serially measured serum SSRI and metabolite concentrations.[39] These results do support drug toxicity rather than drug withdrawal as the cause of clinical signs. Recent authors have suggested the terms "serotonin discontinuation syndrome"[34] or "prenatal antidepressant exposure syndrome."[41]

Although 1 study reported decreased pain reactivity at 2 months of age

in infants with prenatal exposure to SSRIs,[42] several recent reviews have not identified adverse neurodevelopmental outcomes among infants born to women treated with SSRIs during pregnancy.[30,34,43,44] SSRI treatment should be continued during pregnancy at the lowest effective dose, because withdrawal of medication may have harmful effects on the mother-infant dyad. Clinicians should be aware that infants are at risk for manifesting clinical signs of drug toxicity or withdrawal over the first week of life and arrange for early follow-up after the initial hospital discharge. Ideally, recommendations about lactation and breastfeeding should be made in consideration of what is known about the differences among drugs in a therapeutic class vis-à-vis the ratio of human milk to maternal plasma drug concentration, the likely total daily infant drug dose (as a fraction of the daily maternal drug dose normalized for weight), and the ratio of infant to maternal plasma drug concentration. However, in the absence of known adverse effects (eg, diminished suck, sleep disturbances, decreased growth), what constitutes an acceptable fractional drug dose or ratio of plasma concentrations is arbitrary—is 0.10 acceptable but 0.20 not? Paroxetine is the only SSRI for which the ratio of infant to maternal plasma concentrations is low and uniformly <0.10.[45] Fortinguerra et al[46] documented that paroxetine, sertraline, and fluvoxamine are minimally excreted in human milk and provide the infant <10% of the maternal daily dose (normalized for weight). Yet, Weissman et al[45] cite studies in which 6% and 33% of the reported paired infant to maternal plasma concentration ratios for sertraline and fluvoxamine, respectively, are >0.10. A mother on treatment with an SSRI who desires to nurse her infant should be counseled about the benefits of breastfeeding as well as the potential risk that her infant may continue to be exposed to a measureable level of the SSRI with unknown long-term effects.

OPIOIDS

Opioids are a class of natural, endogenous, and synthetic compounds that activate primarily μ-opioid (but also κ- and δ-opioid) receptors in the CNS to produce supraspinal analgesia. Other acute effects include sedation, euphoria, miosis, respiratory depression, and decreased gastrointestinal motility. Prolonged use results in physical and psychological dependence. As a class, opioids demonstrate a narrow therapeutic index. On the other hand, the interpatient range of dose necessary to achieve a similar therapeutic effect is fairly wide because of genetic differences in pharmacokinetics and pharmacodynamics.[47] Morphine is 1 of many natural opioids that can be extracted from the opium poppy. Codeine, heroin (diacetylmorphine), hydromorphone (Dilaudid), fentanyl (Sublimaze), and methadone are examples of synthetic opioids. Endogenous opioids include enkephalins, endorphins, and endomorphins. The term opiate refers to a subclass of alkaloid opioids. Methadone exerts secondary effects by acting as an N-methyl-D-aspartate receptor antagonist, blocking the actions of glutamate, the primary excitatory neurotransmitter in the CNS. Opioids acutely inhibit the release of noradrenaline at synaptic terminals. With chronic opioid exposure, tolerance develops as the rate of noradrenaline release over time increases toward normal. Abrupt discontinuation of exogenous opioids results in supranormal release of noradrenaline and produces the autonomic and behavioral signs and symptoms characteristic of withdrawal.

Opioid abuse in pregnant women presents additional risks for the fetus and newborn. Opioids are small lipophilic molecular weight compounds that cross placental and blood-brain barriers. Active or passive maternal detoxification is associated with increased risk of fetal distress and fetal loss. Maintenance programs with methadone (a full μ-opioid agonist and a Food and Drug Administration [FDA] schedule II controlled substance) for pregnant women can sustain opioid concentrations in the mother and fetus in ranges that minimize opioid craving, suppress abstinence symptomatology, block heroin-induced euphoria, and prevent fetal stress. Other benefits from this once controversial treatment are optimization of prenatal care and general maternal physical and mental health, as well as anticipation of potential withdrawal signs in the newborn infant. Disadvantages of methadone include the extremely unlikely achievement of successful detoxification after delivery and a more severe and prolonged course of NAS compared with heroin exposure. These issues have encouraged the development of other synthetic opioids as alternative treatments to methadone.

Subsequent to the Drug Addiction Treatment Act of 2000 that allowed office-based treatment of addiction by using FDA schedule III to V drugs, the synthetic opioid buprenorphine (a partial μ-opioid agonist) was approved by the FDA in 2002 as a schedule III controlled substance for the treatment of opioid dependence. Neither methadone nor buprenorphine is approved for use in pregnant women, and both are categorized by the FDA as class C pregnancy drugs. Nonetheless, buprenorphine, either alone (Subutex) or in combination with naloxone (Suboxone), has been used both as a first-line treatment of heroin addiction and as a replacement drug for

methadone. Recent results from the Maternal Opioid Treatment: Human Experimental Research study suggest that buprenorphine has some advantages to methadone as a treatment of opioid addiction in pregnant women. Infants born to mothers treated with buprenorphine had shorter hospital stays (10 vs 17.5 days), had shorter treatment durations for NAS (4.1 vs 9.9 days), and required a lower cumulative dose of morphine (1.1 vs 10.4 mg) compared with infants born to mothers on methadone maintenance.[48]

CLINICAL PRESENTATION OF OPIOID WITHDRAWAL

The clinical presentation of NAS varies with the opioid, the maternal drug history (including timing of the most recent use of drug before delivery), maternal metabolism, net transfer of drug across the placenta, placental metabolism (W. Snodgrass, MD, PhD, personal communication, 2008), infant metabolism and excretion, and other factors. In addition, maternal use of other drugs and substances such as cocaine, barbiturates, hypnotics-sedatives, and cigarettes may influence the severity and duration of NAS. Because opioid receptors are concentrated in the CNS and the gastrointestinal tract, the predominant signs and symptoms of pure opioid withdrawal reflect CNS irritability, autonomic overreactivity, and gastrointestinal tract dysfunction (Table 3). Excess environmental stimuli and hunger will exacerbate the perceived severity of NAS.

Onset of signs attributable to neonatal withdrawal from heroin often begins within 24 hours of birth, whereas withdrawal from methadone usually commences around 24 to 72 hours of age.[49] For both opioids, evidence of withdrawal may be delayed until 5 to 7 days of age or later, which is typically after hospital discharge.[50] For

TABLE 3 Clinical Features of the Neonatal Narcotic Abstinence Syndrome

Neurologic Excitability	Gastrointestinal Dysfunction
Tremors	Poor feeding
Irritability	Uncoordinated and constant sucking
Increased wakefulness	Vomiting
High-pitched crying	Diarrhea
Increased muscle tone	Dehydration
Hyperactive deep tendon reflexes	Poor wt gain
Exaggerated Moro reflex	Autonomic signs
Seizures	Increased sweating
Frequent yawning and sneezing	Nasal stuffiness
	Fever
	Mottling
	Temperature instability

infants exposed to buprenorphine, 1 study found that onset of withdrawal peaked at 40 hours and that signs were most severe at 70 hours of age.[51] The different time courses reflect variations in the half-lives of drug elimination. However, if 1 week or longer has elapsed between the last maternal opioid use and delivery of the infant, the incidence of neonatal withdrawal is relatively low.[52] The incidence and severity of NAS are greater in infants exposed to methadone compared with those exposed to buprenorphine[48] or heroin. Still, severe withdrawal has been described in 0 to 50% of buprenorphine-exposed infants.[53–55] In the acute phase, seizures have occurred in 2% to 11% of infants withdrawing from opioids[49,50,56]; however, abnormal EEG results without overt seizure activity have been reported in >30% of neonates.[57,58] Subacute signs of opioid withdrawal may last up to 6 months.[59]

Seizures also may be associated with withdrawal from a variety of non-narcotic drugs (eg, barbiturates,[12,14] alcohol,[14] and sedative-hypnotics[60,61]). The mechanism and significance of seizures associated with withdrawal are unclear. Withdrawal from ethanol begins early, in general, during the first 3 to 12 hours after delivery.[12,15] Diagnosis of sedative withdrawal is more difficult, because classically it appears after the first few days of

life. Barbiturate withdrawal has a median onset of 4 to 7 days, but a wide range from days 1 through 14.[12,13] Other sedative-hypnotics have exhibited even later onset, including as late as day 12 for diazepam[10] and day 21 for chlordiazepoxide.[11]

Studies of the relationship between maternal methadone dose and the incidence and severity of NAS have provided contradictory findings. Some studies demonstrated that larger maternal methadone dosages in late pregnancy were associated with greater neonatal concentrations and increased risk of withdrawal,[8,9,62–68] but others refuted a correlation.[69–74] This lack of consensus is explained in part by different approaches to the management of antenatal methadone maintenance therapy. There were substantial variations in the mean and range of daily methadone dose in the populations studied. Studies that found no correlation tended to enroll infants born to mothers who had been prescribed higher doses of methadone (50–200 mg/day), whereas those that did note a relationship between maternal dose and NAS sequelae reported lower maternal doses (eg, <50 mg/day) or included women undergoing partial detoxification.[67] Another potential explanatory factor is the significant interindividual variability in maternal methadone metabolism.[75] As a result, cumulative fetal exposure can

be expected to vary among infants born to mothers on equivalent methadone regimens.

Methadone concentrations in cord blood and at 48 hours of age,[72] as well as the rate of decline in neonatal serum concentration,[65] appear to correlate with NAS signs. Kuschel et al[72] found that infants who required rescue treatment had lower cord blood methadone concentrations and that, in all but 1 infant, methadone concentrations were undetectable in the serum at 48 hours. Doberczak[65] noted that faster declines in postnatal blood methadone concentrations were associated with more severe CNS withdrawal.

Preterm Infants

Preterm infants have been described as being at lower risk of drug withdrawal with less severe and/or prolonged courses. Infants born at <35 weeks' gestation whose mothers received methadone maintenance had significantly lower total and CNS abstinence scores than did term infants of mothers receiving similar methadone dosages.[64] In a more recent study, lower gestational age correlated with a lower risk of neonatal withdrawal.[68] The apparent decreased severity of signs in preterm infants may relate to developmental immaturity of the CNS, differences in total drug exposure, or lower fat depots of drug. Alternatively, the clinical evaluation of the severity of abstinence may be more difficult in preterm infants, because scoring tools to describe withdrawal were largely developed in term or late preterm infants.[76,77] In a retrospective study, Dysart et al[78] compared the length of hospital stay, duration of medication, and cumulative medication exposure for preterm and term infants born to mothers enrolled in a methadone maintenance program. Infants were evaluated by using an abstinence scoring system[77] and treated uniformly with a neonatal opiate solution. All adverse outcomes were reduced in the preterm cohort.

Abuse of Multiple Drugs

The abuse of multiple drugs during pregnancy is not uncommon,[79] but its effect on the occurrence and severity of neonatal abstinence is controversial. In 1 study, abstinence scores of infants whose mothers abused cocaine and methadone were similar to the scores of infants whose mothers received high-dose maintenance methadone.[64] In another study, the neurobehavioral scores of infants exposed to intrauterine cocaine were similar to those of infants exposed to both cocaine and methadone.[80] Conversely, an unmasked study reported higher abstinence scores in infants exposed to both cocaine and heroin in comparison with those exposed to heroin or cocaine alone.[19] Infants born to mothers maintained on methadone who were also heavy smokers (>20 cigarettes per day) demonstrated higher withdrawal scores that peaked later than infants born to light smokers.[81]

A 1989 case report linked the administration of naloxone for the treatment of apnea in a baby born to a mother with recent methadone ingestion to the onset of seizures. The seizures resolved after morphine treatment but did not respond to administration of phenobarbital or diazepam.[82] For this reason, maternal use of opiates during pregnancy has remained a relative contraindication to the use of naloxone for the treatment of apnea or hypoventilation during the transition period after birth.

DIFFERENTIAL DIAGNOSIS

The presence of maternal characteristics known to be associated with drug abuse during pregnancy can be considered an indication to screen for intrauterine drug exposure. These characteristics include absent, late, or inadequate prenatal care; a previously documented or admitted history of drug abuse; a previous unexplained late fetal demise; precipitous labor; abruptio placentae; hypertensive episodes; severe mood swings; cerebrovascular accidents; myocardial infarction; and repeated spontaneous abortions.[80,83–88] The legal implications of testing and the need for consent from the mother may vary among the states.[89] Each hospital should consider adopting a policy for maternal and newborn screening to avoid discriminatory practices and to comply with local laws.

Withdrawal signs in the newborn may mimic other conditions, such as infection, hypoglycemia, hypocalcemia, hyperthyroidism, intracranial hemorrhage, hypoxic-ischemic encephalopathy, and hyperviscosity.[90] If none of these diagnoses is readily apparent, a detailed maternal drug history should be obtained that includes interviewing the mother about drug use and abuse by her partner, friends, and parents, in addition to queries about the mother's prescription and nonprescription drug use.[90,91] Because maternal self-reporting underestimates drug exposure and maternal urine screening during pregnancy fails to identify many cases of drug use,[83] appropriate neonatal drug screening should be performed. Conversely, no clinical signs should be attributed solely to drug withdrawal on the basis of a positive maternal history without a careful assessment to exclude other causes.

Screening is most commonly accomplished by using neonatal urine specimens. A urine sample must be collected as soon as possible after birth, because many drugs are rapidly metabolized and eliminated.[90,92,93] Even so, a positive urine screening result may only reflect recent drug use. Alcohol is detectable in neonatal urine for 6 to 16 hours after the last maternal ingestion. Amphetamines, benzodiazepines, cocaine metabolites, and opioids are usually cleared within 1 to 3 days after birth. Marijuana and cocaine metabolites may be detectable for weeks, depending on maternal usage.[94]

Drugs that are excreted in the hepatobiliary system as well as drugs excreted by the fetal kidneys into the amniotic fluid are concentrated in meconium. Hence, meconium analysis is most useful when the history and clinical presentation strongly suggest neonatal withdrawal, but the maternal and neonatal urine screening results are negative. Drawbacks of testing for drugs in meconium are that it is not typically performed by hospitals and that results are often not available for days to weeks. Meconium must be collected before it is contaminated by transitional, human milk, or formula stools—otherwise, the assay may not be valid or the reference laboratory may reject the sample. Assay of meconium, although not conclusive if the results are negative, is more likely to identify infants of drug-abusing mothers than is the testing of infant or maternal urine.[95,96] Other specimens that have been tested in research laboratories are maternal and neonatal hair.[97,98] Recently, testing of umbilical cord tissue by using drug class-specific immunoassays was shown to be in concordance with testing of paired meconium specimens at rates of 97%, 95%, 99%, and 91% for the detection of amphetamines, opiates, cocaine, and cannabinoids, respectively.[99] The availability of this tissue from the moment of birth (in contrast to the inherent delay in collecting urine or meconium) may foster the adoption of this method of testing.

ASSESSMENT AND NONPHARMACOLOGIC TREATMENT

Several semiobjective tools are available for quantifying the severity of neonatal withdrawal signs. Clinicians have used discrete or serial scores to assist with therapeutic decisions. The Lipsitz tool, also known as the Neonatal Drug Withdrawal Scoring System,[76] was recommended in the 1998 American Academy of Pediatrics statement "Neonatal Drug Withdrawal,"[100] probably because it is a relatively simple metric with good sensitivity for identifying clinically important withdrawal. The modified Neonatal Abstinence Scoring System (Fig 1),[101] is the predominant tool used in the United States.[102] This more comprehensive instrument assigns a cumulative score based on the interval observation of 21 items relating to signs of neonatal withdrawal.[103] In 1 study, administration of this scoring system with infants verified not to have been exposed to prenatal opiates by meconium analysis resulted in a stable median score of 2 during each of the first 3 days of life, with 95th percentile scores of 5.5 and 7 on days 1 and 2, respectively.[104]

Infants at risk for NAS should be carefully monitored in the hospital for the development of signs consistent with withdrawal. The appropriate duration of hospital observation is variable and depends on a careful assessment of the maternal drug history. An infant born to a mother on a low-dose prescription opiate with a short half-life (eg, hydrocodone; average half-life, 4 hours) may be safely discharged if there are no signs of withdrawal by 3 days of age, whereas an infant born to a mother on an opiate with a prolonged half-life (eg, methadone) should be observed for a minimum of 5 to 7 days. Initial treatment of infants who develop early signs of withdrawal is directed at minimizing environmental stimuli (both light and sound) by placing the infant in a dark, quiet environment; avoiding auto-stimulation by careful swaddling; responding early to an infant's signals;

NEONATAL ABSTINENCE SCORING SYSTEM

SYSTEM	SIGNS AND SYMPTOMS	SCORE	AM				PM						COMMENTS
CENTRAL NERVOUS SYSTEM DISTURBANCES	Continuous High Pitched (or other) Cry	2											Daily Weight:
	Continuous High Pitched (or other) Cry	3											
	Sleeps <1 Hour After Feeding	3											
	Sleeps <2 Hours After Feeding	2											
	Sleeps <3 Hours After Feeding	1											
	Hyperactive Moro Reflex	2											
	Markedly Hyperactive Moro Reflex	3											
	Mild Tremors Disturbed	1											
	Moderate-Severe Tremors Disturbed	2											
	Mild Tremors Undisturbed	3											
	Moderate-Severe Tremors Undisturbed	4											
	Increased Muscle Tone	2											
	Excoriation (Specific Area)	1											
	Myoclonic Jerks	3											
	Generalized Convulsions	5											
METABOLIC/VASOMOTOR/RESPIRATORY DISTURBANCES	Sweating	1											
	Fever 100.4°-101°F (38°-38.3°C)	1											
	Fever > 101°F (38.3°C)	2											
	Frequent Yawning (>3-4 times/interval)	1											
	Mottling	1											
	Nasal Stuffiness	1											
	Sneezing (>3-4 times/interval)	1											
	Nasal Flaring	2											
	Respiratory Rate >60/min	1											
	Respiratory Rate > 60/min with Retractions	2											
GASTRO-INTESTINAL DISTURBANCES	Excessive Sucking	1											
	Poor Feeding	2											
	Regurgitation	2											
	Projectile Vomiting	3											
	Loose Stools	2											
	Watery Stools	3											
	TOTAL SCORE												
	INITIALS OF SCORER												

FIGURE 1
Modified Finnegan's Neonatal Abstinence Scoring Tool. Adapted from ref 101.

adopting appropriate infant positioning and comforting techniques (swaying, rocking); and providing frequent small volumes of hypercaloric formula or human milk to minimize hunger and allow for adequate growth. Caloric needs may be as high as 150 to 250 cal/kg per day because of increased energy expenditure and loss of calories from regurgitation, vomiting, and/or loose stools.[105,106] The infant needs to be carefully observed to recognize fever, dehydration, or weight loss promptly. The goals of therapy are to ensure that the infant achieves adequate sleep and nutrition to establish a consistent pattern of weight gain and begins to integrate into a social environment. Maternal screening for comorbidities, such as HIV or hepatitis C virus infections and polydrug abuse, needs to be performed. Additional supportive care in the form of intravenous fluids, replacement electrolytes, and gavage feedings may be necessary to stabilize the infant's condition in the acute phase and obviate the need for pharmacologic intervention. When possible, and if not otherwise contraindicated, mothers who adhere to a supervised drug treatment program should be encouraged to breastfeed so long as the infant continues to gain weight. Breastfeeding or the feeding of human milk has been associated with less severe NAS that presents later and less frequently requires pharmacologic intervention.[107,108] Methadone is present in very low concentrations in human milk. Cumulative daily intake of methadone in fully breastfed infants has been estimated to range from 0.01 to 0.15 mg/day in the first 30 days of life[109] and 0.15 to 0.30 mg/day between 30 and 180 days of age.[110] Similarly, the amount of buprenorphine excreted in human milk is small. Although more information is needed to evaluate long-term neurodevelopmental outcome of infants exposed to small quantities of buprenorphine, there is no clear reason to discourage breastfeeding in mothers who adhere to methadone or buprenorphine maintenance treatment.[111]

Each nursery should adopt a protocol for the evaluation and management of neonatal withdrawal, and staff should be trained in the correct use of an abstinence assessment tool. In a recent survey of accredited US neonatology fellowship programs, only 55% had implemented a written NAS protocol, and only 69% used a published abstinence scoring system.[102]

RATIONALE AND COMPARATIVE EVIDENCE FOR PHARMACOLOGIC TREATMENT

Drug therapy is indicated to relieve moderate to severe signs of NAS and to prevent complications such as fever, weight loss, and seizures if an infant does not respond to a committed program of nonpharmacologic support. Since the introduction of the abstinence scales in 1975, published reports have documented that the decision to initiate pharmacologic treatment has been based on single or serial withdrawal scores. However, no studies to date have compared the use of different withdrawal score thresholds for initiating pharmacologic intervention on short-term outcomes (eg, severity and duration of withdrawal signs, weight gain, duration of hospitalization, need for pharmacologic treatment, or cumulative drug exposure). Withdrawal from opioids or sedative-hypnotic drugs may be life-threatening, but ultimately, drug withdrawal is a self-limited process. Unnecessary pharmacologic treatment will prolong drug exposure and the duration of hospitalization to the possible detriment of maternal-infant bonding. The only clearly defined benefit of pharmacologic treatment is the short-term amelioration of clinical signs.

Studies have not addressed whether long-term morbidity related to neonatal drug withdrawal is decreased by pharmacologic management of affected infants, or whether continued postnatal drug exposure augments the risk of neurobehavioral and other morbidities. It is possible that pharmacologic therapy of the infant may introduce or reinforce a maternal disposition to rely on drugs for the treatment of infant discomfort or annoying behavior.[112]

Clinicians have treated NAS with a variety of drug preparations, including opioids (tincture of opium, neonatal morphine solution, methadone, and paregoric), barbiturates (phenobarbital), benzodiazepines (diazepam, lorazepam), clonidine, and phenothiazines (chlorpromazine). Information pertinent to the use of these drug preparations in infants is well summarized in the previous American Academy of Pediatrics statement.[100] Recent surveys have documented that, in accord with the recommendations of that statement, 94% of UK and 83% of US clinicians use an opioid (morphine or methadone) as the drug of first choice. The majority of practitioners use phenobarbital as a second drug if the opiate does not adequately control withdrawal signs.[102,113] Daily doses of morphine ranged from 0.24 mg/kg per day to 1.3 mg/kg per day.[113] Paregoric is no longer used, because it contains variable concentrations of other opioids, as well as toxic ingredients such as camphor, anise oil, alcohol, and benzoic acid.[100] The use of diazepam has also fallen into disfavor because of a documented lack of efficacy compared with other agents and because of its adverse effects on infant suck and swallow reflexes.[114–116]

Meta-analyses of published trials regarding the pharmacologic treatment of neonatal withdrawal are available.[117,118] In 2 Cochrane meta-analyses, either an opioid[117] or a sedative[118] drug treatment was compared with a control treatment that could include a nonpharmacologic intervention, a placebo treatment, or another opioid and/or sedative drug. The authors prospectively designated 4 primary outcomes (failure of treatment to control withdrawal signs; incidence of seizures; survival; and neurodevelopmental outcome) for meta-analysis.

Treatment failure was defined variously as the inability of the treatment to maintain abstinence scores within a preset "safe" level and/or the need to add another drug therapy. Some studies did not report primary outcomes and instead quantified secondary outcomes (eg, duration of treatment, duration of hospitalization, rate of weight gain, etc).

Seven studies of opioid treatment that enrolled a total of 585 infants were identified between 1983 and 2004. Methodologic flaws were common and included quasirandom patient allocation; substantial and often unexplained differences in allocation of patients to treatment groups; imbalances in group characteristics after randomization; failure to mask study treatments; and failure to mask outcome measurements. In the single study that assessed oral morphine treatment versus supportive therapy only, 3 consecutive Finnegan scores ≥ 8 prompted institution of the intervention.[119]

No significant effect of morphine was found on the rate of treatment failure. Oral morphine significantly increased the duration of treatment and the length of hospital stay, but it did reduce the number of days required to regain birth weight and duration of supportive care. Four studies compared treatment failures of opioids (paregoric, oral morphine, or methadone) with phenobarbitone.[8,119–121] Neither the meta-analysis nor any individual study identified a significant difference in treatment failure. One study reported a lower incidence of

seizures in the opioid (paregoric) treatment group.[122] No consistent trends in secondary outcomes were observed, although 1 study reported a shorter duration of therapy in the phenobarbitone compared with the paregoric treatment group,[123] and another made the opposite observation when the opioid used was oral morphine.[121] Three studies individually and in combination reported significantly lower rates of treatment failure in infants assigned to opioid (paregoric or methadone) compared with diazepam therapy[8,114,120] but did not define differences in secondary outcomes. No studies reported mortality or neurodevelopmental outcomes.

A second Cochrane review analyzed 6 trials involving 305 infants published between 1969 and 2002 in which sedative treatment of NAS was compared with a nonopioid therapy. Methodologic concerns were similar to the opioid treatment trials. In the sole study of phenobarbitone versus supportive care, no difference in treatment failure was found, but treatment significantly increased the duration of therapy and hospital stay.[119] A small study that allocated infants already treated with diluted tincture of opium (DTO) to phenobarbitone as a second drug versus no additional treatment identified no infants in either group with treatment failure but observed significant reductions in the duration of hospitalization (38 vs 79 days) and the maximal daily dose of opioid in the phenobarbitone-treated infants.[124] Infants were discharged from the hospital once they were no longer taking opioids. However, the mean duration of phenobarbitone treatment was 3.5 months. Of 3 studies that compared phenobarbitone and diazepam treatment, 1 found a significantly lower rate of treatment failure in the phenobarbitone group.[8,114,120] One study of phenobarbitone versus chlorpromazine[125] found

no differences in primary or secondary outcomes.

Since 2004, a number of small studies of varying methodologic quality have compared pharmacologic treatments. In a prospective randomized double-masked study, Langenfeld et al[126] could not identify differences in duration of treatment, duration of hospitalization, or in weight gain (g/day) in infants treated with either DTO or oral morphine drops. A retrospective study found no difference in length of hospitalization in infants with NAS who were treated with methadone or oral morphine solution, but did correlate higher maternal methadone doses with longer lengths of stay.[127] Ebner et al[128] examined the incidence of NAS in infants born to mothers maintained with methadone, morphine, or buprenorphine and compared phenobarbital and oral morphine treatments in affected infants. Sixty-eight percent of infants born to mothers maintained on methadone required pharmacologic treatment at a mean age of 58 hours, compared with 82% of infants at a mean age of 33 hours in the morphine group and 21% of infants at a mean age of 34 hours in the buprenorphine group. The duration of treatment was significantly shorter for infants who received morphine compared with infants who were treated with phenobarbital. A randomized comparison trial of sublingual buprenorphine versus neonatal opium solution for the treatment of NAS showed a nonsignificant reduction in length of treatment and duration of hospitalization in the buprenorphine group.[129] Buprenorphine therapy was well tolerated.

Clonidine is an α_2-adrenergic receptor agonist that has been used in combination with an opioid or other drug in older children and adults to reduce withdrawal symptoms.[130,131] Via a negative feedback mechanism, clonidine reduces CNS sympathetic outflow and palliates symptoms of autonomic overactivity such as tachycardia, hypertension, diaphoresis, restlessness, and diarrhea. Cessation of clonidine treatment can result in a rebound of autonomic activity. Reported experience with clonidine as a primary or adjunctive treatment of NAS is limited but promising. In a small case series, 6 of 7 infants with NAS showed significant resolution of signs when treated with oral clonidine.[132] In a randomized double-masked controlled trial, Agthe et al[133] compared the efficacy and safety of treating NAS with DTO plus oral clonidine (1 μg/kg every 3 hours) versus DTO plus placebo in 80 infants with prenatal exposure to methadone and/or heroin. The combination therapy significantly reduced the median length of treatment of all infants and for infants exposed to methadone, but more infants in the DTO/clonidine group required resumption of DTO after initial discontinuation. The mean total dose of morphine over the treatment course was ~60% lower in the combination therapy group. No clinically significant differences in feeding, weight gain or loss, heart rate, or blood pressure were observed. In another case series, oral clonidine was administered either as a primary or adjunctive therapy for the prevention or treatment of narcotic withdrawal in infants on intravenous fentanyl or infants with antenatal exposure to opiates.[134] In all cases, treatment was successful and clonidine was discontinued without sequelae after a mean duration of 7 days. In a retrospective case series, infants who had evidence of NAS attributable to antenatal methadone exposure had lower severity scores and required fewer days of drug therapy and hospitalization if they had been treated with a combination of clonidine and chloral hydrate rather than a combination of morphine and phenobarbital.[135]

A recently published case series from France that used a historical cohort for a comparison has suggested that the treatment of NAS with the phenothiazine, chlorpromazine, as a single drug may be more effective than treatment with morphine.[136] Infants treated with oral morphine had significantly longer median durations of treatment and hospitalization in comparison with infants treated with chlorpromazine. No adverse affects were reported.

OUTCOME

Assessment of potential long-term morbidity specifically attributable to neonatal drug withdrawal and its treatment is difficult to evaluate. Few studies have followed drug-exposed children beyond the first few years of life. Confounding variables, such as environment and dysfunctional caregivers, complicates the interpretation of outcomes. In a small study, developmental scores on the mental index on the Bayley Scales of Infant Development were not affected by the severity of withdrawal or the treatment chosen.[114] Mean scores on the Bayley Scales of Infant Development were similar for all infants treated for withdrawal, including those receiving phenobarbital, paregoric, or a combination therapy. Scores of infants whose withdrawal was too mild to qualify for pharmacologic intervention were also similar.

Fourteen drug-exposed infants with withdrawal-associated seizures were reported by Doberczak et al.[25] The abstinence scores for 5 of these infants were <7 (the cutoff for treatment); hence, they received no pharmacologic therapy before the onset of seizures. Thirteen of the 14 infants were offspring of mothers enrolled in a methadone treatment program; however, the success of maternal treatment was not described. Of the 14 infants with seizures, 12 were available

for evaluation at 1 year of age; results of neurologic examinations were normal in 9 of the 12 infants evaluated. EEG results were abnormal in 9 neonates; however, subsequent EEGs for 7 of 8 of these infants normalized during follow-up. Mean scores on the Bayley Scales of Infant Development were also normal by 1 year of age, similar to matched controls that were drug exposed, but in whom withdrawal-associated seizures did not develop.[24] Withdrawal-associated seizures seem to be primarily myoclonic, to respond to opiates, and to carry no increased risk of poor outcome. Withdrawal-associated seizures in neonates are different from those associated with other causes. Based on the depression of norepinephrine and dopamine observed with methadone exposure in animal models, withdrawal seizures are speculated to be attributable to lowered levels of neurotransmitters.[137,138] The normalization of the EEG and normal neurologic development are believed to reflect recovery of normal neurotransmitter concentrations during early infancy. Bandstra et al[139] have comprehensively reviewed outcomes of infants and toddlers who were exposed prenatally to opioids and cocaine.

MANAGEMENT OF ACQUIRED OPIOID AND BENZODIAZEPINE DEPENDENCY

One of the cornerstones in caring for critically ill children is to provide adequate and safe analgesia, sedation, amnesia, and anxiolysis by using both pharmacologic and nonpharmacologic measures. Pharmacologic treatment typically includes medications in the opioid and benzodiazepine drug classes. However, if these drugs cannot safely be discontinued within a few days, physical dependence on 1 or both of these classes of medication can develop and manifest with signs and symptoms of withdrawal on acute dosage reduction or cessation of therapy. Infants who undergo complex surgery, who require prolonged medical intensive care for conditions such as respiratory failure or persistent pulmonary hypertension, or who are supported with extracorporeal membrane oxygenation (ECMO) therapy are among those at greatest risk of acquired drug dependency.

Extended treatment with opioids via continuous intravenous infusion results in drug tolerance. Even short-term opioid exposure alters the number and affinity of receptors in key neuronal centers so that an escalation of the opioid infusion rate (which produces an increase in opioid plasma concentrations) becomes necessary to achieve the same physiologic effect.[140] By itself, the development of tolerance does not predict physical dependency or withdrawal.[141] Cumulative exposure to fentanyl, quantified by the total dose in milligrams per kilogram or the number of consecutive days of treatment, correlated with the likelihood of withdrawal.[140,142,143] By using a multiple logistic regression analysis, Arnold et al[140] found that the duration of ECMO therapy was an even more powerful predictor of withdrawal than was cumulative fentanyl exposure. Katz et al[142] reported that among 23 mechanically ventilated children aged 1 week to 22 months (mean, 6 months) who were treated for >24 hours with a continuous fentanyl infusion, 13 of 23 children (57%) developed withdrawal as defined by a Finnegan score ≥8. In this prospective study, a cumulative fentanyl exposure in excess of 2.5 mg/kg or 9 days of therapy was 100% predictive of withdrawal. More recently, in a prospective study of 19 neonates treated with fentanyl for a minimum of 24 hours, Dominquez et al[143] documented that a cumulative fentanyl dose ≥415 µg/kg predicted withdrawal with

70% sensitivity and 78% specificity and that an infusion duration ≥8 days was 90% sensitive and 67% specific for withdrawal. In adults, concomitant treatment with neuromuscular paralytic agents or propofol for >24 hours also increased the likelihood of withdrawal.[144] Signs and symptoms of withdrawal from fentanyl commence within 24 hours of cessation of therapy.

The refinement of pain management in children over the past 2 decades has witnessed an expansion of the use of opioids in the intensive care setting. As a result, more children have been treated for actual or potential withdrawal symptoms as a comorbidity of hospitalization. Fentanyl, a pure µ-opioid receptor antagonist, has become the opioid of choice because of its rapid onset of action, short duration of effect (half-life of 0.5–1 hour), excellent potency, and minimal acute adverse effects. However, fentanyl has not been demonstrated to be safer or more effective than morphine for the provision of long-term analgesia. Indeed, 1 study has reported that patients who were treated prospectively with a continuous morphine infusion during ECMO experienced a significantly lower need for supplemental analgesia, a lower rate of dependency, and a shorter hospital stay compared with a previous group of patients treated with fentanyl during ECMO.[145]

Practitioners have employed a variety of strategies to treat or, in high-risk patients, to prevent signs and symptoms of opioid withdrawal in infants and children. Carr and Todres[146] reported success with a gradual taper of the opioid infusion rate. Children who had received continuous opioid infusions for more than a week required 2 to 3 weeks for complete weaning. One disadvantage of this approach was that intravenous access had to be maintained for the entire course of treatment. Tobias et al[147]

were among the first investigators to describe treatment of opioid withdrawal by conversion to enteral methadone. Methadone was chosen as the opioid of choice because of its excellent oral bioavailability (70%–100%) and long half-life (19–41 hours), which allowed for long intervals between doses.[148] In this initial report, 3 symptomatic patients who had been exposed to continuous or bolus opioids for up to 7 weeks were transitioned to a methadone regimen of 0.1 mg/kg, orally, every 12 hours. Dose reduction by 10% to 20% of the initial dose per week resulted in successful weaning in 4 to 6 weeks.

In 2000, Robertson and et al[149] reported the outcomes of 10 children 6 months to 18 years of age who had received >7 days of opioids (range, 7–53 days). An amount of methadone, equipotent to the existing daily fentanyl or morphine dose, was determined. This amount was reduced by a factor of 6 because of the longer half-life of methadone to calculate the initial total daily methadone dose. Protocols specified 2 different weaning schedules, depending on whether the patient had been treated with opioids (fentanyl or morphine) for either 7 to 14 days or for >14 days. Treatment intervals were gradually lengthened from every 6 hours to every 24 hours when methadone was discontinued. Outcomes of these patients were compared with recent control patients who had also been treated with enteral methadone but not under a standard protocol. Among the protocol patients, there were no treatment failures. Weaning was accomplished in a median of 9 days (range, 5–10 days), which was significantly less than the median of 20 days (range, 9–31 days) observed in the nonprotocol children. Concurrent use of benzodiazepines occurred in 6 of the protocol children, compared with 3 of the nonprotocol group, so that the decreased taper time on protocol was unlikely to have been confounded by other drug therapy. Weaning and discontinuation from benzodiazepines were successful during the methadone taper in all protocol patients.

Meyer et al[150] described a protocol for rescue therapy in 29 patients 1 day to 20 years of age on admission who developed withdrawal during the course of nonstandardized tapers of prolonged continuous fentanyl infusion. Withdrawal was defined as the observation of 3 consecutive Finnegan scores ≥8 obtained at 2-hour intervals. The daily fentanyl dose for the period 24 to 48 hours before withdrawal symptoms was used to calculate an equipotent dose of morphine sulfate. Morphine was administered as a bolus dose every 4 hours and titrated to effect (Finnegan score consistently <8) over 12 to 24 hours. An equipotent amount of methadone was then determined by using the effective morphine dose. Three loading doses of methadone at 12-hour intervals were administered. Afterward, doses were given every 24 hours and weaned by 10% per day. Ten patients were receiving concomitant treatment with a benzodiazepine or chloral hydrate, but these medications were not weaned during the methadone taper. Twenty-five of 29 patients successfully completed this taper over 10 days. Three patients required 21 days, and 1 patient died of sepsis. Sixteen of the patients were discharged from the hospital and completed methadone tapers on an outpatient basis. Nine of the patients had been started on clonidine during the phase of nonstandardized opioid weaning in unsuccessful attempts to prevent withdrawal. A subsequent randomized double-blind follow-up study by the same group of investigators[151]

found that in a group of 37 fentanyl-treated patients, a 5-day methadone taper was as successful as the longer 10-day course (13 of 16 vs 17 of 21 [not significant]) in discontinuing opioid infusions without causing withdrawal. In contrast to their previous study, a standardized taper of lorazepam was allowed in 17 of the 37 patients while on the methadone protocol. Only 1 of these 17 patients who underwent dual tapers required rescue treatment with an increased dose of opioids.

Several factors potentially complicate the adoption of the protocols reported by Robertson, Meyer, and Berens (see Table 4) into routine neonatal clinical practices. Most obvious is that these studies were conducted in a PICU setting; few neonates were included, and their outcomes were not separately analyzed. Other investigators have emphasized that the Finnegan instrument common to all 3 studies has been validated only in term infants undergoing withdrawal secondary to in utero opioid exposure.[152,153] Therefore, the use of this tool may have underestimated withdrawal symptomatology in an older pediatric population. A third concern is that opioids and benzodiazepines are often used concurrently in the same patient, yet symptoms of opioid and benzodiazepine withdrawal overlap to a great extent. Hence, current instruments will not reliably differentiate whether withdrawal symptoms stem from relative opioid or benzodiazepine abstinence.[153] Other scales have been proposed for children and are in various stages of evaluation, including the Opioid and Benzodiazepine Withdrawal Scale,[151] the Sedation Withdrawal Score,[154] and the Sophia Benzodiazepine and Opioid Withdrawal Checklist.[155]

At this time, no optimal pharmacologic regimen for the prevention or treatment of acquired opioid and/or

benzodiazepine dependency can be recommended, because the necessary comparative studies of safety and efficacy are not available.[156] Hence, it is even more incumbent on the practitioner to prescribe pharmacologic interventions with the goal of achieving the desired therapeutic effect by using the fewest drugs at the lowest doses and for the shortest durations possible.

Nonetheless, because many critically ill infants and children do receive treatment with prolonged courses of opioids and benzodiazepines, the following practices are reasonable based on the available evidence:

1. Each clinical unit can establish a threshold level of cumulative exposure to opioids and benzodiazepines above which drug dependency can be expected to occur with a likelihood that justifies anticipatory initiation of a weaning protocol. For example, setting a threshold at a cumulative fentanyl exposure of >2 mg/kg or >7 days' duration would predict a likelihood of dependency >50% but <100%.[141,142]

2. Infants with a cumulative exposure to opioids or benzodiazepines below the thresholds for initiation of weaning protocols can undergo a rapid taper of these medications over a 24- to 48-hour period. Many such children will not subsequently exhibit drug dependency.

3. Signs and symptoms of withdrawal will develop within 24 hours of discontinuation or during the course of a rapid taper of an opioid. If this occurs, 1 of the rescue approaches in Table 4 can be chosen as a guide to facilitate conversion to enteral methadone management and to initiate a weaning strategy, with 2 caveats. Infants on very high daily doses of continuous intravenous opioid may require less than the

TABLE 4 Weaning Protocols by Using Conversion of Continuous Opioid Infusions to Enteral Methadone and for Conversion of Midazolam (Versed) Infusion to Enteral Lorazepam (Ativan)

Robertson et al[149]

Conversion of continuous intravenous fentanyl of 7–14 d duration to enteral methadone:
1. By using the current hourly infusion rate, calculate the 24-h fentanyl dose.
2. Multiply the daily fentanyl dose by a factor of 100 to calculate the equipotent amount of methadone (ratio of potencies assumed to be fentanyl: methadone = 100:1).
3. Divide this amount of methadone by 6 (a correction for the longer half-life of methadone) to calculate an initial total daily dose of methadone, and on day 1 provide this amount orally in 4 divided doses every 6 h for 24 h.
4. Day 2: Provide 80% of original daily dose in 3 divided oral doses every 8 h for 24 h.
5. Day 3: Provide 60% of original daily dose in 3 divided oral doses every 8 h for 24 h.
6. Day 4: Provide 40% of original daily dose in 2 divided oral doses every 12 h for 24 h.
7. Day 5: Provide 20% of original daily dose × 1.
8. Day 6: Discontinue methadone.

Conversion of continuous intravenous fentanyl greater than 14 d duration to enteral methadone:
1. Repeat steps 1–2 above.
2. Days 1–2: Divide the dose of methadone by 6 (a correction for the longer half-life of methadone) and on day 1 provide this amount orally in 4 divided doses every 6 h for 48 h.
3. Days 3–4: Provide 80% of original daily dose in 3 divided oral doses every 8 h for 48 h.
4. Days 5–6: Provide 60% of original daily dose in 3 divided oral doses every 8 h for 48 h.
5. Days 7–8: Provide 40% of original daily dose in 2 divided oral doses every 12 h for 48 h.
6. Days 9–10: Provide 20% of original daily dose once per day for 48 h.
7. Day 11: Discontinue methadone.

For patients on continuous intravenous morphine, proceed as above but do not multiply the daily fentanyl dose by 100, because morphine and methadone are nearly equipotent.

Meyer and Berens[150]

Conversion of continuous intravenous fentanyl to intermittent intravenous morphine:
1. By using the target hourly infusion rate of fentanyl, calculate the 24-h fentanyl dose.
2. Multiply the daily fentanyl dose by a factor of 60 to calculate the equipotent dose of morphine (ratio of potencies assumed to be fentanyl: morphine = 60:1).
3. Divide the dose of morphine by 4 (correcting for the longer half-life of morphine) and on day 1 administer this amount intravenously in 6 divided doses every 4 h.
4. Titrate the morphine dose for adequate effect over 12 to 24 h.

Conversion of intermittent intravenous morphine to enteral methadone:
1. Multiply the dose of morphine given every 4 h by 2 (ratio of potencies assumed to be morphine: methadone = 2:1) to determine an equipotent amount of methadone.
2. Provide this amount of methadone as an oral dose every 12 h for 3 doses.
3. Double this amount of methadone and provide as a single oral dose per day at bedtime.
4. Provide 90% of the initial dose on day 2, 80% on day 3, etc, so that the last dose of methadone (10% of the original dose) is given on day 10.

Protocols at Wolfson Children's Hospital, Jacksonville, Florida

Conversion of continuous intravenous fentanyl >7 d duration to enteral methadone:
1. By using the current hourly infusion rate, calculate the 24-h fentanyl dose.
2. Multiply the daily fentanyl dose by a factor of 100 to calculate the equipotent amount of methadone (ratio of potencies assumed to be fentanyl: methadone = 100:1).
3. Divide this amount of methadone by 8–12 (a correction for the longer half-life of methadone) to calculate an initial total daily dose of methadone (not to exceed 40 mg/day).
4. Days 1–2: Provide the total daily dose of methadone orally in 4 divided doses every 6 h for 48 h. At the time of the second methadone dose, reduce the fentanyl infusion rate to 50%; at the time of the third dose, reduce the fentanyl infusion rate to 25%; and after the fourth methadone dose, discontinue the fentanyl infusion.
5. Days 3–4: Provide 80% of original daily dose in 3 divided oral doses every 8 h for 48 h.
6. Days 5–6: Provide 60% of original daily dose in 3 divided oral doses every 8 h for 48 h.
7. Days 7–8: Provide 40% of original daily dose in 2 divided oral doses every 12 h for 48 h.
8. Days 9–10: Provide 20% of original daily dose once per day for 48 h.
9. Day 11: Discontinue methadone.

Conversion of continuous intravenous midazolam >7 d duration to enteral lorazepam:
1. By using the current hourly infusion rate, calculate the 24-h midazolam dose.
2. Because lorazepam is twice as potent as midazolam and has a sixfold longer half-life, divide the 24 h midazolam dose by 12 to determine the daily lorazepam dose.
3. Divide the calculated lorazepam dose by 4 and initiate every 6 h oral treatments with the intravenous product or an aliquot of a crushed tablet.
4. Wean lorazepam by 10% to 20% per day. The dosage interval can also be increased gradually to every 8 h, then every 12 h, then every 24 h, and then every other day before lorazepam is discontinued.

TABLE 4 Continued

Robertson et al[149]
Summary of Conversion Of Intravenous Opioids to Enteral Methadone

1. Tobias et al[147]: Converted 2 patients on morphine (0.1–0.15 mg/kg q3h) and 1 patient on fentanyl (1–2 μg/kg every 1–2 h) to methadone at a starting dose of 0.2 mg/kg per day.
2. Robertson et al[149]: 1 μg/kg per h fentanyl = 0.4 mg/kg per day methadone.
3. Meyer and Berens[150]: 1 μg/kg per h fentanyl = 0.24 mg/kg per day methadone.
4. Wolfson Children's Hospital: 1 μg/kg per h fentanyl = 0.2–0.3 mg/kg per day methadone.

calculated methadone equivalent to achieve a successful conversion. Also, the rate of weaning should be adjusted on the basis of careful continuing clinical assessment. Eighty percent of children can be successfully weaned from methadone completely within 5 to 10 days.

4. Signs and symptoms of withdrawal from benzodiazepine therapy can be delayed. Intravenous benzodiazepines can be converted to oral lorazepam (Table 4). The required time for weaning can be expected to be proportional to the duration of intravenous benzodiazepine treatment.

5. Infants and children at risk for withdrawal are prudently observed in the hospital for signs and symptoms. Each clinical unit can choose 1 assessment tool and train staff to minimize individual variability in scoring.

6. Discharge from the hospital for infants and very young children is prudently delayed until they are free of withdrawal signs and symptoms for a period of 24 to 48 hours after complete cessation of opioids. Earlier discharge of an older child can be individualized in consideration of the child's overall clinical status, the home environment, and the availability of adequate and prompt follow-up.

7. No clinical studies to date support the premise that initiation of clonidine, chloral hydrate, or continuous intravenous low-dose naloxone[157,158] during the course of continuous opioid infusions will reduce the likelihood or severity of opioid dependency.

CLINICAL HIGHLIGHTS

1) Each nursery that cares for infants with neonatal withdrawal should develop a protocol that defines indications and procedures for screening for maternal substance abuse. In addition, each nursery should develop and adhere to a standardized plan for the evaluation and comprehensive treatment of infants at risk for or showing signs of withdrawal.

2) Screening for maternal substance abuse is best accomplished by using multiple methods, including maternal history, maternal urine testing, and testing of newborn urine and/or meconium specimens that are in compliance with local laws. The screening of biological samples is an adjunct to provide additional information helpful in the ongoing medical care of the infant. The duration of urinary excretion of most drugs is relatively short, and maternal or neonatal urinary screening only addresses drug exposure in the hours immediately before urine collection. Thus, false-negative urine results may occur in the presence of significant intrauterine drug exposure. Although newborn meconium screening also may yield false-negative results, the likelihood is lower than with urinary screening. The more recent availability of testing of umbilical cord samples may be considered a viable screening tool, because it appears to reflect in utero exposures comparable to meconium screening.

3) Drug withdrawal should be considered in the differential diagnosis for infants in whom compatible signs develop. Physicians should be aware of other potential diagnoses that need to be evaluated and, if confirmed, treated appropriately.

4) Nonpharmacologic supportive measures that include minimizing environmental stimuli, promoting adequate rest and sleep, and providing sufficient caloric intake to establish weight gain should constitute the initial approach to therapy.

5) Signs of drug withdrawal can be scored by using a published abstinence assessment tool. Infants with confirmed drug exposure who are unaffected or demonstrating minimal signs of withdrawal do not require pharmacologic therapy. Caution should be exercised before instituting pharmacologic therapy that could lengthen the duration of hospitalization and interfere with maternal-infant bonding.

Together with individualized clinical assessment, the serial and accurate use of a withdrawal assessment tool may facilitate a decision about the institution of pharmacologic therapy and thereafter can provide a quantitative measurement that can be used to adjust drug dosing.

6) The optimal threshold score for the institution of pharmacologic therapy by using any of the published abstinence assessment instruments is unknown.

7) Breastfeeding and the provision of expressed human milk should be encouraged if not contraindicated for other reasons.[111,159]

8) Pharmacologic therapy for withdrawal-associated seizures is indicated. Other causes of neonatal seizures must also be evaluated.

9) Vomiting, diarrhea, or both associated with dehydration and poor weight gain in the absence of other diagnoses are relative indications for treatment, even in the absence of high total withdrawal scores.

10) The limited available evidence from controlled trials of neonatal opioid withdrawal supports the use of oral morphine solution and methadone when pharmacologic treatment is indicated. Growing evidence suggests that oral clonidine is also effective either as a primary or adjunctive therapy, but further prospective trials are warranted. Dosing regimens are listed in Table 5. With respect to other drug treatments

and clinical situations, a number of important caveats apply. Treatment with paregoric is contraindicated, because this preparation contains multiple opiates in addition to morphine, as well as other potentially harmful compounds (alcohol, anise). Morphine prescriptions should be written as milligrams of morphine per kilogram and not as milliliters of DTO per kilogram. Tincture of opium contains a 25-fold higher concentration of morphine than do available oral morphine solutions; hence, it increases the likelihood of drug error and morphine overdose. The relative efficacy and safety of buprenorphine for the treatment of NAS require additional comparative study. The optimal pharmacologic treatment of infants who are withdrawing from sedatives or hypnotics is unknown. Finally, there is also insufficient evidence to state whether an infant born to a mother with multiple drug abuse who meets criteria for pharmacologic therapy of withdrawal signs is best treated with an opioid, a barbiturate, a medication from another drug class, or a combination of drugs from different classes.

11) Physicians need to be aware that the severity of withdrawal signs, including seizures, has not been proven to be associated with differences in long-term outcome after intrauterine drug exposure. Furthermore, treatment of drug withdrawal may not alter the long-term outcome.

12) Given the natural history of withdrawal, it is reasonable for neonates with known antenatal exposure to opioids and benzodiazepines to be observed in the hospital for 4 to 7 days. After discharge, outpatient follow-up should occur early and include reinforcement of the education of the caregiver about the risk of late withdrawal signs.

13) Neonates cared for in ICUs who have developed tolerance to opioids and benzodiazepines as a result of an extended duration of treatment can be converted to an equivalent regimen of oral methadone and lorazepam. Doses may be increased as necessary to achieve patient comfort. These medications can then be reduced by 10% to 20% of the initial dose every 1 to 2 days on the basis of clinical response and serial assessments by using a standardized neonatal abstinence instrument.

14) Significant gaps in knowledge concerning the optimal treatment strategy (including the criteria for instituting pharmacologic therapy, the drug of first choice, and the strategy for weaning) of infants with neonatal withdrawal should be addressed in well-designed randomized controlled studies that are adequately powered to assess short-term outcomes and to provide for long-term follow-up.

LEAD AUTHORS
Mark L. Hudak, MD
Rosemarie C. Tan, MD, PhD

TABLE 5 Drugs Used in the Treatment of Neonatal Narcotic Withdrawal

Drug	Initial Dose	Increment	Maximum Dose	Ref. No.
Oral morphine	0.04 mg/kg every 3–4 h	0.04 mg/kg per dose	0.2 mg/kg per dose	119,121,126,133
Oral methadone	0.05–0.1 mg/kg every 6 h	0.05 mg/kg per dose	To effect	127
Oral clonidine	0.5–1 µg/kg every 3–6 h	Not studied	1 µg/kg every 3 h	132–135

REFERENCES

1. *Results From the 2009 National Survey on Drug Use and Health: Volume I. Summary of National Findings* (Office of Applied Studies, NSDUH Series H-38A, HHS Publication No 10-4856Findings). Rockville, MD: Substance Abuse and Mental Health Services Administration; 2010

2. Bada HS, Das A, Bauer CR, et al. Low birth weight and preterm births: etiologic fraction attributable to prenatal drug exposure. *J Perinatol.* 2005;25(10):631–637

3. Campolongo P, Trezza V, Palmery M, Trabace L, Cuomo V. Developmental exposure to cannabinoids causes subtle and enduring neurofunctional alterations. *Int Rev Neurobiol.* 2009;85:117–133

4. Burns L, Mattick RP. Using population data to examine the prevalence and correlates of neonatal abstinence syndrome. *Drug Alcohol Rev.* 2007;26(5):487–492

5. Kellogg A, Rose CH, Harms RH, Watson WJ. Current trends in narcotic use in pregnancy and neonatal outcomes. Am J Obstet Gynecol. 2011;204:259.e1–e4

6. Harper RG, Solish GI, Purow HM, Sang E, Panepinto WC. The effect of a methadone treatment program upon pregnant heroin addicts and their newborn infants. *Pediatrics.* 1974;54(3):300–305

7. Fricker HS, Segal S. Narcotic addiction, pregnancy, and the newborn. *Am J Dis Child.* 1978;132(4):360–366

8. Madden JD, Chappel JN, Zuspan F, Gumpel J, Mejia A, Davis R. Observation and treatment of neonatal narcotic withdrawal. *Am J Obstet Gynecol.* 1977;127(2):199–201

9. Ostrea EM, Chavez CJ, Strauss ME. A study of factors that influence the severity of neonatal narcotic withdrawal. *J Pediatr.* 1976;88(4 pt 1):642–645

10. Rementería JL, Bhatt K. Withdrawal symptoms in neonates from intrauterine exposure to diazepam. *J Pediatr.* 1977;90(1):123–126

11. Athinarayanan P, Pierog SH, Nigam SK, Glass L. Chloriazepoxide withdrawal in the neonate. *Am J Obstet Gynecol.* 1976;124(2):212–213

12. Bleyer WA, Marshall RE. Barbiturate withdrawal syndrome in a passively addicted infant. *JAMA.* 1972;221(2):185–186

13. Desmond MM, Schwanecke RP, Wilson GS, Yasunaga S, Burgdorff I. Maternal barbiturate utilization and neonatal withdrawal symptomatology. *J Pediatr.* 1972;80(2):190–197

14. Pierog S, Chandavasu O, Wexler I. Withdrawal symptoms in infants with the fetal alcohol syndrome. *J Pediatr.* 1977;90(4):630–633

15. Nichols MM. Acute alcohol withdrawal syndrome in a newborn. *Am J Dis Child.* 1967;113(6):714–715

16. Eyler FD, Behnke M, Garvan CW, Woods NS, Wobie K, Conlon M. Newborn evaluations of toxicity and withdrawal related to prenatal cocaine exposure. *Neurotoxicol Teratol.* 2001;23(5):399–411

17. Bauer CR, Langer JC, Shankaran S, et al. Acute neonatal effects of cocaine exposure during pregnancy. *Arch Pediatr Adolesc Med.* 2005;159(9):824–834

18. Chasnoff IJ, Bussey ME, Savich R, Stack CM. Perinatal cerebral infarction and maternal cocaine use. *J Pediatr.* 1986;108(3):456–459

19. Fulroth R, Phillips B, Durand DJ. Perinatal outcome of infants exposed to cocaine and/or heroin in utero. *Am J Dis Child.* 1989;143(8):905–910

20. Chiriboga CA, Bateman DA, Brust JC, Hauser WA. Neurologic findings in neonates with intrauterine cocaine exposure. *Pediatr Neurol.* 1993;9(2):115–119

21. Hadeed AJ, Siegel SR. Maternal cocaine use during pregnancy: effect on the newborn infant. *Pediatrics.* 1989;84(2):205–210

22. King TA, Perlman JM, Laptook AR, Rollins N, Jackson G, Little B. Neurologic manifestations of in utero cocaine exposure in near-term and term infants. *Pediatrics.* 1995;96(2 pt 1):259–264

23. Brazelton TB. *Neonatal Behavioral Assessment Scale. Clinics in Developmental Medicine. No 88.* 2nd ed. Philadelphia, PA: JB Lippincott Co; 1984

24. Tan-Laxa MA, Sison-Switala C, Rintelman W, Ostrea EM Jr,. Abnormal auditory brainstem response among infants with prenatal cocaine exposure. *Pediatrics.* 2004;113(2):357–360

25. Doberczak TM, Shanzer S, Cutler R, Senie RT, Loucopoulos JA, Kandall SR. One-year follow-up of infants with abstinence-associated seizures. *Arch Neurol.* 1988;45(6):649–653

26. Tronick EZ, Frank DA, Cabral H, Mirochnick M, Zuckerman B. Late dose-response effects of prenatal cocaine exposure on newborn neurobehavioral performance. *Pediatrics.* 1996;98(1):76–83

27. Smith L, Yonekura ML, Wallace T, Berman N, Kuo J, Berkowitz C. Effects of prenatal methamphetamine exposure on fetal growth and drug withdrawal symptoms in infants born at term. *J Dev Behav Pediatr.* 2003;24(1):17–23

28. Billing L, Eriksson M, Steneroth G, Zetterström R. Predictive indicators for adjustment in 4-year-old children whose mothers used amphetamine during pregnancy. *Child Abuse Negl.* 1988;12(4):503–507

29. Cernerud L, Eriksson M, Jonsson B, Steneroth G, Zetterström R. Amphetamine addiction during pregnancy: 14-year follow-up of growth and school performance. *Acta Paediatr.* 1996;85(2):204–208

30. Alwan S, Friedman JM. Safety of selective serotonin reuptake inhibitors in pregnancy. *CNS Drugs.* 2009;23(6):493–509

31. Dahl ML, Olhager E, Ahlner J. Paroxetine withdrawal syndrome in a neonate. *Br J Psychiatry.* 1997;171:391–392

32. Sanz EJ, De-las-Cuevas C, Kiuru A, Bate A, Edwards R. Selective serotonin reuptake inhibitors in pregnant women and neonatal withdrawal syndrome: a database analysis. *Lancet.* 2005;365(9458):482–487

33. Chambers CD, Johnson KA, Dick LM, Felix RJ, Jones KL. Birth outcomes in pregnant women taking fluoxetine. *N Engl J Med.* 1996;335(14):1010–1015

34. Galbally M, Lewis AJ, Lum J, Buist A. Serotonin discontinuation syndrome following in utero exposure to antidepressant medication: prospective controlled study. *Aust N Z J Psychiatry.* 2009;43(9):846–854

35. Haddad PM, Pal BR, Clarke P, Wieck A, Sridhiran S. Neonatal symptoms following maternal paroxetine treatment: serotonin toxicity or paroxetine discontinuation syndrome? *J Psychopharmacol.* 2005;19(5):554–557

36. Nordeng H, Lindemann R, Perminov KV, Reikvam A. Neonatal withdrawal syndrome after in utero exposure to selective serotonin reuptake inhibitors. *Acta Paediatr.* 2001;90(3):288–291

37. Boyer EW, Shannon M. The serotonin syndrome. *N Engl J Med.* 2005;352(11):1112–1120

38. Isbister GK, Dawson A, Whyte IM, Prior FH, Clancy C, Smith AJ. Neonatal paroxetine withdrawal syndrome or actually serotonin syndrome? *Arch Dis Child Fetal Neonatal Ed.* 2001;85(2):F147–F148

39. Laine K, Heikkinen T, Ekblad U, Kero P. Effects of exposure to selective serotonin reuptake inhibitors during pregnancy on serotonergic symptoms in newborns and cord blood monoamine and prolactin concentrations. *Arch Gen Psychiatry.* 2003;60(7):720–726

40. Austin MP. To treat or not to treat: maternal depression, SSRI use in pregnancy and adverse neonatal effects. *Psychol Med.* 2006;36(12):1663–1670

41. Gentile S. On categorizing gestational, birth, and neonatal complications following late pregnancy exposure to antidepressants: the prenatal antidepressant exposure syndrome. *CNS Spectr.* 2010;15(3):167–185

42. Oberlander TF, Grunau RE, Fitzgerald C, Papsdorf M, Rurak D, Riggs W. Pain reactivity in 2-month-old infants after prenatal and postnatal serotonin reuptake inhibitor medication exposure. *Pediatrics.* 2005;115(2):411–425

43. Nordeng H, Spigset O. Treatment with selective serotonin reuptake inhibitors in the third trimester of pregnancy: effects on the infant. *Drug Saf.* 2005;28(7):565–581

44. De las Cuevas C, Sanz EJ. Safety of selective serotonin reuptake inhibitors in pregnancy. *Curr Drug Saf.* 2006;1(1):17–24

45. Weissman AM, Levy BT, Hartz AJ, et al. Pooled analysis of antidepressant levels in lactating mothers, breast milk, and nursing infants. *Am J Psychiatry.* 2004;161(6):1066–1078

46. Fortinguerra F, Clavenna A, Bonati M. Psychotropic drug use during breast-feeding: a review of the evidence. *Pediatrics.* 2009;124(4). Available at: www.pediatrics.org/cgi/content/full/124/4/e547

47. Somogyi AA, Barratt DT, Coller JK. Pharmacogenetics of opioids. *Clin Pharmacol Ther.* 2007;81(3):429–444

48. Jones HE, Kaltenbach K, Heil SH, et al. Neonatal abstinence syndrome after methadone or buprenorphine exposure. *N Engl J Med.* 2010;363(24):2320–2331

49. Zelson C, Rubio E, Wasserman E. Neonatal narcotic addiction: 10 year observation. *Pediatrics.* 1971;48(2):178–189

50. Kandall SR, Gartner LM. Late presentation of drug withdrawal symptoms in newborns. *Am J Dis Child.* 1974;127(1):58–61

51. Lejeune C, Simmat-Durand L, Gourarier L, Aubisson S, ; Groupe d'Etudes Grossesse et Addictions (GEGA). Prospective multicenter observational study of 260 infants born to 259 opiate-dependent mothers on methadone or high-dose buprenophine substitution. *Drug Alcohol Depend.* 2006;82(3):250–257

52. Steg N. Narcotic withdrawal reactions in the newborn. *AMA J Dis Child.* 1957;94(3):286–288

53. Schindler SD, Eder H, Ortner R, Rohrmeister K, Langer M, Fischer G. Neonatal outcome following buprenorphine maintenance during conception and throughout pregnancy. *Addiction.* 2003;98(1):103–110

54. Kayemba-Kay's S, Laclyde JP. Buprenorphine withdrawal syndrome in newborns: a report of 13 cases. *Addiction.* 2003;98(11):1599–1604

55. Lacroix I, Berrebi A, Chaumerliac C, Lapeyre-Mestre M, Montastruc JL, Damase-Michel C. Buprenorphine in pregnant opioid-dependent women: first results of a prospective study. *Addiction.* 2004;99(2):209–214

56. Herzlinger RA, Kandall SR, Vaughan HG Jr,. Neonatal seizures associated with narcotic withdrawal. *J Pediatr.* 1977;91(4):638–641

57. Pinto F, Torrioli MG, Casella G, Tempesta E, Fundarò C. Sleep in babies born to chronically heroin addicted mothers. A follow up study. *Drug Alcohol Depend.* 1988;21(1):43–47

58. van Baar AL, Fleury P, Soepatmi S, Ultee CA, Wesselman PJ. Neonatal behavior after drug dependent pregnancy. *Arch Dis Child.* 1989;64(2):235–240

59. Desmond MM, Wilson GS. Neonatal abstinence syndrome: recognition and diagnosis. *Addict Dis.* 1975;2(1–2):113–121

60. Prenner BM. Neonatal withdrawal syndrome associated with hydroxyzine hydrochloride. *Am J Dis Child.* 1977;131(5):529–530

61. Feld LH, Negus JB, White PF. Oral midazolam preanesthetic medication in pediatric outpatients. *Anesthesiology*. 1990; 73(5):831–834

62. Harper RG, Solish G, Feingold E, Gersten-Woolf NB, Sokal MM. Maternal ingested methadone, body fluid methadone, and the neonatal withdrawal syndrome. *Am J Obstet Gynecol*. 1977;129(4):417–424

63. Strauss ME, Andresko M, Stryker JC, Wardell JN. Relationship of neonatal withdrawal to maternal methadone dose. *Am J Drug Alcohol Abuse*. 1976;3(2):339–345

64. Doberczak TM, Kandall SR, Wilets I. Neonatal opiate abstinence syndrome in term and preterm infants. *J Pediatr*. 1991;118 (6):933–937

65. Doberczak TM, Kandall SR, Friedmann P. Relationship between maternal methadone dosage, maternal-neonatal methadone levels, and neonatal withdrawal. *Obstet Gynecol*. 1993;81(6):936–940

66. Rosen TS, Pippenger CE. Disposition of methadone and its relationship to severity of withdrawal in the newborn. *Addict Dis*. 1975;2(1–2):169–178

67. Dashe JS, Sheffield JS, Olscher DA, Todd SJ, Jackson GL, Wendel GD. Relationship between maternal methadone dosage and neonatal withdrawal. *Obstet Gynecol*. 2002;100(6):1244–1249

68. Liu AJ, Jones MP, Murray H, Cook CM, Nanan R. Perinatal risk factors for the neonatal abstinence syndrome in infants born to women on methadone maintenance therapy. *Aust N Z J Obstet Gynaecol*. 2010;50(3):253–258

69. Brown HL, Britton KA, Mahaffey D, Brizendine E, Hiett AK, Turnquest MA. Methadone maintenance in pregnancy: a reappraisal. *Am J Obstet Gynecol*. 1998;179(2):459–463

70. Mack G, Thomas D, Giles W, Buchanan N. Methadone levels and neonatal withdrawal. *J Paediatr Child Health*. 1991;27 (2):96–100

71. Berghella V, Lim PJ, Hill MK, Cherpes J, Chennat J, Kaltenbach K. Maternal methadone dose and neonatal withdrawal. *Am J Obstet Gynecol*. 2003;189(2):312–317

72. Kuschel CA, Austerberry L, Cornwell M, Couch R, Rowley RS. Can methadone concentrations predict the severity of withdrawal in infants at risk of neonatal abstinence syndrome? *Arch Dis Child Fetal Neonatal Ed*. 2004;89(5):F390–F393

73. Seligman NS, Almario CV, Hayes EJ, Dysart KC, Berghella V, Baxter JK. Relationship between maternal methadone dose at delivery and neonatal abstinence syndrome. *J Pediatr*. 2010;157(3):428–433, e1

74. Cleary BJ, Donnelly J, Strawbridge J, et al. Methadone dose and neonatal abstinence syndrome—systematic review and meta-analysis. *Addiction*. 2010;105(12):2071–2084

75. Drozdick J, III, Berghella V, Hill M, Kaltenbach K. Methadone trough levels in pregnancy. *Am J Obstet Gynecol*. 2002;187 (5):1184–1188

76. Lipsitz PJ. A proposed narcotic withdrawal score for use with newborn infants. A pragmatic evaluation of its efficacy. *Clin Pediatr (Phila)*. 1975;14(6):592–594

77. Finnegan LP, Kron RE, Connaughton JF, Emich JP. Assessment and treatment of abstinence in the infant of the drug-dependent mother. *Int Clin Pharmacol Biopharm*. 1975;12(1–2):19–32

78. Dysart K, Hsieh HC, Kaltenbach K, Greenspan JS. Sequela of preterm versus term infants born to mothers on a methadone maintenance program: differential course of neonatal abstinence syndrome. *J Perinat Med*. 2007;35(4):344–346

79. Johnson K, Gerada C, Greenough A. Treatment of neonatal abstinence syndrome. *Arch Dis Child Fetal Neonatal Ed*. 2003;88(1):F2–F5

80. Chasnoff IJ, Burns WJ, Schnoll SH, Burns KA. Cocaine use in pregnancy. *N Engl J Med*. 1985;313(11):666–669

81. Choo RE, Huestis MA, Schroeder JR, Shin AS, Jones HE. Neonatal abstinence syndrome in methadone-exposed infants is altered by level of prenatal tobacco exposure. *Drug Alcohol Depend*. 2004;75(3):253–260

82. Gibbs J, Newson T, Williams J, Davidson DC. Naloxone hazard in infant of opioid abuser. *Lancet*. 1989;2(8655):159–160

83. Frank DA, Zuckerman BS, Amaro H, et al. Cocaine use during pregnancy: prevalence and correlates. *Pediatrics*. 1988;82 (6):888–895

84. Chasnoff IJ, Burns KA, Burns WJ. Cocaine use in pregnancy: perinatal morbidity and mortality. *Neurotoxicol Teratol*. 1987;9(4):291–293

85. Mitchell M, Sabbagha RE, Keith L, MacGregor S, Mota JM, Minoque J. Ultrasonic growth parameters in fetuses of mothers with primary addiction to cocaine. *Am J Obstet Gynecol*. 1988;159(5):1104–1109

86. Cregler LL, Mark H. Medical complications of cocaine abuse. *N Engl J Med*. 1986;315 (23):1495–1500

87. Chasnoff IJ, Griffith DR, MacGregor S, Dirkes K, Burns KA. Temporal patterns of cocaine use in pregnancy. Perinatal outcome. *JAMA*. 1989;261(12):1741–1744

88. Cocaine abuse: implications for pregnancy. ACOG Committee opinion: Committee on Obstetrics: Maternal and Fetal Medicine number 81—March 1990. *Int J Gynaecol Obstet*. 1991;36(2):164–166

89. Horowitz RM. Drug use in pregnancy: to test, to tell—legal implications for the physician. *Semin Perinatol*. 1991;15(4):324–330

90. Chasnoff IJ. Prenatal substance exposure: maternal screening and neonatal identification and management. *NeoReviews*. 2003;4(9):e228–e235

91. Chasnoff IJ, Neuman K, Thornton C, Callaghan MA. Screening for substance use in pregnancy: a practical approach for the primary care physician. *Am J Obstet Gynecol*. 2001;184(4):752–758

92. Chan D, Klein J, Koren G. New methods for neonatal drug screening. *NeoReviews*. 2003;4(9):e236–e244

93. Beauman SS. Identification and management of neonatal abstinence syndrome. *J Infus Nurs*. 2005;28(3):159–167

94. Reinarz SE, Ecord JS. Drug-of-abuse testing in the neonate. *Neonatal Netw*. 1999;18 (8):55–61

95. Ostrea EM, Jr,Brady MJ, Parks PM, Asensio DC, Naluz A. Drug screening of meconium in infants of drug-dependent mothers: an alternative to urine testing. *J Pediatr*. 1989;115(3):474–477

96. Ryan RM, Wagner CL, Schultz JM, et al. Meconium analysis for improved identification of infants exposed to cocaine in utero. *J Pediatr*. 1994;125(3):435–440

97. Ostrea EM, Jr,Knapp DK, Tannenbaum L, et al. Estimates of illicit drug use during pregnancy by maternal interview, hair analysis, and meconium analysis. *J Pediatr*. 2001;138(3):344–348

98. Vinner E, Vignau J, Thibault D, et al. Neonatal hair analysis contribution to establishing a gestational drug exposure profile and predicting a withdrawal syndrome. *Ther Drug Monit*. 2003;25(4):421–432

99. Montgomery D, Plate C, Alder SC, Jones M, Jones J, Christensen RD. Testing for fetal exposure to illicit drugs using umbilical cord tissue vs meconium. *J Perinatol*. 2006;26(1):11–14

100. American Academy of Pediatrics, Committee on Drugs. Neonatal drug withdrawal. *Pediatrics*. 1998;101(6):1079–1088

101. Finnegan LP. Neonatal abstinence. In: Nelson NM, ed. *Current Therapy in Neonatal–Perinatal Medicine*. 2nd ed. Toronto, Ontario: BC Decker Inc; 1990

102. Sarkar S, Donn SM. Management of neonatal abstinence syndrome in neonatal

intensive care units: a national survey. *J Perinatol.* 2006;26(1):15–17

103. Green M, Suffet F. The Neonatal Narcotic Withdrawal Index: a device for the improvement of care in the abstinence syndrome. *Am J Drug Alcohol Abuse.* 1981;8 (2):203–213

104. Zimmermann-Baer U, Nötzli U, Rentsch K, Bucher HU. Finnegan neonatal abstinence scoring system: normal values for first 3 days and weeks 5-6 in non-addicted infants. *Addiction.* 2010;105(3):524–528

105. Hill RM, Desmond MM. Management of the narcotic withdrawal syndrome in the neonate. *Pediatr Clin North Am.* 1963;10:67–86

106. Wilson GS. Somatic growth effects of perinatal addiction. *Addict Dis.* 1975;2(1–2):333–345

107. Abdel-Latif ME, Pinner J, Clews S, Cooke F, Lui K, Oei J. Effects of breast milk on the severity and outcome of neonatal abstinence syndrome among infants of drug-dependent mothers. *Pediatrics.* 2006;117 (6). Available at: www.pediatrics.org/cgi/content/full/117/6/e1163

108. Isemann B, Meinzen-Derr J, Akinbi H. Maternal and neonatal factors impacting response to methadone therapy in infants treated for neonatal abstinence syndrome. *J Perinatol.* 2011;31(1):25–29

109. Jansson LM, Choo R, Velez ML, et al. Methadone maintenance and breastfeeding in the neonatal period. *Pediatrics.* 2008;121(1):106–114

110. Jansson LM, Choo R, Velez ML, Lowe R, Huestis MA. Methadone maintenance and long-term lactation. *Breastfeed Med.* 2008; 3(1):34–37

111. Jansson LM, ; Academy of Breastfeeding Medicine Protocol Committee. ABM clinical protocol #21: guidelines for breastfeeding and the drug-dependent woman. *Breastfeed Med.* 2009;4(4):225–228

112. Bays J. The care of alcohol- and drug-affected infants. *Pediatr Ann.* 1992;21(8): 485–495

113. O'Grady MJ, Hopewell J, White MJ. Management of neonatal abstinence syndrome: a national survey and review of practice. *Arch Dis Child Fetal Neonatal Ed.* 2009;94(4):F249–F252

114. Kaltenbach K, Finnegan LP. Neonatal abstinence syndrome, pharmacotherapy and developmental outcome. *Neurobehav Toxicol Teratol.* 1986;8(4):353–355

115. Kron RE, Litt M, Eng D, Phoenix MD, Finnegan LP. Neonatal narcotic abstinence: effects of pharmacotherapeutic agents and maternal drug usage on nutritive sucking behavior. *J Pediatr.* 1976;88(4 pt 1):637–641

116. Schiff D, Chan G, Stern L, et al. Diazepam (Valium) for neonatal narcotic withdrawal: a question of safety. *Pediatrics.* 1972;49(6):928–930

117. Osborn DA, Jeffery HE, Cole MJ. Opiate treatment for opiate withdrawal in newborn infants. *Cochrane Database Syst Rev.* 2005;(3):CD002059

118. Osborn DA, Jeffery HE, Cole MJ. Sedatives for opiate withdrawal in newborn infants. *Cochrane Database Syst Rev.* 2005;(3): CD002053

119. Khoo KT. *The Effectiveness of Three Treatment Regimens Used in the Management of Neonatal Abstinence Syndrome* [thesis for PhD]. Melbourne, Australia: University of Melbourne; 1995

120. Finnegan LP, Michael H, Leifer B, Desai S. An evaluation of neonatal abstinence treatment modalities. *NIDA Res Monogr.* 1984;49:282–288

121. Jackson L, Ting A, McKay S, Galea P, Skeoch C. A randomised controlled trial of morphine versus phenobarbitone for neonatal abstinence syndrome. *Arch Dis Child Fetal Neonatal Ed.* 2004;89(4):F300–F304

122. Kandall SR, Doberczak TM, Mauer KR, Strashun RH, Korts DC. Opiate v CNS depressant therapy in neonatal drug abstinence syndrome. *Am J Dis Child.* 1983;137 (4):378–382

123. Carin I, Glass L, Parekh A, Solomon N, Steigman J, Wong S. Neonatal methadone withdrawal. Effect of two treatment regimens. *Am J Dis Child.* 1983;137(12):1166–1169

124. Coyle MG, Ferguson A, Lagasse L, Oh W, Lester B. Diluted tincture of opium (DTO) and phenobarbital versus DTO alone for neonatal opiate withdrawal in term infants. *J Pediatr.* 2002;140(5):561–564

125. Kahn EJ, Neumann LL, Polk GA. The course of the heroin withdrawal syndrome in newborn infants treated with phenobarbital or chlorpromazine. *J Pediatr.* 1969;75 (3):495–500

126. Langenfeld S, Birkenfeld L, Herkenrath P, Müller C, Hellmich M, Theisohn M. Therapy of the neonatal abstinence syndrome with tincture of opium or morphine drops. *Drug Alcohol Depend.* 2005;77(1):31–36

127. Lainwala S, Brown ER, Weinschenk NP, Blackwell MT, Hagadorn JI. A retrospective study of length of hospital stay in infants treated for neonatal abstinence syndrome with methadone versus oral morphine preparations. *Adv Neonatal Care.* 2005;5 (5):265–272

128. Ebner N, Rohrmeister K, Winklbaur B, et al. Management of neonatal abstinence syndrome in neonates born to opioid main-

tained women. *Drug Alcohol Depend.* 2007; 87(2–3):131–138

129. Kraft WK, Gibson E, Dysart K, et al. Sublingual buprenorphine for treatment of neonatal abstinence syndrome: a randomized trial. *Pediatrics.* 2008;122(3). Available at: www.pediatrics.org/cgi/content/full/122/3/e601

130. Gold MS, Redmond DE, Jr,Kleber HD. Clonidine blocks acute opiate-withdrawal symptoms. *Lancet.* 1978;2(8090):599–602

131. Yaster M, Kost-Byerly S, Berde C, Billet C. The management of opioid and benzodiazepine dependence in infants, children, and adolescents. *Pediatrics.* 1996;98(1): 135–140

132. Hoder EL, Leckman JF, Poulsen J, et al. Clonidine treatment of neonatal narcotic abstinence syndrome. *Psychiatry Res.* 1984;13(3):243–251

133. Agthe AG, Kim GR, Mathias KB, et al. Clonidine as an adjunct therapy to opioids for neonatal abstinence syndrome: a randomized, controlled trial. *Pediatrics.* 2009; 123(5). Available at: www.pediatrics.org/cgi/content/123/5/e849

134. Leikin JB, Mackendrick WP, Maloney GE, et al. Use of clonidine in the prevention and management of neonatal abstinence syndrome. *Clin Toxicol (Phila).* 2009;47(6): 551–555

135. Esmaeili A, Keinhorst AK, Schuster T, Beske F, Schlösser R, Bastanier C. Treatment of neonatal abstinence syndrome with clonidine and chloral hydrate. *Acta Paediatr.* 2010;99(2):209–214

136. Mazurier E, Cambonie G, Barbotte E, Grare A, Pinzani V, Picaud JC. Comparison of chlorpromazine versus morphine hydrochloride for treatment of neonatal abstinence syndrome. *Acta Paediatr.* 2008;97 (10):1358–1361

137. Slotkin TA, Whitmore WL, Salvaggio M, Seidler FJ. Perinatal methadone addiction affects brain synaptic development of biogenic amine systems in the rat. *Life Sci.* 1979;24(13):1223–1229

138. McGinty JF, Ford DH. Effects of prenatal methadone on rat brain catecholamines. *Dev Neurosci.* 1980;3(4–6):224–234

139. Bandstra ES, Morrow CE, Mansoor E, Accornero VH. Prenatal drug exposure: infant and toddler outcomes. *J Addict Dis.* 2010;29(2):245–258

140. Arnold JH, Truog RD, Scavone JM, Fenton T. Changes in the pharmacodynamic response to fentanyl in neonates during continuous infusion. *J Pediatr.* 1991;119 (4):639–643

141. Arnold JH, Truog RD, Orav EJ, Scavone JM, Hershenson MB. Tolerance and dependence

in neonates sedated with fentanyl during extracorporeal membrane oxygenation. *Anesthesiology.* 1990;73(6):1136–1140

142. Katz R, Kelly HW, Hsi A. Prospective study on the occurrence of withdrawal in critically ill children who receive fentanyl by continuous infusion. *Crit Care Med.* 1994; 22(5):763–767

143. Dominguez KD, Lomako DM, Katz RW, Kelly HW. Opioid withdrawal in critically ill neonates. *Ann Pharmacother.* 2003;37(4): 473–477

144. Cammarano WB, Pittet JF, Weitz S, Schlobohm RM, Marks JD. Acute withdrawal syndrome related to the administration of analgesic and sedative medications in adult intensive care unit patients. *Crit Care Med.* 1998;26(4):676–684

145. Franck LS, Vilardi J, Durand D, Powers R. Opioid withdrawal in neonates after continuous infusions of morphine or fentanyl during extracorporeal membrane oxygenation. *Am J Crit Care.* 1998;7(5):364–369

146. Carr DB, Todres ID. Fentanyl infusion and weaning in the pediatric intensive care unit: toward science-based practice. *Crit Care Med.* 1994;22(5):725–727

147. Tobias JD, Schleien CL, Haun SE. Methadone as treatment for iatrogenic narcotic dependency in pediatric intensive care unit patients. *Crit Care Med.* 1990;18(11): 1292–1293

148. Anand KJ. Pharmacological approaches to the management of pain in the neonatal intensive care unit. *J Perinatol.* 2007;27 (suppl 1):S4–S11

149. Robertson RC, Darsey E, Fortenberry JD, Pettignano R, Hartley G. Evaluation of an opiate-weaning protocol using methadone in pediatric intensive care unit patients. *Pediatr Crit Care Med.* 2000;1(2):119–123

150. Meyer MM, Berens RJ. Efficacy of an enteral 10-day methadone wean to prevent opioid withdrawal in fentanyl-tolerant pediatric intensive care unit patients. *Pediatr Crit Care Med.* 2001;2(4):329–333

151. Berens RJ, Meyer MT, Mikhailov TA, et al. A prospective evaluation of opioid weaning in opioid-dependent pediatric critical care patients. *Anesth Analg.* 2006;102(4):1045–1050

152. Franck LS, Naughton I, Winter I. Opioid and benzodiazepine withdrawal symptoms in paediatric intensive care patients. *Intensive Crit Care Nurs.* 2004;20(6):344–351

153. Ista E, van Dijk M, Gamel C, Tibboel D, de Hoog M. Withdrawal symptoms in children after long-term administration of sedatives and/or analgesics: a literature review. "Assessment remains troublesome". *Intensive Care Med.* 2007;33(8):1396–1406

154. Cunliffe M, McArthur L, Dooley F. Managing sedation withdrawal in children who undergo prolonged PICU admission after discharge to the ward. *Paediatr Anaesth.* 2004;14(4):293–298

155. Ista E, van Dijk M, Gamel C, Tibboel D, de Hoog M. Withdrawal symptoms in critically ill children after long-term administration of sedatives and/or analgesics: a first evaluation. *Crit Care Med.* 2008;36 (8):2427–2432

156. Simons SH, Anand KJ. Pain control: opioid dosing, population kinetics and side-effects. *Semin Fetal Neonatal Med.* 2006;11(4):260–267

157. Cheung CL, van Dijk M, Green JW, Tibboel D, Anand KJ. Effects of low-dose naloxone on opioid therapy in pediatric patients: a retrospective case-control study. *Intensive Care Med.* 2007;33(1):190–194

158. Darnell CM, Thompson J, Stromberg D, Roy L, Sheeran P. Effect of low-dose naloxone infusion on fentanyl requirements in critically ill children. *Pediatrics.* 2008; 121(5). Available at: www.pediatrics.org/cgi/content/full/121/5/e1363

159. Gartner LM, Morton J, Lawrence RA, et al; American Academy of Pediatrics Section on Breastfeeding. Breastfeeding and the use of human milk. *Pediatrics.* 2005;115 (2):496–506

160. Milhorn HT Jr,. Pharmacologic management of acute abstinence syndromes. *Am Fam Physician.* 1992;45(1):231–239

161. McGowan JD, Altman RE, Kanto WP Jr,. Neonatal withdrawal symptoms after chronic maternal ingestion of caffeine. *South Med J.* 1988;81(9):1092–1094

162. Musa AB, Smith CS. Neonatal effects of maternal clomipramine therapy. *Arch Dis Child.* 1979;54(5):405

163. Rumack BH, Walravens PA. Neonatal withdrawal following maternal ingestion of ethchlorvynol (Placidyl). *Pediatrics.* 1973; 52(5):714–716

164. Reveri M, Pyati SP, Pildes RS. Neonatal withdrawal symptoms associated with glutethimide (Doriden) addiction in the mother during pregnancy. *Clin Pediatr (Phila).* 1977;16(5):424–425

165. Desmond MM, Rudolph AJ, Hill RM, Claghorn JL, Dreesen PR, Burgdorff I. Behavioral alterations in infants born to mothers on psychoactive medication during pregnancy. In: Farrell G, ed. *Congenital Mental Retardation.* Austin, TX: University of Texas Press; 1969:235–244

ERRATA

Hudak ML, Tan RC, The Committee on Drugs and the Committee on Fetus and Newborn. Neonatal Drug Withdrawal. *Pediatrics*. 2012;129;e540.

An error occurred in the Guidance for the Clinician by Hudak ML et al, titled "Neonatal Drug Withdrawal," published in the February 2012 issue of *Pediatrics* (2012;129(2):e540– e560; originally published online January 30, 2012; doi:10.1542/ 2012-3212). On page e547, the formatting of Fig 1 (Modified Finnegan's Neonatal Abstinence Scoring Tool) could be misinterpreted to indicate that 19 rather than 21 independent signs should be scored to assess the clinical severity of neonatal abstinence syndrome. The formatting has been changed (see Table) to differentiate clearly the 21 independent signs.

doi:10.1542/peds.2014-0557

NEONATAL ABSTINENCE SCORING SYSTEM

SYSTEM	SIGNS AND SYMPTOMS	SCORE	AM				PM						COMMENTS
CENTRAL NERVOUS SYSTEM DISTURBANCES (9 domains)	Continuous High Pitched (or other) Cry	2											
	Continuous High Pitched (or other) Cry	3											
	Sleeps <1 Hour After Feeding	3											
	Sleeps <2 Hours After Feeding	2											
	Sleeps <3 Hours After Feeding	1											
	Hyperacti e Moro Reflex	2											
	Markedly Hyperacti e Moro Reflex	3											
	Mild Tremors Disturbed	1											
	Moderate-Se ere Tremors Disturbed	2											
	Mild Tremors Undisturbed	3											
	Moderate-Se ere Tremors Undisturbed	4											
	Increased Muscle Tone	2											
	Excoriation (Specific Area)	1											
	Myoclonic Jerks	3											
	Generalized Con ulsions	5											
METABOLIC/VASOMOTOR/RESPIRATORY DISTURBANCES (8 domains)	Sweating	1											
	Fe er 100.4°-101°F (38°-38.3°C)	1											
	Fe er > 101°F (38.3°C)	2											
	Frequent Yawning (>3-4 times/inter al)	1											
	Mottling	1											
	Nasal Stuffiness	1											
	Sneezing (>3-4 times/inter al)	1											
	Nasal Flaring	2											
	Respiratory Rate >60/min	1											
	Respiratory Rate > 60/min with Retractions	2											
GASTRO-INTESTINAL DISTURBANCES (4 domains)	Excessi e Sucking	1											
	Poor Feeding	2											
	Regurgitation	2											
	Projectile Vomiting	3											
	Loose Stools	2											
	Watery Stools	3											
	TOTAL SCORE												
	INITIALS OF SCORER												

Adapted from: Nelson, Nicholas. Current Therapy in Neonatal-Perinatal Medicine. 2nd ed. Toronto: BC Decker, 1990[101]

CLINICAL REPORT   Guidance for the Clinician in Rendering Pediatric Care

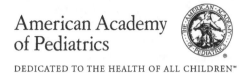

American Academy
of Pediatrics
DEDICATED TO THE HEALTH OF ALL CHILDREN™

Patent Ductus Arteriosus in Preterm Infants

William E. Benitz, MD, FAAP, COMMITTEE ON FETUS AND NEWBORN

abstract

Despite a large body of basic science and clinical research and clinical experience with thousands of infants over nearly 6 decades,[1] there is still uncertainty and controversy about the significance, evaluation, and management of patent ductus arteriosus in preterm infants, resulting in substantial heterogeneity in clinical practice. The purpose of this clinical report is to summarize the evidence available to guide evaluation and treatment of preterm infants with prolonged ductal patency in the first few weeks after birth.

CLINICAL EPIDEMIOLOGY AND NATURAL HISTORY OF PATENT DUCTUS ARTERIOSUS

In term infants, the ductus arteriosus normally constricts after birth and becomes functionally closed by 72 hours of age.[2] In preterm infants, however, closure is delayed, remaining open at 4 days of age in approximately 10% of infants born at 30 through 37 weeks' gestation, 80% of those born at 25 through 28 weeks' gestation, and 90% of those born at 24 weeks' gestation.[3] By day 7 after birth, those rates decline to approximately 2%, 65%, and 87%, respectively. The ductus is likely to close without treatment in infants born at >28 weeks' gestation (73%),[4] in those with birth weight >1000 g (94%),[5] and in infants born at 26 through 29 weeks' gestation who do not have respiratory distress syndrome (93%).[6] Rates of later spontaneous ductal closure among smaller, less mature infants with respiratory distress syndrome are not known because of widespread use of treatments to achieve closure of the patent ductus arteriosus (PDA) in such infants. Data from placebo arms of controlled trials demonstrate that spontaneous ductal closure in these infants is frequent, however. In the Trial of Indomethacin Prophylaxis in Preterms, for example, which included infants with birth weight from 500 to 999 g, 50% of placebo recipients never developed clinical signs of a PDA.[7] In a trial of early versus late indomethacin treatment of infants born at 26 through 31 weeks' gestation in whom PDA was confirmed by echocardiography on day 3, the ductus closed spontaneously by 9 days of age in 78% of those randomized to late intervention.[8]

DOI: 10.1542/peds.2015-3730

PEDIATRICS (ISSN Numbers: Print, 0031-4005; Online, 1098-4275).

Copyright © 2016 by the American Academy of Pediatrics

To cite: Benitz WE and COMMITTEE ON FETUS AND NEWBORN. Patent Ductus Arteriosus in Preterm Infants. *Pediatrics.* 2016;137(1):e20153730

While the ductus remains open, blood typically flows left-to-right from the aorta into the pulmonary arteries. As pulmonary vascular resistance declines over the first several days after birth, the proportion of aortic blood flow that is diverted into the pulmonary circulation correspondingly increases. This "ductal steal" results in excessive blood flow through the lungs, predisposing to development of pulmonary congestion, pulmonary edema, and worsening respiratory failure. Diversion of blood flow from the systemic circulation may exceed capabilities for compensatory increases in total cardiac output, resulting in compromised perfusion of vital organs, including bowel, kidney, and brain. Prolonged patency is associated with numerous adverse outcomes, including prolongation of assisted ventilation and higher rates of death, bronchopulmonary dysplasia (BPD), pulmonary hemorrhage, necrotizing enterocolitis, impaired renal function, intraventricular hemorrhage (IVH), periventricular leukomalacia, and cerebral palsy.[9] The extent to which these adverse outcomes are attributable to the hemodynamic consequences of ductal patency, if at all, has not been established. The strength of these associations led to the hypothesis that intervention to close the ductus might prevent or reduce the severity of these common complications of prematurity. The expectation that this hypothesis would be confirmed, in turn, resulted in widespread adoption of interventions designed to achieve early closure of the ductus in preterm infants.

ASSESSMENT OF HEMODYNAMIC SIGNIFICANCE

The hemodynamic effects of a large left-to-right shunt associated with a PDA may be evident by physical examination, echocardiography, or measurement of serum biomarkers.

In addition to the presence of a classic coarse systolic murmur at the left sternal border, affected infants may have an increased precordial impulse, prominent or bounding arterial pulses, palpable pulses in the palms of the hands, and either low systolic and diastolic blood pressure or low diastolic blood pressure with a widened pulse pressure. Nevertheless, these findings are nonspecific, do not correlate well with echocardiographic findings,[10] and have not been shown to reliably predict responses to treatment or sequelae. In many instances, the presence of a large ductal shunt is suspected only on the basis of respiratory findings, such as radiographic signs of pulmonary congestion, increasing requirements for supplemental oxygen, or inability to reduce mechanical ventilator support. The presence of a PDA is most definitively demonstrated by color Doppler echocardiography, which permits confirmation of ductal patency, measurement of ductal dimensions, and assessment of the direction and velocity of ductal blood flow throughout the cardiac cycle. Substantial ductal shunting may be associated with an increased ratio of left atrial to aortic root dimensions $\geq 1.5:1$, ductal diameter ≥ 1.5 mm, left ventricular volume and pressure loading, and reversal of diastolic flow in the descending aorta or in cerebral or renal arteries.[11,12] Serum concentrations of natriuretic peptides (BNP or N-terminal of the prohormone BNP) are elevated in preterm infants with PDA,[13,14] correlate with echocardiographic measures of shunt volume,[14–16] and decrease after ductal closure.[14,16] Concentrations of troponin T at 48 hours of age are higher in infants with PDA.[17]

The term "hemodynamically significant" is frequently used to differentiate consequential from inconsequential PDA. Neither the best tool nor the optimal thresholds

for identification of infants at greatest risk for adverse sequelae have been delineated. The predictive values of individual echocardiographic measurements are low, but some progress has been made toward correlation of composite scores with risks of adverse long-term outcome, including BPD[18] or neurodevelopmental outcome at 2 years of age.[12] Exploratory studies suggest that elevated concentrations of either N-terminal of the prohormone BNP or troponin T at 48 hours of age may help predict death or severe IVH[19] as well as neurodevelopment at 2 years of age.[12] The presence of a "hemodynamically significant" PDA has been correlated with lower regional cerebral oxygen saturation and higher fractional oxygen extraction[20] and with reduced celiac artery flow,[21] supporting the hypothesis that prolonged ductal patency may have a causal role in substantial and enduring adverse outcomes. Development of an integrated definition of "hemodynamic significance" of PDA will be essential to risk stratification for clinical trials of PDA treatment, but this goal remains elusive.

EVIDENCE FOR BENEFITS OF TREATMENT

Since the early reports of feasibility of surgical closure[22] and efficacy of nonsteroidal antiinflammatory drugs for medical treatment[23,24] of PDA, results have been reported for 50 randomized controlled trials enrolling 4878 preterm infants.[9,25] Although medical and surgical treatments are efficacious in closing the PDA in a large proportion of infants, neither individual clinical trials nor meta-analyses have demonstrated that closing the ductus results in improved long-term outcomes. Odds ratios for the most important outcomes (BPD, necrotizing enterocolitis, neurosensory impairment, death, the combined outcomes of death or BPD and death or neurosensory impairment) indicate that early, routine treatment has no effect, with narrow confidence intervals, so it is unlikely that substantial differences have gone undetected.[9] When given as prophylaxis for IVH beginning within 12 hours of birth, treatment with indomethacin reduces rates of IVH, IVH greater than grade II, and early, severe pulmonary hemorrhage but does not improve long-term neurodevelopmental or respiratory outcomes.[7,26–28] The early neuroprotective effects of indomethacin may not depend on effects on ductal patency and are not replicated with similar use of ibuprofen.[29] In all published trials of prophylaxis or treatment, interventions were initiated within 2 weeks after birth for almost all subjects in the treatment arms, and later backup treatment to achieve ductal closure was common among control subjects.[30,31] The available evidence is therefore insufficient to permit assessment of potential benefits of treatments initiated after 2 weeks of age. The cumulative evidence supports the conclusion that early (in the first 2 weeks after birth), routine (as prophylaxis or for infants with echocardiographic confirmation of ductal patency with or without clinical signs) treatment to close the ductus arteriosus does not improve long-term outcomes for preterm infants. There is insufficient evidence to determine whether there are preterm infants who might benefit from early treatment or that later treatment has no potential benefit. These data also cannot be extrapolated to novel treatments (such as acetaminophen, recently reported to promote ductal closure[32,33]) because the balance between beneficial and adverse effects of new treatments may differ substantially from that for previously studied treatments.

Although surgical ligation is effective for achievement of rapid, complete ductal closure, it is often followed by severe hemodynamic and respiratory collapse, requiring marked escalation in supportive intensive care.[34] The risk of this complication appears to decline substantially over the first 6 weeks after birth.[35] Long-term complications of surgical ligation include paresis of the left vocal cord[36,37] or diaphragm,[38] chylothorax,[38–40] and scoliosis,[41,42] and infants who undergo surgical ligation are more likely to develop BPD,[43–45] retinopathy of prematurity,[45] and neurodevelopmental impairment.[45,46] Treatment with cyclooxygenase inhibitors may lead to impaired renal function,[47] intestinal perforation,[48,49] and altered cerebrovascular regulation.[50] In contrast to prophylactic use, treatment of confirmed PDA with indomethacin is associated with an increased risk of IVH.[9] Treatment to close a patent ductus may therefore not be entirely benign.

Clinical experience with less aggressive strategies for PDA management suggests that a more permissive approach does not result in worse outcomes. Strategies avoiding use of indomethacin or ibuprofen yield outcomes comparable to contemporaneous external benchmarks.[51,52] Less frequent use of surgical ligation in infants with PDA after failure of indomethacin prophylaxis was associated with a lower rate of necrotizing enterocolitis and no increase in rates of other adverse outcomes.[53] Reduced use of indomethacin and ligation at 1 center was associated with an increased rate of the combined outcome of death or chronic lung disease but no increase in rates of individual morbidities or mortality.[54] These experiences indicate that longer periods of exposure to left-to-right ductal shunting may not result in

significantly compromised outcomes, supporting equipoise regarding enrollment of preterm infants into randomized trials designed to assess treatment strategies for preterm infants with PDA.

CLINICAL TRIAL OPPORTUNITIES

As previously noted, evidence-based abandonment of early routine treatment to close the PDA does not preclude other options for management of infants with this condition. First, deciding not to intervene routinely to achieve earlier closure of the ductus should not imply that consequences of ductal patency can be completely ignored.[55] Although many strategies for management of the consequences of PDA have been proposed, none have been subjected to systematic evaluation in clinical trials, which are urgently needed to guide management of these infants. Studies of interventions designed to limit excessive pulmonary blood flow (red cell transfusion, increased positive airway pressure, correction of alkalosis, avoidance of pulmonary vasodilators such as oxygen or nitric oxide), to increase systemic cardiac output (dopamine, captopril, avoidance of hypovolemia), to ameliorate pulmonary edema (fluid restriction, diuretics, correction of hypoproteinemia), or to minimize confounding insults (nephrotoxic drugs, systemic infection/inflammation, hypoxemia, hypocarbia) may be appropriate. Second, early identification of a subset of infants with PDA who are at particular risk on the basis of echocardiographic, serum biomarker, or hemodynamic monitoring (such as measurement of cerebral oxygen saturation or fractional oxygen extraction) may allow more selective treatment in the first 2 weeks after birth. Because few extremely preterm infants (those born at ≤25 weeks, for example) were included in extant trials, they may constitute a high-risk group with potential benefit from early, universal treatment. Similarly, criteria for intervention after the second postnatal week need to be developed. Although early experience suggested that infants more than 10 to 14 days of age are unlikely to respond to medical treatment with ductal closure,[56,57] other analyses have suggested that postmenstrual, not postnatal, age is the critical determinant, with efficacy declining sharply after approximately 33 to 34 weeks' postmenstrual age.[58,59] Therefore, selective treatment of infants born at or before 28 weeks' gestation, who are at highest risk of PDA, may remain an option well beyond 2 weeks' postnatal age. Deferral of treatment may allow avoidance of treatment of those in whom spontaneous closure occurs without seriously compromising the potential efficacy of medical treatment. Delaying ligation may have similar advantages, avoiding surgery in many infants in whom the ductus closes without treatment and reducing the risk of postoperative hemodynamic compromise in those who do require surgery, particularly if surgery can be deferred until after 30 days of age.

Additional research is needed to address 2 broad questions related to prolonged ductal patency in preterm infants. First, the relationship between measures of hemodynamic significance and increased risks for both prolonged patency and adverse clinical outcomes, such as chronic lung disease or neurodevelopmental impairment, needs to be established. Preliminary work using echocardiographic scores and serum biomarkers, described previously, provides a promising foundation for these studies. That information is extremely important for selection of appropriate subjects for enrollment in intervention trials. Second, well-designed and meticulously executed intervention trials, for which the

end points are clinically important long-term outcomes and not simply rates of ductal closure or measures of short-term physiologic changes, are essential. In these trials, both treatment arms must be explicitly defined so that the superior strategy can be replicated in clinical practice and evaluated against alternatives in future trials. If it is not feasible to forgo use of rescue treatment in the control (placebo or late-treatment) arm, strict criteria for both a required time interval and diagnostic thresholds for such treatment are desirable. Without clear demonstration that adverse outcomes can be averted by medical or surgical closure of the ductus, the hypothesis that ductal patency is causal with respect to those outcomes remains unproven.

CONCLUSIONS

A large body of evidence now exists demonstrating that early, routine treatment to induce closure of the ductus in preterm infants, either medically or surgically, in the first 2 weeks after birth does not improve long-term outcomes (level of evidence: 1A[60]). The role of more selective use of medical methods for induction of ductal closure, either for defined high-risk infants in the first 2 postnatal weeks, or more generally, for older infants in whom the ductus remains patent, remains uncertain and requires further study. Prophylactic use of indomethacin may be appropriate in settings where rates of IVH are high or if early, severe pulmonary hemorrhage is common, but may not be justified by expected effects on PDA or by an expectation of better long-term outcomes. There is a lack of evidence to guide management of PDA, necessitating equipoise regarding treatment options and support for parents to permit enrollment of their infants in trials that can expand the available body of evidence.

AAP COMMITTEE ON FETUS AND NEWBORN, 2014–2015

Kristi L. Watterberg, MD, FAAP, Chairperson
Susan Aucott, MD, FAAP
William E. Benitz, MD, FAAP
James J. Cummings, MD, FAAP
Eric C. Eichenwald, MD, FAAP
Jay Goldsmith, MD, FAAP
Brenda B. Poindexter, MD, FAAP
Karen Puopolo, MD, FAAP
Dan L. Stewart, MD, FAAP
Kasper S. Wang, MD, FAAP

LIAISONS

Captain Wanda D. Barfield, MD, MPH, FAAP – *Centers for Disease Control and Prevention*
James Goldberg, MD – *American College of Obstetricians and Gynecologists*
Thierry Lacaze, MD – *Canadian Pediatric Society*
Erin L. Keels, APRN, MS, NNP-BC – *National Association of Neonatal Nurses*
Tonse N.K. Raju, MD, DCH, FAAP – *National Institutes of Health*

STAFF

Jim Couto, MA

ABBREVIATIONS

BPD: bronchopulmonary dysplasia
IVH: intraventricular hemorrhage
PDA: patent ductus arteriosus

REFERENCES

1. Burnard ED. A murmur from the ductus arteriosus in the newborn baby. *BMJ*. 1958;1(5074):806–810

2. Gentile R, Stevenson G, Dooley T, Franklin D, Kawabori I, Pearlman A. Pulsed Doppler echocardiographic determination of time of ductal closure in normal newborn infants. *J Pediatr*. 1981;98(3):443–448

3. Clyman RI, Couto J, Murphy GM. Patent ductus arteriosus: are current neonatal treatment options better or worse than no treatment at all? *Semin Perinatol*. 2012;36(2):123–129

4. Koch J, Hensley G, Roy L, Brown S, Ramaciotti C, Rosenfeld CR. Prevalence of spontaneous closure of the ductus arteriosus in neonates at a birth weight of 1000 grams or less. *Pediatrics*. 2006;117(4):1113–1121

5. Nemerofsky SL, Parravicini E, Bateman D, Kleinman C, Polin RA, Lorenz JM. The ductus arteriosus rarely requires treatment in infants > 1000 grams. *Am J Perinatol.* 2008;25(10):661–666

6. Reller MD, Rice MJ, McDonald RW. Review of studies evaluating ductal patency in the premature infant. *J Pediatr.* 1993;122(6):S59–S62

7. Schmidt B, Davis P, Moddemann D, et al; Trial of Indomethacin Prophylaxis in Preterms Investigators. Long-term effects of indomethacin prophylaxis in extremely-low-birth-weight infants. *N Engl J Med.* 2001;344(26):1966–1972

8. Van Overmeire B, Van de Broek H, Van Laer P, Weyler J, Vanhaesebrouck P. Early versus late indomethacin treatment for patent ductus arteriosus in premature infants with respiratory distress syndrome. *J Pediatr.* 2001;138(2):205–211

9. Benitz WE. Treatment of persistent patent ductus arteriosus in preterm infants: time to accept the null hypothesis? *J Perinatol.* 2010;30(4):241–252

10. Skelton R, Evans N, Smythe J. A blinded comparison of clinical and echocardiographic evaluation of the preterm infant for patent ductus arteriosus. *J Paediatr Child Health.* 1994;30(5):406–411

11. McNamara PJ, Sehgal A. Towards rational management of the patent ductus arteriosus: the need for disease staging. *Arch Dis Child Fetal Neonatal Ed.* 2007;92(6):F424–F427

12. El-Khuffash AF, Slevin M, McNamara PJ, Molloy EJ. Troponin T, N-terminal pro natriuretic peptide and a patent ductus arteriosus scoring system predict death before discharge or neurodevelopmental outcome at 2 years in preterm infants. *Arch Dis Child Fetal Neonatal Ed.* 2011;96(2):F133–F137

13. Choi BM, Lee KH, Eun BL, et al. Utility of rapid B-type natriuretic peptide assay for diagnosis of symptomatic patent ductus arteriosus in preterm infants. *Pediatrics.* 2005;115(3). Available at: www.pediatrics.org/cgi/content/full/115/3/e255

14. Flynn PA, da Graca RL, Auld PA, Nesin M, Kleinman CS. The use of a bedside assay for plasma B-type natriuretic peptide as a biomarker in the management of patent ductus arteriosus in premature neonates. *J Pediatr.* 2005;147(1):38–42

15. El-Khuffash AF, Amoruso M, Culliton M, Molloy EJ. N-terminal pro-B-type natriuretic peptide as a marker of ductal haemodynamic significance in preterm infants: a prospective observational study. *Arch Dis Child Fetal Neonatal Ed.* 2007;92(5):F421–F422

16. Sanjeev S, Pettersen M, Lua J, Thomas R, Shankaran S, L'Ecuyer T. Role of plasma B-type natriuretic peptide in screening for hemodynamically significant patent ductus arteriosus in preterm neonates. *J Perinatol.* 2005;25(11):709–713

17. El-Khuffash AF, Molloy EJ. Influence of a patent ductus arteriosus on cardiac troponin T levels in preterm infants. *J Pediatr.* 2008;153(3):350–353

18. Sehgal A, Paul E, Menahem S. Functional echocardiography in staging for ductal disease severity: role in predicting outcomes. *Eur J Pediatr.* 2013;172(2):179–184

19. El-Khuffash A, Barry D, Walsh K, Davis PG, Molloy EJ. Biochemical markers may identify preterm infants with a patent ductus arteriosus at high risk of death or severe intraventricular haemorrhage. *Arch Dis Child Fetal Neonatal Ed.* 2008;93(6):F407–F412

20. Lemmers PM, Toet MC, van Bel F. Impact of patent ductus arteriosus and subsequent therapy with indomethacin on cerebral oxygenation in preterm infants. *Pediatrics.* 2008;121(1):142–147

21. El-Khuffash A, Higgins M, Walsh K, Molloy EJ. Quantitative assessment of the degree of ductal steal using celiac artery blood flow to left ventricular output ratio in preterm infants. *Neonatology.* 2008;93(3):206–212

22. Gupta JM, Van Vliet PK, Fisk GC, Wright JS. Ductus ligation in respiratory distress syndrome. *J Thorac Cardiovasc Surg.* 1972;63(4):642–647

23. Friedman WF, Hirschklau MJ, Printz MP, Pitlick PT, Kirkpatrick SE. Pharmacologic closure of patent ductus arteriosus in the premature infant. *N Engl J Med.* 1976;295(10):526–529

24. Heymann MA, Rudolph AM, Silverman NH. Closure of the ductus arteriosus in premature infants by inhibition of prostaglandin synthesis. *N Engl J Med.* 1976;295(10):530–533

25. Kluckow M, Jeffery M, Gill A, Evans N. A randomised placebo-controlled trial of early treatment of the patent ductus arteriosus. *Arch Dis Child Fetal Neonatal Ed.* 2014;99(2):F99–F104

26. Ment LR, Vohr B, Allan W, et al. Outcome of children in the indomethacin intraventricular hemorrhage prevention trial. *Pediatrics.* 2000;105(3 pt 1):485–491

27. Rheinlaender C, Helfenstein D, Pees C, et al. Neurodevelopmental outcome after COX inhibitor treatment for patent ductus arteriosus. *Early Hum Dev.* 2010;86(2):87–92

28. Alfaleh K, Smyth JA, Roberts RS, Solimano A, Asztalos EV, Schmidt B; Trial of Indomethacin Prophylaxis in Preterms Investigators. Prevention and 18-month outcomes of serious pulmonary hemorrhage in extremely low birth weight infants: results from the trial of indomethacin prophylaxis in preterms. *Pediatrics.* 2008;121(2). Available at: www.pediatrics.org/cgi/content/full/121/2/e233

29. Ohlsson A, Shah SS. Ibuprofen for the prevention of patent ductus arteriosus in preterm and/or low birth weight infants. *Cochrane Database Syst Rev.* 2011;(7):CD004213

30. Clyman RI, Chorne N. Patent ductus arteriosus: evidence for and against treatment. *J Pediatr.* 2007;150(3):216–219

31. Clyman RI. Recommendations for the postnatal use of indomethacin: an analysis of four separate treatment strategies. *J Pediatr.* 1996;128(5 pt 1):601–607

32. Hammerman C, Bin-Nun A, Markovitch E, Schimmel MS, Kaplan M, Fink D. Ductal closure with paracetamol: a surprising new approach to patent ductus arteriosus treatment. *Pediatrics.* 2011;128(6). Available at: www.pediatrics.org/cgi/content/full/128/6/e1618

33. Oncel MY, Yurttutan S, Erdeve O, et al. Oral paracetamol versus oral ibuprofen in the management of patent ductus arteriosus in preterm infants: a randomized controlled trial. *J Pediatr.* 2014;164(3):510–4.e1

34. Teixeira LS, Shivananda SP, Stephens D, Van Arsdell G, McNamara PJ. Postoperative cardiorespiratory instability following ligation of the preterm ductus arteriosus is related to early need for intervention. *J Perinatol.* 2008;28(12):803–810

35. Teixeira LS, McNamara PJ. Enhanced intensive care for the neonatal ductus arteriosus. *Acta Paediatr.* 2006;95(4):394–403

36. Clement WA, El-Hakim H, Phillipos EZ, Coté JJ. Unilateral vocal cord paralysis following patent ductus arteriosus ligation in extremely low-birth-weight infants. *Arch Otolaryngol Head Neck Surg.* 2008;134(1):28–33

37. Smith ME, King JD, Elsherif A, Muntz HR, Park AH, Kouretas PC. Should all newborns who undergo patent ductus arteriosus ligation be examined for vocal fold mobility? *Laryngoscope.* 2009;119(8):1606–1609

38. Mandhan P, Brown S, Kukkady A, Samarakkody U. Surgical closure of patent ductus arteriosus in preterm low birth weight infants. *Congenit Heart Dis.* 2009;4(1):34–37

39. Gould DS, Montenegro LM, Gaynor JW, et al. A comparison of on-site and off-site patent ductus arteriosus ligation in premature infants. *Pediatrics.* 2003;112(6 pt 1):1298–1301

40. Lippmann M, Nelson RJ, Emmanouilides GC, Diskin J, Thibeault DW. Ligation of patent ductus arteriosus in premature infants. *Br J Anaesth.* 1976;48(4):365–369

41. Roclawski M, Sabiniewicz R, Potaz P, et al. Scoliosis in patients with aortic coarctation and patent ductus arteriosus: does standard posterolateral thoracotomy play a role in the development of the lateral curve of the spine? *Pediatr Cardiol.* 2009;30(7):941–945

42. Shelton JE, Julian R, Walburgh E, Schneider E. Functional scoliosis as a long-term complication of surgical ligation for patent ductus arteriosus

in premature infants. *J Pediatr Surg.* 1986;21(10):855–857

43. Chorne N, Leonard C, Piecuch R, Clyman RI. Patent ductus arteriosus and its treatment as risk factors for neonatal and neurodevelopmental morbidity. *Pediatrics.* 2007;119(6):1165–1174

44. Clyman R, Cassady G, Kirklin JK, Collins M, Philips JB III. The role of patent ductus arteriosus ligation in bronchopulmonary dysplasia: reexamining a randomized controlled trial. *J Pediatr.* 2009;154(6):873–876

45. Kabra NS, Schmidt B, Roberts RS, Doyle LW, Papile L, Fanaroff A; Trial of Indomethacin Prophylaxis in Preterms Investigators. Neurosensory impairment after surgical closure of patent ductus arteriosus in extremely low birth weight infants: results from the Trial of Indomethacin Prophylaxis in Preterms. *J Pediatr.* 2007;150(3):229–234, 234.e1

46. Wickremasinghe AC, Rogers EE, Piecuch RE, et al. Neurodevelopmental outcomes following two different treatment approaches (early ligation and selective ligation) for patent ductus arteriosus. *J Pediatr.* 2012;161(6):1065–1072

47. Fanos V, Benini D, Verlato G, Errico G, Cuzzolin L. Efficacy and renal tolerability of ibuprofen vs. indomethacin in preterm infants with patent ductus arteriosus. *Fundam Clin Pharmacol.* 2005;19(2):187–193

48. Shorter NA, Liu JY, Mooney DP, Harmon BJ. Indomethacin-associated bowel perforations: a study of possible risk factors. *J Pediatr Surg.* 1999;34(3):442–444

49. Watterberg KL, Gerdes JS, Cole CH, et al. Prophylaxis of early adrenal insufficiency to prevent bronchopulmonary dysplasia: a multicenter trial. *Pediatrics.* 2004;114(6):1649–1657

50. Van Bel F, Van de Bor M, Stijnen T, Baan J, Ruys JH. Cerebral blood flow velocity changes in preterm infants after a single dose of indomethacin: duration of its effect. *Pediatrics.* 1989;84(5):802–807

51. Pietz J, Achanti B, Lilien L, Stepka EC, Mehta SK. Prevention of necrotizing

enterocolitis in preterm infants: a 20-year experience. *Pediatrics.* 2007;119(1). Available at: www.pediatrics.org/cgi/content/full/119/1/e164

52. Vanhaesebrouck S, Zonnenberg I, Vandervoort P, Bruneel E, Van Hoestenberghe MR, Theyskens C. Conservative treatment for patent ductus arteriosus in the preterm. *Arch Dis Child Fetal Neonatal Ed.* 2007;92(4):F244–F247

53. Jhaveri N, Moon-Grady A, Clyman RI. Early surgical ligation versus a conservative approach for management of patent ductus arteriosus that fails to close after indomethacin treatment. *J Pediatr.* 2010;157(3):381–387, 387.e1

54. Kaempf JW, Wu YX, Kaempf AJ, Kaempf AM, Wang L, Grunkemeier G. What happens when the patent ductus arteriosus is treated less aggressively in very low birth weight infants? *J Perinatol.* 2012;32(5):344–348

55. Benitz WE. Learning to live with patency of the ductus arteriosus in preterm infants. *J Perinatol.* 2011;31(suppl 1):S42–S48

56. Halliday HL, Hirata T, Brady JP. Indomethacin therapy for large patent ductus arteriosus in the very low birth weight infant: results and complications. *Pediatrics.* 1979;64(2):154–159

57. Smith IJ, Goss I, Congdon PJ. Intravenous indomethacin for patent ductus arteriosus. *Arch Dis Child.* 1984;59(6):537–541

58. Kresch MJ, Moya FR, Ascuitto RJ, Ross-Ascuitto NT, Heusser F. Late closure of the ductus arteriosus using indomethacin in the preterm infant. *Clin Pediatr (Phila).* 1988;27(3):140–143

59. McCarthy JS, Zies LG, Gelband H. Age-dependent closure of the patent ductus arteriosus by indomethacin. *Pediatrics.* 1978;62(5):706–712

60. Oxford Centre for Evidence-based Medicine—Levels of Evidence. 2009. Available at: http://www.cebm.net/oxford-centre-evidence-based-medicine-levels-evidence-march-2009/. Accessed June 25, 2015

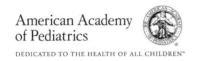

American Academy
of Pediatrics
DEDICATED TO THE HEALTH OF ALL CHILDREN™

TECHNICAL REPORT

Phototherapy to Prevent Severe Neonatal Hyperbilirubinemia in the Newborn Infant 35 or More Weeks of Gestation

abstract

OBJECTIVE: To standardize the use of phototherapy consistent with the American Academy of Pediatrics clinical practice guideline for the management of hyperbilirubinemia in the newborn infant 35 or more weeks of gestation.

METHODS: Relevant literature was reviewed. Phototherapy devices currently marketed in the United States that incorporate fluorescent, halogen, fiber-optic, or blue light-emitting diode light sources were assessed in the laboratory.

RESULTS: The efficacy of phototherapy units varies widely because of differences in light source and configuration. The following characteristics of a device contribute to its effectiveness: (1) emission of light in the blue-to-green range that overlaps the in vivo plasma bilirubin absorption spectrum ($\sim$460$-$490 nm); (2) irradiance of at least 30 μW·cm^{-2}·nm^{-1} (confirmed with an appropriate irradiance meter calibrated over the appropriate wavelength range); (3) illumination of maximal body surface; and (4) demonstration of a decrease in total bilirubin concentrations during the first 4 to 6 hours of exposure.

RECOMMENDATIONS (SEE APPENDIX FOR GRADING DEFINITION): The intensity and spectral output of phototherapy devices is useful in predicting potential effectiveness in treating hyperbilirubinemia (group B recommendation). Clinical effectiveness should be evaluated before and monitored during use (group B recommendation). Blocking the light source or reducing exposed body surface should be avoided (group B recommendation). Standardization of irradiance meters, improvements in device design, and lower-upper limits of light intensity for phototherapy units merit further study. Comparing the in vivo performance of devices is not practical, in general, and alternative procedures need to be explored. *Pediatrics* 2011;128:e1046–e1052

Vinod K. Bhutani, MD, and THE COMMITTEE ON FETUS AND NEWBORN

KEY WORDS
phototherapy, newborn jaundice, hyperbilirubinemia, light treatment

ABBREVIATION
LED—light-emitting diode

This document is copyrighted and is property of the American Academy of Pediatrics and its Board of Directors. All authors have filed conflict of interest statements with the American Academy of Pediatrics. Any conflicts have been resolved through a process approved by the Board of Directors. The American Academy of Pediatrics has neither solicited nor accepted any commercial involvement in the development of the content of this publication.

The guidance in this report does not indicate an exclusive course of treatment or serve as a standard of medical care. Variations, taking into account individual circumstances, may be appropriate.

www.pediatrics.org/cgi/doi/10.1542/peds.2011-1494

doi:10.1542/peds.2011-1494

All technical reports from the American Academy of Pediatrics automatically expire 5 years after publication unless reaffirmed, revised, or retired at or before that time.

PEDIATRICS (ISSN Numbers: Print, 0031-4005; Online, 1098-4275).

INTRODUCTION

Clinical trials have validated the efficacy of phototherapy in reducing excessive unconjugated hyperbilirubinemia, and its implementation has drastically curtailed the use of exchange transfusions.[1] The initiation and duration of phototherapy is defined by a specific range of total bilirubin values based on an infant's postnatal age and the potential risk for bilirubin neurotoxicity.[1] Clinical response to phototherapy depends on the efficacy of the phototherapy device as well as the balance between an infant's rates of bilirubin production and elimination. The active agent in phototherapy is light delivered in measurable doses, which makes phototherapy conceptually similar to pharmacotherapy. This report standardizes the use of phototherapy consistent with the American Academy of Pediatrics clinical practice guideline for the management of hyperbilirubinemia in the newborn infant 35 or more weeks of gestation.

I. COMMERCIAL LIGHT SOURCES

A wide selection of commercial phototherapy devices is available in the United States. A complete discussion of devices is beyond the scope of this review; some are described in Tables 1 and 2. Phototherapy devices can be categorized according to their light source as follows: (1) fluorescent-tube devices that emit different colors (cool white daylight, blue [B], special blue [BB], turquoise, and green) and are straight (F20 T12, 60 cm, 20 W), U-shaped, or spiral-shaped; (2) metal halide bulbs, used in spotlights and incubator lights; (3) light-emitting diodes (LEDs) or metal halide bulbs, used with fiber-optic light guides in pads, blankets, or spotlights; and (4) high-intensity LEDs, used as over- and under-the-body devices.

TABLE 1 Phototherapy Devices Commonly Used in the United States and Their Performance Characteristics

Device	Manufacturer	Distance to Patient (cm)	Footprint Area (Length × Width, cm²)	% Treatable BSA	Spectrum, Total (nm)	Bandwidth* (nm)	Peak (nm)	Footprint Irradiance (μW/cm²/nm)		
								Min	Max	Mean ± SD
Light Emitting Diodes [LED]										
neoBLUE	Natus Medical, San Carlos, CA	30	1152 (48 × 24)	100	420–540	20	462	12	37	30 ± 7
PortaBed	Stanford University, Stanford, CA	≥5	1740 (30 × 58)	100	425–540	27	463	40	76	67 ± 8
Fluorescent										
BiliLite CW/BB	Olympic Medical, San Carlos, CA	45	2928 (48 × 61)	100	380–720	69	578	6	10	8 ± 1
BiliLite BB	Olympic Medical, San Carlos, CA	45	2928 (48 × 61)	100	400–550	35	445	11	22	17 ± 2
BiliLite TL52	Olympic Medical, San Carlos, CA	45	2928 (48 × 61)	100	400–626	69	437	13	23	19 ± 3
BiliBed	Medela, McHenry, IL	0	693 (21 × 33)	71	400–560	80	450	14	59	36 ± 2
Halogen										
MinBiliLite	Olympic Medical, San Carlos, CA	45	490 (25 diam)	54	350–800	190	580	<1	19	7 ± 5
Phototherapy Lite	Philips Inc, Andover, MA	45	490 (25 diam)	54	370–850	200	590	<1	17	5 ± 5
Halogen fiberoptic										
BiliBlanket	Ohmeda, Fairfield, CT	0	150 (10 × 15)	24	390–600	70	533	9	31	20 ± 6
Wallaby II Preterm	Philips, Inc, Andover, MA	0	117 (9 × 13)	19	400–560	45	513	8	30	16 ± 6
Wallaby II Term	Philips, Inc, Andover, MA	0	280 (8 × 35)	53	400–560	45	513	6	11	8 ± 1
SpotLight 1000	Philips, Inc, Andover, MA	45	490 (25 diam)	54	400–560	45	513	1	11	6 ± 3
PEP Model 2000	PEP, Fryeburg, ME	23	1530 (30 × 51)	100	400–717	63	445	12	49	28 ± 11
Bili Soft	GE Healthcare, Laurel, MD	0	825 (25 × 33)	71	400–670	40	453	1	52	25 ± 16

Data in Table 1 are expanded and updated from that previously reported by Vreman et al.[3] The definitions and standards for device assessment are explained below.

EMISSION SPECTRAL QUALITIES: Measured data of the light delivered by each of the light sources are presented as the minimum, maximum and range. Light source emission spectra within the range of 300–700 nm were recorded after the device had reached stable light emission, using a miniature fiberoptic radiometer (IRRAD2000, Ocean Optics, Inc, Dunedin, FL). For precision based device assessment, the spectral bandwidth (*), which is defined as the width of the emission spectrum in nm at 50% of peak light intensity, is the preferred method to distinguish and compare instead of the total range emission spectrum (data usually provided by manufacturers). Emission peak values are also used to characterize the quality of light emitted by a given light source.

IRRADIANCE: Measured data are presented as mean ± standard deviation (SD), representing the irradiance of blue light (including spectral bandwidth), for each device's light footprint at the manufacturer-recommended distance. To compare diverse devices, the spectral irradiance (μW/cm²/nm) measurements were made using calibrated BiliBlanket Meters I and II (Ohmeda, GE Healthcare, Fairfield, CT), which were found to yield identical results with stable output phototherapy devices. This type of meter was selected from the several devices with different photonic characteristics that are commercially available, because it has a wide sensitivity range (400–520 nm with peak sensitivity at 450 nm), which overlaps the bilirubin absorption spectrum and which renders it suitable for the evaluation of narrow and broad wavelength band light sources. The devices have been found exceptionally stable during several years of use and agree closely after each annual calibration.

FOOTPRINT: The minimum and maximum irradiance measured (at the intervals provided or defined) in the given irradiance footprint of the device (length × width). The footprint of a device is that area which is occupied by a patient to receive phototherapy. The irradiance footprint has greater dimensions than the emission surface, which is measured at the point where the light exits a phototherapy device. The minimum and maximum values are shown to indicate the range of irradiances encountered with a device and can be used as an indication of the uniformity of the emitted light. Most devices conform to an international standard to deliver a minimum/maximum footprint light ratio of no lower than 0.4.

BSA: BODY SURFACE AREA refers to percent (%) exposure of either the ventral or dorsal planar surface exposed to light and Irradiance measurements are accurate to ±0.5.

All of the reported devices are marketed in the United States except the PortaBed, which is a non-licensed Stanford-developed research device and the Dutch Crigler-Najjar Association (used by Crigler-Najjar patients).

TABLE 2 Maximum Spectral Irradiance of Phototherapy Devices (Using Commercial Light Meters at Manufacturer Recommended Distances) Compared to Clear-Sky Sunlight

Light Meter [Range, Peak]	Footprint Irradiance, (μW/cm²/nm²)							
	Halogen/Fiberoptic			Fluorescent		LED		Sunlight
	BiliBlanket	Wallaby (Neo)		PEP Bed	Martin/Philips BB	neoBLUE	PortaBed	@ Zenith on 8/31/05
		II	III					
	@ Contact	@ Contact		@ 10 cm	@ 25 cm	@ 30 cm	@ 10 cm	Level Ground
BiliBlanket Meter II [400–520, 450 nm]	34	28	34	40	69	34	76	144
Bili-Meter, Model 22 [425–475, 460 nm]	29	16	32	49	100	25	86	65**
Joey Dosimeter, JD-100 [420–550, 470 nm]	53	51	60	88	174	84	195	304**
PMA-2123 Bilirubin Detector[a] [400–520, 460 nm]	24	24	37	35	70	38	73	81
GoldiLux UVA Photometer, GRP-1[b] [315–400, 365 nm]	<0.04	<0.04	<0.04	<0.04	<0.04	<0.04	<0.04	2489

Data in Table 2 were tested and compiled by Hendrik J. Vreman (June 2007 and reverified December 2010).

** Irradiance presented to this meter exceeded its range. Measurement was made through a stainless-steel screen that attenuated the measured irradiance to 57%, which was subsequently corrected by this factor.

[a] Solar Light Company, Inc., Glenside, PA 19038.

[b] Oriel Instruments, Stratford, CT 06615 and SmartMeter GRP-1 with UV-A probe. GRP-1 measures UV-A light as μW/cm². No artificial light source delivered significant (<0.04 μW/cm²) UV-A radiation at the distances measured.

II. STANDARDS FOR PHOTOTHERAPY DEVICES

Methods for reporting and measuring phototherapy doses are not standardized. Comparisons of commercially available phototherapy devices that use in vitro photodegradation techniques may not accurately predict clinical efficacy.[2] A recent report explored an approach to standardizing and quantifying the magnitude of phototherapy delivered by various devices.[3] Table 1 lists technical data for some of the devices marketed in the United States.[3] Factors to consider in prescribing and implementing phototherapy are (1) emission range of the light source, (2) the light intensity (irradiance), (3) the exposed ("treatable") body surface area illuminated, and (4) the decrease in total bilirubin concentration. A measure of the effectiveness of phototherapy to rapidly configure the bilirubin molecule to less toxic photoisomers (measured in seconds) is not yet clinically available.

A. Light Wavelength

The visible white light spectrum ranges from approximately 350 to 800 nm. Bilirubin absorbs visible light most strongly in the blue region of the spectrum (~460 nm). Absorption of light transforms unconjugated bilirubin molecules bound to human serum albumin in solution into bilirubin photoproducts (predominantly isomers of bilirubin).[2,4,5] Because of the photophysical properties of skin, the most effective light in vivo is probably in the blue-to-green region (~460–490 nm).[2] The first prototype phototherapy device to result in a clinically significant rate of bilirubin decrease used a blue (B) fluorescent-tube light source with 420- to 480-nm emission.[6,7] More effective narrow-band special blue bulbs (F20T12/BB [General Electric, Westinghouse, Sylvania] or TL52/20W [Phillips]) were subsequently used.[8,9] Most recently, commercial compact fluorescent-tube light sources and devices that use LEDs of narrow spectral bandwidth have been used.[9–14] Unless specified otherwise, plastic covers or optical filters need to be used to remove potentially harmful ultraviolet light.

Clinical Context

Devices with maximum emission within the 460- to 490-nm (blue-green) region of the visible spectrum are probably the most effective for treating hyperbilirubinemia.[2,4] Lights with broader emission also will work, although not as effectively. Special blue (BB) fluorescent lights are effective but should not be confused with white lights painted blue or covered with blue plastic sheaths, which should not be used. Devices that contain high-intensity gallium nitride LEDs with emission within the 460- to 490-nm regions are also effective and have a longer lifetime (>20 000 hours), lower heat output, low infrared emission, and no ultraviolet emission.

B. Measuring Light Irradiance

Light intensity or energy output is defined by irradiance and refers to the number of photons (spectral energy) that are delivered per unit area (cm²) of exposed skin.[1] The dose of phototherapy is a measure of the irradiance delivered for a specific duration and adjusted to the exposed body surface area. Determination of an in vivo dose-response relationship is confounded by the optical properties of skin and the rates of bilirubin production and elimination.[1] Irradiance is measured with a radiometer ($W \cdot cm^{-2}$) or spectroradiometer ($\mu W \cdot cm^{-2} \cdot nm^{-1}$) over a given wavelength band. Table 2 compares the spectral irradiance of some of the devices in the US market, as measured with different brands of meters. Often, radiometers measure wavelengths that do not penetrate skin well or that are far from optimal for phototherapy and, therefore, may be of little value for predicting the clinical efficacy of phototherapy units. A direct relationship between irradiance and the rate of in vivo total bilirubin concentration decrease was described in the report of a study of term "healthy" infants with nonhemolytic hyperbilirubinemia (peak values: 15–18 mg/dL) using fluorescent Philips daylight (TL20W/54, TL20W/52) and special blue (TLAK 40W/03) lamps.[15,16] The American Academy of Pediatrics has recommended that the irradiance for intensive phototherapy be at least 30 μW·cm^{-2}·nm^{-1} over the waveband interval 460 to 490 nm.[1] Devices that emit lower irradiance may be supplemented with auxiliary devices. Much higher doses (>65 μW·cm^{-2}·nm^{-1}) might have (as-yet-unidentified) adverse effects. Currently, no single method is in general use for measuring phototherapy dosages. In addition, the calibration methods, wavelength responses, and geometries of instruments are not standardized. Consequently, different radiometers may show different values for the same light source.[2]

Clinical Context

For routine measurements, clinicians are limited by reliance on irradiance meters supplied or recommended by the manufacturer. Visual estimations of brightness and use of ordinary photometric or colorimetric light meters are inappropriate.[1,2] Maximal irradiance can be achieved by bringing the light source close to the infant[1]; however, this should not be done with halogen or tungsten lights, because the heat generated can cause a burn. Furthermore, with some fixtures, increasing the proximity may reduce the exposed body surface area. Irradiance distribution in the illuminated area

(footprint) is rarely uniform; measurements at the center of the footprint may greatly exceed those at the periphery and are variable among phototherapy devices.[1] Thus, irradiance should be measured at several sites on the infant's body surface. The ideal distance and orientation of the light source should be maintained according to the manufacturer's recommendations. The irradiance of all lamps decreases with use; manufacturers may provide useful-lifetime estimates, which should not be exceeded.

C. Optimal Body Surface Area

An infant's total body surface area[17] can be influenced by the disproportionate head size, especially in the more preterm infant. Complete (100%) exposure of the total body surface to light is impractical and limited by use of eye masks and diapers. Circumferential illumination (total body surface exposure from multiple directions) achieves exposure of approximately 80% of the total body surface. In clinical practice, exposure is usually planar: ventral with overhead light sources and dorsal with lighted mattresses. Approximately 35% of the total body surface (ventral or dorsal) is exposed with either method. Changing the infant's posture every 2 to 3 hours may maximize the area exposed to light. Exposed body surface area treated rather than the number of devices (double, triple, etc) used is clinically more important. Maximal skin surface illumination allows for a more intensive exposure and may require combined use of more than 1 phototherapy device.[1]

Clinical Context

Physical obstruction of light by equipment, such as radiant warmers, head covers, large diapers, eye masks that enclose large areas of the scalp, tape, electrode patches, and insulating plastic covers, decrease the exposed skin

surface area. Circumferential phototherapy maximizes the exposed area. Combining several devices, such as fluorescent tubes with fiber-optic pads or LED mattresses placed below the infant or bassinet, will increase the surface area exposed. If the infant is in an incubator, the light rays should be perpendicular to the surface of the incubator to minimize reflectance and loss of efficacy.[1,2]

D. Rate of Response Measured by Decrease in Serum Bilirubin Concentration

The clinical impact of phototherapy should be evident within 4 to 6 hours of initiation with an anticipated decrease of more than 2 mg/dL (34 μmol/L) in serum bilirubin concentration.[1] The clinical response depends on the rates of bilirubin production, enterohepatic circulation, and bilirubin elimination; the degree of tissue bilirubin deposition[15,16,18]; and the rates of the photochemical reactions of bilirubin. Aggressive implementation of phototherapy for excessive hyperbilirubinemia, sometimes referred to as the "crash-cart" approach,[19,20] has been reported to reduce the need for exchange transfusion and possibly reduce the severity of bilirubin neurotoxicity.

Clinical Context

Serial measurements of bilirubin concentration are used to monitor the effectiveness of phototherapy, but the value of these measurements can be confounded by changes in bilirubin production or elimination and by a sudden increase in bilirubin concentration (rebound) if phototherapy is stopped. Periodicity of serial measurements is based on clinical judgment.

III. EVIDENCE FOR EFFECTIVE PHOTOTHERAPY

Light-emission characteristics of phototherapy devices help in predicting

TABLE 3 Practice Considerations for Optimal Administration of Phototherapy

Checklist	Recommendation	Implementation
Light source (nm)	Wavelength spectrum in ~460- 490-nm blue-green light region	Know the spectral output of the light source
Light irradiance ($\mu W \cdot cm^{-2} \cdot nm^{-1}$)	Use optimal irradiance: >30 $\mu W \cdot cm^{-2} \cdot nm^{-1}$ within the 460- to 490-nm waveband	Ensure uniformity over the light footprint area
Body surface area (cm^2)	Expose maximal skin area	Reduce blocking of light
Timeliness of implementation	Urgent or "crash-cart" intervention for excessive hyperbilirubinemia	May conduct procedures while infant is on phototherapy
Continuity of therapy	Briefly interrupt for feeding, parental bonding, nursing care	After confirmation of adequate bilirubin concentration decrease
Efficacy of intervention	Periodically measure rate of response in bilirubin load reduction	Degree of total serum/plasma bilirubin concentration decrease
Duration of therapy	Discontinue at desired bilirubin threshold; be aware of possible rebound increase	Serial bilirubin measurements based on rate of decrease

their effectiveness (group B recommendation) (see Appendix). The clinical effectiveness of the device should be known before and monitored during clinical application (group B recommendation). Local guidelines (instructions) for routine clinical use should be available. Important factors that need to be considered are listed in Table 3. Obstructing the light source and reducing the exposed body surface area must be avoided (group B recommendation).

These recommendations are appropriate for clinical care in high-resource settings. In low-resource settings the use of improvised technologies and affordable phototherapy device choices need to meet minimum efficacy and safety standards.

IV. SAFETY AND PROTECTIVE MEASURES

A clinician skilled in newborn care should assess the neonate's clinical status during phototherapy to ensure adequate hydration, nutrition, and temperature control. Clinical improvement or progression of jaundice should also be assessed, including signs suggestive of early bilirubin encephalopathy such as changes in sleeping pattern, deteriorating feeding pattern, or inability to be consoled while crying.[1] Staff should be educated regarding the importance of safely minimizing the distance of the phototherapy device from the infant. They should be aware that the intensity of light decreases at the outer perimeter of the light footprint and recognize the effects of physical factors that could impede or obstruct light exposure. Staff should be aware that phototherapy does not use ultraviolet light and that exposure to the lights is mostly harmless. Four decades of neonatal phototherapy use has revealed no serious adverse clinical effects in newborn infants 35 or more weeks of gestation. For more preterm infants, who are usually treated with prophylactic rather than therapeutic phototherapy, this may not be true. Informed staff should educate parents regarding the care of their newborn infant undergoing phototherapy. Devices must comply with general safety standards listed by the International Electrotechnical Commission.[21] Other clinical considerations include:

a. Interruption of phototherapy: After a documented decrease in bilirubin concentration, continuous exposure to the light source may be interrupted and the eye mask removed to allow for feeding and maternal-infant bonding.[1]

b. Use of eye masks: Eye masks to prevent retinal damage are used routinely, although there is no evidence to support this recommendation. Retinal damage has been documented in the unpatched eyes of newborn monkeys exposed to phototherapy, but there are no similar data available from human newborns, because eye patches have always been used.[22–24] Purulent eye discharge and conjunctivitis in term infants have been reported with prolonged use of eye patches.[25,26]

c. Use of diapers: Concerns for the long-term effects of continuous phototherapy exposure of the reproductive system have been raised but not substantiated.[27–29] Diapers may be used for hygiene but are not essential.

d. Other protective considerations: Devices used in environments with high humidity and oxygen must meet electrical and fire hazard safety standards.[21] Phototherapy is contraindicated in infants with congenital porphyria or those treated with photosensitizing drugs.[1] Prolonged phototherapy has been associated with increased oxidant stress and lipid peroxidation[30] and riboflavin deficiency.[31] Recent clinical reports of other adverse outcomes (eg, malignant melanoma, DNA damage, and skin changes) have yet to be validated.[1,2,32,33] Phototherapy does not exacerbate hemolysis.[34]

V. RESEARCH NEEDS

Among the gaps in knowledge that remain regarding the use of phototherapy to prevent severe neonatal hyperbilirubinemia, the following are among the most important:

1. The ability to measure the actual wavelength and irradiance delivered by a phototherapy device is urgently needed to assess the efficiency of

phototherapy in reducing total serum bilirubin concentrations.

2. The safety and efficacy of home phototherapy remains a research priority.

3. Further delineation of the short- and long-term consequences of exposing infants with conjugated and unconjugated hyperbilirubinemia to phototherapy is needed.

4. Whether use of phototherapy reduces the risk of bilirubin neurotoxicity in a timely and effective manner needs further exploration.

SUMMARY

Clinicians and hospitals should ensure that the phototherapy devices they use fully illuminate the patient's body surface area, have an irradiance level of $\geq$30 μW·cm^{-2}·nm^{-1} (confirmed with accuracy with an appropriate spectral radiometer) over the waveband of approximately 460 to 490 nm, and are implemented in a timely manner. Standard procedures should be documented for their safe deployment.

LEAD AUTHOR

Vinod K. Bhutani, MD

COMMITTEE ON FETUS AND NEWBORN, 2010–2011

Lu-Ann Papile, MD, Chairperson
Jill E. Baley, MD
Vinod K. Bhutani, MD
Waldemar A. Carlo, MD
James J. Cummings, MD
Praveen Kumar, MD
Richard A. Polin, MD
Rosemarie C. Tan, MD, PhD
Kristi L. Watterberg, MD

FORMER COMMITTEE MEMBER

David H. Adamkin, MD

LIAISONS

CAPT Wanda Denise Barfield, MD, MPH – *Centers for Disease Control and Prevention*
William H. Barth Jr, MD – *American College of Obstetricians and Gynecologists*
Ann L. Jefferies, MD – *Canadian Paediatric Society*
Rosalie O. Mainous, PhD, RNC, NNP – *National Association of Neonatal Nurses*
Tonse N. K. Raju, MD, DCH – *National Institutes of Health*
Kasper S. Wang – *AAP Section on Surgery*

CONSULTANTS

M. Jeffrey Maisels, MBBCh, DSc
Antony F. McDonagh, PhD
David K. Stevenson, MD
Hendrik J. Vreman, PhD

STAFF

Jim Couto, MA

REFERENCES

1. American Academy of Pediatrics, Subcommittee on Hyperbilirubinemia. Management of hyperbilirubinemia in the newborn infant 35 or more weeks of gestation [published correction appears in *Pediatrics*. 2004; 114(4):1138]. *Pediatrics*. 2004;114(1): 297–316

2. McDonagh AF, Agati G, Fusi F, Pratesi R. Quantum yields for laser photocyclization of bilirubin in the presence of human serum albumin: dependence of quantum yield on excitation wavelength. *Photochem Photobiol*. 1989;50(3):305–319

3. Vreman HJ, Wong RJ, Murdock JR, Stevenson DK. Standardized bench method for evaluating the efficacy of phototherapy devices. *Acta Paediatr*. 2008;97(3):308–316

4. Maisels MJ, McDonagh AF. Phototherapy for neonatal jaundice. *N Engl J Med*. 2008; 358(9):920–928

5. McDonagh AF, Lightner DA. Phototherapy and the photobiology of bilirubin. *Semin Liver Dis*. 1988;8(3):272–283

6. Cremer RJ, Perryman PW, Richards DH. Influence of light on the hyperbilirubinaemia of infants. *Lancet*. 1958;1(7030):1094–1097

7. Ennever JF, McDonagh AF, Speck WT. Phototherapy for neonatal jaundice: optimal wavelengths of light. *J Pediatr*. 1983;103(2): 295–299

8. Ennever JF, Sobel M, McDonagh AF, Speck WT. Phototherapy for neonatal jaundice: in vitro comparison of light sources. *Pediatr Res*. 1984;18(7):667–670

9. Nakamura S, Fasol G. InGaN single-quantum-well LEDs. In: *The Blue Laser Diode*. Berlin, Germany: Springer-Verlag; 1997:201–221

10. Vreman HJ, Wong RJ, Stevenson DK, et al. Light-emitting diodes: a novel light source for phototherapy. *Pediatr Res*. 1998;44(5): 804–809

11. Maisels MJ, Kring EA, DeRidder J. Randomized controlled trial of light-emitting diode phototherapy. *J Perinatol*. 2007;27(9): 565–567

12. Seidman DS, Moise J, Ergaz Z, et al. A new blue light-emitting phototherapy device: a prospective randomized controlled study. *J Pediatr*. 2000;136(6):771–774

13. Martins BM, de Carvalho M, Moreira ME, Lopes JM. Efficacy of new microprocessed phototherapy system with five high intensity light emitting diodes (Super LED) [in Portuguese]. *J Pediatr (Rio J)*. 2007;83(3): 253–258

14. Kumar P, Murki S, Malik GK, et al. Light-emitting diodes versus compact fluorescent tubes for phototherapy in neonatal jaundice: a multi-center randomized controlled trial. *Indian Pediatr*. 2010;47(2): 131–137

15. Tan KL. The nature of the dose-response relationship of phototherapy for neonatal hyperbilirubinemia. *J Pediatr*. 1977;90(3): 448–452

16. Tan KL. The pattern of bilirubin response to phototherapy for neonatal hyperbilirubinaemia. *Pediatr Res*. 1982;16(8):670–674

17. Mosteller RD. Simplified calculation of body-surface area. *N Engl J Med*. 1987;317(17): 1098

18. Jährig K, Jährig D, Meisel P. Dependence of the efficiency of phototherapy on plasma bilirubin concentration. *Acta Paediatr Scand*. 1982;71(2):293–299

19. Johnson L, Bhutani VK, Karp K, Sivieri EM, Shapiro SM. Clinical report from the pilot USA Kernicterus Registry (1992 to 2004). *J Perinatol*. 2009;29(suppl 1):S25–S45

20. Hansen TW, Nietsch L, Norman E, et al. Reversibility of acute intermediate phase bilirubin encephalopathy. *Acta Paediatr*. 2009; 98(10):1689–1694

21. International Electrotechnical Commission. International standard: medical electrical equipment part 2-50—particular requirements for the safety of infant phototherapy equipment 60601-2-50, ed2.0. (2009-03-24). Available at: http://webstore.iec.ch/webstore/webstore.nsf/Artnum_PK/42737. Accessed December 21, 2010

22. Ente G, Klein SW. Hazards of phototherapy. *N Engl J Med*. 1970;283(10):544–545

23. Messner KH, Maisels MJ, Leure-DuPree AE. Phototoxicity to the newborn primate retina. *Invest Ophthalmol Vis Sci*. 1978;17(2): 178–182

24. Patz A, Souri EN. Phototherapy and other ocular risks to the newborn. *Sight Sav Rev*. 1972;42(1):29–33

25. Paludetto R, Mansi G, Rinaldi P, Saporito M, De Curtis M, Ciccimarra F. Effects of

different ways of covering the eyes on behavior of jaundiced infants treated with phototherapy. *Biol Neonate*. 1985;47(1): 1–8

26. Fok TF, Wong W, Cheung KL. Eye protection for newborns under phototherapy: comparison between a modified headbox and the conventional eyepatches. *Ann Trop Paediatr*. 1997;17(4):349–354

27. Koç H, Altunhan H, Dilsiz A, et al. Testicular changes in newborn rats exposed to phototherapy. *Pediatr Dev Pathol*. 1999;2(4): 333–336

28. Wurtman RJ. The effects of light on the human body. *Sci Am*. 1975;233(1):69–77

29. Cetinkursun S, Demirbag S, Cincik M, Baykal B, Gunal A. Effects of phototherapy on newborn rat testicles. *Arch Androl*. 2006;52(1): 61–70

30. Lightner DA, Linnane WP, Ahlfors CE. Bilirubin photooxidation products in the urine of jaundiced neonates receiving phototherapy. *Pediatr Res*. 1984;18(8):696–700

31. Sisson TR. Photodegradation of riboflavin in neonates. *Fed Proc*. 1987;46(5): 1883–1885

32. Bauer J, Büttner P, Luther H, Wiecker TS, Möhrle M, Garbe C. Blue light phototherapy of neonatal jaundice does not increase the risk for melanocytic nevus development. *Arch Dermatol*. 2004;140(4):493–494

33. Tatli MM, Minnet C, Kocyigit A, Karadag A. Phototherapy increases DNA damage in lymphocytes of hyperbilirubinemic neonates. *Mutat Res*. 2008;654(1):93–95

34. Maisels MJ, Kring EA. Does intensive phototherapy produce hemolysis in newborns of 35 or more weeks gestation? *J Perinatol*. 2006;26(8):498–500

APPENDIX Definition of Grades for Recommendation and Suggestion for Practice

Grade	Definition	Suggestion for Practice
A	This intervention is recommended. There is a high certainty that the net benefit is substantial	Offer and administer this intervention
B	This intervention is recommended. There is a moderate certainty that the net benefit is moderate to substantial	Offer and administer this intervention
C	This intervention is recommended. There may be considerations that support the use of this intervention in an individual patient. There is a moderate to high certainty that the net benefit is small	Offer and administer this intervention only if other considerations support this intervention in an individual patient
D	This intervention is not recommended. There is a moderate to high certainty that the intervention has no net benefit and that the harms outweigh the benefits	Discourage use of this intervention
I	The current evidence is insufficient to assess the balance of benefits against and harms of this intervention. There is a moderate to high certainty that the intervention has no net benefit and that the harms outweigh the benefits. Evidence is lacking, of poor quality, or conflicting, and the balance of benefits and harms cannot be determined	If this intervention is conducted, the patient should understand the uncertainty about the balance of benefits and harms

US Preventive Services Task Force Grade definitions, May, 2008 (available at www.uspreventiveservicestaskforce.org/3rduspstf/ratings.htm).

American Academy
of Pediatrics

DEDICATED TO THE HEALTH OF ALL CHILDREN®

CLINICAL REPORT

Postdischarge Follow-up of Infants With Congenital Diaphragmatic Hernia

Organizational Principles to Guide and
Define the Child Health Care System and/or
Improve the Health of All Children

Section on Surgery and the Committee on Fetus and Newborn

ABSTRACT

Infants with congenital diaphragmatic hernia often require intensive treatment after birth, have prolonged hospitalizations, and have other congenital anomalies. After discharge from the hospital, they may have long-term sequelae such as respiratory insufficiency, gastroesophageal reflux, poor growth, neurodevelopmental delay, behavior problems, hearing loss, hernia recurrence, and orthopedic deformities. Structured follow-up for these patients facilitates early recognition and treatment of these complications. In this report, follow-up of infants with congenital diaphragmatic hernia is outlined.

www.pediatrics.org/cgi/doi/10.1542/
peds.2007-3282

doi:10.1542/peds.2007-3282

All clinical reports from the American Academy of Pediatrics automatically expire 5 years after publication unless reaffirmed, revised, or retired at or before that time.

The guidance in this report does not indicate an exclusive course of treatment or serve as a standard of medical care. Variations, taking into account individual circumstances, may be appropriate.

Key Words
congenital diaphragmatic hernia, gastroesophageal reflux, pulmonary hypoplasia, follow-up

Abbreviations
CDH—congenital diaphragmatic hernia
ECMO—extracorporeal membrane oxygenation

PEDIATRICS (ISSN Numbers: Print, 0031-4005; Online, 1098-4275). Copyright © 2008 by the American Academy of Pediatrics

INTRODUCTION

Survival rates for patients with congenital diaphragmatic hernia (CDH) have increased during the past decade with the implementation of more "gentle" ventilation and physiology-specific strategies, high-frequency ventilation, extracorporeal membrane oxygenation (ECMO), and improved supportive care.[1–3] Improvement in survival rates has occurred for infants with CDH complicated by severe pulmonary hypoplasia, pulmonary hypertension, and chronic lung disease.[4] However, other significant morbidities, such as neurocognitive delay, gastroesophageal reflux, hearing loss, chest wall deformity, poor growth, hernia recurrence, and complications attributable to associated congenital anomalies, continue to affect the lives of many infants with CDH beyond the neonatal period.[1,5,6]

Coordination of the complex medical and surgical needs of these infants is challenging. Comprehensive multispecialty clinics that aggregate specialty physicians and services are family-friendly and provide for collaborative evaluation and management planning. Same-site multidisciplinary service teams also improve coordination, communication, and support for the medical home pediatrician who is responsible for managing the general health care needs of the infant. Unfortunately, such multispecialty clinics are not available to all infants with CDH. The following information is intended to provide clinicians who care for infants with CDH with a template to organize a comprehensive plan for detection and management of associated morbidities.

PULMONARY MORBIDITY

Survivors with CDH may require treatment beyond the initial hospitalization for chronic lung disease, bronchospasm, pulmonary hypertension, aspiration, pneumonia, and pulmonary hypoplasia. Oxygen treatment beyond the initial hospitalization may be needed for many of these infants, especially those who are treated with ECMO and a prosthetic patch.[7–9] Many survivors not treated with ECMO also receive bronchodilators and inhaled steroids.[8] At least 4% of survivors require a long-term tracheostomy.[9,10] Nearly one fourth of infants with CDH who survive have obstructive airway disease at 5 years of age,[10,11] and some have pulmonary hypertension that persists for months or years. Pulmonary hypertension that persists for more than the first few weeks after birth is a risk factor for early death.[12] Persistent abnormalities in lung function also have been demonstrated on ventilation/perfusion scans.[8,12–15]

Pneumonia occurs in approximately 7% of infants with CDH during the first year after birth.[5,16,17] Aspiration-associated pneumonia and bronchospasm may be reduced in frequency by avoiding oral feeding if oromotor incoordination is significant and by early detection and treatment of gastroesophageal reflux. Pneumonia may be prevented in part by treatment for chronic lung disease, effective management of pulmonary secretions, and immunization with recommended childhood vaccines (such as pneumococcal, influenza, and other recommended vaccines). Palivizumab (respiratory syncytial virus monoclonal antibody; Synagis [MedImmune, Inc, Gaithersburg,

MD]) also is suggested for infants with CDH who have chronic lung disease, as described in the "Revised Indications for the Use of Palivizumab and Respiratory Syncytial Virus Immune Globulin Intravenous for the Prevention of Respiratory Syncytial Virus Infections" technical report and policy statement by the American Academy of Pediatrics.[18,19]

Although the incidence of chronic lung disease is 33% to 52% at discharge, most infants who survive CDH have clinical improvement over time.[6,16,17] Nevertheless, nearly 50% of adult survivors have impairment on pulmonary function testing.[16]

GASTROESOPHAGEAL REFLUX/FOREGUT DYSMOTILITY

Gastroesophageal reflux or some form of foregut dysmotility occurs in 45% to 90% of infants with CDH.[20-24] Abnormal hiatal anatomy at the gastroesophageal junction, lack of an angle of His in some patients, and herniation of the stomach into the chest with distortion are possible mechanisms to explain this high incidence of gastroesophageal reflux. Esophageal dilation or ectasia also has been described in some infants with CDH, and as many as 70% of such infants have severe gastroesophageal reflux.[21] The incidence of gastroesophageal reflux also correlates with defect size and need for patch repair.[20,25] Pulmonary morbidity may be worsened by aspiration associated with gastroesophageal reflux. Importantly, a high incidence of esophagitis in adult survivors with CDH suggests that long-term surveillance is needed.[26] For all patients with CDH, it is important to have a high index of suspicion for gastroesophageal reflux. Antireflux surgery may be an option for patients with failed medical therapy, although the long-term success rate of this procedure has yet to be proven.

GROWTH FAILURE

Many survivors with CDH fail to grow as well as healthy term infants do and require close nutritional surveillance and intervention.[6,9,20] Infants with CDH and chronic lung disease often have poor oral feeding skills. Gastroesophageal reflux is common, and oral aversion is frequent; both contribute to growth deficiency. In 1 clinical series, more than 50% of infants with CDH had weight below the 25th percentile.[20] Gastrostomy tube placement was performed in 33% of infants in this series. Van Meurs et al[6] showed that more than 40% of CDH survivors had weight below the 5th percentile at 2 years of age. Gastrostomy tube feeding is suggested by some experts who hypothesize that nasogastric or orogastric tube feeding impairs oral feeding. Others suggest use of nasogastric or orogastric tube feeding for a period of time, especially when success with oral feeding is anticipated within several months. Despite controversy about the most appropriate mode of feeding the infant with CDH at discharge, almost 33% do not orally feed enough fluid volume to support growth and receive feedings through nasogastric or gastrostomy tubes.[6,20] Early recognition and intervention is essential for optimizing both somatic and alveolar growth and long-term outcomes for infants with CDH.

NEUROCOGNITIVE DELAY AND BEHAVIORAL DISORDERS

Significant developmental delay and behavioral disorders have been reported for a large number of infants with CDH. The infant with a large diaphragmatic defect or need for ECMO is at greatest risk.[27-36] Nobuhara et al[27] reported developmental delay in more than 33% of their CDH survivors. McGahren et al[30] described neurologic abnormalities in 67% of infants with CDH who were treated with ECMO compared with 24% of infants with CDH who were not as ill and did not receive ECMO.

The critical illness and physiologic disruption of high-risk infants with CDH places them at risk of neurologic and developmental disabilities. Many infants who present with symptoms of CDH soon after birth are clinically unstable and hypoxemic and require high levels of extraordinary life support such as ECMO and other invasive therapies. Although severity of illness is most predictive of long-term outcome, complications associated with invasive therapies may contribute to morbidity in CDH survivors. In a study by Bernbaum et al[37] of survivors receiving ECMO, infants with CDH treated with ECMO had a higher risk of significant neurodevelopmental delays than did infants without CDH. The higher risk of disability in ECMO-treated survivors with CDH compared with ECMO-treated survivors without CDH suggests that at least 3 potential factors may contribute to neurodevelopmental disability in infants with CDH: (1) an intrinsic neurologic abnormality, (2) greater number and severity of morbidities that impair development in infants who require ECMO, (3) and a greater number of ECMO-associated complications.

HEARING LOSS

Sensorineural hearing loss has been described in a number of case series of CDH survivors[27,28,33,35] and seems to occur in infants regardless of whether they were treated with ECMO. The cause remains unknown, but it is speculated to be related to treatments for respiratory failure (such as hyperventilation, ototoxic medications, or neuromuscular blockade).[38] Severe hypoxemia, prolonged ventilation, and ECMO also are risk factors. Approximately half of infants with initially normal hearing assessments develop hearing loss later in infancy.[39-41]

HERNIA RECURRENCE

Recurrent diaphragmatic hernias have been reported in 8% to 50% of patients with CDH. The single-most important predictor of hernia recurrence is the presence of a large defect that requires a patch to repair.[2,6,42,43] Recurrences can present from months to years after the initial hospitalization, or the patient can remain asymptomatic. Detection of recurrences may be discovered incidentally on chest radiographs performed for surveillance or other reasons.[6,43] The lifetime risk of recurrence for a patient with a patch repair is unknown.

ORTHOPEDIC DEFORMITIES

Pectus deformities and progressive asymmetry of the chest wall have been described in CDH survivors.[27,28,44] The incidence of these orthopedic disorders ranges from

TABLE 1 Recommended Schedule of Follow-up for Infants With CDH

	Before Discharge	1–3 mo After Birth	4–6 mo After Birth	9–12 mo After Birth	15–18 mo After Birth	Annual Through 16 y
Weight, length, occipital-frontal circumference	X	X	X	X	X	X
Chest radiograph	X	If patched	If patched	If patched	If patched	If patched
Pulmonary function testing			If indicated		If indicated	If indicated
Childhood immunizations	As indicated throughout childhood	X	X	X	X	X
RSV prophylaxis	RSV season during first 2 years after birth (if evidence of chronic lung disease)	X	X	X	X	X
Echocardiogram and cardiology follow-up	X	If previously abnormal or if on supplemental oxygen	If previously abnormal or if on supplemental oxygen	If previously abnormal or if on supplemental oxygen	If previously abnormal or if on supplemental oxygen	If previously abnormal or if on supplemental oxygen
Head computed tomography or MRI	If (1) abnormal finding on head ultrasound; (2) seizures/abnormal neurologic findings[a]; or (3) ECMO or patch repair	As indicated	As indicated	As indicated	As indicated	As indicated
Hearing evaluation[44]	Auditory brainstem evoked response or otoacoustic emissions screen	X	X	X	X	Every 6 mo to age 3 y, then annually to age 5 y
Developmental screening evaluation	X	X	X	X		Annually to age 5 y
Neurodevelopmental evaluation	X			X		Annually to age 5 y
Assessment for oral feeding problems	X	X	If oral feeding problems	If oral feeding problems	If oral feeding problems	If oral feeding problems
Upper gastrointestinal study, pH probe, and/or gastric scintiscan	Consider for all patients	If symptoms	If symptoms	Consider for all patients	If symptoms	If symptoms
Esophagoscopy		If symptoms	If symptoms	If symptoms or if abnormal gastrointestinal evaluations	If symptoms	If symptoms
Scoliosis and chest wall deformity screening (physical examination, chest radiograph, and/or computed tomography of the chest)				X		X

The neurosensory tests performed and frequency of surveillance may differ among infants with CDH because of variability in neurologic, developmental, and physiologic impairments. Follow-up should be tailored to each infant. RSV indicates respiratory syncytial virus.

[a] Muscle weakness, hypotonia, hypertonia, or other abnormal neurologic sign or symptom.

21% to 48%. Many of them are mild and do not require surgical intervention. Scoliosis also has been found in these patients, with an incidence of 10% to 27%.[27,44] The incidence of both of these morbidities is higher in patients who have large defects and a patch repair. Periodic and regular follow-up is suggested to detect and prevent development of functionally significant deformities from developing.

OTHER CONGENITAL ABNORMALITIES

Additional congenital anomalies are present in approximately 40% of infants with CDH.[45–48] Congenital heart lesions account for nearly two thirds of these anomalies and have a major effect on risk of mortality.[45,48] Anomalies of the central nervous system, esophageal atresia, and omphalocele also are relatively prevalent compared with other organ systems. A number of syndromes and chromosomal anomalies (such as trisomies 21, 13, and 18; Fryns syndrome; Brachmann-de Lange syndrome; and Pallister-Killian syndrome) include CDH as one of the associated anomalies. Each of these anomalies and syndromes adds to the complexity and specialty care needs for affected infants. The care requirements for such infants necessitate individualized, multidisciplinary care plans.

SUMMARY

Survivors with CDH are at risk of a number of morbidities that may affect development and function. Infants with large defects, those who have received ECMO, or those with a patch repair are at highest risk. These unique patients, especially those at highest risk, require long-term periodic follow-up by a multidisciplinary team of medical, surgical, and developmental specialists to identify and treat morbidities before additional disability results. Preventive pediatric health care according to guidelines developed by the American Academy of Pediatrics is recommended for all children, including those with CDH.[49–52] To emphasize the importance of follow-up for specific morbidities associated with CDH, additional suggestions are provided (Table 1). These are most applicable to children with extraordinary medical and surgical complications associated with CDH and should be individualized depending on the specific needs of each infant.

SECTION ON SURGERY, 2006–2007

Kurt D. Newman, MD, Chairperson
Mary Lynn Brandt, MD
Richard R. Ricketts, MD
Robert C. Schamberger, MD
Brad W. Warner, MD
*Kevin P. Lally, MD

STAFF

Aleksandra Stolic, MPH

COMMITTEE ON FETUS AND NEWBORN, 2006–2007

Ann R. Stark, MD, Chairperson
David H. Adamkin, MD
Daniel G. Batton, MD

Edward F. Bell, MD
Vinod K. Bhutani, MD
Susan E. Denson, MD
Gilbert I. Martin, MD
Kristi L. Watterberg, MD
*William Engle, MD

LIAISONS

Keith J. Barrington, MD
    Canadian Paediatric Society
Gary D. V. Hankins, MD
    American College of Obstetrics and Gynecology
Tonse N. K. Raju, MD
    National Institutes of Health
Kay M. Tomashek, MD
    Centers for Disease Control and Prevention
Carol Wallman, MSN
    National Association of Neonatal Nurses and
    Association of Women's Health, Obstetric and
    Neonatal Nurses

STAFF

Jim Couto, MA

*Lead authors

REFERENCES

1. Muratore CS, Wilson JM. Congenital diaphragmatic hernia: where are we and where do we go from here? *Semin Perinatol.* 2000;24(6):418–428
2. Ssemakula N, Stewart DL, Goldsmith LJ, Cook LN, Bond SJ. Survival of patients with congenital diaphragmatic hernia during the ECMO era: an 11-year experience. *J Pediatr Surg.* 1997;32(12):1683–1689
3. Wilson JM, Lund DP, Lillehei CW, Vacanti JP. Congenital diaphragmatic hernia: a tale of two cities—the Boston experience. *J Pediatr Surg.* 1997;32(3):401–405
4. Lally KP, Lally PA, Van Meurs KP, et al. Treatment evolution in high-risk congenital diaphragmatic hernia: ten years' experience with diaphragmatic agenesis. *Ann Surg.* 2006;244(4): 505–513
5. Davis PJ, Firmin RK, Manktelow B, et al. Long-term outcome following extracorporeal membrane oxygenation for congenital diaphragmatic hernia: the UK experience. *J Pediatr.* 2004; 144(3):309–315
6. Van Meurs KP, Robbins ST, Reed VL, et al. Congenital diaphragmatic hernia: long-term outcome in neonates treated with extracorporeal membrane oxygenation. *J Pediatr.* 1993; 122(6):893–899
7. Ijsselstijn H, Tibboel D, Hop WJ, Molenaar JC, de Jongste JC. Long-term pulmonary sequelae in children with congenital diaphragmatic hernia. *Am J Respir Crit Care Med.* 1997;155(1): 174–180
8. Muratore CS, Kharasch V, Lund DP, et al. Pulmonary morbidity in 100 survivors of congenital diaphragmatic hernia monitored in a multidisciplinary clinic. *J Pediatr Surg.* 2001;36(1): 133–140
9. Jaillard SM, Pierrat V, Dubois A, et al. Outcome at 2 years of infants with congenital diaphragmatic hernia: a population-based study. *Ann Thorac Surg.* 2003;75(1):250–256
10. Bagolan P, Casaccia G, Crescenzi F, Nahom A, Trucchi A, Giorlandino C. Impact of a current treatment protocol on outcome of high-risk congenital diaphragmatic hernia. *J Pediatr Surg.* 2004;39(3):313–318

11. Wischermann A, Holschneider AM, Hubner U. Long-term follow-up of children with diaphragmatic hernia. *Eur J Pediatr Surg.* 1995;5(1):13–18

12. Dillon PW, Cilley R, Mauger D, Zachary C, Meier A. The relationship between pulmonary artery pressures and survival in congenital diaphragmatic hernia. *J Pediatr Surg.* 2004;39(3): 307–312

13. Okuyama H, Kubota A, Kawahara H, Oue T, Kitayama Y, Yagi M. Correlation between lung scintigraphy and long-term outcome in survivors of congenital diaphragmatic hernia. *Pediatr Pulmonol.* 2006;41(9):882–886

14. Arena F, Baldari S, Centorrino A, et al. Mid- and long-term effects on pulmonary perfusion, anatomy and diaphragmatic motility in survivors of congenital diaphragmatic hernia [published correction appears in *Pediatr Surg Int.* 2006;22(3):304]. *Pediatr Surg Int.* 2005;21(12):954–959

15. Falconer AR, Brown RA, Helms P, Gordon I, Baron JA. Pulmonary sequelae in survivors of congenital diaphragmatic hernia. *Thorax.* 1990;45(2):126–119

16. Vanamo K, Rintala R, Sovijärvi A, et al. Long-term pulmonary sequelae in survivors of congenital diaphragmatic defects. *J Pediatr Surg.* 1996;31(8):1096–1100

17. Bos AP, Hussain SM, Hazebroek FW, Tibboel D, Meradji M, Molenaar JC. Radiographic evidence of bronchopulmonary dysplasia in chronic lung disease survivors. *Pediatr Pulmonol.* 1993;15(4):231–234

18. Meissner HC, Long SS; American Academy of Pediatrics Committee on Infectious Diseases and Committee on Fetus and Newborn. Revised indications for the use of palivizumab and respiratory syncytial virus immune globulin intravenous for the prevention of respiratory syncytial virus infections [technical report]. *Pediatrics.* 2003;112(6 pt 1):1447–1452

19. American Academy of Pediatrics Committee on Infectious Diseases and Committee on Fetus and Newborn. Revised indications for the use of palivizumab and respiratory syncytial virus immune globulin intravenous for the prevention of respiratory syncytial virus infections [policy statement]. *Pediatrics.* 2003; 112(6 pt 1):1442–1446

20. Muratore CS, Utter S, Jaksic T, Lund DP, Wilson JM. Nutritional morbidity in survivors of congenital diaphragmatic hernia. *J Pediatr Surg.* 2001;36(8):1171–1176

21. Stolar CJ, Levy JP, Dillon PW, Reyes C, Belamarich P, Berdon WE. Anatomic and functional abnormalities of the esophagus in infants surviving congenital diaphragmatic hernia. *Am J Surg.* 1990;159(2):204–207

22. Fasching G, Huber A, Uray E, Sorantin E, Lindbichler F, Mayr J. Gastroesophageal reflux and diaphragmatic motility after repair of congenital diaphragmatic hernia. *Eur J Pediatr Surg.* 2000;10(6):360–364

23. Koot VCM, Bergmeijer JH, Bos AP, Molenaar JC. Incidence and management of gastroesophageal reflux after repair of congenital diaphragmatic hernia. *J Pediatr Surg.* 1993;28(1): 48–52

24. Kieffer J, Sapin E, Berg A, Beaudoin S, Bargy F, Helardot PG. Gastroesophageal reflux after repair of congenital diaphragmatic hernia. *J Pediatr Surg.* 1995;30(9):1330–1333

25. Sigalet DL, Nguyen LT, Aldolph V, Laberge JM, Hong AR, Guttman FM. Gastroesophageal reflux associated with large diaphragmatic hernias. *J Pediatr Surg.* 1994;29(9):1262–1265

26. Vanamo K, Rintala RJ, Lindahl H, Louhimo I. Long-term gastrointestinal morbidity in patients with congenital diaphragmatic defects. *J Pediatr Surg.* 1996;31(4):551–554

27. Nobuhara KK, Lund DP, Mitchell J, Karasch V, Wilson JM. Long-term outlook for survivors of congenital diaphragmatic hernia. *Clin Perinatol.* 1996;23(4):873–887

28. Lund DP, Mitchell J, Kharasch V, Quigley S, Kuehn M, Wilson JM. Congenital diaphragmatic hernia: the hidden morbidity. *J Pediatr Surg.* 1994;29(2):258–264

29. Bouman NH, Koot HM, Tibboel D, Hazebroek FW. Children with congenital diaphragmatic hernia are at risk for lower levels of cognitive functioning and increased emotional and behavioral problems. *Eur J Pediatr Surg.* 2000;10(1):3–7

30. McGahren ED, Mallik K, Rodgers BM. Neurological outcome is diminished in survivors of congenital diaphragmatic hernia requiring extracorporeal membrane oxygenation. *J Pediatr Surg.* 1997;32(8):1216–1220

31. Hunt RW, Kean MJ, Stewart MJ, Inder TE. Patterns of cerebral injury in a series of infants with congenital diaphragmatic hernia utilizing magnetic resonance imaging. *J Pediatr Surg.* 2004;39(1):31–36

32. Davenport M, Rivlin E, D'Souza SW, Bianchi A. Delayed surgery for congenital diaphragmatic hernia: neurodevelopmental outcome in late childhood. *Arch Dis Child.* 1992;67(11): 1353–1356

33. Rasheed A, Tindall S, Cueny DL, Klein MD, Delaney-Black V. Neurodevelopmental outcome after congenital diaphragmatic hernia: extracorporeal membrane oxygenation before and after surgery. *J Pediatr Surg.* 2001;36(4):539–544

34. Stolar CJ, Crisafi MA, Driscoll YT. Neurocognitive outcome for neonates treated with extracorporeal membrane oxygenation: are infants with congenital diaphragmatic hernia different? *J Pediatr Surg.* 1995;30(2):366–371; discussion 371–372

35. Cortes RA, Keller RL, Townsend T, et al. Survival of severe congenital diaphragmatic hernia has morbid consequences. *J Pediatr Surg.* 2005;40(1):36–45; discussion 45–46

36. Crankson SJ, Al Jadaan SA, Namshan MA, Al-Rabeeah AA, Oda O. The immediate and long-term outcomes of newborns with congenital diaphragmatic hernia. *Pediatr Surg Int.* 2006; 22(4):335–340

37. Bernbaum J, Schwartz IP, Gerdes M, D'Agostino JA, Coburn CE, Polin RA. Survivors of extracorporeal membrane oxygenation at 1 year of age: the relationship of primary diagnosis with health and neurodevelopmental sequelae. *Pediatrics.* 1995;96(5 pt 1):907–913

38. Cheung PY, Tyebkhan JM, Peliowski A, Ainsworth W, Robertson CM. Prolonged use of pancuronium bromide and sensorineural hearing loss in childhood survivors of congenital diaphragmatic hernia. *J Pediatr.* 1999;135(2 pt 1):233–239

39. Robertson CM, Tyebkhan JM, Hagler ME, Cheung PY, Peliowski A, Etches PC. Late-onset, progressive sensorineural hearing loss after severe neonatal respiratory failure. *Otol Neurotol.* 2002;23(3):353–356

40. Masi R, Capolupo I, Casaccia G, et al. Sensorineural hearing loss is frequent and progressive in infants with high risk congenital diaphragmatic hernia not treated with extracorporeal membrane oxygenation [abstr]. Presented at the 53rd annual congress of the British Association of Paediatric Surgeons; July 18–21, 2006; Stockholm, Sweden. Abstract 072

41. Fligor BJ, Neault MW, Mullen CH, Feldman HA, Jones DT. Factors associated with sensorineural hearing loss among survivors of extracorporeal membrane oxygenation therapy. *Pediatrics.* 2005;115(6):1519–1528

42. Lally KP, Paranka MS, Roden J, et al. Congenital diaphragmatic hernia: stabilization and repair on ECMO. *Ann Surg.* 1992; 216(5):569–573

43. Moss RL, Chen CM, Harrison MR. Prosthetic patch durability in congenital diaphragmatic hernia: a long-term follow-up study. *J Pediatr Surg.* 2001;36(1):152–154

44. Vanamo K, Peltonen J, Rintala R, Lindahl H, Jaaskelainen J, Louhimo I. Chest wall and spinal deformities in adults with congenital diaphragmatic defects. *J Pediatr Surg.* 1996;31(6): 851–854

45. Cohen MS, Rychik J, Bush DM, et al. Influence of congenital

heart disease on survival in children with congenital diaphragmatic hernia. *J Pediatr.* 2002;141(1):25–30

46. Fauza DO, Wilson JM. Congenital diaphragmatic hernia and associated anomalies: their incidence, identification, and impact on prognosis. *J Pediatr Surg.* 1994;29(8):1113–1117

47. Hartman GE. Diaphragmatic hernia. In: Behrman RE, Kliegman RM, Jenson HB, eds. *Nelson Textbook of Pediatrics.* 17th ed. Philadelphia, PA: WB Saunders; 2004:1353–1355

48. Graziano JN; Congenital Diaphragmatic Hernia Study Group. Cardiac anomalies in patients with congenital diaphragmatic hernia and their prognosis: a report from the Congenital Diaphragmatic Hernia Study Group. *J Pediatr Surg.* 2005;40(6): 1045–1049

49. American Academy of Pediatrics. *Bright Futures: Guidelines for Health Supervision of Infants, Children, and Adolescents.* 3rd ed. Elk Grove Village, IL: American Academy of Pediatrics; 2007

50. American Academy of Pediatrics, Committee on Practice and Ambulatory Medicine. Recommendations for preventive pediatric health care. *Pediatrics.* 2000;105(3):645–646

51. Follow-up care of high-risk infants. *Pediatrics.* 2004;114(5 suppl): 1377–1397

52. Joint Committee on Infant Hearing. Year 2000 position statement: principles and guidelines for early hearing detection and intervention programs. *Pediatrics.* 2000;106(4): 798–817

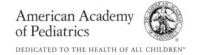

American Academy of Pediatrics
DEDICATED TO THE HEALTH OF ALL CHILDREN™

Guidance for the Clinician in
Rendering Pediatric Care

Clinical Report—Postnatal Glucose Homeostasis in Late-Preterm and Term Infants

David H. Adamkin, MD and COMMITTEE ON FETUS AND NEWBORN

KEY WORDS
newborn, glucose, neonatal hypoglycemia, late-preterm infant

ABBREVIATIONS
NH—neonatal hypoglycemia
$D_{10}W$—dextrose 10% in water

www.pediatrics.org/cgi/doi/10.1542/peds.2010-3851

doi:10.1542/peds.2010-3851

All clinical reports from the American Academy of Pediatrics automatically expire 5 years after publication unless reaffirmed, revised, or retired at or before that time.

PEDIATRICS (ISSN Numbers: Print, 0031-4005; Online, 1098-4275).

abstract

This report provides a practical guide and algorithm for the screening and subsequent management of neonatal hypoglycemia. Current evidence does not support a specific concentration of glucose that can discriminate normal from abnormal or can potentially result in acute or chronic irreversible neurologic damage. Early identification of the at-risk infant and institution of prophylactic measures to prevent neonatal hypoglycemia are recommended as a pragmatic approach despite the absence of a consistent definition of hypoglycemia in the literature. *Pediatrics* 2011;127:575–579

INTRODUCTION

This clinical report provides a practical guide for the screening and subsequent management of neonatal hypoglycemia (NH) in at-risk late-preterm (34–36⁶⁄₇ weeks' gestational age) and term infants. An expert panel convened by the National Institutes of Health in 2008 concluded that there has been no substantial evidence-based progress in defining what constitutes clinically important NH, particularly regarding how it relates to brain injury, and that monitoring for, preventing, and treating NH remain largely empirical.[1] In addition, the simultaneous occurrence of other medical conditions that are associated with brain injury, such as hypoxia-ischemia or infection, could alone, or in concert with NH, adversely affect the brain.[2–5] For these reasons, this report does not identify any specific value or range of plasma glucose concentrations that potentially could result in brain injury. Instead, it is a pragmatic approach to a controversial issue for which evidence is lacking but guidance is needed.

BACKGROUND

Blood glucose concentrations as low as 30 mg/dL are common in healthy neonates by 1 to 2 hours after birth; these low concentrations, seen in all mammalian newborns, usually are transient, asymptomatic, and considered to be part of normal adaptation to postnatal life.[6–8] Most neonates compensate for "physiologic" hypoglycemia by producing alternative fuels including ketone bodies, which are released from fat.

Clinically significant NH reflects an imbalance between supply and use of glucose and alternative fuels and may result from a multitude of disturbed regulatory mechanisms. A rational definition of NH must account for the fact that acute symptoms and long-term neurologic sequelae occur within a continuum of low plasma glucose values of varied duration and severity.

The authors of several literature reviews have concluded that there is not a specific plasma glucose concentration or duration of hypoglycemia that can predict permanent neurologic injury in high-risk infants.[3,9,10] Data that have linked plasma glucose concentration with adverse long-term neurologic outcomes are confounded by variable definitions of hypoglycemia and its duration (seldom reported), the omission of control groups, the possible inclusion of infants with confounding conditions, and the small number of asymptomatic infants who were followed.[3,11,12] In addition, there is no single concentration or range of plasma glucose concentrations that is associated with clinical signs. Therefore, there is no consensus regarding when screening should be performed and which concentration of glucose requires therapeutic intervention in the asymptomatic infant. The generally adopted plasma glucose concentration that defines NH for all infants (<47 mg/dL) is without rigorous scientific justification.[1,3,4,9,12]

WHICH INFANTS TO SCREEN

Because plasma glucose homeostasis requires glucogenesis and ketogenesis to maintain normal rates of fuel use,[13] NH most commonly occurs in infants with impaired glucogenesis and/or ketogenesis,[14,15] which may occur with excessive insulin production, altered counterregulatory hormone production, an inadequate substrate supply,[14–16] or a disorder of fatty acid oxidation.[15] NH occurs most commonly in infants who are small for gestational age, infants born to mothers who have diabetes, and late-preterm infants. It remains controversial whether otherwise normal infants who are large for gestational age are at risk of NH, largely because it is difficult to exclude maternal diabetes or maternal hyperglycemia (prediabe-

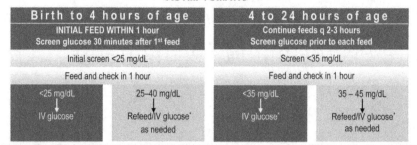

Screening and Management of Postnatal Glucose Homeostasis in Late Preterm and Term SGA, IDM/LGA Infants
[(LPT) Infants 34 – 36⁶ᐟ⁷ weeks and SGA (screen 0-24 hrs); IDM and LGA ≥34 weeks (screen 0-12 hrs)]

Symptomatic and <40 mg/dL ⟶ IV glucose

ASYMPTOMATIC

Birth to 4 hours of age	4 to 24 hours of age
INITIAL FEED WITHIN 1 hour Screen glucose 30 minutes after 1st feed	Continue feeds q 2-3 hours Screen glucose prior to each feed
Initial screen <25 mg/dL	Screen <35 mg/dL
Feed and check in 1 hour	Feed and check in 1 hour

| <25 mg/dL → IV glucose* | 25–40 mg/dL → Refeed/IV glucose* as needed | <35 mg/dL → IV glucose* | 35–45 mg/dL → Refeed/IV glucose* as needed |

Target glucose screen ≥45 mg/dL prior to routine feeds
* Glucose dose = 200 mg/kg (dextrose 10% at 2 mL/kg) and/or IV infusion at 5–8 mg/kg per min (80–100 mL/kg per d). Achieve plasma glucose level of 40-50 mg/dL.

Symptoms of hypoglycemia include: Irritability, tremors, jitteriness, exaggerated Moro reflex, high-pitched cry, seizures, lethargy, floppiness, cyanosis, apnea, poor feeding.

FIGURE 1

Screening for and management of postnatal glucose homeostasis in late-preterm (LPT 34–36⁶ᐟ⁷ weeks) and term small-for-gestational age (SGA) infants and infants who were born to mothers with diabetes (IDM)/large-for-gestational age (LGA) infants. LPT and SGA (screen 0–24 hours), IDM and LGA ≥34 weeks (screen 0–12 hours). IV indicates intravenous.

tes) with standard glucose-tolerance tests.

A large number of additional maternal and fetal conditions may also place infants at risk of NH. Clinical signs are common with these conditions, and it is likely that patients with such a condition are already being monitored and that plasma glucose analyses are being performed.[13,17] Therefore, for practicality, "at risk" in the management approach outlined in Fig 1 includes only infants who are small for gestational age, infants who are large for gestational age, infants who were born to mothers who have diabetes, and late-preterm infants. Routine screening and monitoring of blood glucose concentration is not needed in healthy term newborn infants after an entirely normal pregnancy and delivery. Blood glucose concentration should only be measured in term infants who have clinical manifestations or who are known to be at risk. Plasma or blood glucose concentration should be measured as soon as possible (min-

utes, not hours) in any infant who manifests clinical signs (see "Clinical Signs") compatible with a low blood glucose concentration (ie, the symptomatic infant).

Breastfed term infants have lower concentrations of plasma glucose but higher concentrations of ketone bodies than do formula-fed infants.[13,17] It is postulated that breastfed infants tolerate lower plasma glucose concentrations without any clinical manifestations or sequelae of NH because of the increased ketone concentrations.[8,12–14]

WHEN TO SCREEN

Neonatal glucose concentrations decrease after birth, to as low as 30 mg/dL during the first 1 to 2 hours after birth, and then increase to higher and relatively more stable concentrations, generally above 45 mg/dL by 12 hours after birth.[6,7] Data on the optimal timing and intervals for glucose screening are limited. It is controversial whether to screen the asymptomatic at-risk infant for NH during this normal physiologic nadir. No studies have demonstrated harm from a few hours of asymptomatic hypoglycemia during this normal postnatal period of establishing "physiologic glucose homeostasis."[9]

Infants born to mothers with diabetes may develop asymptomatic NH as early as 1 hour after birth[18] and usually by 12 hours of age.[18] In contrast, infants who are large for gestational age or small for gestational age may develop low plasma glucose concentrations at as early as 3 hours of age,[19] and these infants may be at risk of NH for up to 10 days after birth.[20] Therefore, at-risk infants should be screened for NH with a frequency and duration related to risk factors specific to the individual infant.[5] Screening the asymptomatic at-risk infant can be performed within the first hours of birth and continued through multiple feed-fast cycles. Late-preterm infants and infants who are small for gestational age should be fed every 2 to 3 hours and screened before each feeding for at least the first 24 hours. After 24 hours, repeated screening before feedings should be continued if plasma glucose concentrations remain lower than 45 mg/dL.

LABORATORY DATA

When NH is suspected, the plasma or blood glucose concentration must be determined immediately by using one of the laboratory enzymatic methods (eg, glucose oxidase, hexokinase, or dehydrogenase method). Plasma blood glucose values tend to be approximately 10% to 18% higher than whole-blood values because of the higher water content of plasma.[21,22]

Although a laboratory determination is the most accurate method of measuring the glucose concentration, the results may not be available quickly enough for rapid diagnosis of NH, which thereby delays the initiation of treatment.[23] Bedside reagent test-strip

glucose analyzers can be used if the test is performed carefully and the clinician is aware of the limited accuracy of these devices. Rapid measurement methods available at the bedside include the handheld reflectance colorimeter and electrode methods. The blood sample is usually obtained from a warmed heel.

Test-strip results demonstrate a reasonable correlation with actual plasma glucose concentrations, but the variation from the actual level may be as much as 10 to 20 mg/dL.[24–27] Unfortunately, this variation is greatest at low glucose concentrations. There is no point-of-care method that is sufficiently reliable and accurate in the low range of blood glucose to allow it to be used as the sole method for screening for NH.

Because of limitations with "rapid" bedside methods, the blood or plasma glucose concentration must be confirmed by laboratory testing ordered stat. A long delay in processing the specimen can result in a falsely low concentration as erythrocytes in the sample metabolize the glucose in the plasma. This problem can be avoided by transporting the blood in tubes that contain a glycolytic inhibitor such as fluoride.

Screening of the at-risk infant for NH and institution of prophylactic measures to prevent prolonged or symptomatic NH is a reasonable goal. Treatment of suspected NH should not be postponed while waiting for laboratory confirmation. However, there is no evidence to show that such rapid treatment will mitigate neurologic sequelae.

CLINICAL SIGNS

The clinical signs of NH are not specific and include a wide range of local or generalized manifestations that are common in sick neonates.[12,13,17] These signs include jitteriness, cyanosis, seizures, apneic episodes, tachypnea,

weak or high-pitched cry, floppiness or lethargy, poor feeding, and eye-rolling. It is important to screen for other possible underlying disorders (eg, infection) as well as hypoglycemia. Such signs usually subside quickly with normalization of glucose supply and plasma concentration.[9,13] Coma and seizures may occur with prolonged NH (plasma or blood glucose concentrations lower than 10 mg/dL range) and repetitive hypoglycemia. The more serious signs (eg, seizure activity) usually occur late in severe and protracted cases of hypoglycemia and are not easily or rapidly reversed with glucose replacement and normalization of plasma glucose concentrations.[28–30] Development of clinical signs may be ameliorated by the presence of alternative substrates.[31]

Because avoidance and treatment of cerebral energy deficiency is the principal concern, greatest attention should be paid to neurologic signs. To attribute signs and symptoms to NH, Cornblath et al[12] have suggested that the Whipple triad be fulfilled: (1) a low blood glucose concentration; (2) signs consistent with NH; and (3) resolution of signs and symptoms after restoring blood glucose concentrations to normal values.[12]

MANAGEMENT

Any approach to management needs to account for the overall metabolic and physiologic status of the infant and should not unnecessarily disrupt the mother-infant relationship and breastfeeding. The definition of a plasma glucose concentration at which intervention is indicated needs to be tailored to the clinical situation and the particular characteristics of a given infant. For example, further investigation and immediate intravenous glucose treatment might be instituted for an infant with clinical signs and a plasma glucose concentration of less than 40 mg/

dL, whereas an at-risk but asymptomatic term formula-fed infant may only require an increased frequency of feeding and would receive intravenous glucose only if the glucose values decreased to less than 25 mg/dL (birth to 4 hours of age) or 35 mg/dL (4–24 hours of age).[32] Follow-up glucose concentrations and clinical evaluation must always be obtained to ensure that postnatal glucose homeostasis is achieved and maintained.

Because severe, prolonged, symptomatic hypoglycemia may result in neuronal injury,[27,28,32] prompt intervention is necessary for infants who manifest clinical signs and symptoms. A reasonable (although arbitrary) cutoff for treating symptomatic infants is 40 mg/dL. This value is higher than the physiologic nadir and higher than concentrations usually associated with clinical signs. A plasma sample for a laboratory glucose determination needs to be obtained just before giving an intravenous "minibolus" of glucose (200 mg of glucose per kg, 2 mL/kg dextrose 10% in water [$D_{10}W$], intravenously) and/or starting a continuous infusion of glucose ($D_{10}W$ at 80–100 mL/kg per day). A reasonable goal is to maintain plasma glucose concentrations in symptomatic infants between 40 and 50 mg/dL.

Figure 1 is a guideline for the screening and management of NH in late-preterm infants and term infants who were born to mothers with diabetes, small for gestational age, or large for gestational age. In developing a pragmatic approach to the asymptomatic at-risk infant during the first 24 hours after birth, mode of feeding, risk factors, and hours of age were considered. This strategy is based on the following observations from Cornblath and Ichord[13]: (1) almost all infants with proven symptomatic NH during the first hours of life have plasma glucose concentrations lower than 20 to 25 mg/dL; (2) persistent or recurrent NH syndromes present with equally low plasma glucose concentrations; and (3) little or no evidence exists to indicate that asymptomatic NH at any concentration of plasma glucose in the first days of life results in any adverse sequelae in growth or neurologic development.[13]

Figure 1 is divided into 2 time periods (birth to 4 hours and 4–12 hours) and accounts for the changing values of glucose that occur over the first 12 hours after birth. The recommended values for intervention are intended to provide a margin of safety over concentrations of glucose associated with clinical signs. The intervention recommendations also provide a range of values over which the clinician can decide to refeed or provide intravenous glucose. The target glucose concentration is greater than 45 mg/dL before each feeding. At-risk infants should be fed by 1 hour of age and screened 30 minutes after the feeding. This recommendation is consistent with that of the World Health Organization. Gavage feeding may be considered in infants who are not nippling well. Glucose screening should continue until 12 hours of age for infants born to mothers with diabetes and those who are large for gestational age and maintain plasma glucose concentrations of greater than 40 mg/dL. Late-preterm infants and infants who are small for gestational age require glucose monitoring for at least 24 hours after birth, because they may be more vulnerable to low glucose concentrations, especially if regular feedings or intravenous fluids are not yet established.[20] If inadequate postnatal glucose homeostasis is documented, the clinician must be certain that the infant can maintain normal plasma glucose concentrations on a routine diet for a reasonably extended period (through at least 3 feed-fast periods) before discharge. It is recommended that the at-risk asymptomatic infant who has glucose concentrations of less than 25 mg/dL (birth to 4 hours of age) or less than 35 mg/dL (4–24 hours of age) be refed and that the glucose value be rechecked 1 hour after refeeding. Subsequent concentrations lower than 25 mg/dL, or lower than 35 mg/dL, respectively, after attempts to refeed, necessitate treatment with intravenous glucose. Persistent hypoglycemia can be treated with a minibolus (200 mg/kg [2 mL/kg] $D_{10}W$) and/or intravenous infusion of $D_{10}W$ at 5 to 8 mg/kg per minute, 80 to 100 mL/kg per day; the goal is to achieve a plasma glucose concentration of 40 to 50 mg/dL (higher concentrations will only stimulate further insulin secretion). If it is not possible to maintain blood glucose concentrations of greater than 45 mg/dL after 24 hours of using this rate of glucose infusion, consideration should be given to the possibility of hyperinsulinemic hypoglycemia, which is the most common cause of severe persistent hypoglycemia in the newborn period. A blood sample should be sent for measurement of insulin along with a glucose concentration at the time when a bedside blood glucose concentration is less than 40 mg/dL, and an endocrinologist should be consulted.

SUMMARY

Current evidence does not support a specific concentration of glucose that can discriminate euglycemia from hypoglycemia or can predict that acute or chronic irreversible neurologic damage will result. Therefore, similar to the Canadian Paediatric Society guidelines, a significantly low concentration of glucose in plasma should be reliably established and treated to restore glucose values to a normal physiologic range.[5] Recognizing infants at risk of disturbances in postnatal glucose homeostasis and providing a margin of safety by early measures to prevent (feeding) and treat (feeding and intravenous glucose infusion) low concentrations are primary goals. Follow-up glucose measurements are always indicated to be sure an infant can maintain normal glucose concentrations over several feed-fast cycles. This will also permit recognition of infants with persistent hyperinsulinemic hypoglycemia and infants with fatty acid oxidation disorders.

LEAD AUTHOR

David H. Adamkin, MD

COMMITTEE ON FETUS AND NEWBORN, 2009–2010

Lu-Ann Papile, MD, Chairperson
David H. Adamkin, MD
Jill E. Baley, MD
Vinod K. Bhutani, MD
Waldemar A. Carlo, MD
Praveen Kumar, MD
Richard A. Polin, MD
Rosemarie C. Tan, MD, PhD
Kasper S. Wang, MD

Kristi L. Watterberg, MD

LIAISONS

Capt Wanda Denise Barfield, MD, MPH –
Centers for Disease Control and Prevention
William H. Barth Jr, MD – *American College of
Obstetricians and Gynecologists*
Ann L. Jefferies, MD
Rosalie O. Mainous, PhD, RNC, NNP – *National
Association of Neonatal Nurses*
Tonse N. K. Raju, MD, DCH – *National Institutes
of Health*

STAFF

Jim Couto, MA

REFERENCES

1. Hay W Jr, Raju TK, Higgins RD, Kalhan SC, Devaskar SU. Knowledge gaps and research needs for understanding and treating neonatal hypoglycemia: workshop report from Eunice Kennedy Shriver National Institute of Child Health and Human Development. *J Pediatr*. 2009;155(5):612–617

2. Adamkin DH. Update on neonatal hypoglycemia. *Arch Perinat Med*. 2005;11(3):13–15

3. Sinclair JC. Approaches to definition of neonatal hypoglycemia. *Acta Paediatr Jpn*. 1997;39(suppl 1):S17–S20

4. McGowan JE. Commentary, neonatal hypoglycemia. Fifty years later, the questions remain the same. *Neoreviews*. 2004;5(9): e363–e364

5. Canadian Paediatric Society. Screening guidelines for newborns at risk for low blood glucose. *Paediatr Child Health*. 2004; 9(10):723–729

6. Srinivasan G, Pildes RS, Cattamanchi G, Voora S, Lilien LD. Plasma glucose values in normal neonates: a new look. *J Pediatr*. 1986;109(1):114–117

7. Heck LJ, Erenberg A. Serum glucose levels in term neonates during the first 48 hours of life. *J Pediatr*. 1987;110(1):119–122

8. Hoseth E, Joergensen A, Ebbesen F, Moeller M. Blood glucose levels in a population of healthy, breast fed, term infants of appropriate size for gestational age. *Arch Dis Child Fetal Neonatal Ed*. 2000;83(2):F117–F119

9. Rozance PJ, Hay W. Hypoglycemia in newborn infants: features associated with adverse outcomes. *Biol Neonate*. 2006;90(2):74–86

10. Sinclair JC, Steer PA. Neonatal hypoglycemia and subsequent neurodevelopment: a critique of follow-up studies. Presented at: CIBA Foundation discussion meeting: Hypoglycemia in Infancy; October 17, 1989; London, England

11. Boluyt N, van Kempen A, Offringa M. Neurodevelopment after neonatal hypoglycemia:

a systematic review and design of an optimal future study. *Pediatrics*. 2006;117(6): 2231–2243

12. Cornblath M, Hawdon JM, Williams AF, et al. Controversies regarding definition of neonatal hypoglycemia: suggested operational thresholds. *Pediatrics*. 2000;105(5): 1141–1145

13. Cornblath M, Ichord R. Hypoglycemia in the neonate. *Semin Perinatol*. 2000;24(2): 136–149

14. Hawdon JM, Ward Platt MP, Aynsley-Green A. Patterns of metabolic adaptation for preterm and term infants in the first neonatal week. *Arch Dis Child*. 1992;67(4 spec No.): 357–365

15. Kalhan S, Parmimi P. Gluconeogenesis in the fetus and neonate. *Semin Perinatol*. 2000;24(2):94–106

16. Swenne I, Ewald U, Gustafsson J, Sandberg F, Ostenson C. Inter-relationship between serum concentrations of glucose, glucagon and insulin during the first two days of life in healthy newborns. *Acta Paediatr*. 1994; 83(9):915–919

17. Williams AF. Hypoglycaemia of the newborn: a review. *Bull World Health Organ*. 1997; 75(3):261–290

18. Agrawal RK, Lui K, Gupta JM. Neonatal hypoglycemia in infants of diabetic mothers. *J Paediatr Child Health*. 2000;36(4):354–356

19. Holtrop PC. The frequency of hypoglycemia in full-term large and small for gestational age newborns. *Am J Perinatol*. 1993;10(2): 150–154

20. Hume R, McGeechan A, Burchell A. Failure to detect preterm infants at risk of hypoglycemia before discharge. *J Pediatr*. 1999; 134(4):499–502

21. Burrin JM, Alberti KGMM. What is blood glucose: can it be measured? *Diabet Med*. 1990;7(3):199–206

22. Aynsley-Green A. Glucose: a fuel for thought! *J Paediatr Child Health*. 1991;27(1):21–30

23. Cornblath M, Schwartz R. Hypoglycemia in the neonate. *J Pediatr Endocrinol*. 1993; 6(2):113–129

24. Altimier L, Roberts W. One Touch II hospital system for neonates: correlation with serum glucose values. *Neonatal Netw*. 1996; 15(2):15–18

25. Giep TN, Hall RT, Harris K, Barrick B, Smith S. Evaluation of neonatal whole blood versus plasma glucose concentration by ion-selective electrode technology and comparison with two whole blood chromogen test strip methods. *J Perinatol*. 1996;16(4):244–249

26. Maisels MJ, Lee C. Chemstrip glucose test strips: correlation with true glucose values less than 80 mg/dL. *Crit Care Med*. 1983; 11(4):293–295

27. Hussain K, Sharief N. The inaccuracy of venous and capillary blood glucose measurement using reagent strips in the newborn period and the effect of haematocrit. *Early Hum Dev*. 2000;57(2):111–121

28. de Lonlay P, Touati G, Robert JJ, Saudubray JM. Persistent hyperinsulinaemic hypoglycaemia. *Semin Neonatol*. 2002;7(1):95–100

29. Meissner T, Brune W, Mayatepek E. Persistent hyperinsulinaemic hypoglycaemia of infancy: therapy, clinical outcome and mutational analysis. *Eur J Pediatr*. 1997; 156(10):754–757

30. Menni F, deLonlay P, Sevin C, et al. Neurologic outcomes of 90 neonates and infants with persistent hyperinsulinemic hypoglycemia. *Pediatrics*. 2001;107(3):476–479

31. Adam PA, Raiha N, Rahiala EL, Kekomaki M. Oxidation of glucose and D-B-OH-butyrate by the early human fetal brain. *Acta Paediatr Scand*. 1975;64(1):17–24

32. Kalhan S, Peter-Wohl S. Hypoglycemia: what is it for the neonate? *Am J Perinatol*. 2000; 17(1):11–18

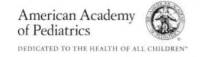

American Academy of Pediatrics

DEDICATED TO THE HEALTH OF ALL CHILDREN™

Guidance for the Clinician in
Rendering Pediatric Care

Clinical Report—Premedication for Nonemergency Endotracheal Intubation in the Neonate

abstract

Endotracheal intubation is a common procedure in newborn care. The purpose of this clinical report is to review currently available evidence on use of premedication for intubation, identify gaps in knowledge, and provide guidance for making decisions about the use of premedication. *Pediatrics* 2010;125:608–615

Praveen Kumar, MD, Susan E. Denson, MD, Thomas J. Mancuso, MD, COMMITTEE ON FETUS AND NEWBORN, SECTION ON ANESTHESIOLOGY AND PAIN MEDICINE

KEY WORDS
neonate, endotracheal intubation, premedication

ABBREVIATION
LMA—laryngeal mask airway

The guidance in this report does not indicate an exclusive course of treatment or serve as a standard of medical care. Variations, taking into account individual circumstances, may be appropriate.

This document is copyrighted and is property of the American Academy of Pediatrics and its Board of Directors. All authors have filed conflict of interest statements with the American Academy of Pediatrics. Any conflicts have been resolved through a process approved by the Board of Directors. The American Academy of Pediatrics has neither solicited nor accepted any commercial involvement in the development of the content of this publication.

INTRODUCTION

Endotracheal intubation is a common procedure in NICUs and should be performed expeditiously in as controlled an environment as possible to reduce complications. Several studies that evaluated the success rate of neonatal endotracheal intubations have reported that successful intubations frequently require more than 1 attempt and are rarely accomplished within the currently recommended time frame.[1–3] Many failed attempts can be attributed to suboptimal intubating conditions. Excellent intubating conditions are characterized by good jaw relaxation, open and immobile vocal cords, and suppression of pharyngeal and laryngeal reflexes assessed by the absence of coughing or diaphragmatic movements in response to intubation.[4] Several trials have demonstrated that the use of premedication for intubation of the newborn significantly improves intubating conditions, decreases the time and number of attempts needed to complete the intubation procedure, and minimizes the potential for intubation-related airway trauma.[5–10]

The alleviation of pain in neonates should be the goal of all caregivers, because repeated painful experiences have the potential for deleterious consequences.[11] The experience of being intubated is unpleasant and painful and seriously disturbs physiologic homeostasis.[12,13] A consensus statement from the International Evidence-Based Group for Neonatal Pain concluded that "tracheal intubation without the use of analgesia or sedation should be performed only for resuscitation in the delivery room or for life-threatening situations associated with the unavailability of intravenous access."[14] Subsequently, in a recent policy statement the American Academy of Pediatrics also recommended that every health care facility caring for neonates implement an effective pain-prevention program and use pharmacologic and nonpharmacologic therapies for the prevention of pain associated with procedures.[11] Despite these recommendations, there remains wide variation in the frequency of use of premedication before intubation, and in the medications used for premedication.[15,16] Some of the reasons offered for not using premedications before intubation are concern for ad-

www.pediatrics.org/cgi/doi/10.1542/peds.2009-2863

doi:10.1542/peds.2009-2863

All clinical reports from the American Academy of Pediatrics automatically expire 5 years after publication unless reaffirmed, revised, or retired at or before that time.

PEDIATRICS (ISSN Numbers: Print, 0031-4005; Online, 1098-4275).

Copyright © 2010 by the American Academy of Pediatrics

verse reactions and/or toxic effects of the medications, inadequate time for administration of medications in emergency situations, and the perception that risk/benefit ratios are worsened by using premedications.[13] This report will address some of these issues, including the choices of available medications, the circumstances for the use of medications, the risks of these medications, and the appropriate precautions to take while adopting these procedures.

PHYSIOLOGIC RESPONSES TO INTUBATION

The process of intubation may cause hypoxemia,[17] bradycardia,[18] intracranial hypertension,[19] systemic hypertension,[17] and pulmonary hypertension.[20] Hypoxemia seems to be related either to apnea at the time of intubation or possible airway obstruction associated with positioning.[17] Bradycardia is presumed to be vagal in origin, because the very rapid onset is suggestive of a reflexive etiology[17] and is not prevented by preoxygenation and the avoidance of hypoxemia.[18] The increase in intracranial pressure may be a result of coughing and struggling of the infant that can result in venous stasis with an increase in cerebral blood volume.[19,21] Systemic arterial hypertension has been investigated in adults and seems to be caused by an increase in systemic vascular resistance, which is probably caused by catecholamine release.[22] Pulmonary hypertension leading to right ventricular failure has been described in adults,[23] and although pulmonary artery pressures have not been measured in newborn infants undergoing intubation, endotracheal suctioning is known to cause an increase in pulmonary artery pressure postoperatively in infants with congenital heart disease[20] and is presumed to occur with intubation. In addition, improperly performed direct laryngoscopy can cause traumatic injuries to the face, eyes, tongue, and gums, and placement of the endotracheal tube can dislodge the arytenoids or damage other glottic structures. These injuries can be avoided by improved technique that can be enhanced by the use of premedication.[24]

CHARACTERISTICS OF AN IDEAL STRATEGY

An ideal strategy for premedication for intubation eliminates the pain, discomfort, and physiologic abnormalities of the procedure, helps to carry out intubation expeditiously, minimizes the chances for traumatic injury to the newborn, and has no adverse effects. An individual skilled in the use of bag-mask ventilation should be present to ensure adequate ventilation after the use of premedication and before the intubation. An ideal approach would be to administer supplemental oxygen, as needed, via a properly sized face mask, then a vagolytic agent, followed by analgesic and/or hypnotic medications before infusion of a muscle relaxant. The vagolytic drug prevents bradycardia, the analgesic and/or hypnotic drug can control pain and may render the infant unconscious and minimize adverse hemodynamic responses to laryngoscopy, and the muscle relaxant provides the best possible intubating conditions. Nonpharmacologic interventions, including swaddling and comfortable positioning, would contribute to the infant's comfort as well.

Analgesia

Premedication with an analgesic reduces the pain and discomfort of intubation. An ideal analgesic agent would have a rapid onset, be of short duration, have no adverse effects on respiratory mechanics, and possess predictable pharmacokinetic properties. None of the currently available agents fit this profile.

Opioids are the most commonly used medications for analgesia in the neonate. The mechanism of action of the individual opioids involves interaction at various receptor sites in both the central and peripheral nervous system to modify transmission of painful signals and diminish pain perception.[25] Morphine is the most frequently used opiate for pain control in the neonate. It has been used for acute postoperative pain control and as a continuous infusion for ventilated infants. The use of morphine for premedication for intubation was studied in a randomized, controlled trial of 34 premature infants in which infants were given either morphine alone or placebo 5 minutes before the intubation. There was no effect on the severity of physiologic disturbances during intubation including the duration of severe hypoxemia, incidence of bradycardia, and change in mean blood pressure.[26] This lack of effect is thought to be because of the delayed onset of action of morphine[27] related to the relative hydrophilic nature of the drug. Intravenous morphine has a mean onset of action at 5 minutes and peak effect at 15 minutes.[25] Another randomized, controlled trial of 20 preterm infants compared the use of morphine and midazolam versus remifentanil and midazolam for intubation.[8] No differences were noted between the groups with regard to pain control or hemodynamic variables, but the probability of having excellent intubation conditions was significantly higher with remifentanil than with morphine. All infants pretreated with remifentanil and midazolam were intubated at first attempt compared with only 60% of the infants in the morphine and midazolam group.[8] In another study, when morphine was used in combination with a vagolytic and a paralytic agent, the time needed to intubate was reduced and bradycardia was decreased.[24] However, these effects may be related to the vagolytic and paralytic agents used in the study, not to morphine effects. Furthermore, the status of pain control was not assessed in that study. For these reasons, morphine alone would not be the most appropriate choice for premedication for intubations. Meperidine is rarely used in neonates because of its slow onset of action, variability in metabolism, and risk of toxic effects of its metabolites; as a result, it is not recommended.[27]

Fentanyl is the most frequently used synthetic opioid in the neonate. This drug may be preferable to morphine for pain control for intubation because of a more rapid onset of action related to its more lipophilic nature.[25] Fentanyl's impact on some of the physiologic disturbances during intubation has been studied. In older infants and children this drug blunts physiologic disturbances during endotracheal suctioning and, in patients after surgery, decreases pulmonary arterial pressure and systemic hypertension.[20,23] It is likely that such responses may occur during intubation too. Its impact on cerebral and systemic hemodynamics was studied with a short-term infusion in 15 preterm infants, and there were no significant changes in the systemic or cerebral perfusion or pressure.[28] Although fentanyl as a single agent in intubation has not been studied, a cohort study of 33 preterm and term infants intubated after a combination of atropine, fentanyl, and a paralytic agent showed that fentanyl had no significant adverse effects.[7] Remifentanil, another synthetic opiate, has a rapid onset of action and an ultrashort duration of action and has been shown to be a useful drug for neonatal intubation.[8,29] A primary concern with synthetic opioid use is the risk of chest wall rigidity, but this risk can be reduced by slow administration and can be treated with either naloxone or muscle relaxants.[30] However, it is important to remember that the use of naloxone, a competitive antagonist at all opioid receptors, will also reverse the analgesic effects of these drugs.

Sedation

Sedatives do not always reduce pain but can sedate or render individuals unconscious or amnestic depending on the dose and individual response. Benzodiazepines have been frequently used for sedation before elective intubations but may not be appropriate in many cases. Midazolam is the most commonly used medication in this category[31] in the United States, but it has not been shown to reduce any physiologic changes during intubation. In a randomized, double-blind trial (stopped after only 16 intubations because of adverse events and reported in a letter to the editor), preterm infants who received midazolam and atropine for intubation had more desaturations, and 29% required cardiopulmonary resuscitation compared with those in the groups that received either atropine alone or no premedication.[32] Midazolam can cause hypotension in both preterm and term infants,[33–36] decreased cardiac output in older children,[37] and decreased cerebral blood flow velocity in premature infants.[33,38] The studies that demonstrated these effects were not performed as part of premedication for intubation, and the results may not be applicable to the circumstances necessitating endotracheal intubation. However, kinetic studies in preterm and term infants have shown that the serum half-life of midazolam given as continuous infusion or by repetitive dosing can exceed 22 hours.[38,39] Further concern in the use of midazolam for preterm infants is the exposure to the preservative benzyl alcohol.[40,41] For these reasons, midazolam should not be used in preterm infants, but it can be considered for use in the term or older infant as part of the premedication sequence for elective intubation in the NICU.

Elective intubation of patients before surgery is often accomplished with a sedative-hypnotic agent such as a barbiturate and a muscle relaxant. Barbiturates have been used for induction of anesthesia for decades; however, barbiturates are poor analgesics.[42] Barbiturates such as thiopental and methohexital have a rapid onset and short duration of action. In a randomized, placebo-controlled trial in term infants, thiopental was shown to reduce changes in heart rate and blood pressure during intubation and to shorten the time to intubation.[43] In a small cohort study of term and preterm infants, methohexital facilitated intubation with rapid onset within 1 minute of sedation and recovery within 10 minutes.[44] However, more studies are necessary before methohexital can be recommended for use.

Propofol is a nonbarbiturate anesthetic that is frequently used for induction of anesthesia in older children and adults but has not been well evaluated in newborns. Propofol is lipophilic and rapidly equilibrates between plasma and brain with quick loss of consciousness and also has a short duration of action after a single-bolus dose.[25] In a randomized, controlled trial in 63 premature infants, propofol was shown to be a more effective induction agent than the morphine, atropine, and suxamethonium regimen to facilitate neonatal intubation.[9] Oxygenation during intubation was maintained better in the propofol group and was attributed to the maintenance of spontaneous respiration in infants who received propofol. Twenty-three percent of the infants in the morphine, atropine, and suxamethonium group and 6% of the infants in the propofol group sustained intubation-related trauma. No other adverse events were noted in the propofol group. Although the results of this study are encouraging, more research confirming these initial findings is necessary before propofol can be recommended as a single premedication agent for neonatal intubation. Propofol can only be administered intravenously, and pain at the site of injection that may sometimes be moderately severe has been reported with intravenous injection of propofol in 10% to 20% of patients.[45]

Vagolytic Agents

Vagolytic agents prevent bradycardia during intubation and decrease bronchial and salivary secretions but are infrequently used for neonatal intubation.[46] One reason for their sparse use has been the concern that vagolytic agents mask hypoxia-induced bradycardia during intubation; however, most episodes of bradycardia during intubation are secondary to vagal stimulation, not hypoxia. Glycopyrrolate and atropine are both effective vagolytic agents, and although they have not been directly compared in neonates, they have been studied in infants and children. In a randomized, controlled trial in 90 older infants and children that compared the use of glycopyrrolate and atropine at anesthetic induction, none had bradycardia, but more subjects who received atropine developed sinus tachycardia than those who received glycopyrrolate.[47] Glycopyrrolate is widely used in pediatric intensive care and anesthesia; however, its pharmacokinetics in small preterm infants is not known.

Muscle Relaxants

The ideal muscle relaxant for intubation would have a rapid onset, short duration of action, and minimal or no deleterious effect on heart rate and blood pressure. None of the currently available agents meet all these criteria for neonates, but use of a muscle relaxant to facilitate intubation can eliminate or minimize the increase in intracranial pressure that occurs during awake intubation. This has been demonstrated with both succinylcholine in preterm infants[48] and pancuronium in preterm and term infants.[18]

Succinylcholine, the only depolarizing agent in clinical use, blocks neuromuscular transmission by binding to the acetylcholine receptors of the muscle membrane and depolarizing the membrane. It has both a rapid onset and a short duration of action. In a randomized, controlled trial in preterm infants, succinylcholine given with morphine and atropine was compared with awake intubation. This combination resulted in faster intubation with less bradycardia and less trauma as defined by less blood in the oral and nasal passages.[48]

The nondepolarizing muscle relaxants compete with acetylcholine for receptors on the motor endplate but do not result in depolarization of the membrane. Of these agents, pancuronium is widely used in newborns and has few adverse effects but is slower in onset of action and longer acting compared with the other available muscle relaxants. Pancuronium has a vagolytic effect that helps minimize the reflex bradycardia that often accompanies laryngoscopy. In a randomized, controlled trial, infants who received pancuronium and atropine showed less hypoxia during intubation and less increase in intracranial pressure compared with infants who received no premedication or atropine alone.[18]

Mivacurium, another nondepolarizing agent, is no longer commercially available because of its adverse effect of · histamine release and associated bronchospasm. Cisatracurium has been introduced to replace mivacurium and seems to have similar physiologic effects but has not yet been tested in a neonatal population. Vecuronium and rocuronium, 2 other nondepolarizing muscle relaxants in wide use in pediatric anesthesia and PICUs, are characterized by their minimal effects on blood pressure or heart rate. Rocuronium is a metabolic derivative of vecuronium and has quicker onset to paralysis and shorter duration of action compared with vecuronium.

ADVERSE EFFECTS

Concern for adverse effects has been a barrier to implementing premedication for intubation,[49] but most reports and randomized, controlled trials have not demonstrated serious adverse effects. A large multicenter observational study showed no increase in the frequency of adverse effects when infants were premedicated.[31] When used alone, fentanyl and other synthetic opioids have been associated with acute chest wall rigidity in both preterm and term infants, which can significantly impair ventilation.[30] However, this adverse effect may be related to dose and rapid delivery and can be prevented by slow infusion of an appropriate dose and overcome with muscle relaxant[50] or reversed with naloxone.[30]

Succinylcholine has been reported to have rare serious adverse effects in children, including hyperkalemia, myoglobinemia, and cardiac arrhythmias. Atropine seems to protect against bradyarrhythmias induced by succinylcholine.[51] Hyperkalemia is also unlikely, because marked elevations have been reported only in clinical circumstances associated with significant tissue destruction.[51] Succinylcholine is a known trigger of malignant hyperthermia, a skeletal muscle disorder inherited as an autosomal dominant trait. The incidence of malignant hyperthermia is estimated to be 0.4 to 0.5 in 10 000 in the general population.[52] Diagnosis and management of malignant hyperthermia is beyond the scope of this report. Succinylcholine should not be used in the presence of hyperkalemia and/or a family history of malignant hyperthermia.[53]

CLINICAL CIRCUMSTANCES FOR INTUBATION WITHOUT PREMEDICATION

Intubation without premedication may be acceptable during resuscitation or after acute deterioration or critical illness at a later age. The risk/benefit ratio may also support intubation without premedication in infants with upper airway anomalies such as Pierre Robin sequence. Intubation of infants with severely abnormal airways can be difficult, and the infant's own respiratory effort may be essential for maintaining an open airway. If intubation attempts are unsuccessful in these infants, the use of laryngeal mask airway (LMA) or anticipatory transfer to a center with a team of personnel, including a neonatologist, pediatric otolaryngologist, and pediatric anesthesiologist, experienced in managing infants with structurally abnormal airways should be considered. It is important to note that LMA is a temporary airway device and should be used only as a last resort while preparations for a secure airway are in progress. One might also consider the use of a fiber-optic bronchoscope for intubation if personnel experienced in its use are available.[54]

GAPS IN KNOWLEDGE

Many unanswered questions remain regarding the practice of premedication for nonemergent intubation in the newborn.

- The optimal pharmaceutical agents have not been developed for use in newborns, and appropriate drug doses of currently available agents based on gestational age are currently unknown.
- The pharmacokinetic and pharmacodynamic characteristics of many drugs used in premedication have not been well studied in newborns.

- An ideal combination and/or sequence of premedications have not been established.
- Alternative routes of administration of premedications have not been systematically studied.
- Long-term benefits and adverse effects of premedications are unknown.

Further research must continue to answer these and other questions.

CLINICAL IMPLICATIONS

- Preparation should include having appropriate equipment such as an oxygen source, appropriately sized bags, face masks, endotracheal tubes, stylet, laryngoscope, and suction.
- All support staff assisting with the procedure should have clearly preassigned responsibilities during the procedure.
- Infants should have cardiorespiratory, oxygen saturation, and noninvasive blood pressure monitoring during nonemergent intubation, and an end-tidal carbon dioxide detector should be available. Intravenous access should preferably be established, and the stomach should be decompressed.
- All personnel who intubate neonates should acquire training with LMAs, because this device may prove to be an effective bridge to intubation in some cases in which bag-mask ventilation is suboptimal.[55,56] Appropriately sized LMAs should be available for all intubations, particularly when any difficulty is anticipated. LMAs have been used successfully in late-preterm and term newborns weighing more than 2500 g.
- Individuals who perform intubations should be experienced in the use of bag-mask ventilation and be knowledgeable about the effects of the procedure of laryngoscopy and intubation, as well as risks and benefits of premedications. Ascertainment of appropriate endotracheal tube position immediately after intubation should be done by auscultation and end-tidal carbon dioxide monitoring.
- Except for emergent intubation during resuscitation either in the delivery room or after acute deterioration or critical illness at a later age, premedication should be used for all endotracheal intubations in newborns. Medications with rapid onset and short duration of action are preferable (Table 1).
  - Analgesic agents or anesthetic dose of a hypnotic drug should be given.
  - Vagolytic agents and rapid-onset muscle relaxants should be considered.
  - Use of sedatives alone such as benzodiazepines without analgesic agents should be avoided.
  - A muscle relaxant without an analgesic agent should not be used.
- Each unit should develop protocols and lists of preferred medications to improve compliance and minimize medication errors and adverse effects.
- For circumstances in which intravenous access is not available, alternative routes such as intramuscular administration can be considered.

TABLE 1 Medications for Premedication for Nonemergency Intubation

Drug	Route/Dose	Onset of Action	Duration of Action	Common Adverse Effects	Comments[a]
Analgesic					
Fentanyl	IV or IM[b]/1–4 μg/kg	IV, almost immediate; IM, 7–15 min	IV, 30–60 min; IM, 1–2 h	Apnea, hypotension, CNS depression, chest wall rigidity	Preferred analgesic Effects reversible with naloxone Give slowly (preferably over 3–5 min, at least over 1–2 min) to avoid chest wall rigidity Chest wall rigidity can be treated with naloxone and muscle relaxants
Remifentanil	IV/1–3 μg/kg May repeat in 2–3 min if needed	IV, almost immediate	IV, 3–10 min	Apnea, hypotension, CNS depression, chest wall rigidity	Acceptable analgesic Short duration of action and limited experience in neonates Effects reversible with naloxone Give slowly over 1–2 min to avoid chest wall rigidity Chest wall rigidity can be treated with naloxone and muscle relaxants
Morphine	IV or IM/0.05–0.1 mg/kg	IV, 5–15 min; IM, 10–30 min	IV, 3–5 h; IM, 3–5 h	Apnea, hypotension, CNS depression	Acceptable analgesic agent Use only if other opioids are not available; if selected, must wait at least 5 min for onset of action Effects reversible with naloxone
Hypnotic/sedative					
Midazolam	IV or IM/0.05–0.1 mg/kg	IV, 1–5 min; IM, within 5–15 min	IV, 20–30 min; IM, 1–6 h	Apnea, hypotension, CNS depression	Acceptable sedative for use in term infants in combination with analgesic agents Hypotension more likely when used in combination with fentanyl Not recommended in premature infants Effects reversible with flumazenil
Thiopental	IV/3–4 mg/kg	IV, 30–60 s	IV, 5–30 min	Histamine release, apnea, hypotension, bronchospasm	Acceptable hypnotic agent Hypotension more likely when used in combination with fentanyl and/or midazolam
Propofol	IV/2.5 mg/kg	Within 30 s	3–10 min	Histamine release, apnea, hypotension, bronchospasm, bradycardia; often causes pain at injection site	Acceptable hypnotic agent Limited experience in newborns Neonatal dosing has not been well established
Muscle relaxant					
Pancuronium	IV/0.05–0.10 mg/kg	1–3 min	40–60 min	Mild histamine release, hypertension, tachycardia, bronchospasm, excessive salivation	Acceptable muscle relaxant Relatively longer duration of action Effects reversible with atropine and neostigmine
Vecuronium	IV/0.1 mg/kg	2–3 min	30–40 min	Mild histamine release, hypertension/hypotension, tachycardia, arrhythmias, bronchospasm	Preferred muscle relaxant Effects reversible with atropine and neostigmine
Rocuronium	IV/0.6–1.2 mg/kg	1–2 min	20–30 min	Mild histamine release, hypertension/hypotension, tachycardia, arrhythmias, bronchospasm	Preferred muscle relaxant Effects reversible with atropine and neostigmine
Succinylcholine	IV/1–2 mg/kg; IM[b]/2 mg/kg	IV, 30–60 s; IM, 2–3 min	IV, 4–6 min; IM, 10–30 min	Hypertension/hypotension, tachycardia, arrhythmias, bronchospasm, hyperkalemia, myoglobinemia, malignant hyperthermia	Acceptable muscle relaxant Contraindicated in presence of hyperkalemia and family history of malignant hyperthermia
Vagolytic					
Atropine	IV or IM/0.02 mg/kg	1–2 min	0.5–2 h	Tachycardia, dry hot skin	Preferred vagolytic agent
Glycopyrrolate	IV/4–10 μg/kg	1–10 min	~6 h	Tachycardia, arrhythmias, bronchospasm	Acceptable vagolytic agent Limited experience in newborns Contains benzyl alcohol as preservative

Most of these drugs have limited pharmacokinetics data from newborns and are not approved for use in the newborn, but they have been used in newborns. IV indicates intravenously; IM, intramuscularly; CNS, central nervous system.

[a] Preferred and acceptable designation of medications is based on consensus opinion after review of available evidence.

[b] Consider only if no intravenous access.

REFERENCES

1. Lane B, Finer N, Rich W. Duration of intubation attempts during neonatal resuscitation. *J Pediatr.* 2004;145(1):67–70

2. Leone TA, Rich W, Finer NN. Neonatal intubation: success of pediatric trainees. *J Pediatr.* 2005;146(5):638–641

3. O'Donnell CPF, Kamlin COF, Davis PG, Morley CJ. Endotracheal intubation attempts during neonatal resuscitation: success rates, duration, and adverse effects. *Pediatrics.* 2006; 117(1). Available at: www.pediatrics.org/cgi/content/full/117/1/e16

4. Skinner HJ, Biswas A, Mahajan RP. Evaluation of intubating conditions with rocuronium and either propofol or etomidate for rapid sequence induction. *Anaesthesia.* 1998;53(7):702–710

5. Roberts KD, Leone TA, Edwards WH, Rich WD, Finer NN. Premedication for nonemergent neonatal intubations: a randomized controlled trial comparing atropine and fentanyl to atropine, fentanyl and mivacurium. *Pediatrics.* 2006;118(4):1583–1591

6. Lemyre B, Cheng R, Gaboury I. Atropine, fentanyl and succinylcholine for non-urgent intubations in newborns. *Arch Dis Child Fetal Neonatal Ed.* 2009;94(6):F439–F442

7. Dempsey EM, Al Hazzani F, Faucher D, Barrington KJ. Facilitation of neonatal endotracheal intubation with mivacurium and fentanyl in the neonatal intensive care unit. *Arch Dis Child Fetal Neonatal Ed.* 2006;91(4): F279–F282

8. Pereira e Silva Y, Gomez RS, Marcatto J, Maximo TA, Barbosa RF, Simões e Silva AC. Morphine versus remifentanil for intubating preterm neonates. *Arch Dis Child Fetal Neonatal Ed.* 2007;92(4):F293–F294

9. Ghanta S, Abdel-Latif ME, Lui K, Ravindranathan H, Awad J, Oei J. Propofol compared with the morphine, atropine, and suxamethonium regimen as induction agents for neonatal endotracheal intubation: a randomized controlled trial. *Pediatrics.* 2007;119(6). Available at: www.pediatrics.org/cgi/content/full/119/6/e1248

10. Carbajal R, Eble B, Anand KJS. Premedication for tracheal intubation in neonates: confusion or controversy? *Semin Perinatol.* 2007;31(5):309–317

11. American Academy of Pediatrics, Committee on Fetus and Newborn; American Academy of Pediatrics, Section on Surgery; Canadian Paediatric Society, Fetus and Newborn Committee. Prevention and management of pain in the neonate: an update [published correction appears in *Pediatrics.* 2007; 119(2):425]. *Pediatrics.* 2006;118(5): 2231–2241

12. Topulos GP, Lansing RW, Banzett RB. The experience of complete neuromuscular blockade in awake humans. *J Clin Anesth.* 1993; 5(5):369–374

13. Porter F, Wolf C, Gold J, Lotsoff D, Miller J. Pain and pain management in newborn infants: a survey of physicians and nurses. *Pediatrics.* 1997;100(4):626–632

14. Anand KJS; International Evidence-Based Group for Neonatal Pain. Consensus statement for the prevention and management of pain in the newborn. *Arch Pediatr Adolesc Med.* 2001;155(2):173–180

15. Whyte S, Birrell G, Wyllie J, Woolf A. Premedication before intubation in UK neonatal units. *Arch Dis Child Fetal Neonatal Ed.* 2000; 82(1):F38–F41

16. Sarkar S, Schumaker RE, Baumgart S, Donn SM. Are newborns receiving premedication before elective intubation? *J Perinatol.* 2006;26(5):286–289

17. Marshall TA, Deeder R, Pai S, Berkowitz GP, Austin TL. Physiologic changes associated with endotracheal intubation in preterm infants. *Crit Care Med.* 1984;12(6):501–503

18. Kelly M, Finer NN. Nasotracheal intubation in the neonate: physiologic responses and effects of atropine and pancuronium. *J Pediatr.* 1984;105(2):303–309

19. Friesen RH, Honda AT, Thieme RE. Changes in anterior fontanel pressure in preterm neonates during tracheal intubation. *Anesth Analg.* 1987;66(9):874–878

20. Hickey PR, Hansen DD, Wessel D, Lang P, Jonas RA, Elixson EM. Blunting of stress responses in the pulmonary circulation of infants by fentanyl. *Anesth Analg.* 1985;64(12): 1137–1142

21. Raju TNN, Vidyasagar D, Torres C, Grundy D, Bennett EJ. Intracranial pressure during intubation and anesthesia in infants. *J Pediatr.* 1980;96(5):860–862

22. Xie A, Skatrud J, Puleo D, Morgan B. Exposure to hypoxia produces long-lasting sympathetic activation in humans. *J Appl Physiol.* 2001;91(4):1555–1562

23. Hickey PR, Retzack SM. Acute right ventricular failure after pulmonary hypertensive responses to airway instrumentation: effect

of fentanyl dose. *Anesthesiology.* 1993; 78(2):372–376

24. Oei J, Hari R, Butha T, Lui K. Facilitation of neonatal nasotracheal intubation with premedication: a randomized controlled trial. *J Paediatr Child Health.* 2002;38(2): 146–150

25. Brunson LL, Lazo JS, Parker KL, eds. *Goodman and Gilman's The Pharmacological Basis of Therapeutics.* 11th ed. New York, NY: McGraw Hill; 2006

26. Lemyre B, Doucette J, Kalyn A, Gray S, Marrin M. Morphine for elective endotracheal intubation in neonates: a randomized trial. *BMC Pediatr.* 2004;4:20

27. Bhatt-Mehta V. Current guidelines for the treatment of acute pain in children. *Drugs.* 1996;51(5):760–776

28. Hamon I, Hascoet JM, Debbiche A, Vert P. Effects of fentanyl administration on general and cerebral haemodynamics in sick newborn infants. *Acta Paediatr.* 1996;85(3): 361–365

29. Crawford MW, Hayes J, Tan JM. Dose-response of remifentanil for tracheal intubation in infants. *Anesth Analg.* 2005;100(6): 1599–1604

30. Fahnenstich H, Steffan J, Kau N, Bartmann P. Fentanyl-induced chest wall rigidity and laryngospasm in preterm and term infants. *Crit Care Med.* 2000;28(3):836–839

31. Simon L, Trifa M, Mokhtari M, Hamza J, Treluyer JM. Premedication for tracheal intubation: a prospective survey in 75 neonatal and pediatric intensive care units. *Crit Care Med.* 2004;32(2):565–568

32. Attardi DM, Paul DA, Tuttle DJ, Greenspan JS. Premedication for intubation in neonates. *Arch Dis Child Fetal Neonatal Ed.* 2000;83(2):F161

33. Harte GJ, Gray PH, Lee TC, Steer PA, Charles BG. Haemodynamic responses and population pharmacokinetics of midazolam following administration to ventilated, preterm neonates. *J Paediatr Child Health.* 1997; 33(4):335–338

34. Jacqz-Aigrain E, Daoud P, Burtin P, Desplanques L, Beaufils F. Placebo-controlled trial of midazolam sedation in mechanically

ventilated newborn babies. *Lancet.* 1994; 344(8923):646–650

35. van Straaten HL, Rademaker CM, de Vries LS. Comparison of the effect of midazolam or vecuronium on blood pressure and cerebral blood flow velocity in the premature newborn. *Dev Pharmacol Ther.* 1992;19(4): 191–195

36. McCarver-May D, Kang J, Aouthmany M, et al. Comparison of chloral hydrate and midazolam for sedation of neonates for neuroimaging studies. *J Pediatr.* 1996;128(4): 573–576

37. Shekerdemian L, Bush A, Redington A. Cardiovascular effects of intravenous midazolam after open heart surgery. *Arch Dis Child.* 1997;76(1):57–61

38. Lee TC, Charles BG, Harte GJ, Gray PH, Steer PA, Flenady VJ. Population pharmacokinetic modeling in very premature infants receiving midazolam during mechanical ventilation: midazolam neonatal pharmacokinetics. *Anesthesiology.* 1999;90(2):451–457

39. Jacqz-Aigrain E, Daoud P, Burtin P, Maherzi S, Beaufils F. Pharmacokinetics of midazolam during continuous infusion in critically ill neonates. *Eur J Clin Pharmacol.* 1992; 42(3):329–332

40. Centers for Disease Control and Prevention. Neonatal deaths associated with use of benzyl alcohol: United States. *MMWR Morb Mortal Wkly Rep.* 1982;31(22):290–291

41. Hiller JL, Benda GI, Rahatzad M, et al. Benzyl alcohol toxicity: impact on mortality and intraventricular hemorrhage among very low birth weight infants. *Pediatrics.* 1986;77(4): 500–506

42. White PF. Clinical pharmacology of intravenous induction drugs. *Int Anesthesiol Clin.* 1988;26(2):98–104

43. Bhutada A, Sahni R, Rastogi S, Wung JT. Randomised controlled trial of thiopental for intubation in neonates. *Arch Dis Child Fetal Neonatal Ed.* 2000;82(1):F34–F37

44. Naulaers G, Deloof E, Vanhole C, Kola E, Devlieger H. Use of methohexital for elective intubation in neonates. *Arch Dis Child Fetal Neonatal Ed.* 1997;77(1):F61–F64

45. Barbi E, Marchetti T, Gerarduzzi E, et al. Pretreatment with intravenous ketamine re-

duces propofol injection pain. *Paediatr Anesth.* 2003;13(9):764–768

46. Rautakorpi P, Manner T, Kanto J. A survey of current usage of anticholinergic drugs in paediatric anaesthesia in Finland. *Acta Anaesth Scand.* 1999;43(10):1057–1059

47. Desalu I, Kushimo OT, Bode CO. A comparative study of the haemodynamic effects of atropine and glycopyrrolate at induction of anaesthesia in children. *West Afr J Med.* 2005;24(2):115–119

48. Barrington KJ, Finer NN, Etches PC. Succinylcholine and atropine for premedication of the newborn infant before nasotracheal intubation: a randomized, controlled trial. *Crit Care Med.* 1989;17(12):1293–1296

49. Ziegler JW, Todres ID. Intubation of newborns. *Am J Dis Child.* 1992;146(2):147–149

50. Barrington KJ, Byrne PJ. Premedication for neonatal intubation. *Am J Perinatol.* 1998; 15(4):213–216

51. Davis PJ, Lerman J, Tofovic SP, Cook DR. Pharmacology of pediatric anesthesia. In: Motoyama EK, Davis PJ, eds. *Smith's Anesthesia for Infants and Children. Pharmacology of Pediatric Anesthesia.* 7th ed. Philadelphia, PA: Mosby/Elsevier; 2005:215–219

52. Ording H. Incidence of malignant hyperthermia in Denmark. *Anesth Analg.* 1985;64(7): 700–704

53. Mancuso TJ. Neuromuscular disorders. In: *Practical Aspects of Pediatric Anesthesia.* Philadelphia, PA: Wolters Kluwer/Lippincott, Williams & Wilkins; 2008:547

54. Scheller JG, Schulman SR. Fiber-optic bronchoscopic guidance for intubating a neonate with Pierre-Robin syndrome. *J Clin Anesth.* 1991;3(1):45–47

55. Paterson SJ, Byrne PJ, Molesky MG, Seal RF, Finucane BT. Neonatal resuscitation using the laryngeal mask airway. *Anesthesiology.* 1994;80(6):1248–1253

56. American Society of Anesthesiologists. Practice guidelines for the management of the difficult airway: an updated report by the American Society of Anesthesiologists Task Force on Management of Difficult Airway. *Anesthesiology.* 2003;98(5):1269–1277

POLICY STATEMENT   Organizational Principles to Guide and Define the Child Health
Care System and/or Improve the Health of all Children

American Academy
of Pediatrics

DEDICATED TO THE HEALTH OF ALL CHILDREN™

Prevention and Management of Procedural Pain in the Neonate: An Update

COMMITTEE ON FETUS AND NEWBORN and SECTION ON ANESTHESIOLOGY AND PAIN MEDICINE

abstract

The prevention of pain in neonates should be the goal of all pediatricians and health care professionals who work with neonates, not only because it is ethical but also because repeated painful exposures have the potential for deleterious consequences. Neonates at greatest risk of neurodevelopmental impairment as a result of preterm birth (ie, the smallest and sickest) are also those most likely to be exposed to the greatest number of painful stimuli in the NICU. Although there are major gaps in knowledge regarding the most effective way to prevent and relieve pain in neonates, proven and safe therapies are currently underused for routine minor, yet painful procedures. Therefore, every health care facility caring for neonates should implement (1) a pain-prevention program that includes strategies for minimizing the number of painful procedures performed and (2) a pain assessment and management plan that includes routine assessment of pain, pharmacologic and nonpharmacologic therapies for the prevention of pain associated with routine minor procedures, and measures for minimizing pain associated with surgery and other major procedures.

DOI: 10.1542/peds.2015-4271

PEDIATRICS (ISSN Numbers: Print, 0031-4005; Online, 1098-4275).

To cite: AAP COMMITTEE ON FETUS AND NEWBORN and SECTION ON ANESTHESIOLOGY AND PAIN MEDICINE. Prevention and Management of Procedural Pain in the Neonate: An Update. *Pediatrics.* 2016;137(2):e20154271

Previous guidance from the American Academy of Pediatrics (AAP) and the Canadian Pediatric Society addressed the need to assess neonatal pain, especially during and after diagnostic and therapeutic procedures.[1,2] These organizations also provided recommendations on preventing or minimizing pain in newborn infants and treating unavoidable pain promptly and adequately.[1,2] This statement updates previous recommendations with new evidence on the prevention, assessment, and treatment of neonatal procedural pain.

BACKGROUND

Neonates are frequently subjected to painful procedures, with the most immature infants receiving the highest number of painful events.[3–5]

Despite recommendations from the AAP and other experts, neonatal pain continues to be inconsistently assessed and inadequately managed.[2,3] A large prospective study from France in 2008 found that specific pharmacologic or nonpharmacologic analgesia was given before painful procedures in only 21% of infants, and ongoing analgesia was given in an additional 34%.[3] Thus, infants received analgesia for approximately half of the procedures performed, with wide variation among facilities.

The prevention and alleviation of pain in neonates, particularly preterm infants, is important not only because it is ethical but also because exposure to repeated painful stimuli early in life is known to have short- and long-term adverse sequelae. These sequelae include physiologic instability, altered brain development, and abnormal neurodevelopment, somatosensory, and stress response systems, which can persist into childhood.[5-15] Nociceptive pathways are active and functional as early as 25 weeks' gestation and may elicit a generalized or exaggerated response to noxious stimuli in immature newborn infants.[16]

Researchers have demonstrated that a procedure-related painful stimulus that results in increased excitability of nociceptive neurons in the dorsal horn of the spinal cord accentuates the infant's sensitivity to subsequent noxious and nonnoxious sensory stimuli (ie, sensitization).[17,18] This persistent sensory hypersensitivity can be physiologically stressful, particularly in preterm infants.[19-22] Investigators have demonstrated increased stress-related markers and elevated free radicals after even simple procedures, such as routine heel punctures or tape removal from central venous catheters,[23,24] which can adversely affect future pain perception.[8] Specific cortical pain processing occurs even in preterm infants; however, multiple factors interact to influence the nociceptive processing and/or behavioral responses to pain.[14,16,25-27] Noxious stimuli activate these signaling pathways but also activate the central inhibitory circuits, thus altering the balance between the excitatory and inhibitory feedback mechanisms. The immaturity of the dorsal horn synaptic connectivity and descending inhibitory circuits in neonates results in poor localization and discrimination of sensory input and poor noxious inhibitory modulation, thus facilitating central nervous system sensitization to repeated noxious stimuli.[25]

ASSESSMENT OF PAIN AND STRESS IN THE NEONATE

Reliable neonatal pain assessment tools are essential for the rating and management of neonatal pain, and their use has been strongly recommended by the AAP and by international researchers, including the International Evidence-Based Group for Neonatal Pain.[1,2,28] However, the effective management of pain in the neonate remains problematic because of the inability of the infant to report his or her own pain and the challenges of assessing pain in extremely premature, ill, and neurologically compromised neonates.[29] Thus, pain assessment tools reflect surrogate measures of physiologic and behavioral responses to pain. Although numerous neonatal pain scales exist (Table 1), only 5 pain scales have been subjected to rigorous psychometric testing with the patients serving as their own controls, measuring their physiologic and behavioral responses by using the scale in question (Neonatal Facial Coding System,[30,31] Premature Infant Pain Profile [PIPP],[32-34] Neonatal Pain and Sedation Scale,[35,36] Behavioral Infant Pain Profile,[37] and Douleur Aiguë du Nouveau-né[38]). Many of the current pain assessment tools have been tested against existing or newly developed tools and against each other to determine which is more reliable for a particular population and application, but more research is needed.[29,39]

Contextual factors such as gestational age and behavioral state may play a significant role in pain assessment and are beginning to be included in some assessment tools (eg, the PIPP-Revised).[40,41] New and emerging technologies to measure pain responses, such as near-infrared spectroscopy, amplitude-integrated electroencephalography, functional MRI, skin conductance, and heart rate variability assessment, are being investigated.[53,54] These innovations hold promise in the development of neurophysiologically based methods for assessing noxious stimuli processing at the cortical level in neonates while they are awake, sedated, or anesthetized. If the neurophysiologic measures prove to be reliable and quantifiable, these measures could be used in the future to simultaneously correlate with the physiologic and behavioral pain assessment scales to determine the most clinically useful tool(s).

Many of the tools developed to measure acute pain in neonates are multidimensional in nature and include a combination of physiologic and behavioral signs. These tools were most commonly developed to assess unventilated infants; only a few scales are validated to assess pain in infants who are ventilated through an endotracheal tube or receiving nasal continuous positive airway pressure.[42,55] Recently, investigators reported that 2 behaviorally based, one-dimensional pain assessment tools (the Behavioral Indicators of Infant Pain and the Neonatal Facial Coding System) were more sensitive in detecting behavioral cues related to pain in term neonates than the PIPP.[56]

It is unlikely that a single, comprehensive pain assessment

TABLE 1 Pain Assessment Tools for Neonates

Pain Assessment Tool	Number and GA of Infants Studied	Indicators	Intervention Studied	Validation Methodology	Intended Use
Neonatal Facial Coding System (NFCS)[30,31] (1998, 2003)	N = 40 24–32 wk GA 5–56 DOL	Brow lowering Eye squeeze Nasolabial furrowing Lip opening Vertical mouth stretch Horizontal mouth stretch Taut tongue Chin quiver Lip pursing	Postoperative abdominal or thoracic surgery	Patients served as controls Interrater reliability: 0.86 Construct validity: demonstrated Feasibility: established	Acute pain Prolonged pain Postoperative pain
Premature Infant Pain Profile (PIPP)[32–34] (1996, 1999)	N = 211, 43, 24 Age: 28–40 wk GA	GA Behavioral state Maximum HR % Decrease in O_2 sat Brow bulge Eye squeeze Nasolabial furrow	Heel lance	Patients served as controls Internal consistency: 0.71 Construct validity: established Interrater reliability: 0.93–0.96 Intrarater reliability: 0.94–0.98	Acute pain
Neonatal Pain Agitation and Sedation Scale (NPASS)[35,36] (2010) (http://www.n-pass.com/research.html)	N = 42 Age: 23–40 wk GA 1–100 DOL	Crying Behavioral state Facial expressions Extremities/tone Vital signs (HR, BP, RR, O_2 sat)	Heel lance	Validated against PIPP Interrater reliability: 0.86–0.93 Internal consistency: 0.84–0.89 Construct (discriminate) validity: established Convergent validity: correlation with the PIPP scores Spearman rank correlation coefficient of 0.75 and 0.72 Test-retest reliability: 0.87	Acute pain Prolonged pain Level of sedation
Behavioral Indicators of Infant Pain (BIIP)[37] (2007)	N = 92 Age: 24–32 wk GA	Behavioral state Facial expressions Hand movements	Heel lance	Validated against NIPS Internal consistency: 0.82 Interrater reliability: 0.80–0.92 Construct validity: 85.9 Concurrent validity: correlations between the BIIP and NIPS = 0.64. Correlations between the BIIP and mean HR also remained moderate between GAs: earlier born = 0.33, $P < .05$; later born, $r = 0.50$, $P < .001$	Acute pain
Douleur Aiguë du Nouveau-né (DAN)[38] (1997)	N = 42 Age: 24–41 wk GA	Facial movements Limb movements Vocal expression	Heel lance Venipuncture	Patients served as controls Internal consistency: 0.88 Interrater reliability: 91.2 (Krippendorf)	Procedural pain
Premature Infant Pain Profile—Revised (PIPP-R)[40,41] (2014)	N = 52, 85, 31 Age: 25–40 wk GA	Maximum HR % Decrease in O_2 sat Brow bulge Eye squeeze Nasolabial furrow GA and behavioral state assessed if pain response detected	Retrospective comparison of PIPP and PIPP-R scores	Validated against PIPP Construct validity: established Feasibility: established	Acute pain

TABLE 1 Continued

Pain Assessment Tool	Number and GA of Infants Studied	Indicators	Intervention Studied	Validation Methodology	Intended Use
Faceless Acute Neonatal Pain Scale (FANS)[42] (2010)	$N = 53$ Age: 30–35 wk GA	HR change Acute discomfort (bradycardia, desat) Limb movements Vocal expression (must be nonintubated)	Heel lance	Validated against DAN Interrater reliability: 0.92 (0.9–0.98) Internal consistency: Cronbach's $\alpha = 0.72$ The ICC between the FANS and DAN scores was 0.88 (0.76–0.93)	Acute pain Developed for use when the neonate's face is not completely visible related to respiratory devices
Neonatal Infant Pain Scale (NIPS)[43] (1993)	$N = 38$ Age: 26–47 wk GA	Facial expression Crying Breathing patterns Arm movements Leg movements State of arousal	Needle insertion	Validated against VAS Concurrent validity: correlations with VAS ranged from 0.53 to 0.84. Interrater reliability: 0.92–0.97 Internal consistency: Cronbach's α's were 0.95, 0.87, and 0.88 for before, during, and after the procedures, respectively	Acute pain Postoperative pain
Crying Requires Increased oxygen administration, Increased vital signs, Expression, Sleeplessness (CRIES)[44] (1995)	$N = 24$ Age: 32–60 wk GA 1382 observations	Crying Requires O_2 to maintain sat at 95% Increased blood pressure, HR Expression Sleep state	Postoperative pain	Validated against the Objective Pain Score Interrater reliability: 0.72 Construct validity: yes Discriminant validity: yes	Prolonged pain Postoperative pain
COMFORTneo[45] (2009)	$N = 286$ Age: 24.6–42.6 wk GA 3600 assessments	Alertness Calmness/agitation Respiratory response in ventilated patient Crying in spontaneously breathing patient Body movement Facial tension Body muscle tone	Tertiary NICU care, including ventilation	Validated against Numeric Rating Scale Internal consistency: Cronbach's $\alpha = 0.88$ for nonventilated, 0.84 for ventilated patients Interrater reliability: 0.79 Concurrent validity: Pearson product-moment correlation coefficient between COMFORTneo and NRS-pain = 0.54 Correlation coefficient: 0.75 (95% confidence interval: 0.70–0.79; $P < 0001$)	Persistent or prolonged pain Level of sedation
COVERS Neonatal pain scale[46] (2010)	$N = 21$ Age: 27–40 wk GA	Crying F_{IO_2} requirement Vital signs (HR, BP, frequency of apnea/bradycardia Facial expression Resting state Body movements	Heel lance	Validated different GAs against CRIES, NIPS, and PIPP Concurrent validity: premature infants PIPP versus COVERS, $r = 0.84$; full-term infants NIPS versus COVERS, $r = 0.95$ Construct validity: baseline ($P < .05$); heel stick ($P < .05$); recovery ($P < .05$)	Acute pain

TABLE 1 Continued

Pain Assessment Tool	Number and GA of Infants Studied	Indicators	Intervention Studied	Validation Methodology	Intended Use
Pain Assessment in Neonates (PAIN)[47] (2002)	N = 196 neonates Age: 26–47 wk GA	Facial expression Cry Breathing pattern Extremity movement State of arousal F_{IO_2} required for sat >95% Increase in HR	Heel lance, suctioning, IV placement, circumcision, NG tube insertion, tape or IV removal	Adapted from NIPS and CRIES Inter-rater reliability: not established Correlation between the total scores on the two scales (NIPS and PAIN) was 0.93 ($P < .001$).	Acute pain
Pain Assessment Tool (PAT)[48,49] (2005)	N = 144 Age: 27–40 wk GA	Posture/tone Cry Sleep pattern Expression Color Respirations HR O_2 sat BP Nurse's perception	Ventilated and postoperative neonates	Validated against CRIES and VAS Interrater reliability: 0.85 Correlation between PAT and CRIES scores (r = 0.76) and (0.38) between the PAT score and VAS	Prolonged pain
Scale for Use in Newborns (SUN)[50] (1998)	N = 33 Age: 24–40 wk GA 0–214 DOL 68 procedures	CNS state Breathing Movement Tone Face HR changes Mean BP changes	Intubation PIV insertion	Validated against NIPS and COMFORT Coefficient of variation: 33 ± 8%	Acute pain
Échelle Douleur Inconfort Nouveau-Né (EDIN)[51] (2001)	N = 76 Age: 25–36 wk GA	Facial activity Body movements Quality of sleep Quality of contact with nurses Consolability	Acute and chronic ventilation; NEC, postoperative for PDA ligation	Patients served as controls Interrater reliability: coefficient range of 0.59–0.74 Internal consistency: Cronbach's α coefficients ranged from 0.86 to 0.94	Prolonged pain
Bernese Pain Scale for Neonates (BPSN)[52] (2004)	N = 12 Age: 27–41 wk GA 288 pain assessments	Alertness Duration of crying Time to calm Skin color Eyebrow bulge with eye squeeze Posture Breathing pattern	Heel lance	Validated against VAS and PIPP Concurrent and convergent validity: compared with VAS and PIPP was r = 0.86 and r = 0.91, respectively ($P < .0001$) Interrater reliability: r = 0.86–0.97 Intrarater reliability: r = 0.98–0.99	Acute pain

BP, blood pressure; CNS, central nervous system; desat, desaturation; DOL, days of life; F_{IO_2}, fraction of inspired oxygen; GA, gestational age; HR, heart rate; ICC, intraclass correlation coefficient; IV, intravenous (catheter); NEC, necrotizing enterocolitis; NG, nasogastric; PDA, patent ductus arteriosus; PIV, peripheral intravenous (line); RR, respiratory rate; sat, saturation; VAS, visual analog scale.

tool will be satisfactory for assessing neonatal pain for all situations and in infants of all gestational ages,[39,57] although initial validation studies have been published for the PIPP-Revised in infants with a gestational age of 25 to 41 weeks.[40,41] More research needs to be performed to assess the intensity of both acute and chronic pain at the bedside, to differentiate signs and symptoms of pain from those attributable to other causes, and to understand the significance of situations when there is no perceptible response to pain.[40,41] However, even with those limitations, one can use the available evidence to choose a pain assessment tool that is appropriate for the type of pain assessed (acute, prolonged, postoperative) and advocate for the competency of the neonatal care provider team with the specific use of that tool.[58] Table 1 lists commonly used pain assessment tools and the evidence used to test them.

NONPHARMACOLOGIC TREATMENT STRATEGIES

Pediatricians and health care professionals who work with neonates have the difficult task of balancing the need for appropriate monitoring, testing, and treatment versus minimizing pain and stress to the patient. Nonpharmacologic strategies for pain management, such as swaddling combined with positioning, facilitated tucking (holding the infant in a flexed position with arms close to the trunk) with or without parental assistance, nonnutritive sucking, and massage, have all shown variable effectiveness in reducing pain and/or stress-related behaviors related to mild to moderately painful or stressful interventions.[59–63] A meta-analysis of 51 studies of nonpharmacologic interventions used during heel lance and intravenous catheter insertion found that sucking-related and swaddling/facilitated-tucking interventions were beneficial for

preterm neonates and that sucking-related and rocking/holding interventions were beneficial for term neonates, but that no benefit was evident among older infants.[64]

Skin-to-skin care (SSC), with or without sucrose or glucose administration, has been shown to decrease some measures of pain in preterm and term infants.[65] An analysis of 19 studies examining the effects of SSC on neonatal pain caused by single needle-related procedures found no statistical benefit for physiologic indicators of pain but did show benefit for composite pain score items.[65] However, some investigators have reported decreased cortisol concentrations and decreased autonomic indicators of pain in preterm infants during SSC, suggestive of a physiologic benefit.[66,67]

The effects of breastfeeding on pain response have also been investigated. A Cochrane systematic review published in 2012 found that breastfeeding during a heel lance or venipuncture was associated with significantly lower pain responses in term neonates (eg, smaller increases in heart rate and shorter crying time), compared with other nonpharmacologic interventions such as positioning, rocking, or maternal holding. Breastfeeding showed similar effectiveness to oral sucrose or glucose solutions.[68] This meta-analysis of 20 randomized controlled trials (RCTs)/quasi-RCTs also found that providing supplemental human milk via a pacifier or syringe seems to be as effective as providing sucrose or glucose for pain relief in term neonates.

Sensorial stimulation (SS), a method of gently stimulating the tactile, gustatory, auditory, and visual systems simultaneously, has shown effectiveness at decreasing pain during minor procedures such as heel lance.[69] SS is achieved by looking at and gently talking to the infant, while stroking or massaging the face

or back, and providing oral sucrose or glucose solution before a painful procedure. A systematic review of 16 studies found that SS was more effective than sucrose when all elements of SS were used,[69] and 1 study suggested that SS may play an important role in nonpharmacologic management of procedural pain for neonates.[70]

PHARMACOLOGIC TREATMENT STRATEGIES

Sucrose and Glucose

Oral sucrose is commonly used to provide analgesia to infants during mild to moderately painful procedures. It has been extensively studied for this purpose, yet many gaps in knowledge remain, including appropriate dosing, mechanism of action, soothing versus analgesic effects, and long-term consequences.[71–73] A meta-analysis of 57 studies including >4730 infants with gestational ages ranging from 25 to 44 weeks concluded that sucrose is safe and effective for reducing procedural pain from a single event.[74]

Maximum reductions in physiologic and behavioral pain indicators have been noted when sucrose was administered ~2 minutes before a painful stimulus, and the effects lasted ~4 minutes.[74–76] Procedures of longer duration, such as ophthalmologic examinations or circumcision, may require multiple doses of sucrose to provide continual analgesic effect.[76] In animal studies, the analgesic effects of sucrose appear to be a sweet-taste-mediated response of opiate, endorphin, and possibly dopamine or acetylcholine pathways; however, the mechanism of action is not well understood in human neonates.[72,77–81] An additive analgesic effect has been noted when sucrose is used in conjunction with other nonpharmacologic measures, such as nonnutritive sucking and swaddling, especially for procedures such as ophthalmologic examinations and immunizations.[74,78] Although the evidence that oral sucrose alleviates procedurally related pain and stress, as judged by clinical pain scores, appears to be strong, a small RCT found no difference in either nociceptive brain activity on electroencephalography or spinal nociceptive reflex withdrawal on electromyography between sucrose or sterile water administered to term infants before a heel lance.[73] This masked study did find, however, that clinical pain scores were decreased in the infants receiving sucrose, and several methodologic concerns limit the conclusions that can be drawn from the trial.[74]

Sucrose use is common in most nurseries; however, doses vary widely.[82] Although an optimal dose has not been determined,[74] an oral dose of 0.1 to 1 mL of 24% sucrose (or 0.2–0.5 mL/kg) 2 minutes before a painful procedure has been recommended, taking into account gestational age, severity of illness, and procedure to be performed.[71] The role and safety of long-term sucrose use for persistent, ongoing pain have not been systematically studied. One study in 107 preterm infants of <31 weeks' gestation found worse neurodevelopmental scores at 32, 36, and 40 weeks' gestational age in infants who had received >10 doses of sucrose over a 24-hour period in the first week of life, raising concerns about frequent dosing in newly born preterm infants.[83,84] In addition, 1 infant in that study developed hyperglycemia coincident with frequent sucrose dosing, which may have been related to the sucrose or to subsequently diagnosed sepsis.[83] When sucrose is used as a pain management strategy, it should be prescribed and tracked as a medication. More research is needed to better understand the effects of sucrose use for analgesia.[71,81,84]

Glucose has also been found to be effective in decreasing response to brief painful procedures. A meta-analysis of 38 RCTs that included 3785 preterm and term neonates found that the administration of 20% to 30% glucose solutions reduced pain scores and decreased crying during heel lance and venipuncture compared with water or no intervention. The authors concluded that glucose could be used as an alternative to sucrose solutions, although no recommendations about dose or timing of administration could be made.[85] As described for sucrose, however, glucose may not be effective for longer procedures. For example, an RCT found no effect of glucose on pain response during ophthalmologic examinations.[86]

Opioids, Benzodiazepines, and Other Drugs

The most common pharmacologic agents used for pain relief in newborns are opioids, with fentanyl and morphine most often used, especially for persistent pain. Analgesics and sedatives are known to be potent modulators of several G-protein–linked receptor signaling pathways in the developing brain that are implicated in the critical regulation of neural tissue proliferation, survival, and differentiation. Studies of appropriate dosing and long-term effects of these analgesics given during the neonatal period are woefully lacking and/or conflicting.[87,88] However, in their absence, it remains critical to achieve adequate pain control in newborns, both as an ethical duty and because painful experiences in the NICU can have long-term adverse effects.[7,10,19,20,89]

Studies evaluating pharmacologic prevention and treatment of mild to moderate pain have generally been limited to a specific procedure such as intubation. The AAP recommends routine pain management during procedures such as circumcision,[90] chest drain insertion and removal,[2] and nonemergency intubations.[91]

However, effective management strategies for pain and sedation during mechanical ventilation remain elusive. A recent systematic review reported limited favorable effect with selective rather than routine use of opioids for analgesia in mechanically ventilated infants.[92] Concerns have been raised for adverse short- and long-term neurodevelopmental outcomes related to the use of morphine infusions in preterm neonates.[92,93] However, a follow-up study in ninety 8- to 9-year-olds who had previously participated in 1 RCT comparing continuous morphine infusion with placebo found that low-dose morphine infusion did not affect cognition or behavior and may have had a positive effect on everyday executive functions for these children.[87]

A 2008 Cochrane systematic review found insufficient evidence to recommend the routine use of opioids in mechanically ventilated infants.[94] Although there appeared to be a reduction in pain, there were no long-term benefits favoring the treatment groups; and concerns for adverse effects, such as respiratory depression, increase in the duration of mechanical ventilation, and development of dependence and tolerance, were raised. Other short-term physiologic adverse effects of concern included hypotension, constipation, and urinary retention for morphine and bradycardia and chest wall rigidity for fentanyl.[94] Remifentanil, a shorter-acting fentanyl derivative, may be an alternative for short-term procedures and surgeries because it is not cleared by liver metabolism, but there are no studies examining its long-term effects.[95,96]

Benzodiazepines, most commonly midazolam, are frequently used in the NICU for sedation. However, because there is evidence of only minor additional analgesic effect, they may not provide much benefit. These agents can potentiate the respiratory depression and hypotension that can occur with opioids, and infants receiving them should be carefully monitored.[97] Midazolam was associated with adverse short-term effects in the NOPAIN (Neonatal Outcome and Prolonged Analgesia in Neonates) trial.[98] A systematic review in 2012 found insufficient evidence to recommend midazolam infusions for sedation in the NICU and raised safety concerns, particularly regarding neurotoxicity.[97]

Alternative medications, such as methadone,[99] ketamine, propofol, and dexmedetomidine, have been proposed for pain management in neonates; however, few, if any, studies of these agents have been performed in this population, and caution should be exercised when considering them for use because of concerns about unanticipated adverse effects and potential neurotoxic effects.[100] Although the potential benefits of using methadone for the treatment of neonatal pain include satisfactory analgesic effects and enteral bioavailability as well as prolonged duration of action related to its long half-life and lower expense compared with other opiates, safe and effective dosing regimens have yet to be developed.[101] Ketamine is a dissociative anesthetic that, in lower doses, provides good analgesia, amnesia, and sedation.[102] Although ketamine has been well studied in older populations, further research is needed to establish safety profiles for use in neonates because of concerns regarding possible neurotoxicity.[103] Propofol has been used for short procedural sedation in children because of its rapid onset and clearance. The clearance of propofol in the neonatal population is inversely related to postmenstrual age, with significant variability in its pharmacokinetics in preterm and term neonates.[104] It has also been associated with bradycardia, desaturations, and

prolonged hypotension in newborn infants.[105] Limited experience with dexmedetomidine in preterm and term infants suggests that it may provide effective sedation and analgesia. Preliminary pharmacokinetic data showed decreased clearance in preterm infants compared with term infants and a favorable safety profile over a 24-hour period.[106]

The use of oral or intravenous acetaminophen has been limited to postoperative pain control. Although intravenous acetaminophen has not been approved by the US Food and Drug Administration, preliminary data on its safety and efficacy are promising in neonates and infants and it may decrease the total amount of morphine needed to treat postoperative pain.[107–109] Nonsteroidal antiinflammatory medication use has been restricted to pharmacologic closure of patent ductus arteriosus because of concerns regarding renal insufficiency, platelet dysfunction, and the development of pulmonary hypertension.[110] An animal study suggests that cyclooxygenase-1 inhibitors are less effective in immature compared with mature animals, probably because of decreased cyclooxygenase-1 receptor expression in the spinal cord.[110] This decrease in receptor expression may explain the lack of efficacy of nonsteroidal antiinflammatory drugs in human infants.[111]

Topical Anesthetic Agents

Topical anesthesia may provide pain relief during some procedures. The most commonly studied and used topical agents in the neonatal population are tetracaine gel and Eutectic Mixture of Local Anesthetics (EMLA), a mixture of 2.5% lidocaine and 2.5% prilocaine. These agents have been found to decrease measures of pain during venipuncture, percutaneous central venous catheter insertion, and

peripheral arterial puncture.[112–114] EMLA did not decrease pain-related measures during heel lance[113] but may decrease pain measures during lumbar puncture,[115] particularly if the patient is concurrently provided with oral sucrose or glucose solution.[116] Concerns related to the use of topical anesthetics include methemaglobinemia, prolonged application times to allow absorption for optimal effectiveness, local skin irritation, and toxicity, especially in preterm infants.[117,118]

CONCLUSIONS AND RECOMMENDATIONS

In summary, there are significant research gaps regarding the assessment, management, and outcomes of neonatal pain; and there is a continuing need for studies evaluating the effects of neonatal pain and pain-prevention strategies on long-term neurodevelopmental, behavioral, and cognitive outcomes. The use of pharmacologic treatments for pain prevention and management in neonates continues to be hampered by the paucity of data on the short- and long-term safety and efficacy of these agents. At the same time, repetitive pain in the NICU has been associated with adverse neurodevelopmental, behavioral, and cognitive outcomes, calling for more research to address gaps in knowledge.[5,8,22,89,119–122] Despite incomplete data, the pediatrician and other health care professionals who care for neonates face the need to weigh both of these concerns in assessing pain and the need for pain prevention and management on a continuing basis throughout the infant's hospitalization.

Recommendations

1. Preventing or minimizing pain in neonates should be the goal of pediatricians and other health care professionals who care for neonates. To facilitate this goal, each institution should

have written guidelines, based on existing and emerging evidence, for a stepwise pain-prevention and treatment plan, which includes judicious use of procedures, routine assessment of pain, use of both pharmacologic and nonpharmacologic therapies for the prevention of pain associated with routine minor procedures, and effective medications to minimize pain associated with surgery and other major procedures.

2. Despite the significant challenges of assessing pain in this population, currently available, validated neonatal pain assessment tools should be consistently used before, during, and after painful procedures to monitor the effectiveness of pain relief interventions. In addition, the need for pain prevention and management should be assessed on a continuing basis throughout the infant's hospitalization.

3. Nonpharmacologic strategies, such as facilitated tucking, nonnutritive sucking, provision of breastfeeding or providing expressed human milk, or SS have been shown to be useful in decreasing pain scores during short-term mild to moderately painful procedures and should be consistently used.

4. Oral sucrose and/or glucose solutions can be effective in neonates undergoing mild to moderately painful procedures, either alone or in combination with other pain relief strategies. When sucrose or glucose is used as a pain management strategy, it should be prescribed and tracked as a medication; evidence-based protocols should be developed and implemented in nurseries, and more research should be conducted to better understand the effects of sucrose use for analgesia.

5. The pediatrician and other health care professionals who care for neonates must weigh potential and actual benefits and burdens when using pharmacologic treatment methods based on available evidence. Some medications can potentiate the respiratory depression and hypotension that can occur with opioids, and infants receiving them should be carefully monitored. Caution should be exercised when considering newer medications for which data in neonates are sparse or nonexistent.

6. Pediatricians, other neonatal health care providers, and family members should receive continuing education regarding the recognition, assessment, and management of pain in neonates, including new evidence as it becomes available.

7. To address the gaps in knowledge, more research should be conducted on pain assessment tools and pharmacologic and nonpharmacologic strategies to prevent or ameliorate pain. Studies on pharmacokinetics and pharmacodynamics of newer medications are needed to prevent therapeutic misadventures in the most vulnerable patients in pediatric practice.

LEAD AUTHORS

Erin Keels, APRN, MS, NNP-BC
Navil Sethna, MD, FAAP

COMMITTEE ON FETUS AND NEWBORN, 2015–2016

Kristi L. Watterberg, MD, FAAP, Chairperson
James J. Cummings, MD, FAAP
William E. Benitz, MD, FAAP
Eric C. Eichenwald, MD, FAAP
Brenda B. Poindexter, MD, FAAP
Dan L. Stewart, MD, FAAP
Susan W. Aucott, MD, FAAP
Jay P. Goldsmith, MD, FAAP
Karen M. Puopolo, MD, PhD, FAAP
Kasper S. Wang, MD, FAAP

LIAISONS

Tonse N.K. Raju, MD, DCH, FAAP — *National Institutes of Health*
Captain Wanda D. Barfield, MD, MPH, FAAP — *Centers for Disease Control and Prevention*
Erin L. Keels, APRN, MS, NNP-BC — *National Association of Neonatal Nurses*
Thierry Lacaze, MD — *Canadian Pediatric Society*
Maria Mascola, MD — *American College of Obstetricians and Gynecologists*

STAFF

Jim Couto, MA

SECTION ON ANESTHESIOLOGY AND PAIN MEDICINE EXECUTIVE COMMITTEE, 2014–2015

Joseph D. Tobias, MD, FAAP, Chairperson
Rita Agarwal, MD, FAAP, Chairperson-Elect
Corrie T.M. Anderson, MD, FAAP
Courtney A. Hardy, MD, FAAP
Anita Honkanen, MD, FAAP
Mohamed A. Rehman, MD, FAAP
Carolyn F. Bannister, MD, FAAP

LIAISONS

Randall P. Flick, MD, MPH, FAAP — *American Society of Anesthesiologists Committee on Pediatrics*
Constance S. Houck, MD, FAAP — *AAP Committee on Drugs*

STAFF

Jennifer Riefe, MEd

ABBREVIATIONS

AAP: American Academy of Pediatrics
PIPP: Premature Infant Pain Profile
RCT: randomized controlled trial
SS: sensorial stimulation
SSC: skin-to-skin care

REFERENCES

1. American Academy of Pediatrics Committee on Fetus and Newborn, Committee on Drugs, Section on Anesthesiology, Section on Surgery; Canadian Paediatric Society Fetus and Newborn Committee. Prevention and management of pain and stress in the neonate. *Pediatrics*. 2000;105(2):454–461

2. Batton DG, Barrington KJ, Wallman C; American Academy of Pediatrics

Committee on Fetus and Newborn; American Academy of Pediatrics Section on Surgery; Canadian Paediatric Society Fetus and Newborn Committee. Prevention and management of pain in the neonate: an update. *Pediatrics.* 2006;118(5):2231–2241

3. Carbajal R, Rousset A, Danan C, et al. Epidemiology and treatment of painful procedures in neonates in intensive care units. *JAMA.* 2008;300(1):60–70

4. Simons SH, van Dijk M, Anand KS, Roofthooft D, van Lingen RA, Tibboel D. Do we still hurt newborn babies? A prospective study of procedural pain and analgesia in neonates. *Arch Pediatr Adolesc Med.* 2003;157(11):1058–1064

5. Anand KJ, Aranda JV, Berde CB, et al. Summary proceedings from the neonatal pain-control group. *Pediatrics.* 2006;117(3 Suppl 1):S9–S22

6. Anand KJ. Clinical importance of pain and stress in preterm neonates. *Biol Neonate.* 1998;73(1):1–9

7. Vinall J, Grunau RE. Impact of repeated procedural pain-related stress in infants born very preterm. *Pediatr Res.* 2014;75(5):584–587

8. Doesburg SM, Chau CM, Cheung TP, et al. Neonatal pain-related stress, functional cortical activity and visual-perceptual abilities in school-age children born at extremely low gestational age. *Pain.* 2013;154(10):1946–1952

9. Hermann C, Hohmeister J, Demirakça S, Zohsel K, Flor H. Long-term alteration of pain sensitivity in school-aged children with early pain experiences. *Pain.* 2006;125(3):278–285

10. Grunau RE, Whitfield MF, Petrie-Thomas J, et al. Neonatal pain, parenting stress and interaction, in relation to cognitive and motor development at 8 and 18 months in preterm infants. *Pain.* 2009;143(1–2):138–146

11. Walker SM, Franck LS, Fitzgerald M, Myles J, Stocks J, Marlow N. Long-term impact of neonatal intensive care and surgery on somatosensory perception in children born extremely preterm. *Pain.* 2009;141(1–2):79–87

12. Beggs S, Torsney C, Drew LJ, Fitzgerald M. The postnatal reorganization of primary afferent input and dorsal horn cell receptive fields in the rat spinal cord is an activity-dependent process. *Eur J Neurosci.* 2002;16(7):1249–1258

13. Jennings E, Fitzgerald M. Postnatal changes in responses of rat dorsal horn cells to afferent stimulation: a fibre-induced sensitization. *J Physiol.* 1998;509(pt 3):859–868

14. Schmelzle-Lubiecki BM, Campbell KA, Howard RH, Franck L, Fitzgerald M. Long-term consequences of early infant injury and trauma upon somatosensory processing. *Eur J Pain.* 2007;11(7):799–809

15. Ranger M, Chau CM, Garg A, et al. Neonatal pain-related stress predicts cortical thickness at age 7 years in children born very preterm. *PLoS One.* 2013;8(10):e76702

16. Slater R, Cantarella A, Gallella S, et al. Cortical pain responses in human infants. *J Neurosci.* 2006;26(14):3662–3666

17. Ingram RA, Fitzgerald M, Baccei ML. Developmental changes in the fidelity and short-term plasticity of GABAergic synapses in the neonatal rat dorsal horn. *J Neurophysiol.* 2008;99(6):3144–3150

18. Walker SM, Meredith-Middleton J, Lickiss T, Moss A, Fitzgerald M. Primary and secondary hyperalgesia can be differentiated by postnatal age and ERK activation in the spinal dorsal horn of the rat pup. *Pain.* 2007;128(1–2):157–168

19. Holsti L, Grunau RE, Oberlander TF, Whitfield MF. Prior pain induces heightened motor responses during clustered care in preterm infants in the NICU. *Early Hum Dev.* 2005;81(3):293–302

20. Grunau RE, Holsti L, Haley DW, et al. Neonatal procedural pain exposure predicts lower cortisol and behavioral reactivity in preterm infants in the NICU. *Pain.* 2005;113(3):293–300

21. Cignacco E, Hamers J, van Lingen RA, et al. Neonatal procedural pain exposure and pain management in ventilated preterm infants during the first 14 days of life. *Swiss Med Wkly.* 2009;139(15–16):226–232

22. Bouza H. The impact of pain in the immature brain. *J Matern Fetal Neonatal Med.* 2009;22(9):722–732

23. Bellieni CV, Iantorno L, Perrone S, et al. Even routine painful procedures can be harmful for the newborn. *Pain.* 2009;147(1–3):128–131

24. Slater L, Asmerom Y, Boskovic DS, et al. Procedural pain and oxidative stress in premature neonates. *J Pain.* 2012;13(6):590–597

25. Fitzgerald M. The development of nociceptive circuits. *Nat Rev Neurosci.* 2005;6(7):507–520

26. Hohmeister J, Demirakça S, Zohsel K, Flor H, Hermann C. Responses to pain in school-aged children with experience in a neonatal intensive care unit: cognitive aspects and maternal influences. *Eur J Pain.* 2009;13(1):94–101

27. Grunau RE, Whitfield MF, Fay TB. Psychosocial and academic characteristics of extremely low birth weight (< or =800 g) adolescents who are free of major impairment compared with term-born control subjects. *Pediatrics.* 2004;114(6). Available at: www.pediatrics.org/cgi/content/full/114/6/e725

28. Anand KJ; International Evidence-Based Group for Neonatal Pain. Consensus statement for the prevention and management of pain in the newborn. *Arch Pediatr Adolesc Med.* 2001;155(2):173–180

29. Hummel P, van Dijk M. Pain assessment: current status and challenges. *Semin Fetal Neonatal Med.* 2006;11(4):237–245

30. Grunau RE, Oberlander T, Holsti L, Whitfield MF. Bedside application of the Neonatal Facial Coding System in pain assessment of premature neonates. *Pain.* 1998;76(3):277–286

31. Peters JW, Koot HM, Grunau RE, et al. Neonatal Facial Coding System for assessing postoperative pain in infants: item reduction is valid and feasible. *Clin J Pain.* 2003;19(6):353–363

32. Stevens B, Johnston C, Petryshen P, Taddio A. Premature Infant Pain Profile: development and initial validation. *Clin J Pain.* 1996;12(1):13–22

33. Ballantyne M, Stevens B, McAllister M, Dionne K, Jack A. Validation of the premature infant pain profile in the clinical setting. *Clin J Pain.* 1999;15(4):297–303

34. Jonsdottir RB, Kristjansdottir G. The sensitivity of the Premature Infant Pain Profile—PIPP to measure pain in hospitalized neonates. *J Eval Clin Pract.* 2005;11(6):598–605

35. Hummel P, Puchalski M, Creech SD, Weiss MG. Clinical reliability and validity of the N-PASS: neonatal pain, agitation and sedation scale with prolonged pain. *J Perinatol.* 2008;28(1):55–60

36. Hummel P, Lawlor-Klean P, Weiss MG. Validity and reliability of the N-PASS assessment tool with acute pain. *J Perinatol.* 2010;30(7):474–478

37. Holsti L, Grunau RE. Initial validation of the Behavioral Indicators of Infant Pain (BIIP). *Pain.* 2007;132(3):264–272

38. Carbajal R, Paupe A, Hoenn E, Lenclen R, Olivier-Martin M. [APN: evaluation behavioral scale of acute pain in newborn infants.] [Article in French]. *Arch Pediatr.* 1997;4(7):623–628

39. Cong X, McGrath JM, Cusson RM, Zhang D. Pain assessment and measurement in neonates: an updated review. *Adv Neonatal Care.* 2013;13(6):379–395

40. Stevens BJ, Gibbins S, Yamada J, et al. The premature infant pain profile-revised (PIPP-R): initial validation and feasibility. *Clin J Pain.* 2014;30(3):238–243

41. Gibbins S, Stevens BJ, Yamada J, et al. Validation of the Premature Infant Pain Profile-Revised (PIPP-R). *Early Hum Dev.* 2014;90(4):189–193

42. Milesi C, Cambonie G, Jacquot A, et al. Validation of a neonatal pain scale adapted to the new practices in caring for preterm newborns. *Arch Dis Child Fetal Neonatal Ed.* 2010;95(4):F263–F266

43. Lawrence J, Alcock D, McGrath P, Kay J, MacMurray SB, Dulberg C. The development of a tool to assess neonatal pain. *Neonatal Netw.* 1993;12(6):59–66

44. Krechel SW, Bildner J. CRIES: a new neonatal postoperative pain measurement score. Initial testing of validity and reliability. *Paediatr Anaesth.* 1995;5(1):53–61

45. van Dijk M, Roofthooft DW, Anand KJ, et al. Taking up the challenge of measuring prolonged pain in (premature) neonates: the COMFORTneo scale seems promising. *Clin J Pain.* 2009;25(7):607–616

46. Hand I, Noble L, Geiss D, Wozniak L, Hall C. COVERS Neonatal Pain Scale: development and validation. *Int J Pediatr.* 2010. Available at: www.hindawi.com/journals/ijpedi/2010/496719/. Accessed December 17, 2014

47. Hudson-Barr D, Capper-Michel B, Lambert S, Palermo TM, Morbeto K, Lombardo S. Validation of the Pain Assessment in Neonates (PAIN) scale with the Neonatal Infant Pain Scale (NIPS). *Neonatal Netw.* 2002;21(6):15–21

48. Hodgkinson K, Bear M, Thorn J, Van Blaricum S. Measuring pain in neonates: evaluating an instrument and developing a common language. *Aust J Adv Nurs.* 1994;12(1):17–22

49. Spence K, Gillies D, Harrison D, Johnston L, Nagy S. A reliable pain assessment tool for clinical assessment in the neonatal intensive care unit. *J Obstet Gynecol Neonatal Nurs.* 2005;34(1):80–86

50. Blauer T, Gerstmann D. A simultaneous comparison of three neonatal pain scales during common NICU procedures. *Clin J Pain.* 1998;14(1):39–47

51. Debillon T, Zupan V, Ravault N, Magny JF, Dehan M. Development and initial validation of the EDIN scale, a new tool for assessing prolonged pain in preterm infants. *Arch Dis Child Fetal Neonatal Ed.* 2001;85(1):F36–F41

52. Cignacco E, Mueller R, Hamers JP, Gessler P. Pain assessment in the neonate using the Bernese Pain Scale for Neonates. *Early Hum Dev.* 2004;78(2):125–131

53. Slater R, Cantarella A, Franck L, Meek J, Fitzgerald M. How well do clinical pain assessment tools reflect pain in infants? *PLoS Med.* 2008;5(6):e129

54. Smith GC, Gutovich J, Smyser C, et al. Neonatal intensive care unit stress is associated with brain development in preterm infants. *Ann Neurol.* 2011;70(4):541–549

55. Hünseler C, Merkt V, Gerloff M, Eifinger F, Kribs A, Roth B. Assessing pain in ventilated newborns and infants: validation of the Hartwig score. *Eur J Pediatr.* 2011;170(7):837–843

56. Arias MC, Guinsburg R. Differences between uni-and multidimensional scales for assessing pain in term newborn infants at the bedside. *Clinics (Sao Paulo).* 2012;67(10):1165–1170

57. Ahn Y, Jun Y. Measurement of pain-like response to various NICU stimulants for high-risk infants. *Early Hum Dev.* 2007;83(4):255–262

58. Walden M, Gibbins S. *Pain Assessment and Management: Guidelines for Practice.* 2nd ed. Glenview, IL: National Association of Neonatal Nurses; 2010

59. Morrow C, Hidinger A, Wilkinson-Faulk D. Reducing neonatal pain during routine heel lance procedures. *MCN Am J Matern Child Nurs.* 2010;35(6):346–354; quiz: 354–356

60. Axelin A, Salanterä S, Kirjavainen J, Lehtonen L. Oral glucose and parental holding preferable to opioid in pain management in preterm infants. *Clin J Pain.* 2009;25(2):138–145

61. Obeidat H, Kahalaf I, Callister LC, Froelicher ES. Use of facilitated tucking for nonpharmacological pain management in preterm infants: a systematic review. *J Perinat Neonatal Nurs.* 2009;23(4):372–377

62. Liaw JJ, Yang L, Katherine Wang KW, Chen CM, Chang YC, Yin T. Non-nutritive sucking and facilitated tucking relieve preterm infant pain during heel-stick procedures: a prospective, randomised controlled crossover trial. *Int J Nurs Stud.* 2012;49(3):300–309

63. Abdallah B, Badr LK, Hawwari M. The efficacy of massage on short and long term outcomes in preterm infants. *Infant Behav Dev.* 2013;36(4):662–669

64. Pillai Riddell RR, Racine NM, Turcotte K, et al. Non-pharmacological management of infant and young child procedural pain. *Cochrane Database Syst Rev.* 2011;20115(10):CD006275

65. Johnston C, Campbell-Yeo M, Fernandes A, Inglis D, Streiner D, Zee R. Skin-to-skin care for procedural pain

in neonates. *Cochrane Database Syst Rev.* 2014;1(1):CD008435

66. Cong X, Cusson RM, Walsh S, Hussain N, Ludington-Hoe SM, Zhang D. Effects of skin-to-skin contact on autonomic pain responses in preterm infants. *J Pain.* 2012;13(7):636–645

67. Cong X, Ludington-Hoe SM, Walsh S. Randomized crossover trial of kangaroo care to reduce biobehavioral pain responses in preterm infants: a pilot study. *Biol Res Nurs.* 2011;13(2):204–216

68. Shah PS, Herbozo C, Aliwalas LL, Shah VS. Breastfeeding or breast milk for procedural pain in neonates. *Cochrane Database Syst Rev.* 2012;12(12):CD004950

69. Bellieni CV, Tei M, Coccina F, Buonocore G. Sensorial saturation for infants' pain. *J Matern Fetal Neonatal Med.* 2012;25(suppl 1):79–81

70. Gitto E, Pellegrino S, Manfrida M, et al. Stress response and procedural pain in the preterm newborn: the role of pharmacological and non-pharmacological treatments. *Eur J Pediatr.* 2012;171(6):927–933

71. Harrison D, Beggs S, Stevens B. Sucrose for procedural pain management in infants. *Pediatrics.* 2012;130(5):918–925

72. Slater R, Cornelissen L, Fabrizi L, et al. Oral sucrose as an analgesic drug for procedural pain in newborn infants: a randomised controlled trial. *Lancet.* 2010;376(9748):1225–1232

73. Wilkinson DJ, Savulescu J, Slater R. Sugaring the pill: ethics and uncertainties in the use of sucrose for newborn infants. *Arch Pediatr Adolesc Med.* 2012;166(7):629–633

74. Stevens B, Yamada J, Lee GY, Ohlsson A. Sucrose for analgesia in newborn infants undergoing painful procedures. *Cochrane Database Syst Rev.* 2013;1(1):CD001069

75. Lefrak L, Burch K, Caravantes R, et al. Sucrose analgesia: identifying potentially better practices. *Pediatrics.* 2006;118(2 suppl 2):S197–S202

76. Johnston CC, Stremler R, Horton L, Friedman A. Effect of repeated doses of sucrose during heel stick procedure in preterm neonates. *Biol Neonate.* 1999;75(3):160–166

77. Fernandez M, Blass EM, Hernandez-Reif M, Field T, Diego M, Sanders C. Sucrose attenuates a negative electroencephalographic response to an aversive stimulus for newborns. *J Dev Behav Pediatr.* 2003;24(4):261–266

78. Blass EM, Watt LB. Suckling- and sucrose-induced analgesia in human newborns. *Pain.* 1999;83(3):611–623

79. Shide DJ, Blass EM. Opioidlike effects of intraoral infusions of corn oil and polycose on stress reactions in 10-day-old rats. *Behav Neurosci.* 1989;103(6):1168–1175

80. Anseloni VC, Ren K, Dubner R, Ennis M. A brainstem substrate for analgesia elicited by intraoral sucrose. *Neuroscience.* 2005;133(1):231–243

81. Holsti L, Grunau RE. Considerations for using sucrose to reduce procedural pain in preterm infants. *Pediatrics.* 2010;125(5):1042–1047

82. Taddio A, Yiu A, Smith RW, Katz J, McNair C, Shah V. Variability in clinical practice guidelines for sweetening agents in newborn infants undergoing painful procedures. *Clin J Pain.* 2009;25(2):153–155

83. Johnston CC, Filion F, Snider L, et al. Routine sucrose analgesia during the first week of life in neonates younger than 31 weeks' postconceptional age. *Pediatrics.* 2002;110(3):523–528

84. Johnston CC, Filion F, Snider L, et al. How much sucrose is too much sucrose [letter]? *Pediatrics.* 2007;119(1):226

85. Bueno M, Yamada J, Harrison D, et al. A systematic review and meta-analyses of nonsucrose sweet solutions for pain relief in neonates. *Pain Res Manag.* 2013;18(3):153–161

86. Costa MC, Eckert GU, Fortes BG, Fortes Filho JB, Silveira RC, Procianoy RS. Oral glucose for pain relief during examination for retinopathy of prematurity: a masked randomized clinical trial. *Clinics (Sao Paulo).* 2013;68(2):199–204

87. de Graaf J, van Lingen RA, Valkenburg AJ, et al. Does neonatal morphine use affect neuropsychological outcomes at 8 to 9 years of age? *Pain.* 2013;154(3):449–458

88. Rozé JC, Denizot S, Carbajal R, et al. Prolonged sedation and/or analgesia

and 5-year neurodevelopment outcome in very preterm infants: results from the EPIPAGE cohort. *Arch Pediatr Adolesc Med.* 2008;162(8):728–733

89. Whitfield MF, Grunau RE. Behavior, pain perception, and the extremely low-birth weight survivor. *Clin Perinatol.* 2000;27(2):363–379

90. American Academy of Pediatrics, Task Force on Circumcision. Circumcision policy statement. *Pediatrics.* 1999;103(3):686–693

91. Kumar P, Denson SE, Mancuso TJ; Committee on Fetus and Newborn, Section on Anesthesiology and Pain Medicine. Premedication for nonemergency endotracheal intubation in the neonate. *Pediatrics.* 2010;125(3):608–615

92. Bellù R, de Waal K, Zanini R. Opioids for neonates receiving mechanical ventilation: a systematic review and meta-analysis. *Arch Dis Child Fetal Neonatal Ed.* 2010;95(4):F241–F251

93. Anand KJ, Hall RW, Desai N, et al; NEOPAIN Trial Investigators Group. Effects of morphine analgesia in ventilated preterm neonates: primary outcomes from the NEOPAIN randomised trial. *Lancet.* 2004;363(9422):1673–1682

94. Bellù R, de Waal KA, Zanini R. Opioids for neonates receiving mechanical ventilation. *Cochrane Database Syst Rev.* 2008;1:CD004212

95. Choong K, AlFaleh K, Doucette J, et al. Remifentanil for endotracheal intubation in neonates: a randomised controlled trial. *Arch Dis Child Fetal Neonatal Ed.* 2010;95(2):F80–F84

96. Lago P, Tiozzo C, Boccuzzo G, Allegro A, Zacchello F. Remifentanil for percutaneous intravenous central catheter placement in preterm infant: a randomized controlled trial. *Paediatr Anaesth.* 2008;18(8):736–744

97. Ng E, Taddio A, Ohlsson A. Intravenous midazolam infusion for sedation of infants in the neonatal intensive care unit. *Cochrane Database Syst Rev.* 2012;6(6):CD002052

98. Anand KJ, Barton BA, McIntosh N, et al. Analgesia and sedation in preterm neonates who require ventilatory support: results from the NOPAIN trial. Neonatal Outcome and Prolonged

Analgesia in Neonates. *Arch Pediatr Adolesc Med.* 1999;153(4):331–338

99. Anand KJ. Pharmacological approaches to the management of pain in the neonatal intensive care unit. *J Perinatol.* 2007;27(suppl 1):S4–S11

100. Durrmeyer X, Vutskits L, Anand KJ, Rimensberger PC. Use of analgesic and sedative drugs in the NICU: integrating clinical trials and laboratory data. *Pediatr Res.* 2010;67(2):117–127

101. Chana SK, Anand KJ. Can we use methadone for analgesia in neonates? *Arch Dis Child Fetal Neonatal Ed.* 2001;85(2):F79–F81

102. Nemergut ME, Yaster M, Colby CE. Sedation and analgesia to facilitate mechanical ventilation. *Clin Perinatol.* 2013;40(3):539–558

103. Cravero JP, Havidich JE. Pediatric sedation—evolution and revolution. *Paediatr Anaesth.* 2011;21(7):800–809

104. Allegaert K, Peeters MY, Verbesselt R, et al. Inter-individual variability in propofol pharmacokinetics in preterm and term neonates. *Br J Anaesth.* 2007;99(6):864–870

105. Vanderhaegen J, Naulaers G, Van Huffel S, Vanhole C, Allegaert K. Cerebral and systemic hemodynamic effects of intravenous bolus administration of propofol in neonates. *Neonatology.* 2010;98(1):57–63

106. Chrysostomou C, Schulman SR, Herrera Castellanos M, et al. A phase II/III, multicenter, safety, efficacy, and pharmacokinetic study of dexmedetomidine in preterm and term neonates. *J Pediatr.* 2014;164(2):276–282

107. Allegaert K, van den Anker J. Pharmacokinetics and pharmacodynamics of intravenous acetaminophen in neonates. *Expert Rev Clin Pharmacol.* 2011;4(6):713–718

108. Ceelie I, de Wildt SN, van Dijk M, et al. Effect of intravenous paracetamol on postoperative morphine requirements in neonates and infants undergoing major noncardiac surgery: a randomized controlled trial. *JAMA.* 2013;309(2):149–154

109. Ohlsson A, Shah PS. Paracetamol (acetaminophen) for prevention or treatment of pain in newborns. *Cochrane Database Syst Rev.* 2015;6(6):CD011219

110. Ohlsson A, Walia R, Shah S. Ibuprofen for the treatment of patent ductus arteriosus in preterm and/or low birth weight infants. *Cochrane Database Syst Rev.* 2008;1:CD003481

111. Ririe DG, Prout HD, Barclay D, Tong C, Lin M, Eisenach JC. Developmental differences in spinal cyclooxygenase 1 expression after surgical incision. *Anesthesiology.* 2006;104(3):426–431

112. Taddio A, Ohlsson A, Einarson TR, Stevens B, Koren G. A systematic review of lidocaine-prilocaine cream (EMLA) in the treatment of acute pain in neonates. *Pediatrics.* 1998;101(2):e1

113. Kapellou O. Blood sampling in infants (reducing pain and morbidity). 2011;Apr 5: 2011. pii: 0313

114. Hall RW, Anand KJ. Pain management in newborns. *Clin Perinatol.* 2014;41(4):895–924

115. Kaur G, Gupta P, Kumar A. A randomized trial of eutectic mixture of local anesthetics during lumbar puncture in newborns. *Arch Pediatr Adolesc Med.* 2003;157(11):1065–1070

116. Biran V, Gourrier E, Cimerman P, Walter-Nicolet E, Mitanchez D, Carbajal R. Analgesic effects of EMLA cream and oral sucrose during venipuncture in preterm infants. *Pediatrics.* 2011;128(1). Available at: www.pediatrics.org/cgi/content/full/128/1/e63

117. Foster JP, Taylor C, Bredemeyer SL. Topical anaesthesia for needle-related pain in newborn infants. *Cochrane Database Syst Rev.* 2013; (1):CD010331

118. Maulidi H, McNair C, Seller N, Kirsh J, Bradley TJ, Greenway SC, Tomlinson C. Arrhythmia associated with tetracaine in an extremely low birth weight premature infant. *Pediatrics.* 2012;130(6). Available at: www.pediatrics.org/cgi/content/full/130/6/e1704

119. Harrison D, Yamada J, Stevens B. Strategies for the prevention and management of neonatal and infant pain. *Curr Pain Headache Rep.* 2010;14(2):113–123

120. Grunau R. Early pain in preterm infants: a model of long-term effects. *Clin Perinatol.* 2002;29(3):373–394, vii–viii

121. Taddio A, Shah V, Gilbert-MacLeod C, Katz J. Conditioning and hyperalgesia in newborns exposed to repeated heel lances. *JAMA.* 2002;288(7):857–861

122. Anand KJ, Johnston CC, Oberlander TF, Taddio A, Lehr VT, Walco GA. Analgesia and local anesthesia during invasive procedures in the neonate. *Clin Ther.* 2005;27(6):844–876

SECTION 7
Safe Sleep

CLINICAL REPORT Guidance for the Clinician in Rendering Pediatric Care

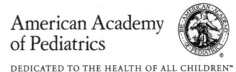

American Academy
of Pediatrics

DEDICATED TO THE HEALTH OF ALL CHILDREN™

Safe Sleep and Skin-to-Skin Care in the Neonatal Period for Healthy Term Newborns

Lori Feldman-Winter, MD, MPH, FAAP, Jay P. Goldsmith, MD, FAAP, COMMITTEE ON FETUS AND NEWBORN, TASK FORCE ON SUDDEN INFANT DEATH SYNDROME

abstract

Skin-to-skin care (SSC) and rooming-in have become common practice in the newborn period for healthy newborns with the implementation of maternity care practices that support breastfeeding as delineated in the World Health Organization's "Ten Steps to Successful Breastfeeding." SSC and rooming-in are supported by evidence that indicates that the implementation of these practices increases overall and exclusive breastfeeding, safer and healthier transitions, and improved maternal-infant bonding. In some cases, however, the practice of SSC and rooming-in may pose safety concerns, particularly with regard to sleep. There have been several recent case reports and case series of severe and sudden unexpected postnatal collapse in the neonatal period among otherwise healthy newborns and near fatal or fatal events related to sleep, suffocation, and falls from adult hospital beds. Although these are largely case reports, there are potential dangers of unobserved SSC immediately after birth and throughout the postpartum hospital period as well as with unobserved rooming-in for at-risk situations. Moreover, behaviors that are modeled in the hospital after birth, such as sleep position, are likely to influence sleeping practices after discharge. Hospitals and birthing centers have found it difficult to develop policies that will allow SSC and rooming-in to continue in a safe manner. This clinical report is intended for birthing centers and delivery hospitals caring for healthy newborns to assist in the establishment of appropriate SSC and safe sleep policies.

This document is copyrighted and is property of the American Academy of Pediatrics and its Board of Directors. All authors have filed conflict of interest statements with the American Academy of Pediatrics. Any conflicts have been resolved through a process approved by the Board of Directors. The American Academy of Pediatrics has neither solicited nor accepted any commercial involvement in the development of the content of this publication.

Clinical reports from the American Academy of Pediatrics benefit from expertise and resources of liaisons and internal (AAP) and external reviewers. However, clinical reports from the American Academy of Pediatrics may not reflect the views of the liaisons or the organizations or government agencies that they represent.

The guidance in this report does not indicate an exclusive course of treatment or serve as a standard of medical care. Variations, taking into account individual circumstances, may be appropriate.

All clinical reports from the American Academy of Pediatrics automatically expire 5 years after publication unless reaffirmed, revised, or retired at or before that time.

DOI: 10.1542/peds.2016-1889

PEDIATRICS (ISSN Numbers: Print, 0031-4005; Online, 1098-4275).

Copyright © 2016 by the American Academy of Pediatrics

FINANCIAL DISCLOSURE: The authors have indicated they do not have a financial relationship relevant to this article to disclose.

FUNDING: No external funding.

POTENTIAL CONFLICT OF INTEREST: The authors have indicated they have no potential conflicts of interest to disclose.

To cite: Feldman-Winter L, Goldsmith JP, AAP COMMITTEE ON FETUS AND NEWBORN, AAP TASK FORCE ON SUDDEN INFANT DEATH SYNDROME. Safe Sleep and Skin-to-Skin Care in the Neonatal Period for Healthy Term Newborns. *Pediatrics*. 2016;138(3):e20161889

INTRODUCTION

Definition of Skin-to-Skin Care and Rooming-In

Skin-to-skin care (SSC) is defined as the practice of placing infants in direct contact with their mothers or other caregivers with the ventral skin of the infant facing and touching the ventral skin of the mother/

caregiver (chest-to-chest). The infant is typically naked or dressed only in a diaper to maximize the surface-to-surface contact between mother/caregiver and the infant, and the dyad is covered with prewarmed blankets, leaving the infant's head exposed. SSC is recommended for all mothers and newborns, regardless of feeding or delivery method, immediately after birth (as soon as the mother is medically stable, awake, and able to respond to her newborn) and to continue for at least 1 hour, as defined by the World Health Organization's (WHO's) "Ten Steps to Successful Breastfeeding."[1,2] SSC is also a term used to describe continued holding of the infant in the manner described above and beyond the immediate delivery period and lasting throughout infancy, whenever the mother/caregiver and infant have the opportunity. For mothers planning to breastfeed, SSC immediately after delivery and continued throughout the postpartum period also involves encouraging mothers to recognize when their infants are ready to breastfeed and providing help if needed.[2] Additional recommendations by the WHO, as part of the Baby-Friendly Hospital Initiative and endorsed by the American Academy of Pediatrics (AAP) in 2009, include the following specifications for the period of time immediately after delivery: routine procedures such as assessments and Apgar scores are conducted while SSC is underway, and procedures that may be painful or require separation should be delayed until after the first hour; if breastfeeding, these procedures should occur after the first breastfeeding is completed.[3] The AAP further delineates that the administration of vitamin K and ophthalmic prophylaxis can be delayed for at least 1 hour and up to 4 hours after delivery. The Baby-Friendly Hospital Initiative encourages continued SSC throughout the hospital stay while rooming-in.[4]

Unless there is a medical reason for separation, such as resuscitation, SSC may be provided for all newborns. In the case of cesarean deliveries, SSC may also be provided when the mother is awake and able to respond to her infant. In some settings, SSC may be initiated in the operating room following cesarean deliveries, while in other settings SSC may begin in the recovery room. SSC for healthy newborns shall be distinguished from "kangaroo care" in this clinical report, because the latter applies to preterm newborns or infants cared for in the NICU.[5] This report is intended for mothers and infants who are well, are being cared for in the routine postpartum or mother-infant setting, and have not required resuscitation. Although sick or preterm newborns may benefit from SSC, this review is intended only for healthy term newborns. Late preterm infants (defined as a gestational age of 34–37 weeks) may also benefit from early SSC but are at increased risk of a number of early neonatal morbidities.[6]

Rooming-in is defined as allowing mothers and infants to remain together 24 hours per day while in the delivery hospital. This procedure is recommended for all mothers and their healthy newborns, regardless of feeding or delivery method, and in some cases applies to older late preterm (>35 weeks' gestation) or early term (37–39 weeks' gestation) newborns who are otherwise healthy and receiving routine care, who represent up to 70% of this population.[7] Mothers are expected to be more involved with routine care, such as feeding, holding, and bathing. Newborns may remain with their mothers unless there is a medical reason for separation for either the mother or the infant. Procedures that can be performed at the bedside can be performed while the infant is preferably being held skin-to-skin or at least in the room with the mother. Being held skin-to-skin by the mother has been shown to decrease pain in newborns undergoing painful procedures such as blood draws.[8,9] Mothers may nap, shower, or leave the room with the expectation that the mother-infant staff members monitor the newborn at routine intervals. Mothers are encouraged to use call bells for assistance with their own care or that of their newborns.

Evidence for SSC and Rooming-In

SSC has been researched extensively as a method to provide improved physiologic stability for newborns and potential benefits for mothers. SSC immediately after birth stabilizes the newborn body temperature and can help prevent hypothermia.[10,11] SSC also helps stabilize blood glucose concentrations, decreases crying, and provides cardiorespiratory stability, especially in late preterm newborns.[12] SSC has been shown in numerous studies as a method to decrease pain in newborns being held by mothers[13-16] and fathers.[17] In preterm infants, SSC has been shown to result in improved autonomic and neurobehavioral maturation and gastrointestinal adaptation, more restful sleep patterns, less crying, and better growth.[18-21] Although not specifically studied in full-term infants, it is likely that these infants also benefit in similar ways.

SSC also benefits mothers. Immediately after birth, SSC decreases maternal stress and improves paternal perception of stress in their relationship.[22] A recent study suggested that SSC and breastfeeding within 30 minutes of birth reduce postpartum hemorrhage.[23] Experimental models indicate that mother-infant separation causes significant stress, and the consequences of this stress on the hypothalamic-pituitary-adrenal axis persist.[24] In a randomized trial examining the relationship between SSC and maternal depression and stress, both depression scores and salivary cortisol concentrations were lower over the first month among postpartum mothers providing SSC compared with mothers who were provided no guidance about SSC.[22] For breastfeeding mother-infant dyads, SSC enhances the opportunity for an early first breastfeeding, which, in turn, leads to more readiness to breastfeed, an organized breastfeeding suckling pattern, and more success in exclusive and overall breastfeeding,[12,25,26] even after cesarean deliveries.[27] Further evidence shows a benefit for mothers after cesarean deliveries who practice SSC as soon as the mother is alert and responsive in increased breastfeeding initiation, decreased time to the first breastfeeding, reduced formula supplementation, and increased bonding and maternal satisfaction.[28] Increasing rates of breastfeeding ultimately have short- and long-term health benefits, such as decreased risk of infections, obesity, cancer, and sudden infant death syndrome.[3]

The evidence for rooming-in also extends beyond infant feeding practices and is consistent with contemporary models of family-centered care.[29] Rooming-in and the maternity care practices aligned with keeping mothers and newborns together in a hospital setting were defined as best practice but not fully implemented in the post–World War II era, largely because of nursing culture and the presumption that newborns were safer in a sterile nursery environment.[30] Rooming-in leads to improved patient satisfaction.[31,32] Integrated mother-infant care leads to optimal outcomes for healthy mothers and infants, including those with neonatal abstinence syndrome.[33] Rooming-in also provides more security, may avoid newborn abductions or switches, leads to decreased infant abandonment,[34] and provides more

opportunity for supervised maternal-newborn interactions.[35] Hospital staff members caring for mother-infant dyads have more opportunities to empower mothers to care for their infants than when infant care is conducted without the mother and in a separate nursery. For the breastfeeding mother-infant dyad, rooming-in may help to support cue-based feeding, leading to increased frequency of breastfeeding, especially in the first few days[36]; decreased hyperbilirubinemia; and increased likelihood of continued breastfeeding up to 6 months.[37]

SSC and rooming-in are 2 of the important steps in the WHO's "Ten Steps to Successful Breastfeeding" and serve as the basic tenets for a baby-friendly–designated delivery hospital.[1,38,39] The Ten Steps include practices that also improve patient safety and outcomes by supporting a more physiologic transition immediately after delivery; maintaining close contact between the mother and her newborn, which decreases the risk of infection and sepsis; increasing the opportunity for the development of a protective immunologic environment; decreasing stress responses by the mother and her infant; and enhancing sleep patterns in the mother.[40–42]

SAFETY CONCERNS REGARDING IMMEDIATE SSC

Rarely are there contraindications to providing SSC; however, there are potential safety concerns to address. A newborn requiring positive-pressure resuscitation should be continuously monitored, and SSC should be postponed until the infant is stabilized.[43] Furthermore, certain conditions, such as low Apgar scores (less than 7 at 5 minutes) or medical complications from birth, may require careful observation and monitoring of the newborn during SSC and in some cases may prevent SSC.[11] Other

safety concerns are attributable to the lack of standardization in the approach, discontinuous observation of the mother-infant dyad (with lapses exceeding 10 to 15 minutes during the first few hours of life), lack of education and skills among staff supporting the dyad during transition while skin-to-skin, and unfamiliarity with the potential risks of unsafe positioning and methods of assessment that may avert problems.[44] The main concerns regarding immediate postnatal SSC include sudden unexpected postnatal collapse (SUPC), which includes any condition resulting in temporary or permanent cessation of breathing or cardiorespiratory failure.[45–48] Many, but not all, of these events are related to suffocation or entrapment. In addition, falls may occur during SSC, particularly if unobserved, and other situations or conditions may occur that prevent SSC from continuing safely.[44,49]

SUPC is a rare but potentially fatal event in otherwise healthy-appearing term newborns. The definition of SUPC varies slightly depending on the author and population studied. One definition offered by the British Association of Perinatal Medicine[50] includes any term or near-term (defined as >35 weeks' gestation in this review) infant who meets the following criteria: (1) is well at birth (normal 5-minute Apgar and deemed well enough for routine care), (2) collapses unexpectedly in a state of cardiorespiratory extremis such that resuscitation with intermittent positive-pressure ventilation is required, (3) collapses within the first 7 days of life, and (4) either dies, goes on to require intensive care, or develops encephalopathy. Other potential medical conditions should be excluded (eg, sepsis, cardiac disease) for SUPC to be diagnosed. The incidence of SUPC in the first hours to days of life varies widely because of different definitions, inclusion and exclusion criteria of newborns being described, and lack of standardized reporting and may be higher in certain settings. The incidence is estimated to be 2.6 to 133 cases per 100 000 newborns. In 1 case series, the authors described one-third of SUPC events occurring in the first 2 hours of life, one-third occurring between 2 and 24 hours of life, and the final third occurring between 1 and 7 days of life.[51] Other authors suggested that 73% of SUPC events occur in the first 2 hours of life.[52] In the case series by Pejovic and Herlenius,[51] 15 of the 26 cases of SUPC were found to have occurred during SSC in a prone position. Eighteen were in primiparous mothers, 13 occurred during unsupervised breastfeeding at <2 hours of age, and 3 occurred during smart cellular phone use by the mother. Five developed grade 2 hypoxic-ischemic encephalopathy (moderate encephalopathy), with 4 requiring hypothermia treatment. Twenty-five of the 26 cases had favorable neurologic outcomes in 1 series; however, in another review, mortality was as high as 50%, and among survivors, 50% had neurologic sequelae.[53] Experimental models suggest that autoresuscitation of breathing after hypoxic challenge takes longer with lower postnatal age and decreased core body temperature.[54]

SUPC, in some definitions, includes acute life-threatening episodes; however, the latter is presumed to be more benign. An apparent life-threatening episode, or what may be referred to as a brief resolved unexplained event, may be low risk and require simple interventions such as positional changes, brief stimulation, or procedures to resolve airway obstruction.[46,53]

Falls are another concern in the immediate postnatal period. Mothers who are awake and able to respond to their newborn infant immediately after birth may become suddenly and unexpectedly sleepy, ill, or unable to continue holding their infant. Fathers or other support people providing SSC may also suddenly become unable to continue to safely hold the newborn because of lightheadedness, fatigue, incoordination, or other factors. If a hospital staff member is not immediately available to take over, unsafe situations may occur, and newborns may fall to the floor or may be positioned in a manner that obstructs their airway.

SUGGESTIONS TO IMPROVE SAFETY IMMEDIATELY AFTER DELIVERY

Several authors have suggested mechanisms for standardizing the procedure of immediate postnatal SSC to prevent sentinel events; however, none of the checklists or procedures developed have been proven to reduce the risk. Frequent and repetitive assessments, including observation of newborn breathing, activity, color, tone, and position, may avert positions that obstruct breathing or events leading to sudden collapse.[41] In addition, continuous monitoring by trained staff members and the use of checklists may improve safety.[35] Some have suggested continuous pulse oximetry; however, there is no evidence that this practice would improve safety, and it may be impractical. Given the occurrence of events in the first few hours of life, it is prudent to consider staffing the delivery unit to permit continuous staff observation with frequent recording of neonatal vital signs. A procedure manual that is implemented in a standardized fashion and practiced with simulation drills may include sequential steps identified in Box 1.[55]

BOX 1: PROCEDURE FOR IMMEDIATE SKIN-TO-SKIN CARE

1. Delivery of newborn
2. Dry and stimulate for first breath/cry, and assess newborn
3. If the newborn is stable, place skin to skin with cord attached (with option to milk cord), clamp cord after 1 minute or after placenta delivered, and reassess newborn to permit physiological circulatory transition[56]
4. Continue to dry entire newborn except hands to allow the infant to suckle hands bathed in amniotic fluid (which smells and tastes similar to colostrum), which facilitates rooting and first breastfeeding[57]
5. Cover head with cap (optional) and place prewarmed blankets to cover body of newborn on mother's chest, leaving face exposed[58]
6. Assess Apgar scores at 1 and 5 minutes
7. Replace wet blankets and cap with dry warm blankets and cap
8. Assist and support to breastfeed

Risk stratification and associated monitoring and care may avert SUPC, falls, and suffocation.[59] High-risk situations may include infants who required resuscitation (ie, any positive-pressure ventilation), those with low Apgar scores, late preterm and early term (37–39 weeks' gestation) infants, difficult delivery, mother receiving codeine[60] or other medications that may affect the newborn (eg, general anesthesia or magnesium sulfate), sedated mother, and excessively sleepy mothers and/or newborns. Mothers may be assessed to determine their level of fatigue and sleep deprivation.[61] In situations such as those described, increased staff vigilance with continuous monitoring, as described previously, is important to assist with SSC throughout the immediate postpartum period.[62] Additional suggestions to improve safety include enhancements to the environment, such as stabilizing the ambient temperature,[63] use of appropriate lighting so that the infant's color and condition can be easily assessed, and facilitating an unobstructed view of the newborn (Box 2). Additional support persons, such as doulas and family members, may augment but not replace staff monitoring. Furthermore, staff education, appropriate staffing, and awareness of genetic risks may limit sentinel events such as SUPC. These suggestions, however, have not yet been tested in prospective studies to determine efficacy.

BOX 2. COMPONENTS OF SAFE POSITIONING FOR THE NEWBORN WHILE SKIN-TO-SKIN[62]:

1. Infant's face can be seen

2. Infant's head is in "sniffing" position

3. Infant's nose and mouth are not covered

4. Infant's head is turned to one side

5. Infant's neck is straight, not bent

6. Infant's shoulders and chest face mother

7. Infant's legs are flexed

8. Infant's back is covered with blankets

9. Mother-infant dyad is monitored continuously by staff in the delivery environment and regularly on the postpartum unit

10. When mother wants to sleep, infant is placed in bassinet or with another support person who is awake and alert

SSC may be continued while moving a mother from a delivery surface (either in a delivery room or operating room) to the postpartum maternal bed. Transitions of mother-infant dyads throughout this period, and from delivery settings to postpartum settings,

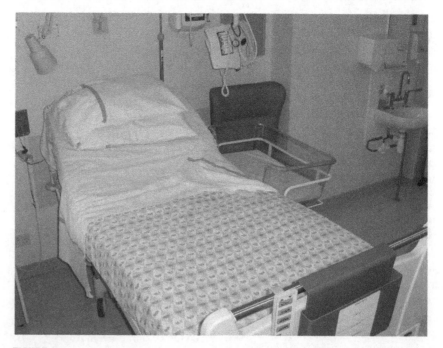

FIGURE 1
Side-car bassinet for in-hospital use. Photo courtesy of Kristin Tully, PhD.

facilitate continued bonding, thermoregulation, and increased opportunities for breastfeeding. These transitions may be accomplished safely with skilled staff members by using a standardized procedure.[64] A newborn who is not properly secured may pose a risk for falls or unsafe positioning, leading to suffocation.

SAFETY CONCERNS REGARDING ROOMING-IN

Despite all of the advantages of rooming-in, there are specific conditions that pose risks for the newborn. Many of the same concerns that occur during SSC in the immediate postnatal period continue to be of concern while rooming-in, especially if the mother and infant are sleeping together in the mother's bed on the postpartum unit.[65] In addition, breastfeeding mothers may fall asleep unintentionally while breastfeeding in bed, which can result in suffocation.[66] Infant falls may be more common in the postpartum setting because of less frequent

monitoring and increased time that a potentially fatigued mother is alone with her newborn(s).[67] The Oregon Patient Safety Review evaluated 7 hospitals that were part of 1 larger health system and identified 9 cases of newborn falls (from 22 866 births), for a rate of 3.94 falls per 10 000 births over a 2-year period from 2006 to 2007, which is higher than previous reports of 1.6 per 100 000.[68-70] It is not clear whether this higher incidence was attributable to an actual increase or better reporting. For hospitals transitioning to mother-infant dyad care (1 nurse providing care for both mother and infant) or separate mother-newborn care while rooming-in, it is important to communicate to staff that the same level of attention and care is necessary to provide optimal safety. Mothers will be naturally exhausted and potentially sleep-deprived or may sleep in short bursts.[61] They may also be unable to adjust their position or ambulate safely while carrying a newborn. The postpartum period provides unique challenges regarding falls/drops and is understudied compared with falls in the neurologically impaired or elderly patient. Checklists and scoring tools may be appropriate and have the potential to decrease these adverse events, particularly if geared to the unique needs of the postpartum period, such as short-term disability from numbness or pain, sleepiness or lethargy related to pregnancy and delivery, and effects from medication.[71]

Even though mothers and family members may be educated about the avoidance of bed-sharing, falling asleep while breastfeeding or holding the newborn during SSC is common. Staff can educate support persons and/or be immediately available to safely place newborns on a close but separate sleep surface when mothers fall asleep. Mothers may be reassured that they or their support persons can safely provide SSC and that staff will be available to assist with the transition to a safe sleep surface as needed. Mothers who have had cesarean deliveries are particularly at risk because of limited mobility and effects of anesthesia and warrant closer monitoring.[72]

Several studies examining safety while rooming-in have been conducted. Sixty-four mother-infant dyads were studied in the United Kingdom and randomly assigned to have newborns sleep in a stand-alone bassinet, a side-car bassinet (Fig 1), or the mother's bed to determine perception of safety (by video monitoring) and breastfeeding outcomes.[73] Breastfeeding was more frequent among those sharing a bed and using a side-car than a separate bassinet, but there were more hazards associated with bed-sharing than using a side-car or bassinet. Although there were no adverse events in this study, the authors concluded that the side-car provided the best opportunities for breastfeeding with the safest conditions. In a similar study

examining dyads after cesarean delivery, more hazards were associated with stand-alone bassinets than side-car bassinets. However, side-car technology for hospital beds is not yet well established in the United States, and safety data are not yet available. Given the level of disability in mothers who have had a cesarean delivery, side-car technology holds promise for improvement in the safety of the rooming-in environment.[74]

SUGGESTIONS TO IMPROVE SAFETY WHILE ROOMING-IN

Healthy mother-infant dyads are safest when kept together and cared for as a unit in a mother-infant setting. Staffing ratios are determined to meet the needs of both the mother and her newborn(s) and to ensure the best possible outcomes. The Association of Women's Health, Obstetric and Neonatal Nurses' recommendations are to have no more than 3 dyads assigned to 1 nurse to avoid situations in which nursing staff are not immediately available and able to regularly monitor the mother-infant dyads throughout the postpartum period.[75] These ratios may permit routine monitoring, rapid response to call bells, and adequate time for teaching; however, nursing staff extenders, such as health educators and nursing assistants, may augment care. Mothers and families who are informed of the risks of bed-sharing and guided to place newborns on separate sleep surfaces for sleep are more likely to follow these recommendations while in the hospital and after going home. Family members and staff can be available to assist mothers with transitioning the newborn to a safe sleep location, and regular staff supervision facilitates the recognition of sleepy family members and safer placement of the newborns in bassinets or side-cars.

SUGGESTIONS FOR ROOMING-IN

1. Use a patient safety contract with a particular focus on high-risk situations (see parent handout Newborn Safety Information for Parents[68] and sample contract[71]).

2. Monitor mothers according to their risk assessment: for example, observing every 30 minutes during nighttime and early morning hours for higher-risk dyads.[69]

3. Use fall risk assessment tools.[76]

4. Implement maternal egress testing (a modification of a tool originally designed to transfer obese patients from bed to stand, chair, or ambulation by using repetition to verify stability), especially if the mother is using medications that may affect stability in ambulating.[69]

5. Review mother-infant equipment to ensure proper function and demonstrate the appropriate use of equipment, such as bed rails and call bells, with mothers and families.

6. Publicize information about how to prevent newborn falls throughout the hospital system.

7. Use risk assessment tools to avoid hazards of SSC and rooming-in practices.[77]

TRANSITIONING TO HOME AND SAFE SLEEP BEYOND DISCHARGE

Information provided to parents at the time of hospital discharge should include anticipatory guidance about breastfeeding and sleep safety.[3,78,79] Pediatricians, hospitals, and other clinical staff should abide by AAP recommendations/guidance on breastfeeding and safe sleep, pacifier introduction, maternal smoking, use of alcohol, sleep positioning, bed-sharing, and appropriate sleep surfaces, especially when practicing SSC.[79] In addition, the AAP recommends the avoidance of practices that increase the risk of sudden and unexpected infant death, such as smoking, the use of alcohol, placing the infant in a nonsupine position for sleep, nonexclusive breastfeeding, and placing the infant to sleep (with or without another person) on sofas or chairs.[79,80] To facilitate continued exclusive breastfeeding, the coordination of postdischarge support is recommended to enable the best opportunity to meet breastfeeding goals. Mothers may be referred to peer support groups and trained lactation specialists if breastfeeding problems occur. Community support is optimized by coordination with the medical home.[81]

CONCLUSIONS

Pediatricians and other providers have important roles in the implementation of safe SSC and rooming-in practices. Safe implementation with the use of a standardized approach may prevent adverse events such as SUPC and falls.

The following suggestions support safe implementation of these practices:

1. Develop standardized methods and procedures of providing immediate and continued SSC with attention to continuous monitoring and assessment.

2. Standardize the sequence of events immediately after delivery to promote safe transition, thermoregulation, uninterrupted SSC, and direct observation of the first breastfeeding session.

3. Document maternal and newborn assessments and any changes in conditions.

4. Provide direct observation of the mother-infant dyad while in the delivery room setting.

5. Position the newborn in a manner that provides an unobstructed airway.

6. Conduct frequent assessments and monitoring of the mother-infant dyad during postpartum rooming-in settings, with particular attention to high-risk situations such as nighttime and early morning hours.

7. Assess the level of maternal fatigue periodically. If the mother is tired or sleepy, move the infant to a separate sleep surface (eg, side-car or bassinet) next to the mother's bed.

8. Avoid bed-sharing in the immediate postpartum period by assisting mothers to use a separate sleep surface for the infant.

9. Promote supine sleep for all infants. SSC may involve the prone or side position of the newborn, especially if the dyad is recumbent; therefore, it is imperative that the mother/caregiver who is providing SSC be awake and alert.

10. Train all health care personnel in standardized methods of providing immediate SSC after delivery, transitioning the mother-infant dyad, and monitoring the dyad during SSC and rooming-in throughout the delivery hospital period.

LEAD AUTHORS

Lori Feldman-Winter, MD, MPH, FAAP
Jay P. Goldsmith, MD, FAAP

TASK FORCE ON SUDDEN INFANT DEATH SYNDROME

Rachel Y. Moon, MD, FAAP, Chairperson
Robert A. Darnall, MD
Lori Feldman-Winter, MD, MPH, FAAP
Michael H. Goodstein, MD, FAAP
Fern R. Hauck, MD, MS

CONSULTANTS

Marian Willinger, PhD – *Eunice Kennedy Shriver National Institute for Child Health and Human Development*
Carrie K. Shapiro-Mendoza, PhD, MPH – *Centers for Disease Control and Prevention*

COMMITTEE ON FETUS AND NEWBORN, 2015–2016

Kristi L. Watterberg, MD, FAAP, Chairperson
James J. Cummings, MD, FAAP
William E. Benitz, MD, FAAP
Eric C. Eichenwald, MD, FAAP
Brenda B. Poindexter, MD, FAAP
Dan L. Stewart, MD, FAAP
Susan W. Aucott, MD, FAAP
Jay P. Goldsmith, MD, FAAP
Karen M. Puopolo, MD, PhD, FAAP
Kasper S. Wang, MD, FAAP

LIAISONS

Tonse N.K. Raju, MD, DCH, FAAP – *National Institutes of Health*
Wanda D. Barfield, MD, MPH, FAAP – *Centers for Disease Control and Prevention*
Erin L. Keels, APRN, MS, NNP-BC – *National Association of Neonatal Nurses*
Thierry Lacaze, MD – *Canadian Pediatric Society*
Maria Mascola, MD – *American College of Obstetricians and Gynecologists*

STAFF

Jim Couto, MA

ABBREVIATIONS

AAP: American Academy of Pediatrics
SIDS: sudden infant death syndrome
SSC: skin-to-skin care
SUPC: sudden unexpected postnatal collapse
WHO: World Health Organization

REFERENCES

1. World Health Organization. Evidence for the ten steps to successful breastfeeding. Geneva, Switzerland: World Health Organization; 1998. Available at: www.who.int/nutrition/publications/evidence_ten_step_eng.pdf. Accessed May 5, 2016

2. World Health Organization; UNICEF. Baby-Friendly Hospital Initiative: revised, updated, and expanded for integrated care. 2009. Available at: http://apps.who.int/iris/bitstream/10665/43593/1/9789241594967_eng.pdf. Accessed May 5, 2016

3. Eidelman AI, Schanler RJ; Section on Breastfeeding. Breastfeeding and the use of human milk. *Pediatrics.*

2012;129(3). Available at: www.pediatrics.org/cgi/content/full/129/3/e827

4. Baby-Friendly USA. Guidelines and evaluation criteria for facilities seeking Baby-Friendly designation. 2012. Available at: https://www.babyfriendlyusa.org/get-started/the-guidelines-evaluation-criteria. Accessed May 5, 2016

5. World Health Organization. Kangaroo mother care: a practical guide. 2003. Available at: http://apps.who.int/iris/bitstream/10665/42587/1/9241590351.pdf. Accessed May 5, 2016

6. Baley J, ; Committee on Fetus and Newborn. Skin-to-skin care for term and preterm infants in the neonatal ICU. *Pediatrics*. 2015;136(3):596–599

7. Horgan MJ. Management of the late preterm infant: not quite ready for prime time. *Pediatr Clin North Am*. 2015;62(2):439–451

8. Codipietro L, Ceccarelli M, Ponzone A. Breastfeeding or oral sucrose solution in term neonates receiving heel lance: a randomized, controlled trial. *Pediatrics*. 2008;122(3). Available at: www.pediatrics.org/cgi/content/full/122/3/e716

9. Gray L, Miller LW, Philipp BL, Blass EM. Breastfeeding is analgesic in healthy newborns. *Pediatrics*. 2002;109(4):590–593

10. Nimbalkar SM, Patel VK, Patel DV, Nimbalkar AS, Sethi A, Phatak A. Effect of early skin-to-skin contact following normal delivery on incidence of hypothermia in neonates more than 1800 g: randomized control trial. *J Perinatol*. 2014;34(5):364–368

11. Moore ER, Anderson GC. Randomized controlled trial of very early mother-infant skin-to-skin contact and breastfeeding status. *J Midwifery Womens Health*. 2007;52(2):116–125

12. Moore ER, Anderson GC, Bergman N, Dowswell T. Early skin-to-skin contact for mothers and their healthy newborn infants. *Cochrane Database Syst Rev*. 2012;5:CD003519

13. Johnston C, Campbell-Yeo M, Fernandes A, Inglis D, Streiner D, Zee R. Skin-to-skin care for procedural pain in neonates. *Cochrane Database Syst Rev*. 2014;1:CD008435

14. Kostandy R, Anderson GC, Good M. Skin-to-skin contact diminishes pain from hepatitis B vaccine injection in healthy full-term neonates. *Neonatal Netw*. 2013;32(4):274–280

15. Okan F, Ozdil A, Bulbul A, Yapici Z, Nuhoglu A. Analgesic effects of skin-to-skin contact and breastfeeding in procedural pain in healthy term neonates. *Ann Trop Paediatr*. 2010;30(2):119–128

16. Castral TC, Warnock F, Leite AM, Haas VJ, Scochi CG. The effects of skin-to-skin contact during acute pain in preterm newborns. *Eur J Pain*. 2008;12(4):464–471

17. Erlandsson K, Dsilna A, Fagerberg I, Christensson K. Skin-to-skin care with the father after cesarean birth and its effect on newborn crying and prefeeding behavior. *Birth*. 2007;34(2):105–114

18. Feldman R, Eidelman AI, Sirota L, Weller A. Comparison of skin-to-skin (kangaroo) and traditional care: parenting outcomes and preterm infant development. *Pediatrics*. 2002;110(1 pt 1):16–26

19. Feldman R, Weller A, Sirota L, Eidelman AI. Skin-to-skin contact (Kangaroo care) promotes self-regulation in premature infants: sleep-wake cyclicity, arousal modulation, and sustained exploration. *Dev Psychol*. 2002;38(2):194–207

20. Feldman R, Eidelman AI. Skin-to-skin contact (kangaroo care) accelerates autonomic and neurobehavioural maturation in preterm infants. *Dev Med Child Neurol*. 2003;45(4):274–281

21. Chwo M-J, Anderson GC, Good M, Dowling DA, Shiau S-HH, Chu D-M. A randomized controlled trial of early kangaroo care for preterm infants: effects on temperature, weight, behavior, and acuity. *J Nurs Res*. 2002;10(2):129–142

22. Mörelius E, Örtenstrand A, Theodorsson E, Frostell A. A randomised trial of continuous skin-to-skin contact after preterm birth and the effects on salivary cortisol, parental stress, depression, and breastfeeding. *Early Hum Dev*. 2015;91(1):63–70

23. Saxton A, Fahy K, Rolfe M, Skinner V, Hastie C. Does skin-to-skin contact and breast feeding at birth affect the rate of primary postpartum haemorrhage: results of a cohort study. *Midwifery*. 2015;31(11):1110–1117

24. Vetulani J. Early maternal separation: a rodent model of depression and a prevailing human condition. *Pharmacol Rep*. 2013;65(6):1451–1461

25. Dani C, Cecchi A, Commare A, Rapisardi G, Breschi R, Pratesi S. Behavior of the newborn during skin-to-skin. *J Hum Lact*. 2015;31(3):452–457

26. Dumas L, Lepage M, Bystrova K, Matthiesen A-S, Welles-Nyström B, Widström A-M. Influence of skin-to-skin contact and rooming-in on early mother-infant interaction: a randomized controlled trial. *Clin Nurs Res*. 2013;22(3):310–336

27. Beiranvand S, Valizadeh F, Hosseinabadi R, Pournia Y. The effects of skin-to-skin contact on temperature and breastfeeding successfulness in full-term newborns after cesarean delivery. *Int J Pediatr*. 2014;2014:846486

28. Stevens J, Schmied V, Burns E, Dahlen H. Immediate or early skin-to-skin contact after a Caesarean section: a review of the literature. *Matern Child Nutr*. 2014;10(4):456–473

29. Phillips CR. *Family-Centered Maternity Care*. Sudbury, MA: Jones & Bartlett Learning; 2003

30. Silberman SL. Pioneering in family-centered maternity and infant care: Edith B. Jackson and the Yale rooming-in research project. *Bull Hist Med*. 1990;64(2):262–287

31. Mullen K, Conrad L, Hoadley G, Iannone D. Family-centered maternity care: one hospital's quest for excellence. *Nurs Womens Health*. 2007;11(3):282–290

32. Martell LK. Postpartum women's perceptions of the hospital environment. *J Obstet Gynecol Neonatal Nurs*. 2003;32(4):478–485

33. Ordean A, Kahan M, Graves L, Abrahams R, Kim T. Obstetrical and neonatal outcomes of methadone-maintained pregnant women: a Canadian multisite cohort study. *J Obstet Gynaecol Can*. 2015;37(3):252–257

34. Lvoff NM, Lvoff V, Klaus MH. Effect of the baby-friendly initiative on

infant abandonment in a Russian hospital. *Arch Pediatr Adolesc Med.* 2000;154(5):474–477

35. O'Connor S, Vietze PM, Sherrod KB, Sandler HM, Altemeier WA III. Reduced incidence of parenting inadequacy following rooming-in. *Pediatrics.* 1980;66(2):176–182

36. Jaafar SH, Lee KS, Ho JJ. Separate care for new mother and infant versus rooming-in for increasing the duration of breastfeeding. *Cochrane Database Syst Rev.* 2012;9:CD006641

37. Chiou ST, Chen LC, Yeh H, Wu SR, Chien LY. Early skin-to-skin contact, rooming-in, and breastfeeding: a comparison of the 2004 and 2011 National Surveys in Taiwan. *Birth.* 2014;41(1):33–38

38. Merewood A, Patel B, Newton KN, et al Breastfeeding duration rates and factors affecting continued breastfeeding among infants born at an inner-city US Baby-Friendly hospital. *J Hum Lact.* 2007;23(2):157–164

39. Aghdas K, Talat K, Sepideh B. Effect of immediate and continuous mother-infant skin-to-skin contact on breastfeeding self-efficacy of primiparous women: a randomised control trial. *Women Birth.* 2014;27(1):37–40

40. Montgomery-Downs HE, Clawges HM, Santy EE. Infant feeding methods and maternal sleep and daytime functioning. *Pediatrics.* 2010;126(6). Available at: www.pediatrics.org/cgi/content/full/126/6/e1562

41. Takahashi Y, Tamakoshi K, Matsushima M, Kawabe T. Comparison of salivary cortisol, heart rate, and oxygen saturation between early skin-to-skin contact with different initiation and duration times in healthy, full-term infants. *Early Hum Dev.* 2011;87(3):151–157

42. Daschner FD. Nosocomial infections in maternity wards and newborn nurseries: rooming-in or not? *J Hosp Infect.* 1986;7(1):1–3

43. Swanson JR, Sinkin RA. Transition from fetus to newborn. *Pediatr Clin North Am.* 2015;62(2):329–343

44. Davanzo R, De Cunto A, Paviotti G, et al. Making the first days of life safer: preventing sudden unexpected postnatal collapse while promoting breastfeeding. *J Hum Lact.* 2015;31(1):47–52

45. Poets A, Steinfeldt R, Poets CF. Sudden deaths and severe apparent life-threatening events in term infants within 24 hours of birth. *Pediatrics.* 2011;127(4). Available at: www.pediatrics.org/cgi/content/full/127/4/e869

46. Andres V, Garcia P, Rimet Y, Nicaise C, Simeoni U. Apparent life-threatening events in presumably healthy newborns during early skin-to-skin contact. *Pediatrics.* 2011;127(4). Available at: www.pediatrics.org/cgi/content/full/127/4/e1073

47. Dageville C, Pignol J, De Smet S. Very early neonatal apparent life-threatening events and sudden unexpected deaths: incidence and risk factors. *Acta Paediatr.* 2008;97(7):866–869

48. Leow JY, Platt MP. Sudden, unexpected and unexplained early neonatal deaths in the North of England. *Arch Dis Child Fetal Neonatal Ed.* 2011;96(6):F440–F442

49. Goldsmith JP. Hospitals should balance skin-to-skin contact with safe sleep policies. *AAP News.* 2013;34(11):22

50. Nassi N, Piumelli R, Nardini V, et al. Sudden unexpected perinatal collapse and sudden unexpected early neonatal death. *Early Hum Dev.* 2013;89(suppl 4):S25–S26

51. Pejovic NJ, Herlenius E. Unexpected collapse of healthy newborn infants: risk factors, supervision and hypothermia treatment. *Acta Paediatr.* 2013;102(7):680–688

52. Becher JC, Bhushan SS, Lyon AJ. Unexpected collapse in apparently healthy newborns—a prospective national study of a missing cohort of neonatal deaths and near-death events. *Arch Dis Child Fetal Neonatal Ed.* 2012;97(1):F30–F34

53. Herlenius E, Kuhn P. Sudden unexpected postnatal collapse of newborn infants: a review of cases, definitions, risks, and preventive measures. *Transl Stroke Res.* 2013;4(2):236–247

54. Fewell JE. Protective responses of the newborn to hypoxia. *Respir Physiol Neurobiol.* 2005;149(1–3):243–255

55. Schoch DE, Lawhon G, Wicker LA, Yecco G. An interdisciplinary multidepartmental educational program toward baby friendly hospital designation. *Adv Neonatal Care.* 2014;14(1):38–43

56. Niermeyer S, Velaphi S. Promoting physiologic transition at birth: re-examining resuscitation and the timing of cord clamping. *Semin Fetal Neonatal Med.*2013;18(6):385–392

57. Widström AM, Lilja G, Aaltomaa-Michalias P, Dahllöf A, Lintula M, Nissen E. Newborn behaviour to locate the breast when skin-to-skin: a possible method for enabling early self-regulation. *Acta Paediatr.* 2011;100(1):79–85

58. Christensson K, Siles C, Moreno L, et al. Temperature, metabolic adaptation and crying in healthy full-term newborns cared for skin-to-skin or in a cot. *Acta Paediatr.* 1992;81(6–7):488–493

59. Abike F, Tiras S, Dunder I, Bahtiyar A, Akturk Uzun O, Demircan O. A new scale for evaluating the risks for in-hospital falls of newborn infants: a failure modes and effects analysis study. *Int J Pediatr.* 2010;2010:547528

60. Madadi P, Ross CJ, Hayden MR, et al. Pharmacogenetics of neonatal opioid toxicity following maternal use of codeine during breastfeeding: a case-control study. *Clin Pharmacol Ther.* 2009;85(1):31–35

61. Rychnovsky J, Hunter LP. The relationship between sleep characteristics and fatigue in healthy postpartum women. *Womens Health Issues.* 2009;19(1):38–44

62. Ludington-Hoe Sm MK, Morgan K. Infant assessment and reduction of sudden unexpected postnatal collapse risk during skin-to-skin contact. *Newborn Infant Nurs Rev.* 2014;14(1):28–33

63. Delavar M, Akbarianrad Z, Mansouri M, Yahyapour M. Neonatal hypothermia and associated risk factors at baby friendly hospital in Babol, Iran. *Ann Med Health Sci Res.* 2014;4(8, suppl 2):S99–S103

64. Elliott-Carter N, Harper J. Keeping mothers and newborns together after cesarean: how one hospital made the change. *Nurs Womens Health.* 2012;16(4):290–295

65. Thach BT. Deaths and near deaths of healthy newborn infants while bed sharing on maternity wards. *J Perinatol.* 2014;34(4):275–279

66. Feldman K, Whyte RK. Two cases of apparent suffocation of newborns during side-lying breastfeeding. *Nurs Womens Health.* 2013;17(4):337–341

67. Wallace SC; Pennsylvania Patient Safety Authority. Balancing family bonding with newborn safety. *Pennsylvania Patient Safety Advisory.* 2014;11(3). Available at: http://patientsafetyauth ority.org/ADVISORIES/AdvisoryLibrary/ 2014/Sep;11(3)/Pages/102.aspx

68. Helsley L, McDonald JV, Stewart VT. Addressing in-hospital "falls" of newborn infants. *Jt Comm J Qual Patient Saf.* 2010;36(7):327–333

69. Gaffey AD. Fall prevention in our healthiest patients: assessing risk and preventing injury for moms and babies. *J Healthc Risk Manag.* 2015;34(3):37–40

70. Monson SA, Henry E, Lambert DK, Schmutz N, Christensen RD. In-hospital falls of newborn infants: data from a multihospital health care system. *Pediatrics.* 2008;122(2). Available at: www.pediatrics.org/cgi/content/full/ 122/2/e277

71. Lockwood S, Anderson K. Postpartum safety: a patient-centered approach to fall prevention. *MCN Am J Matern Child Nurs.* 2013;38(1):15–18, quiz 19–20

72. Mahlmeister LR. Couplet care after cesarean delivery: creating a safe environment for mother and baby. *J Perinat Neonatal Nurs.* 2005;19(3):212–214

73. Ball HL, Ward-Platt MP, Heslop E, Leech SJ, Brown KA. Randomised trial of infant sleep location on the postnatal ward. *Arch Dis Child.* 2006;91(12):1005–1010

74. Tully KP, Ball HL. Postnatal unit bassinet types when rooming-in after cesarean birth: implications for breastfeeding and infant safety. *J Hum Lact.* 2012;28(4):495–505

75. Scheich B, Bingham D; AWHONN Perinatal Staffing Data Collaborative. Key findings from the AWHONN perinatal staffing data collaborative. *J Obstet Gynecol Neonatal Nurs.* 2015;44(2):317–328

76. Heafner L, Suda D, Casalenuovo N, Leach LS, Erickson V, Gawlinski A. Development of a tool to assess risk for falls in women in hospital obstetric units. *Nurs Womens Health.* 2013;17(2):98–107

77. Slogar A, Gargiulo D, Bodrock J. Tracking 'near misses' to keep newborns safe from falls. *Nurs Womens Health.* 2013;17(3):219–223

78. American Academy of Pediatrics. Education in quality improvement for pediatric practice: safe and healthy beginnings. 2012. Available at: https:// www.aap.org/en-us/professional- resources/quality-improvement/ Quality-Improvement-Innovation- Networks/Pages/Safe-and-Healthy- Beginnings-Improvement-Project.aspx. Accessed May 5, 2016

79. Moon RY; Task Force on Sudden Infant Death Syndrome. SIDS and other sleep- related infant deaths: expansion of recommendations for a safe infant sleeping environment. *Pediatrics.* 2011;128(5). Available at: www.pediatrics. org/cgi/content/full/128/5/e1341

80. Hauck FR, Thompson JM, Tanabe KO, Moon RY, Vennemann MM. Breastfeeding and reduced risk of sudden infant death syndrome: a meta-analysis. *Pediatrics.* 2011;128(1):103–110

81. Turchi RM, Antonelli RC, Norwood KW, et al; Council on Children with Disabilities and Medical Home Implementation Project Advisory Committee. Patient- and family- centered care coordination: a framework for integrating care for children and youth across multiple systems. *Pediatrics.* 2014;133(5). Available at: www.pediatrics.org/cgi/ content/full/133/5/e1451

American Academy
of Pediatrics

DEDICATED TO THE HEALTH OF ALL CHILDREN™

Skin-to-Skin Care for Term and Preterm Infants in the Neonatal ICU

Jill Baley, MD, COMMITTEE ON FETUS AND NEWBORN

abstract

"Kangaroo mother care" was first described as an alternative method of caring for low birth weight infants in resource-limited countries, where neonatal mortality and infection rates are high because of overcrowded nurseries, inadequate staffing, and lack of equipment. Intermittent skin-to-skin care (SSC), a modified version of kangaroo mother care, is now being offered in resource-rich countries to infants needing neonatal intensive care, including those who require ventilator support or are extremely premature. SSC significantly improves milk production by the mother and is associated with a longer duration of breastfeeding. Increased parent satisfaction, better sleep organization, a longer duration of quiet sleep, and decreased pain perception during procedures have also been reported in association with SSC. Despite apparent physiologic stability during SSC, it is prudent that infants in the NICU have continuous cardiovascular monitoring and that care be taken to verify correct head positioning for airway patency as well as the stability of the endotracheal tube, arterial and venous access devices, and other life support equipment.

www.pediatrics.org/cgi/doi/10.1542/peds.2015-2335

DOI: 10.1542/peds.2015-2335

PEDIATRICS (ISSN Numbers: Print, 0031-4005; Online, 1098-4275).

BACKGROUND

"Kangaroo mother care" (KMC) was first described as an alternative method of caring for low birth weight infants in resource-limited countries, where neonatal mortality and infection rates are high because of overcrowded nurseries, inadequate staffing, and lack of equipment. In the original version of KMC, the infant is placed in continuous skin-to-skin contact in a vertical position between the mother's breasts and beneath her clothes and is exclusively (or nearly exclusively) breastfed. A meta-analysis of 988 infants enrolled in 3 randomized controlled trials of continuous KMC begun in the first postnatal week in low- or middle-income countries found a 51% reduction in mortality among infants with a birth weight <2000 g (relative risk: 0.49 [95% confidence interval: 0.29–0.82]).[1] Although the methods of this review have come under question,[2] a Cochrane meta-analysis of 18 trials of continuous KMC begun before postnatal day 10 in infants with a birth weight <2500 g also showed significantly reduced mortality and morbidity at discharge or 40 to 41 weeks' postmenstrual age and at follow-up; it also found a decreased incidence of health care–related sepsis and an improvement in some measures of infant growth, breastfeeding, and mother-infant attachment.[3] Thirteen of these 18 studies were conducted in low- to middle-income countries.

Intermittent skin-to-skin care (SSC) in NICUs in resource-rich countries differs from traditional KMC in that it is usually used for varying, shorter periods of time; can be offered to less stable and technology-supported infants; and can be performed by both parents. Intermittent SSC in resource-rich countries has not been associated with decreased mortality, although data are currently insufficient to determine an effect.[3] However, it is widely offered to parents for other perceived benefits, such as enhancing attachment, parental self-esteem, and breastfeeding.[4,5]

EVIDENCE

Benefits

The most substantial evidence of benefit from SSC is for breastfeeding. Individual randomized controlled trials and a systematic review have shown that intermittent SSC is associated with longer and more exclusive breastfeeding and higher volumes of expressed milk.[6,7] The systematic review reported that short periods of SSC (up to 1 hour at all visits) increased the duration of any breastfeeding, variably reported by different studies as 1 month after discharge (relative risk: 4.76 [95% confidence interval: 1.19–19.10]) or for more than 6 weeks (relative risk: 1.95 [95% confidence interval: 1.03–3.70]) among clinically stable infants in industrialized nations.[7] A number of studies have also indicated that SSC may improve a mother's attachment or bonding and her feeling of being needed by or comfortable with her infant.[3,8–12]

In addition, SSC promotes the participation of the mother and father in the infant's care, strengthens the family role in the care of a fragile infant, and decreases feelings of helplessness.[10] Mothers report less stress and more satisfaction with NICU care, and both parents are more responsive to their infant's cues.[3,8–12]

The evidence is less clear for a beneficial effect regarding sleep and neurobehavioral maturation. One report found increased frontal brain activity during both quiet and active sleep, which is thought to be predictive of improved neurobehavioral outcomes.[13] Other studies using electroencephalography and polysomnography data indicate that preterm infants who receive SSC have more mature sleep organization, with increased total and quiet sleep, decreased REM sleep and arousals from sleep, and an improvement in sleep cycling.[14,15] They also appeared more alert and observant and spent less time crying. Two cohort studies found that infants receiving SSC demonstrated better autonomic regulation and maternal–infant interactions at term gestation, as well as higher scores on the Bayley Scales of Infant Development–Second Edition at 6 or 12 months of age.[8,16] Of the infants enrolled in the second study, 117 were followed up to 10 years of age, and the authors reported that those who received SSC showed attenuated stress response, improved autonomic functioning, better-organized sleep, and better cognitive control.[17]

SSC has also been advocated for the nonpharmacologic management of procedural pain. A Cochrane review of the effect of SSC for relief of procedural pain concluded that it seemed to be effective for a single painful procedure such as a heel lance, as measured by using composite pain indicators.[18] The review found that behavioral indicators of pain tended to favor SSC, whereas physiologic indicators were

generally not affected, suggesting possible observer bias in scoring behavioral indicators. However, small studies have reported reduced cortisol concentrations and decreased autonomic indicators of pain in preterm infants during SSC.[19,20] The authors of the Cochrane review recommend confirmatory studies of previous findings and call for new studies examining optimal duration of SSC, use in different gestational age groups, effects of repeated use, and long-term effects.[18]

Risks

Investigators initially postulated that continuous KMC would promote colonization with maternal flora rather than resistant hospital flora. Consistent with this hypothesis, meta-analyses of randomized controlled trials in resource-limited countries have exhibited fewer episodes of sepsis, necrotizing enterocolitis, and pneumonia.[1,3] However, infections may be spread among mothers, infants, and caregivers, particularly in multiple-bed units, as has been reported for respiratory syncytial virus and tuberculosis.[21,22] Although a recent report described an association between SSC and development of methicillin-resistant *Staphylococcus aureus* infections among infants in 1 NICU (particularly those with very low birth weights), the authors did not believe that there was a causal relationship.[23] Parents should be monitored for skin infections and might need cleansing of the skin before infant contact. Some experts consider infants with open lesions (eg, open neural tube defects, abdominal wall defects) to be particularly at risk.

Most studies of physiologic stability during SSC have been performed on stable, nonintubated infants. One meta-analysis reported a statistically but not clinically significant increase in body temperature (0.22°C) and a decrease in oxygen saturation (0.60%) in 190 term and 326 preterm infants receiving SSC compared with incubator care.[24] These effects were most pronounced in nurseries in low- and middle-income settings and in cold environments. There was no change in heart rate before, during, or after SSC, and no difference was noted between preterm and term infants. Although 1 study of 22 infants reported an increase in desaturation and bradycardia during SSC,[25] other studies have shown no significant increase in desaturation, bradycardic or apneic events, or in oxygen consumption.[26–28] Despite apparent physiologic stability during SSC, it is prudent that infants in the NICU be continuously monitored and that care be taken to verify correct head positioning for airway patency as well as the stability of the endotracheal tube, arterial and venous access devices, and other life support equipment. Any infant who requires careful temperature regulation or a high-humidity environment might have SSC delayed until he or she is more stable.

There may be resistance among health care providers regarding offering SSC. This resistance could stem from fear of harm to the infant or from lack of experience, time, or assistance to transfer the infant to the parent and/or monitor the infant's well-being. A nursing simulation training program may help promote acceptance of SSC.[29] Multiple guidelines for the provision of SSC have been published,[30–33] and each facility needs to consider staffing, experience, and resources in the development of its institutional guidelines. Because SSC has been shown to be feasible and safe in the NICU in infants as young as 26 weeks' gestation,[34] with benefits for both parents and infants, facilities are encouraged to offer this care when possible.

IMPLICATIONS FOR CLINICAL PRACTICE

1. It has been shown that skin-to-skin care results in improved breastfeeding, milk production, parental satisfaction, and bonding.

2. Both parents can be encouraged to provide skin-to-skin care, with appropriate guidelines and protocols, for both preterm and term infants in the NICU.

3. Despite apparent physiologic stability during skin-to-skin care, it is prudent that infants in the NICU have continuous cardiovascular monitoring and that care be taken to monitor correct head positioning for airway patency as well as the stability of the endotracheal tube, arterial and venous access devices, and other life support equipment.

LEAD AUTHOR

Jill Baley, MD

COMMITTEE ON FETUS AND NEWBORN, 2014–2015

Kristi Watterberg, MD, Chairperson
James Cummings, MD
Eric Eichenwald, MD
Brenda Poindexter, MD
Dan L. Stewart, MD
Susan W. Aucott, MD
Karen M. Puopolo, MD
Jay P. Goldsmith, MD

LIAISONS

William Benitz, MD – *AAP Section on Perinatal Pediatrics*
Kasper S. Wang, MD – *AAP Section on Surgery*
Thierry Lacaze, MD – *Canadian Pediatric Society*
Jeffrey L. Ecker, MD – *American College of Obstetricians and Gynecologists*
Tonse N.K. Raju, MD, DCH – *National Institutes of Health*
Wanda Barfield, MD, MPH – *Centers for Disease Control and Prevention*
Erin Keels, MS, APRN, NNP-BC – *National Association of Neonatal Nurses*

STAFF

Jim Couto, MA
Address correspondence to: KWatterberg@salud.unm.edu

ABBREVIATIONS

KMC: kangaroo mother care
SSC: skin-to-skin care

REFERENCES

1. Lawn JE, Mwansa-Kambafwile J, Horta BL, Barros FC, Cousens S. 'Kangaroo mother care' to prevent neonatal deaths due to preterm birth complications. *Int J Epidemiol.* 2010;39 (suppl 1):i144–i154

2. Sloan NL, Ahmed S, Anderson GC, Moore E. Comment on: 'kangaroo mother care' to prevent neonatal deaths due to preterm birth complications. *Int J Epidemiol.* 2011;40(2):521–525

3. Conde-Agudelo A, Díaz-Rossello JL. Kangaroo mother care to reduce morbidity and mortality in low birthweight infants. *Cochrane Database Syst Rev.* 2014;4(4):CD002771

4. Franck LS, Bernal H, Gale G. Infant holding policies and practices in neonatal units. *Neonatal Netw.* 2002; 21(2):13–20

5. Field T, Hernandez-Reif M, Feijo L, Freedman J. Prenatal, perinatal and neonatal stimulation: a survey of neonatal nurseries. *Infant Behav Dev.* 2006;29(1):24–31

6. Hake-Brooks SJ, Anderson GC. Kangaroo care and breastfeeding of mother-preterm infant dyads 0-18 months: a randomized, controlled trial. *Neonatal Netw.* 2008;27(3):151–159

7. Renfrew MJ, Craig D, Dyson L, et al. Breastfeeding promotion for infants in neonatal units: a systematic review and economic analysis. *Health Technol Assess.* 2009;13(40):1–146, iii–iv

8. Ohgi S, Fukuda M, Moriuchi H, et al. Comparison of kangaroo care and standard care: behavioral organization, development, and temperament in healthy, low-birth-weight infants through 1 year. *J Perinatol.* 2002;22(5):374–379

9. Charpak N, Ruiz JG, Zupan J, et al. Kangaroo mother care: 25 years after. *Acta Paediatr.* 2005;94(5):514–522

10. Nyqvist KH, Anderson GC, Bergman N, et al. Towards universal kangaroo mother care: recommendations and report from the first European conference and Seventh International Workshop on kangaroo mother care. *Acta Paediatr.* 2010;99(6):820–826

11. Johnson AN. The maternal experience of kangaroo holding. *J Obstet Gynecol Neonatal Nurs.* 2007;36(6):568–573

12. Tessier R, Charpak N, Giron M, Cristo M, de Calume ZF, Ruiz-Peláez JG. Kangaroo mother care, home environment and father involvement in the first year of life: a randomized controlled study. *Acta Paediatr.* 2009;98(9):1444–1450

13. Welch MG, Myers MM, Grieve PG, et al; FNI Trial Group. Electroencephalographic activity of preterm infants is increased by Family Nurture Intervention: a randomized controlled trial in the NICU. *Clin Neurophysiol.* 2014;125(4):675–684

14. Ludington-Hoe SM, Johnson MW, Morgan K, et al. Neurophysiologic assessment of neonatal sleep organization: preliminary results of a randomized, controlled trial of skin contact with preterm infants. *Pediatrics.* 2006;117(5). Available at: www.pediatrics.org/cgi/content/full/117/5/e909

15. Feldman R, Eidelman AI. Skin-to-skin contact (kangaroo care) accelerates autonomic and neurobehavioural maturation in preterm infants. *Dev Med Child Neurol.* 2003;45(4):274–281

16. Feldman R, Eidelman AI, Sirota L, Weller A. Comparison of skin-to-skin (kangaroo) and traditional care: parenting outcomes and preterm infant development. *Pediatrics.* 2002;110(1 pt 1):16–26

17. Feldman R, Rosenthal Z, Eidelman AI. Maternal-preterm skin-to-skin contact enhances child physiologic organization and cognitive control across the first 10 years of life. *Biol Psychiatry.* 2014;75(1):56–64

18. Johnston C, Campbell-Yeo M, Fernandes A, Inglis D, Streiner D, Zee R. Skin-to-skin care for procedural pain in neonates. *Cochrane Database Syst Rev.* 2014;1(1):CD008435

19. Cong X, Ludington-Hoe SM, Walsh S. Randomized crossover trial of kangaroo care to reduce biobehavioral pain responses in preterm infants: a pilot study. *Biol Res Nurs.* 2011;13(2):204–216

20. Cong X, Cusson RM, Walsh S, Hussain N, Ludington-Hoe SM, Zhang D. Effects of skin-to-skin contact on autonomic pain responses in preterm infants. *J Pain.* 2012;13(7):636–645

21. Visser A, Delport S, Venter M. Molecular epidemiological analysis of a nosocomial outbreak of respiratory syncytial virus associated pneumonia in a kangaroo mother care unit in South Africa. *J Med Virol.* 2008;80(4):724–732

22. Heyns L, Gie RP, Goussard P, Beyers N, Warren RM, Marais BJ. Nosocomial transmission of Mycobacterium tuberculosis in kangaroo mother care units: a risk in tuberculosis-endemic areas. *Acta Paediatr.* 2006;95(5):535–539

23. Sakaki H, Nishioka M, Kanda K, Takahashi Y. An investigation of the risk factors for infection with methicillin-resistant Staphylococcus aureus among patients in a neonatal intensive care unit. *Am J Infect Control.* 2009;37(7):580–586

24. Mori R, Khanna R, Pledge D, Nakayama T. Meta-analysis of physiological effects of skin-to-skin contact for newborns and mothers. *Pediatr Int.* 2010;52(2):161–170

25. Bohnhorst B, Gill D, Dördelmann M, Peter CS, Poets CF. Bradycardia and desaturation during skin-to-skin care: no relationship to hyperthermia. *J Pediatr.* 2004;145(4):499–502

26. Bauer J, Sontheimer D, Fischer C, Linderkamp O. Metabolic rate and energy balance in very low birth weight infants during kangaroo holding by their mothers and fathers. *J Pediatr.* 1996;129(4):608–611

27. Heimann K, Vaessen P, Peschgens T, Stanzel S, Wenzl TG, Orlikowsky T. Impact of skin to skin care, prone and supine positioning on cardiorespiratory parameters and thermoregulation in premature infants. *Neonatology.* 2010;97(4):311–317

28. Ludington-Hoe SM, Anderson GC, Swinth JY, Thompson C, Hadeed AJ. Randomized controlled trial of kangaroo care: cardiorespiratory and thermal effects on healthy preterm infants. *Neonatal Netw.* 2004;23(3):39–48

29. Hendricks-Munoz KD, Mayers RM. A neonatal nurse training program in kangaroo mother care (KMC) decreases barriers to KMC utilization in the NICU. *Am J Perinatol.* 2014;31(11):987–992

30. Kledzik T. Holding the very low birth weight infant: skin-to-skin techniques. *Neonatal Netw.* 2005;24(1):7–14

31. DiMenna L. Considerations for implementation of a neonatal kangaroo care protocol. *Neonatal Netw.* 2006;25(6):405–412

32. Welch MG, Hofer MA, Stark RI, et al; FNI Trial Group. Randomized controlled trial of family nurture intervention in the NICU: assessments of length of stay, feasibility and safety. *BMC Pediatr.* 2013;13:148–162

33. Ludington-Hoe SM, Ferreira C, Swinth J, Ceccardi JJ. Safe criteria and procedure for kangaroo care with intubated preterm infants. *J Obstet Gynecol Neonatal Nurs.* 2003;32(5):579–588

34. Bier JA, Ferguson AE, Morales Y, et al. Comparison of skin-to-skin contact with standard contact in low-birth-weight infants who are breast-fed. *Arch Pediatr Adolesc Med.* 1996;150(12):1265–1269

SECTION 8
Sudden Infant Death Syndrome/Infant Death

POLICY STATEMENT
Organizational Principles to Guide and Define the Child Health
Care System and/or Improve the Health of all Children

American Academy
of Pediatrics

DEDICATED TO THE HEALTH OF ALL CHILDREN™

SIDS and Other Sleep-Related Infant Deaths: Updated 2016 Recommendations for a Safe Infant Sleeping Environment

TASK FORCE ON SUDDEN INFANT DEATH SYNDROME

abstract

Approximately 3500 infants die annually in the United States from sleep-related infant deaths, including sudden infant death syndrome (SIDS; International Classification of Diseases, 10th Revision [ICD-10], R95), ill-defined deaths (ICD-10 R99), and accidental suffocation and strangulation in bed (ICD-10 W75). After an initial decrease in the 1990s, the overall death rate attributable to sleep-related infant deaths has not declined in more recent years. Many of the modifiable and nonmodifiable risk factors for SIDS and other sleep-related infant deaths are strikingly similar. The American Academy of Pediatrics recommends a safe sleep environment that can reduce the risk of all sleep-related infant deaths. Recommendations for a safe sleep environment include supine positioning, the use of a firm sleep surface, room-sharing without bed-sharing, and the avoidance of soft bedding and overheating. Additional recommendations for SIDS reduction include the avoidance of exposure to smoke, alcohol, and illicit drugs; breastfeeding; routine immunization; and use of a pacifier. New evidence is presented for skin-to-skin care for newborn infants, use of bedside and in-bed sleepers, sleeping on couches/armchairs and in sitting devices, and use of soft bedding after 4 months of age. The recommendations and strength of evidence for each recommendation are included in this policy statement. The rationale for these recommendations is discussed in detail in the accompanying technical report (www.pediatrics.org/cgi/doi/10.1542/peds.2016-2940).

DOI: 10.1542/peds.2016-2938

PEDIATRICS (ISSN Numbers: Print, 0031-4005; Online, 1098-4275).

Copyright © 2016 by the American Academy of Pediatrics

FINANCIAL DISCLOSURE: The author has indicated she does not have a financial relationship relevant to this article to disclose.

FUNDING: No external funding.

POTENTIAL CONFLICT OF INTEREST: The author has indicated she has no potential conflicts of interest to disclose.

To cite: AAP TASK FORCE ON SUDDEN INFANT DEATH SYNDROME. SIDS and Other Sleep-Related Infant Deaths: Updated 2016 Recommendations for a Safe Infant Sleeping Environment. *Pediatrics.* 2016;138(5):e20162938

BACKGROUND

Sudden unexpected infant death (SUID), also known as sudden unexpected death in infancy, or SUDI, is a term used to describe any sudden and unexpected death, whether explained or unexplained

TABLE 1 Definitions of Terms

Bed-sharing: Parent(s) and infant sleeping together on any surface (bed, couch, chair).
Caregivers: Throughout the document, "parents" are used, but this term is meant to indicate any infant caregivers.
Cosleeping: This term is commonly used, but the task force finds it confusing, and it is not used in this document. When used, authors need to make clear whether they are referring to sleeping in close proximity (which does not necessarily entail bed-sharing) or bed-sharing.
Room-sharing: Parent(s) and infant sleeping in the same room on separate surfaces.
Sleep-related infant death: SUID that occurs during an observed or unobserved sleep period.
Sudden infant death syndrome (SIDS): Cause assigned to infant deaths that cannot be explained after a thorough case investigation, including a scene investigation, autopsy, and review of the clinical history.[1]
Sudden unexpected infant death (SUID), or sudden unexpected death in infancy (SUDI): A sudden and unexpected death, whether explained or unexplained (including SIDS), occurring during infancy.

TABLE 2 Summary of Recommendations With Strength of Recommendation

A-level recommendations
  Back to sleep for every sleep.
  Use a firm sleep surface.
  Breastfeeding is recommended.
  Room-sharing with the infant on a separate sleep surface is recommended.
  Keep soft objects and loose bedding away from the infant's sleep area.
  Consider offering a pacifier at naptime and bedtime.
  Avoid smoke exposure during pregnancy and after birth.
  Avoid alcohol and illicit drug use during pregnancy and after birth.
  Avoid overheating.
  Pregnant women should seek and obtain regular prenatal care.
  Infants should be immunized in accordance with AAP and CDC recommendations.
  Do not use home cardiorespiratory monitors as a strategy to reduce the risk of SIDS.
  Health care providers, staff in newborn nurseries and NICUs, and child care providers should endorse and model the SIDS risk-reduction recommendations from birth.
  Media and manufacturers should follow safe sleep guidelines in their messaging and advertising.
  Continue the "Safe to Sleep" campaign, focusing on ways to reduce the risk of all sleep-related infant deaths, including SIDS, suffocation, and other unintentional deaths. Pediatricians and other primary care providers should actively participate in this campaign.
B-level recommendations
  Avoid the use of commercial devices that are inconsistent with safe sleep recommendations.
  Supervised, awake tummy time is recommended to facilitate development and to minimize development of positional plagiocephaly.
C-level recommendations
  Continue research and surveillance on the risk factors, causes, and pathophysiologic mechanisms of SIDS and other sleep-related infant deaths, with the ultimate goal of eliminating these deaths entirely.
  There is no evidence to recommend swaddling as a strategy to reduce the risk of SIDS.

The following levels are based on the Strength-of-Recommendation Taxonomy (SORT) for the assignment of letter grades to each of its recommendations (A, B, or C).[2] Level A: There is good-quality patient-oriented evidence. Level B: There is inconsistent or limited-quality patient-oriented evidence. Level C: The recommendation is based on consensus, disease-oriented evidence, usual practice, expert opinion, or case series for studies of diagnosis, treatment, prevention, or screening. Note: "patient-oriented evidence" measures outcomes that matter to patients: morbidity, mortality, symptom improvement, cost reduction, and quality of life; "disease-oriented evidence" measures immediate, physiologic, or surrogate end points that may or may not reflect improvements in patient outcomes (eg, blood pressure, blood chemistry, physiologic function, pathologic findings). CDC, Centers for Disease Control and Prevention.

(including sudden infant death syndrome [SIDS] and ill-defined deaths), occurring during infancy. After case investigation, SUID can be attributed to suffocation, asphyxia, entrapment, infection, ingestions, metabolic diseases, arrhythmia-associated cardiac channelopathies, and trauma (unintentional or nonaccidental). SIDS is a subcategory of SUID and is a cause assigned to infant deaths that cannot be explained after a thorough case investigation, including a scene investigation, autopsy, and review of the clinical history.[1] (See Table 1 for definitions of terms.) The distinction between SIDS and other SUIDs, particularly those that occur during an unobserved sleep period (sleep-related infant deaths), such as unintentional suffocation, is challenging, cannot be determined by autopsy alone, and may remain unresolved after a full case investigation. Many of the modifiable and nonmodifiable risk factors for SIDS and suffocation are strikingly similar. This document focuses on the subset of SUIDs that occur during sleep.

The recommendations outlined herein were developed to reduce the risk of SIDS and sleep-related suffocation, asphyxia, and entrapment among infants in the general population. As defined by epidemiologists, risk refers to the probability that an outcome will occur given the presence of a particular factor or set of factors. Although all 19 recommendations are intended for all who care for infants, the last 4 recommendations also are directed toward health policy makers, researchers, and professionals who care for or work on behalf of infants. In addition, because certain behaviors, such as smoking, can increase risk for the infant, some recommendations are directed toward women who are pregnant or may become pregnant in the near future.

Table 2 summarizes each recommendation and provides the strength of the recommendation, which is based on the Strength-of-Recommendation Taxonomy.[2] It should be noted that there are no randomized controlled trials with regard to SIDS and other sleep-related deaths; instead, case-control studies are the standard.

The recommendations are based on epidemiologic studies that include infants up to 1 year of age. Therefore, recommendations for sleep position and the sleep environment, unless otherwise specified, are for the first year after birth. The evidence-based recommendations that follow are provided to guide health care providers in conversations with parents and others who care for infants. Health care providers are encouraged to have open and nonjudgmental conversations with families about their sleep practices. Individual medical conditions may warrant that a health care provider recommend otherwise after weighing the relative risks and benefits.

For the background literature review and data analyses on which this policy statement and recommendations are based, refer to the accompanying technical report, "SIDS and Other Sleep-Related Infant Deaths: Evidence Base for 2016 Updated Recommendations for a Safe Infant Sleeping Environment," available in the electronic pages of this issue (www.pediatrics.org/cgi/doi/10.1542/peds.2016-2940).[3]

RECOMMENDATIONS TO REDUCE THE RISK OF SIDS AND OTHER SLEEP-RELATED INFANT DEATHS

1. Back to sleep for every sleep.

To reduce the risk of SIDS, infants should be placed for sleep in a supine position (wholly on the back) for every sleep by every caregiver until the child reaches 1 year of age.[4–8] Side sleeping is not safe and is not advised.[5,7]

The supine sleep position does not increase the risk of choking and aspiration in infants, even those with gastroesophageal reflux, because infants have airway anatomy and mechanisms that protect against aspiration.[9,10] The American Academy of Pediatrics (AAP) concurs with the North American Society for Pediatric Gastroenterology and Nutrition that "the risk of SIDS outweighs the benefit of prone or lateral sleep position on GER [gastroesophageal reflux]; therefore, in most infants from birth to 12 months of age, supine positioning during sleep is recommended. ...Therefore, prone positioning is acceptable if the infant

is observed and awake, particularly in the postprandial period, but prone positioning during sleep can only be considered in infants with certain upper airway disorders in which the risk of death from GERD [gastroesophageal reflux disease] may outweigh the risk of SIDS."[11] Examples of such upper airway disorders are those in which airway-protective mechanisms are impaired, including infants with anatomic abnormalities, such as type 3 or 4 laryngeal clefts, who have not undergone antireflux surgery. There is no evidence to suggest that infants receiving nasogastric or orogastric feeds are at an increased risk of aspiration if placed in the supine position. Elevating the head of the infant's crib is ineffective in reducing gastroesophageal reflux[12] and is not recommended; in addition, elevating the head of the crib may result in the infant sliding to the foot of the crib into a position that may compromise respiration.

Preterm infants should be placed supine as soon as possible. Preterm infants are at increased risk of SIDS,[13,14] and the association between prone sleep position and SIDS among low birth weight and preterm infants is equal to, or perhaps even stronger than, the association among those born at term.[15] The task force concurs with the AAP Committee on Fetus and Newborn that "preterm infants should be placed supine for sleeping, just as term infants should, and the parents of preterm infants should be counseled about the importance of supine sleeping in preventing SIDS. Hospitalized preterm infants should be kept predominantly in the supine position, at least from the postmenstrual age of 32 weeks onward, so that they become acclimated to supine sleeping before discharge."[16] NICU personnel should endorse safe sleeping guidelines with parents of infants from the time of admission to the NICU.

As stated in the AAP clinical report, "skin-to-skin care is recommended for all mothers and newborns, regardless of feeding or delivery method, immediately following birth (as soon as the mother is medically stable, awake, and able to respond to her newborn), and to continue for at least an hour."[17] Thereafter, or when the mother needs to sleep or take care of other needs, infants should be placed supine in a bassinet. There is no evidence that placing infants on their side during the first few hours after delivery promotes clearance of amniotic fluid and decreases the risk of aspiration. Infants in the newborn nursery and infants who are rooming in with their parents should be placed in the supine position as soon as they are ready to be placed in the bassinet.

Although data to make specific recommendations as to when it is safe for infants to sleep in the prone or side position are lacking, studies establishing prone and side sleeping as risk factors for SIDS include infants up to 1 year of age. Therefore, the best evidence suggests that infants should continue to be placed supine until 1 year of age. Once an infant can roll from supine to prone and from prone to supine, the infant can be allowed to remain in the sleep position that he or she assumes. Because rolling into soft bedding is an important risk factor for SUID after 3 months of age,[18] parents and caregivers should continue to keep the infant's sleep environment clear of soft or loose bedding.

2. Use a firm sleep surface.

Infants should be placed on a firm sleep surface (eg, mattress in a safety-approved crib) covered by a fitted sheet with no other bedding or soft objects to reduce the risk of SIDS and suffocation.

A firm surface maintains its shape and will not indent or conform to the shape of the infant's head when the infant is placed on the surface.

Soft mattresses, including those made from memory foam, could create a pocket (or indentation) and increase the chance of rebreathing or suffocation if the infant is placed in or rolls over to the prone position.[19,20]

A crib, bassinet, portable crib, or play yard that conforms to the safety standards of the Consumer Product Safety Commission (CPSC), including those for slat spacing less than 2-3/8 inches, snugly fitting and firm mattresses, and no drop sides, is recommended.[21] In addition, parents and providers should check to make sure that the product has not been recalled. This is particularly important for used cribs. Cribs with missing hardware should not be used, nor should the parent or provider attempt to fix broken components of a crib, because many deaths are associated with cribs that are broken or with missing parts (including those that have presumably been fixed). Local organizations throughout the United States can help to provide low-cost or free cribs or play yards for families with financial constraints.

Bedside sleepers are attached to the side of the parental bed. The CPSC has published safety standards for these products,[22] and they may be considered by some parents as an option. However, there are no CPSC safety standards for in-bed sleepers. The task force cannot make a recommendation for or against the use of either bedside sleepers or in-bed sleepers, because there have been no studies examining the association between these products and SIDS or unintentional injury and death, including suffocation.

Only mattresses designed for the specific product should be used. Mattresses should be firm and should maintain their shape even when the fitted sheet designated for that model is used, such that there are no gaps between the mattress and the wall of the crib, bassinet, portable crib, or play yard. Pillows or cushions should not be used as substitutes for mattresses or in addition to a mattress. Mattress toppers, designed to make the sleep surface softer, should not be used for infants younger than 1 year.

There is no evidence that special crib mattresses and sleep surfaces that claim to reduce the chance of rebreathing carbon dioxide when the infant is in the prone position reduce the risk of SIDS. However, there is no disadvantage to the use of these mattresses if they meet the safety standards as described previously.

Soft materials or objects, such as pillows, quilts, comforters, or sheepskins, even if covered by a sheet, should not be placed under a sleeping infant. If a mattress cover to protect against wetness is used, it should be tightly fitting and thin.

Infants should not be placed for sleep on beds, because of the risk of entrapment and suffocation.[23,24] In addition, portable bed rails should not be used with infants, because of the risk of entrapment and strangulation.

The infant should sleep in an area free of hazards, such as dangling cords, electric wires, and window-covering cords, because these may present a strangulation risk.

Sitting devices, such as car seats, strollers, swings, infant carriers, and infant slings, are not recommended for routine sleep in the hospital or at home, particularly for young infants.[25-30] Infants who are younger than 4 months are particularly at risk, because they may assume positions that can create a risk of suffocation or airway obstruction or may not be able to move out of a potentially asphyxiating situation. When infant slings and cloth carriers are used for carrying, it is important to ensure that the infant's head is up and above the fabric, the face is visible, and the nose and mouth are clear of obstructions.[31] After nursing, the infant should be repositioned in the sling so that the head is up, is clear of fabric, and is not against the adult's body or the sling. If an infant falls asleep in a sitting device, he or she should be removed from the product and moved to a crib or other appropriate flat surface as soon as is safe and practical. Car seats and similar products are not stable on a crib mattress or other elevated surfaces.[32-36] Infants should not be left unattended in car seats and similar products, nor should they be placed or left in car seats and similar products with the straps unbuckled or partially buckled.[30]

3. Breastfeeding is recommended.

Breastfeeding is associated with a reduced risk of SIDS.[37-39] Unless contraindicated, mothers should breastfeed exclusively or feed with expressed milk (ie, not offer any formula or other nonhuman milk-based supplements) for 6 months, in alignment with recommendations of the AAP.[40]

The protective effect of breastfeeding increases with exclusivity.[39] However, any breastfeeding has been shown to be more protective against SIDS than no breastfeeding.[39]

4. It is recommended that infants sleep in the parents' room, close to the parents' bed, but on a separate surface designed for infants, ideally for the first year of life, but at least for the first 6 months.

There is evidence that sleeping in the parents' room but on a separate surface decreases the risk of SIDS by as much as 50%.[6,8,41,42] In addition, this arrangement is most likely to prevent suffocation, strangulation, and entrapment that may occur when the infant is sleeping in the adult bed.

The infant's crib, portable crib, play yard, or bassinet should be placed in the parents' bedroom until the child's first birthday. Although there is no specific evidence for moving an infant to his or her own room before 1 year of age, the first 6 months are particularly critical, because the rates of SIDS and other sleep-related deaths, particularly those occurring in bed-sharing situations, are highest in the first 6 months. Placing the crib close to the parents' bed so that the infant is within view and reach can facilitate feeding, comforting, and monitoring of the infant. Room-sharing reduces SIDS risk and removes the possibility of suffocation, strangulation, and entrapment that may occur when the infant is sleeping in the adult bed.

There is insufficient evidence to recommend for or against the use of devices promoted to make bed-sharing "safe." There is no evidence that these devices reduce the risk of SIDS or suffocation or are safe. Some products designed for in-bed use (in-bed sleepers) are currently under study but results are not yet available. Bedside sleepers, which attach to the side of the parental bed and for which the CPSC has published standards,[22] may be considered by some parents as an option. There are no CPSC safety standards for in-bed sleepers. The task force cannot make a recommendation for or against the use of either bedside sleepers or in-bed sleepers, because there have been no studies examining the association between these products and SIDS or unintentional injury and death, including suffocation.

Infants who are brought into the bed for feeding or comforting should be returned to their own crib or bassinet when the parent is ready to return to sleep.[7,43]

Couches and armchairs are extremely dangerous places for infants. Sleeping on couches and armchairs places infants at extraordinarily high risk of infant death, including SIDS,[4,6,7,42,43] suffocation through entrapment or wedging between seat cushions, or overlay if another person is also sharing this surface.[44] Therefore, parents and other caregivers should be especially vigilant as to their wakefulness when feeding infants or lying with infants on these surfaces.

Infants should never be placed on a couch or armchair for sleep.

The safest place for an infant to sleep is on a separate sleep surface designed for infants close to the parents' bed. However, the AAP acknowledges that parents frequently fall asleep while feeding the infant. Evidence suggests that it is less hazardous to fall asleep with the infant in the adult bed than on a sofa or armchair, should the parent fall asleep. It is important to note that a large percentage of infants who die of SIDS are found with their head covered by bedding. Therefore, no pillows, sheets, blankets, or any other items that could obstruct infant breathing or cause overheating should be in the bed. Parents should also follow safe sleep recommendations outlined elsewhere in this statement. Because there is evidence that the risk of bed-sharing is higher with longer duration, if the parent falls asleep while feeding the infant in bed, the infant should be placed back on a separate sleep surface as soon as the parent awakens.

There are specific circumstances that, in case-control studies and case series, have been shown to substantially increase the risk of SIDS or unintentional injury or death while bed-sharing, and these should be avoided at all times:

- Bed-sharing with a term normal-weight infant younger than 4 months[6,8,42,43,45,46] and infants born preterm and/or with low birth weight,[47] regardless of parental smoking status. Even for breastfed infants, there is an increased risk of SIDS when bed-sharing if younger than 4 months.[48] This appears to be a particularly vulnerable time, so if parents choose to feed their infants younger than 4 months in bed, they should be especially vigilant to not fall asleep.

- Bed-sharing with a current smoker (even if he or she does not smoke in bed) or if the mother smoked during pregnancy.[6,7,46,49,50]

- Bed-sharing with someone who is impaired in his or her alertness or ability to arouse because of fatigue or use of sedating medications (eg, certain antidepressants, pain medications) or substances (eg, alcohol, illicit drugs).[8,48,51,52]

- Bed-sharing with anyone who is not the infant's parent, including nonparental caregivers and other children.[4]

- Bed-sharing on a soft surface, such as a waterbed, old mattress, sofa, couch, or armchair.[4,6,7,42,43]

- Bed-sharing with soft bedding accessories, such as pillows or blankets.[4,53]

- The safety and benefits of cobedding for twins and higher-order multiples have not been established. It is prudent to provide separate sleep surfaces and avoid cobedding for twins and higher-order multiples in the hospital and at home.[54]

5. **Keep soft objects and loose bedding away from the infant's sleep area to reduce the risk of SIDS, suffocation, entrapment, and strangulation.**

Soft objects,[19,20,55–58] such as pillows and pillow-like toys, quilts, comforters, sheepskins, and loose bedding,[4,7,59–64] such as blankets and nonfitted sheets, can obstruct an infant's nose and mouth. An obstructed airway can pose a risk of suffocation, entrapment, or SIDS.

Infant sleep clothing, such as a wearable blanket, is preferable to blankets and other coverings to keep the infant warm while reducing the chance of head covering or entrapment that could result from blanket use.

Bumper pads or similar products that attach to crib slats or sides were originally intended to prevent injury or death attributable to head entrapment. Cribs manufactured to newer standards have a narrower distance between slats to prevent head entrapment. Because bumper pads have been implicated as a factor contributing to deaths from suffocation, entrapment, and strangulation[65,66] and because they are not necessary to prevent head entrapment with new safety standards for crib slats, they are not recommended for infants.[65,66]

6. Consider offering a pacifier at nap time and bedtime.

Although the mechanism is yet unclear, studies have reported a protective effect of pacifiers on the incidence of SIDS.[67,68] The protective effect of the pacifier is observed even if the pacifier falls out of the infant's mouth.[69,70]

The pacifier should be used when placing the infant for sleep. It does not need to be reinserted once the infant falls asleep. If the infant refuses the pacifier, he or she should not be forced to take it. In those cases, parents can try to offer the pacifier again when the infant is a little older.

Because of the risk of strangulation, pacifiers should not be hung around the infant's neck. Pacifiers that attach to infant clothing should not be used with sleeping infants.

Objects, such as stuffed toys and other items that may present a suffocation or choking risk, should not be attached to pacifiers.

For breastfed infants, pacifier introduction should be delayed until breastfeeding is firmly established.[40] Infants who are not being directly breastfed can begin pacifier use as soon as desired.

There is insufficient evidence that finger sucking is protective against SIDS.

7. Avoid smoke exposure during pregnancy and after birth.

Both maternal smoking during pregnancy and smoke in the infant's environment after birth are major risk factors for SIDS.

Mothers should not smoke during pregnancy or after the infant's birth.[71-74]

There should be no smoking near pregnant women or infants. Encourage families to set strict rules for smoke-free homes and cars and to eliminate secondhand tobacco smoke from all places in which children and other nonsmokers spend time.[75,76]

The risk of SIDS is particularly high when the infant bed-shares with an adult smoker, even when the adult does not smoke in bed.[6,7,46,49,50,77]

8. Avoid alcohol and illicit drug use during pregnancy and after birth.

There is an increased risk of SIDS with prenatal and postnatal exposure to alcohol or illicit drug use.

Mothers should avoid alcohol and illicit drugs periconceptionally and during pregnancy.[78-85]

Parental alcohol and/or illicit drug use in combination with bed-sharing places the infant at particularly high risk of SIDS.[8,51]

9. Avoid overheating and head covering in infants.

Although studies have shown an increased risk of SIDS with overheating,[86-89] the definition of overheating in these studies varies. Therefore, it is difficult to provide specific room temperature guidelines to avoid overheating.

In general, infants should be dressed appropriately for the environment, with no greater than 1 layer more than an adult would wear to be comfortable in that environment.

Parents and caregivers should evaluate the infant for signs of overheating, such as sweating or the infant's chest feeling hot to the touch.

Overbundling and covering of the face and head should be avoided.[90]

There is currently insufficient evidence to recommend the use of a fan as a SIDS risk-reduction strategy.

10. Pregnant women should obtain regular prenatal care.

There is substantial epidemiologic evidence linking a lower risk of SIDS for infants whose mothers obtain

regular prenatal care.[71-74] Pregnant women should follow guidelines for frequency of prenatal visits.[91]

11. Infants should be immunized in accordance with recommendations of the AAP and Centers for Disease Control and Prevention.

There is no evidence that there is a causal relationship between immunizations and SIDS.[92-95] Indeed, recent evidence suggests that vaccination may have a protective effect against SIDS.[96-98]

12. Avoid the use of commercial devices that are inconsistent with safe sleep recommendations.

Be particularly wary of devices that claim to reduce the risk of SIDS. Examples include, but are not limited to, wedges and positioners and other devices placed in the adult bed for the purpose of positioning or separating the infant from others in the bed. Crib mattresses also have been developed to improve the dispersion of carbon dioxide in the event that the infant ends up in the prone position during sleep. Although data do not support the claim of carbon dioxide dispersion unless there is an active dispersal component,[99] there is no harm in using these mattresses if they meet standard safety requirements. However, there is no evidence that any of these devices reduce the risk of SIDS. Importantly, the use of products claiming to increase sleep safety does not diminish the importance of following recommended safe sleep practices. Information about a specific product can be found on the CPSC Web site (www.cpsc.gov). The AAP concurs with the US Food and Drug Administration and the CPSC that manufacturers should not claim that a product or device protects against SIDS unless there is scientific evidence to that effect.

13. Do not use home cardiorespiratory monitors as a strategy to reduce the risk of SIDS.

The use of cardiorespiratory monitors has not been documented to decrease the incidence of SIDS.[100–103] These devices are sometimes prescribed for use at home to detect apnea or bradycardia and, when pulse oximetry is used, decreases in oxyhemoglobin saturation for infants at risk of these conditions. In addition, routine in-hospital cardiorespiratory monitoring before discharge from the hospital has not been shown to detect infants at risk of SIDS. There are no data that other commercial devices that are designed to monitor infant vital signs reduce the risk of SIDS.

14. Supervised, awake tummy time is recommended to facilitate development and to minimize development of positional plagiocephaly.

Although there are no data to make specific recommendations as to how often and how long it should be undertaken, the task force concurs with the AAP Committee on Practice and Ambulatory Medicine and Section on Neurologic Surgery that "a certain amount of prone positioning, or 'tummy time,' while the infant is awake and being observed is recommended to help prevent the development of flattening of the occiput and to facilitate development of the upper shoulder girdle strength necessary for timely attainment of certain motor milestones."[104]

Diagnosis, management, and other prevention strategies for positional plagiocephaly, such as avoidance of excessive time in car seats and changing the infant's orientation in the crib, are discussed in detail in the AAP clinical report on positional skull deformities.[104]

15. There is no evidence to recommend swaddling as a strategy to reduce the risk of SIDS.

Swaddling, or wrapping the infant in a light blanket, is often used as a strategy to calm the infant and encourage the use of the supine position. There is a high risk of death if a swaddled infant is

placed in or rolls to the prone position.[88,105,106] If infants are swaddled, they should always be placed on the back. Swaddling should be snug around the chest but allow for ample room at the hips and knees to avoid exacerbation of hip dysplasia. When an infant exhibits signs of attempting to roll, swaddling should no longer be used.[88,105,106] There is no evidence with regard to SIDS risk related to the arms swaddled in or out. These decisions about swaddling should be made on an individual basis, depending on the physiologic needs of the infant.

16. Health care professionals, staff in newborn nurseries and NICUs, and child care providers should endorse and model the SIDS risk-reduction recommendations from birth.[107–109]

Staff in NICUs should model and implement all SIDS risk-reduction recommendations as soon as the infant is medically stable and well before anticipated discharge.

Staff in newborn nurseries should model and implement these recommendations beginning at birth and well before anticipated discharge.

All physicians, nurses, and other health care providers should receive education on safe infant sleep. Health care providers should screen for and recommend safe sleep practices at each visit for infants up to 1 year old. Families who do not have a safe sleep space for their infant should be provided with information about low-cost or free cribs or play yards.

Hospitals should ensure that hospital policies are consistent with updated safe sleep recommendations and that infant sleep spaces (bassinets, cribs) meet safe sleep standards.

All state regulatory agencies should require that child care providers receive education on safe infant sleep and implement safe sleep practices. It is preferable that they have written policies.

17. Media and manufacturers should follow safe sleep guidelines in their messaging and advertising.

Media exposures (including movie, television, magazines, newspapers, and Web sites), manufacturer advertisements, and store displays affect individual behavior by influencing beliefs and attitudes.[107,109] Media and advertising messages contrary to safe sleep recommendations may create misinformation about safe sleep practices.[110]

18. Continue the "Safe to Sleep" campaign, focusing on ways to reduce the risk of all sleep-related infant deaths, including SIDS, suffocation, and other unintentional deaths. Pediatricians and other primary care providers should actively participate in this campaign.

Public education should continue for all who care for infants, including parents, child care providers, grandparents, foster parents, and babysitters, and should include strategies for overcoming barriers to behavior change.

The campaign should continue to have a special focus on the black and American Indian/Alaskan Native populations because of the higher incidence of SIDS and other sleep-related infant deaths in these groups.

The campaign should specifically include strategies to increase breastfeeding while decreasing bed-sharing, and eliminating tobacco smoke exposure. The campaign should also highlight the circumstances that substantially increase the risk of SIDS or unintentional injury or death while bed-sharing, as listed previously.

These recommendations should be introduced before pregnancy and ideally in secondary school curricula to both males and females and incorporated into courses developed to train teenaged and adult babysitters. The importance of maternal preconceptional health, infant breastfeeding, and the avoidance of substance use (including alcohol and smoking) should be included in this training.

Safe sleep messages should be reviewed, revised, and reissued at least every 5 years to address the next generation of new parents and products on the market.

19. **Continue research and surveillance on the risk factors, causes, and pathophysiologic mechanisms of SIDS and other sleep-related infant deaths, with the ultimate goal of eliminating these deaths altogether.**

Education campaigns need to be evaluated, and innovative intervention methods need to be encouraged and funded.

Continued research and improved surveillance on the etiology and pathophysiologic basis of SIDS should be funded.

Standardized protocols for death scene investigations, as per Centers for Disease Control and Prevention protocol, should continue to be implemented. Comprehensive autopsies, including full external and internal examination of all major organs and tissues including the brain; complete radiographs; metabolic testing; and toxicology screening should be performed. Training about how to conduct a comprehensive death scene investigation offered to medical examiners, coroners, death scene investigators, first responders, and law enforcement should continue; and resources to maintain training and conduct of these investigations need to be allocated. In addition, child death reviews, with involvement of pediatricians and other primary care providers, should be supported and funded.

Improved and widespread surveillance of SIDS and SUID cases should be implemented and funded.

Federal and private funding agencies should remain committed to all

aspects of the aforementioned research.

ACKNOWLEDGMENTS

We acknowledge the contributions provided by others to the collection and interpretation of data examined in preparation of this report. We are particularly grateful for the independent biostatistical report submitted by Robert W. Platt, PhD.

LEAD AUTHOR

Rachel Y. Moon, MD, FAAP

TASK FORCE ON SUDDEN INFANT DEATH SYNDROME

Rachel Y. Moon, MD, FAAP, Chairperson
Robert A. Darnall, MD
Lori Feldman-Winter, MD, MPH, FAAP
Michael H. Goodstein, MD, FAAP
Fern R. Hauck, MD, MS

CONSULTANTS

Marian Willinger, PhD – Eunice Kennedy Shriver *National Institute for Child Health and Human Development*
Carrie K. Shapiro-Mendoza, PhD, MPH – *Centers for Disease Control and Prevention*

STAFF

James Couto, MA

ABBREVIATIONS

AAP: American Academy of Pediatrics
CPSC: Consumer Product Safety Commission
SIDS: sudden infant death syndrome
SUID: sudden unexpected infant death

REFERENCES

1. Willinger M, James LS, Catz C. Defining the sudden infant death syndrome (SIDS): deliberations of an expert panel convened by the National Institute of Child Health and Human Development. *Pediatr Pathol.* 1991;11(5):677–684

2. Ebell MH, Siwek J, Weiss BD, et al. Strength of recommendation taxonomy (SORT): a patient-centered approach to grading evidence in the medical literature. *Am Fam Physician.* 2004;69(3):548–556

3. Moon RY; AAP Task Force on Sudden Infant Death Syndrome. SIDS and other sleep-related infant deaths: Evidence base for 2016 updated recommendations for a safe infant sleeping environment. *Pediatrics.* 2016;138(5):e20162940

4. Hauck FR, Herman SM, Donovan M, et al. Sleep environment and the risk of sudden infant death syndrome in an urban population: the Chicago Infant Mortality Study. *Pediatrics.* 2003; 111(5 pt 2):1207–1214

5. Li DK, Petitti DB, Willinger M, et al. Infant sleeping position and the risk of sudden infant death syndrome in California, 1997-2000. *Am J Epidemiol.* 2003;157(5):446–455

6. Blair PS, Fleming PJ, Smith IJ, et al; CESDI SUDI Research Group. Babies sleeping with parents: case-control study of factors influencing the risk of the sudden infant death syndrome. *BMJ.* 1999;319(7223):1457–1461

7. Fleming PJ, Blair PS, Bacon C, et al; Confidential Enquiry into Stillbirths and Deaths Regional Coordinators and Researchers. Environment of infants during sleep and risk of the sudden infant death syndrome: results of 1993-5 case-control study for confidential inquiry into stillbirths and deaths in infancy. *BMJ.* 1996;313(7051):191–195

8. Carpenter RG, Irgens LM, Blair PS, et al. Sudden unexplained infant death in 20 regions in Europe: case control study. *Lancet.* 2004;363(9404):185–191

9. Malloy MH. Trends in postneonatal aspiration deaths and reclassification of sudden infant death syndrome: impact of the "Back to Sleep" program. *Pediatrics.* 2002;109(4):661–665

10. Tablizo MA, Jacinto P, Parsley D, Chen ML, Ramanathan R, Keens TG. Supine sleeping position does not cause clinical aspiration in neonates in hospital newborn nurseries. *Arch Pediatr Adolesc Med.* 2007;161(5):507–510

11. Vandenplas Y, Rudolph CD, Di Lorenzo C, et al; North American Society

for Pediatric Gastroenterology Hepatology and Nutrition; European Society for Pediatric Gastroenterology Hepatology and Nutrition. Pediatric gastroesophageal reflux clinical practice guidelines: joint recommendations of the North American Society for Pediatric Gastroenterology, Hepatology, and Nutrition (NASPGHAN) and the European Society for Pediatric Gastroenterology, Hepatology, and Nutrition (ESPGHAN). *J Pediatr Gastroenterol Nutr.* 2009;49(4):498–547

12. Tobin JM, McCloud P, Cameron DJ. Posture and gastro-oesophageal reflux: a case for left lateral positioning. *Arch Dis Child.* 1997;76(3):254–258

13. Malloy MH, Hoffman HJ. Prematurity, sudden infant death syndrome, and age of death. *Pediatrics.* 1995;96(3 pt 1):464–471

14. Sowter B, Doyle LW, Morley CJ, Altmann A, Halliday J. Is sudden infant death syndrome still more common in very low birthweight infants in the 1990s? *Med J Aust.* 1999;171(8):411–413

15. Oyen N, Markestad T, Skaerven R, et al. Combined effects of sleeping position and prenatal risk factors in sudden infant death syndrome: the Nordic Epidemiological SIDS Study. *Pediatrics.* 1997;100(4):613–621

16. American Academy of Pediatrics Committee on Fetus and Newborn. Hospital discharge of the high-risk neonate. *Pediatrics.* 2008;122(5):1119–1126

17. Winter-Feldman L, Golsmith JP; American Academy of Pediatrics Committee on Fetus and Newborn. Safe sleep and skin-to-skin care in the neonatal period for healthy term newborns. *Pediatrics.* 2016;138(3):e20161889

18. Colvin JD, Collie-Akers V, Schunn C, Moon RY. Sleep environment risks for younger and older infants. *Pediatrics.* 2014;134(2):e406–e412

19. Kemp JS, Nelson VE, Thach BT. Physical properties of bedding that may increase risk of sudden infant death syndrome in prone-sleeping infants. *Pediatr Res.* 1994;36(1 pt 1): 7–11

20. Kemp JS, Livne M, White DK, Arfken CL. Softness and potential to cause rebreathing: differences in bedding used by infants at high and low risk for sudden infant death syndrome. *J Pediatr.* 1998;132(2):234–239

21. US Consumer Product Safety Commission. *Crib Safety Tips: Use Your Crib Safely,* CPSC Document 5030. Washington, DC: US Consumer Product Safety Commission; 2006

22. US Consumer Product Safety Commission. Safety standard for bedside sleepers. *Fed Reg.* 2014;79(10):2581–2589

23. Ostfeld BM, Perl H, Esposito L, et al. Sleep environment, positional, lifestyle, and demographic characteristics associated with bed sharing in sudden infant death syndrome cases: a population-based study. *Pediatrics.* 2006;118(5):2051–2059

24. Scheers NJ, Rutherford GW, Kemp JS. Where should infants sleep? A comparison of risk for suffocation of infants sleeping in cribs, adult beds, and other sleeping locations. *Pediatrics.* 2003;112(4):883–889

25. Bass JL, Bull M. Oxygen desaturation in term infants in car safety seats. *Pediatrics.* 2002;110(2 pt 1):401–402

26. Kornhauser Cerar L, Scirica CV, Stucin Gantar I, Osredkar I don'D, Neubauer D, Kinane TB. A comparison of respiratory patterns in healthy term infants placed in car safety seats and beds. *Pediatrics.* 2009;124(3). Available at: www.pediatrics.org/cgi/content/full/124/3/e396

27. Côté A, Bairam A, Deschenes M, Hatzakis G. Sudden infant deaths in sitting devices. *Arch Dis Child.* 2008;93(5):384–389

28. Merchant JR, Worwa C, Porter S, Coleman JM, deRegnier RA. Respiratory instability of term and near-term healthy newborn infants in car safety seats. *Pediatrics.* 2001;108(3):647–652

29. Willett LD, Leuschen MP, Nelson LS, Nelson RM Jr. Risk of hypoventilation in premature infants in car seats. *J Pediatr.* 1986;109(2):245–248

30. Batra EK, Midgett JD, Moon RY. Hazards associated with sitting and carrying devices for children

two years and younger. *J Pediatr.* 2015;167(1):183–187

31. US Consumer Product Safety Commission. Safety Standard for Sling Carriers. *Fed Reg.* 2014;79(141):42724–42734

32. Desapriya EB, Joshi P, Subzwari S, Nolan M. Infant injuries from child restraint safety seat misuse at British Columbia Children's Hospital. *Pediatr Int.* 2008;50(5):674–678

33. Graham CJ, Kittredge D, Stuemky JH. Injuries associated with child safety seat misuse. *Pediatr Emerg Care.* 1992;8(6):351–353

34. Parikh SN, Wilson L. Hazardous use of car seats outside the car in the United States, 2003-2007. *Pediatrics.* 2010;126(2):352–357

35. Pollack-Nelson C. Fall and suffocation injuries associated with in-home use of car seats and baby carriers. *Pediatr Emerg Care.* 2000;16(2):77–79

36. Wickham T, Abrahamson E. Head injuries in infants: the risks of bouncy chairs and car seats. *Arch Dis Child.* 2002;86(3):168–169

37. Ip S, Chung M, Raman G, Trikalinos TA, Lau J. A summary of the Agency for Healthcare Research and Quality's evidence report on breastfeeding in developed countries. *Breastfeed Med.* 2009;4(suppl 1):S17–S30

38. Vennemann MM, Bajanowski T, Brinkmann B, et al; GeSID Study Group. Does breastfeeding reduce the risk of sudden infant death syndrome? *Pediatrics.* 2009;123(3). Available at: www.pediatrics.org/cgi/content/full/123/3/e406

39. Hauck FR, Thompson JM, Tanabe KO, Moon RY, Vennemann MM. Breastfeeding and reduced risk of sudden infant death syndrome: a meta-analysis. *Pediatrics.* 2011;128(1):103–110

40. Eidelman AI, Schanler RJ; Section on Breastfeeding. Breastfeeding and the use of human milk. *Pediatrics.* 2012;129(3). Available at: www.pediatrics.org/cgi/content/full/129/3/e827

41. Mitchell EA, Thompson JMD. Co-sleeping increases the risk of SIDS, but sleeping in the parents' bedroom lowers it. In: Rognum TO,

ed. *Sudden Infant Death Syndrome: New Trends in the Nineties*. Oslo, Norway: Scandinavian University Press; 1995:266–269

42. Tappin D, Ecob R, Brooke H. Bedsharing, roomsharing, and sudden infant death syndrome in Scotland: a case-control study. *J Pediatr.* 2005;147(1):32–37

43. McGarvey C, McDonnell M, Chong A, O'Regan M, Matthews T. Factors relating to the infant's last sleep environment in sudden infant death syndrome in the Republic of Ireland. *Arch Dis Child.* 2003;88(12):1058–1064

44. Rechtman LR, Colvin JD, Blair PS, Moon RY. Sofas and infant mortality. *Pediatrics.* 2014;134(5). Available at: www.pediatrics.org/cgi/content/full/134/5/e1293

45. McGarvey C, McDonnell M, Hamilton K, O'Regan M, Matthews T. An 8 year study of risk factors for SIDS: bed-sharing versus non-bed-sharing. *Arch Dis Child.* 2006;91(4):318–323

46. Vennemann MM, Hense HW, Bajanowski T, et al Bed sharing and the risk of sudden infant death syndrome: can we resolve the debate? *J Pediatr.* 2012;160(1):44–48, e42

47. Blair PS, Platt MW, Smith IJ, Fleming PJ; CESDI SUDI Research Group. Sudden infant death syndrome and sleeping position in pre-term and low birth weight infants: an opportunity for targeted intervention. *Arch Dis Child.* 2006;91(2):101–106

48. Carpenter R, McGarvey C, Mitchell EA, et al. Bed sharing when parents do not smoke: is there a risk of SIDS? An individual level analysis of five major case-control studies. *BMJ Open.* 2013;3(5):e002299

49. Arnestad M, Andersen M, Vege A, Rognum TO. Changes in the epidemiological pattern of sudden infant death syndrome in southeast Norway, 1984-1998: implications for future prevention and research. *Arch Dis Child.* 2001;85(2):108–115

50. Scragg R, Mitchell EA, Taylor BJ, et al; New Zealand Cot Death Study Group. Bed sharing, smoking, and alcohol in the sudden infant death syndrome. *BMJ.* 1993;307(6915):1312–1318

51. Blair PS, Sidebotham P, Evason-Coombe C, Edmonds M, Heckstall-Smith EM, Fleming P. Hazardous cosleeping environments and risk factors amenable to change: case-control study of SIDS in south west England. *BMJ.* 2009;339:b3666

52. Blair PS, Sidebotham P, Pease A, Fleming PJ. Bed-sharing in the absence of hazardous circumstances: is there a risk of sudden infant death syndrome? An analysis from two case-control studies conducted in the UK. *PLoS One.* 2014;9(9):e107799

53. Fu LY, Moon RY, Hauck FR. Bed sharing among black infants and sudden infant death syndrome: interactions with other known risk factors. *Acad Pediatr.* 2010;10(6):376–382

54. Tomashek KM, Wallman C; American Academy of Pediatrics Committee on Fetus and Newborn. Cobedding twins and higher-order multiples in a hospital setting. *Pediatrics.* 2007;120(6):1359–1366

55. Chiodini BA, Thach BT. Impaired ventilation in infants sleeping facedown: potential significance for sudden infant death syndrome. *J Pediatr.* 1993;123(5):686–692

56. Sakai J, Kanetake J, Takahashi S, Kanawaku Y, Funayama M. Gas dispersal potential of bedding as a cause for sudden infant death. *Forensic Sci Int.* 2008;180(2–3):93–97

57. Patel AL, Harris K, Thach BT. Inspired CO(2) and O(2) in sleeping infants rebreathing from bedding: relevance for sudden infant death syndrome. *J Appl Physiol (1985).* 2001;91(6):2537–2545

58. Kanetake J, Aoki Y, Funayama M. Evaluation of rebreathing potential on bedding for infant use. *Pediatr Int.* 2003;45(3):284–289

59. Brooke H, Gibson A, Tappin D, Brown H. Case-control study of sudden infant death syndrome in Scotland, 1992-5. *BMJ.* 1997;314(7093):1516–1520

60. L'Hoir MP, Engelberts AC, van Well GTJ, et al. Risk and preventive factors for cot death in The Netherlands, a low-incidence country. *Eur J Pediatr.* 1998;157(8):681–688

61. Markestad T, Skadberg B, Hordvik E, Morild I, Irgens LM. Sleeping position and sudden infant death syndrome (SIDS): effect of an intervention programme to avoid prone sleeping. *Acta Paediatr.* 1995;84(4):375–378

62. Ponsonby A-L, Dwyer T, Couper D, Cochrane J. Association between use of a quilt and sudden infant death syndrome: case-control study. *BMJ.* 1998;316(7126):195–196

63. Beal SM, Byard RW. Accidental death or sudden infant death syndrome? *J Paediatr Child Health.* 1995;31(4):269–271

64. Wilson CA, Taylor BJ, Laing RM, Williams SM, Mitchell EA. Clothing and bedding and its relevance to sudden infant death syndrome: further results from the New Zealand Cot Death Study. *J Paediatr Child Health.* 1994;30(6):506–512

65. Thach BT, Rutherford GW Jr, Harris K. Deaths and injuries attributed to infant crib bumper pads. *J Pediatr.* 2007;151(3):271–274, 274.e1–274.e3

66. Scheers NJ, Woodard DW, Thach BT. Crib bumpers continue to cause infant deaths: a need for a new preventive approach. *J Pediatr.* 2016;169:93–97, e91

67. Hauck FR, Omojokun OO, Siadaty MS. Do pacifiers reduce the risk of sudden infant death syndrome? A meta-analysis. *Pediatrics.* 2005;116(5). Available at: www.pediatrics.org/cgi/content/full/116/5/e716

68. Li DK, Willinger M, Petitti DB, Odouli R, Liu L, Hoffman HJ. Use of a dummy (pacifier) during sleep and risk of sudden infant death syndrome (SIDS): population-based case-control study. *BMJ.* 2006;332(7532):18–22

69. Franco P, Scaillet S, Wermenbol V, Valente F, Groswasser J, Kahn A. The influence of a pacifier on infants' arousals from sleep. *J Pediatr.* 2000;136(6):775–779

70. Weiss PP, Kerbl R. The relatively short duration that a child retains a pacifier in the mouth during sleep: implications for sudden infant death syndrome. *Eur J Pediatr.* 2001;160(1):60–70

71. Getahun D, Amre D, Rhoads GG, Demissie K. Maternal and obstetric risk factors for sudden infant death syndrome in the United States. *Obstet Gynecol.* 2004;103(4):646–652

72. Kraus JF, Greenland S, Bulterys M. Risk factors for sudden infant death syndrome in the US Collaborative Perinatal Project. *Int J Epidemiol.* 1989;18(1):113–120

73. Paris CA, Remler R, Daling JR. Risk factors for sudden infant death syndrome: changes associated with sleep position recommendations. *J Pediatr.* 2001;139(6):771–777

74. Stewart AJ, Williams SM, Mitchell EA, Taylor BJ, Ford RP, Allen EM. Antenatal and intrapartum factors associated with sudden infant death syndrome in the New Zealand Cot Death Study. *J Paediatr Child Health.* 1995;31(5):473–478

75. Farber HJ, Walley SC, Groner JA, Nelson KE; Section on Tobacco Control. Clinical practice policy to protect children from tobacco, nicotine, and tobacco smoke [policy statement]. *Pediatrics.* 2015;136(5):1008–1017

76. Farber HJ, Groner J, Walley S, Nelson K; Section on Tobacco Control. Protecting children from tobacco, nicotine, and tobacco smoke [technical report]. *Pediatrics.* 2015;136(5). Available at: www.pediatrics.org/cgi/content/full/136/5/e1439

77. Zhang K, Wang X. Maternal smoking and increased risk of sudden infant death syndrome: a meta-analysis. *Leg Med (Tokyo).* 2013;15(3):115–121

78. Rajegowda BK, Kandall SR, Falciglia H. Sudden unexpected death in infants of narcotic-dependent mothers. *Early Hum Dev.* 1978;2(3):219–225

79. Chavez CJ, Ostrea EM Jr, Stryker JC, Smialek Z. Sudden infant death syndrome among infants of drug-dependent mothers. *J Pediatr.* 1979;95(3):407–409

80. Durand DJ, Espinoza AM, Nickerson BG. Association between prenatal cocaine exposure and sudden infant death syndrome. *J Pediatr.* 1990;117(6):909–911

81. Ward SL, Bautista D, Chan L, et al. Sudden infant death syndrome in infants of substance-abusing mothers. *J Pediatr.* 1990;117(6):876–881

82. Rosen TS, Johnson HL. Drug-addicted mothers, their infants, and SIDS. *Ann N Y Acad Sci.* 1988;533:89–95

83. Kandall SR, Gaines J, Habel L, Davidson G, Jessop D. Relationship of maternal substance abuse to subsequent sudden infant death syndrome in offspring. *J Pediatr.* 1993;123(1):120–126

84. Fares I, McCulloch KM, Raju TN. Intrauterine cocaine exposure and the risk for sudden infant death syndrome: a meta-analysis. *J Perinatol.* 1997;17(3):179–182

85. O'Leary CM, Jacoby PJ, Bartu A, D'Antoine H, Bower C. Maternal alcohol use and sudden infant death syndrome and infant mortality excluding SIDS. *Pediatrics.* 2013;131(3). Available at: www.pediatrics.org/cgi/content/full/131/3/e770

86. Fleming PJ, Gilbert R, Azaz Y, et al. Interaction between bedding and sleeping position in the sudden infant death syndrome: a population based case-control study. *BMJ.* 1990;301(6743):85–89

87. Ponsonby A-L, Dwyer T, Gibbons LE, Cochrane JA, Jones ME, McCall MJ. Thermal environment and sudden infant death syndrome: case-control study. *BMJ.* 1992;304(6822):277–282

88. Ponsonby A-L, Dwyer T, Gibbons LE, Cochrane JA, Wang Y-G. Factors potentiating the risk of sudden infant death syndrome associated with the prone position. *N Engl J Med.* 1993;329(6):377–382

89. Iyasu S, Randall LL, Welty TK, et al. Risk factors for sudden infant death syndrome among northern plains Indians. *JAMA.* 2002;288(21):2717–2723

90. Blair PS, Mitchell EA, Heckstall-Smith EM, Fleming PJ. Head covering—a major modifiable risk factor for sudden infant death syndrome: a systematic review. *Arch Dis Child.* 2008;93(9):778–783

91. American Academy of Pediatrics Committee on Fetus and Newborn; ACOG Committee on Obstetric Practice. *Guidelines for Perinatal Care.* 7th ed. Elk Grove Village, IL: American Academy of Pediatrics; 2012

92. Immunization Safety Review Committee. Stratton K, Almario DA, Wizemann TM, McCormick MC, eds. *Immunization Safety Review: Vaccinations and Sudden Unexpected Death in Infancy.* Washington, DC: National Academies Press; 2003

93. Moro PL, Arana J, Cano M, Lewis P, Shimabukuro TT. Deaths reported to the Vaccine Adverse Event Reporting System, United States, 1997-2013. *Clin Infect Dis.* 2015;61(6):980–987

94. Miller ER, Moro PL, Cano M, Shimabukuro TT. Deaths following vaccination: what does the evidence show? *Vaccine.* 2015;33(29):3288–3292

95. Moro PL, Jankosky C, Menschik D, et al. Adverse events following Haemophilus influenzae type b vaccines in the Vaccine Adverse Event Reporting System, 1990-2013. *J Pediatr.* 2015;166(4):992–997

96. Mitchell EA, Stewart AW, Clements M, Ford RPK; New Zealand Cot Death Study Group. Immunisation and the sudden infant death syndrome. *Arch Dis Child.* 1995;73(6):498–501

97. Jonville-Béra AP, Autret-Leca E, Barbeillon F, Paris-Llado J; French Reference Centers for SIDS. Sudden unexpected death in infants under 3 months of age and vaccination status—a case-control study. *Br J Clin Pharmacol.* 2001;51(3):271–276

98. Fleming PJ, Blair PS, Platt MW, Tripp J, Smith IJ, Golding J. The UK accelerated immunisation programme and sudden unexpected death in infancy: case-control study. *BMJ.* 2001;322(7290):822

99. Carolan PL, Wheeler WB, Ross JD, Kemp RJ. Potential to prevent carbon dioxide rebreathing of commercial products marketed to reduce sudden infant death syndrome risk. *Pediatrics.* 2000;105(4 pt 1):774–779

100. Hodgman JE, Hoppenbrouwers T. Home monitoring for the sudden infant death syndrome: the case against. *Ann N Y Acad Sci.* 1988;533:164–175

101. Ward SL, Keens TG, Chan LS, et al. Sudden infant death syndrome in infants evaluated by apnea programs in California. *Pediatrics.* 1986;77(4):451–458

102. Monod N, Plouin P, Sternberg B, et al. Are polygraphic and cardiopneumographic respiratory patterns useful tools for predicting the risk for sudden infant death syndrome? A 10-year study. *Biol Neonate.* 1986;50(3):147–153

103. Ramanathan R, Corwin MJ, Hunt CE, et al; Collaborative Home Infant Monitoring Evaluation (CHIME) Study Group. Cardiorespiratory events recorded on home monitors: comparison of healthy infants with those at increased risk for SIDS. *JAMA.* 2001;285(17):2199–2207

104. Laughlin J, Luerssen TG, Dias MS; Committee on Practice and Ambulatory Medicine; Section on Neurological Surgery. Prevention and management of positional skull deformities in infants. *Pediatrics.* 2011;128(6):1236–1241

105. van Sleuwen BE, Engelberts AC, Boere-Boonekamp MM, Kuis W, Schulpen TW, L'Hoir MP. Swaddling: a systematic review. *Pediatrics.* 2007;120(4). Available at: www.pediatrics.org/cgi/content/full/120/4/e1097

106. McDonnell E, Moon RY. Infant deaths and injuries associated with wearable blankets, swaddle wraps, and swaddling. *J Pediatr.* 2014;164(5):1152–1156

107. Willinger M, Ko C-W, Hoffman HJ, Kessler RC, Corwin MJ. Factors associated with caregivers' choice of infant sleep position, 1994-1998: the National Infant Sleep Position Study. *JAMA.* 2000;283(16):2135–2142

108. Brenner RA, Simons-Morton BG, Bhaskar B, et al. Prevalence and predictors of the prone sleep position among inner-city infants. *JAMA.* 1998;280(4):341–346

109. Von Kohorn I, Corwin MJ, Rybin DV, Heeren TC, Lister G, Colson ER. Influence of prior advice and beliefs of mothers on infant sleep position. *Arch Pediatr Adolesc Med.* 2010;164(4):363–369

110. Joyner BL, Gill-Bailey C, Moon RY. Infant sleep environments depicted in magazines targeted to women of childbearing age. *Pediatrics.* 2009;124(3):e416–e422

TECHNICAL REPORT

American Academy
of Pediatrics

DEDICATED TO THE HEALTH OF ALL CHILDREN™

SIDS and Other Sleep-Related Infant Deaths: Evidence Base for 2016 Updated Recommendations for a Safe Infant Sleeping Environment

Rachel Y. Moon, MD, FAAP, TASK FORCE ON SUDDEN INFANT DEATH SYNDROME

abstract

Approximately 3500 infants die annually in the United States from sleep-related infant deaths, including sudden infant death syndrome (SIDS), ill-defined deaths, and accidental suffocation and strangulation in bed. After an initial decrease in the 1990s, the overall sleep-related infant death rate has not declined in more recent years. Many of the modifiable and nonmodifiable risk factors for SIDS and other sleep-related infant deaths are strikingly similar. The American Academy of Pediatrics recommends a safe sleep environment that can reduce the risk of all sleep-related infant deaths. Recommendations for a safe sleep environment include supine positioning, use of a firm sleep surface, room-sharing without bed-sharing, and avoidance of soft bedding and overheating. Additional recommendations for SIDS risk reduction include avoidance of exposure to smoke, alcohol, and illicit drugs; breastfeeding; routine immunization; and use of a pacifier. New evidence and rationale for recommendations are presented for skin-to-skin care for newborn infants, bedside and in-bed sleepers, sleeping on couches/armchairs and in sitting devices, and use of soft bedding after 4 months of age. In addition, expanded recommendations for infant sleep location are included. The recommendations and strength of evidence for each recommendation are published in the accompanying policy statement, "SIDS and Other Sleep-Related Infant Deaths: Updated 2016 Recommendations for a Safe Infant Sleeping Environment," which is included in this issue.

This document is copyrighted and is property of the American Academy of Pediatrics and its Board of Directors. All authors have filed conflict of interest statements with the American Academy of Pediatrics. Any conflicts have been resolved through a process approved by the Board of Directors. The American Academy of Pediatrics has neither solicited nor accepted any commercial involvement in the development of the content of this publication.

Technical reports from the American Academy of Pediatrics benefit from expertise and resources of liaisons and internal (AAP) and external reviewers. However, technical reports from the American Academy of Pediatrics may not reflect the views of the liaisons or the organizations or government agencies that they represent.

The guidance in this report does not indicate an exclusive course of treatment or serve as a standard of medical care. Variations, taking into account individual circumstances, may be appropriate.

All technical reports from the American Academy of Pediatrics automatically expire 5 years after publication unless reaffirmed, revised, or retired at or before that time.

DOI: 10.1542/peds.2016-2940

PEDIATRICS (ISSN Numbers: Print, 0031-4005; Online, 1098-4275).

FINANCIAL DISCLOSURE: The author has indicated she does not have a financial relationship relevant to this article to disclose.

FUNDING: No external funding.

POTENTIAL CONFLICT OF INTEREST: The author has indicated she has no potential conflicts of interest to disclose.

To cite: Moon RY and AAP TASK FORCE ON SUDDEN INFANT DEATH SYNDROME. SIDS and Other Sleep-Related Infant Deaths: Evidence Base for 2016 Updated Recommendations for a Safe Infant Sleeping Environment. *Pediatrics.* 2016;138(5): e20162940

SEARCH STRATEGY AND METHODOLOGY

Literature searches with the use of PubMed were conducted for each of the topics in the technical report, concentrating on articles published since 2011 (when the last technical report and policy statement were published[1,2]). All iterations of the search terms were used for each topic area. For example, the pacifier topic search combined either "SIDS,"

"SUID," "sudden death," or "cot death" with "pacifier," "dummy," "soother," and "sucking." A total of 63 new studies were judged to be of sufficiently high quality to be included in this technical report. In addition, because the data regarding bed-sharing have been conflicting, the independent opinion of a biostatistician with special expertise in perinatal epidemiology was solicited. The strength of evidence for recommendations, using the Strength-of-Recommendation Taxonomy,[3] was determined by the task force members. A draft version of the policy statement and technical report was submitted to relevant committees and sections of the American Academy of Pediatrics (AAP) for review and comment. After the appropriate revisions were made, a final version was submitted to the AAP Executive Committee for final approval.

SUDDEN UNEXPECTED INFANT DEATH AND SUDDEN INFANT DEATH SYNDROME: DEFINITIONS AND DIAGNOSTIC ISSUES

Sudden unexpected infant death (SUID), also known as sudden unexpected death in infancy (SUDI), is a term used to describe any sudden and unexpected death, whether explained or unexplained (including sudden infant death syndrome [SIDS] and ill-defined deaths), occurring during infancy. After case investigation, SUID can be attributed to causes of death such as suffocation, asphyxia, entrapment, infection, ingestions, metabolic diseases, and trauma (unintentional or nonaccidental). SIDS is a subcategory of SUID and is a cause assigned to infant deaths that cannot be explained after a thorough case investigation including autopsy, a scene investigation, and review of clinical history.[4] (See Table 1 for definitions of terms.) The distinction between SIDS and other SUIDs, particularly those that

TABLE 1 Definitions of Terms

Caregivers: Throughout the document, "parents" are used, but this term is meant to indicate any infant caregivers.

Bed-sharing: Parent(s) and infant sleeping together on any surface (bed, couch, chair).

Cosleeping: This term is commonly used, but the task force finds it confusing and it is not used in this document. When used, authors need to make clear whether they are referring to sleeping in close proximity (which does not necessarily entail bed-sharing) or bed-sharing.

Room-sharing: Parent(s) and infant sleeping in the same room on separate surfaces.

Sleep-related infant death: SUID that occurs during an observed or unobserved sleep period.

Sudden infant death syndrome (SIDS): Cause assigned to infant deaths that cannot be explained after a thorough case investigation including a scene investigation, autopsy, and review of the clinical history.[4]

Sudden unexpected infant death (SUID), or sudden unexpected death in infancy (SUDI): A sudden and unexpected death, whether explained or unexplained (including SIDS), occurring during infancy.

occur during an unobserved sleep period (ie, sleep-related infant deaths), such as unintentional suffocation, is challenging, cannot be determined by autopsy alone, and may remain unresolved after a full case investigation. A few deaths that are diagnosed as SIDS are found, with further specialized investigations, to be attributable to metabolic disorders or arrhythmia-associated cardiac channelopathies.

Although standardized guidelines for conducting thorough case investigations have been developed (http://www.cdc.gov/sids/pdf/suidi-form2-1-2010.pdf),[5] these guidelines have not been uniformly adopted across the >2000 US medical examiner and coroner jurisdictions.[6] Information from emergency responders, scene investigators, and caregiver interviews may provide additional evidence to assist death certifiers (ie, medical examiners and coroners) in accurately determining the cause of death. However, death certifiers represent a diverse group with varying levels of skill and education. In addition, there are diagnostic preferences. Recently, much attention has focused on reporting differences among death certifiers. On one extreme, some certifiers have abandoned the use of SIDS as a cause-of-death explanation.[6] At the other extreme, some certifiers will not classify a death as suffocation in the absence of a pathologic marker of asphyxia at autopsy (ie, pathologic findings

diagnostic of oronasal occlusion or chest compression[7]), even with strong evidence from the scene investigation suggesting a probable unintentional suffocation.

US Trends in SIDS, Other SUIDs, and Postneonatal Mortality

To monitor trends in SIDS and other SUIDs nationally, the United States classifies diseases and injuries according to the International Statistical Classification of Diseases (ICD) diagnostic codes. In the United States, the National Center for Health Statistics assigns a SIDS diagnostic code (International Classification of Diseases, 10th Revision [ICD-10] R95) if the death is classified with terminology such as SIDS (including presumed, probable, or consistent with SIDS), sudden infant death, sudden unexplained death in infancy, sudden unexpected infant death, SUID, or SUDI on the certified death certificate.[8,9] A death will be coded "other ill-defined and unspecified causes of mortality" (ICD-10 R99) if the cause of the death is reported as unknown or unspecified.[8] A death is coded "accidental suffocation and strangulation in bed" (ICD-10 W75) when the terms asphyxia, asphyxiated, asphyxiation, strangled, strangulated, strangulation, suffocated, or suffocation are reported, along with the terms bed or crib. This code also includes deaths while sleeping on couches and armchairs.

SIDS AND OTHER SLEEP-RELATED INFANT DEATHS:
EVIDENCE BASE FOR 2016 UPDATED RECOMMENDATIONS FOR A SAFE INFANT SLEEPING ENVIRONMENT

377

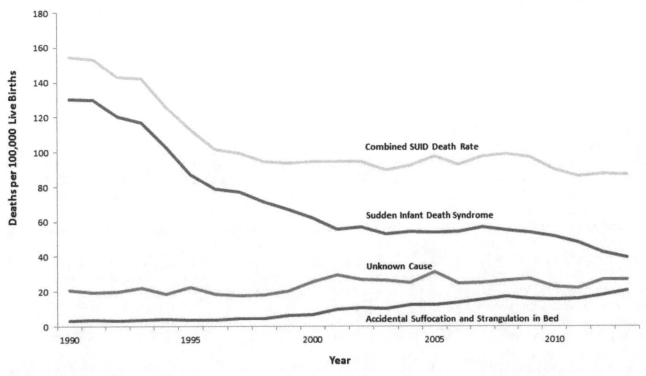

FIGURE 1

Trends in SUID by cause, 1990–2013. Source: Centers for Disease Control and Prevention/National Center for Health Statistics, National Vital Statistics System, compressed mortality file. (Figure duplicated from http://www.cdc.gov/sids/data.htm.)

Although SIDS was defined somewhat loosely until the mid-1980s, there was minimal change in the incidence of SIDS in the United States until the early 1990s. In 1992, in response to epidemiologic reports from Europe and Australia, the AAP recommended that infants be placed for sleep in a nonprone position as a strategy to reduce the risk of SIDS.[10] The "Back to Sleep" campaign (which is now known as the "Safe to Sleep" campaign[11]) was initiated in 1994 under the leadership of the National Institute of Child Health and Human Development (now the *Eunice Kennedy Shriver* National Institute of Child Health and Human Development) as a joint effort of the Maternal and Child Health Bureau of the Health Resources and Services Administration, the AAP, the SIDS Alliance (now First Candle), and the Association of SIDS and Infant Mortality Programs. Between 1992 and 2001, the SIDS rate declined,

with the most dramatic declines in the years immediately after the first nonprone sleep position recommendations, and this decline was consistent with the steady increase in the prevalence of supine sleeping (Fig 1).[12] The US SIDS rate decreased from 120 deaths per 100 000 live births in 1992 to 56 deaths per 100 000 live births in 2001, representing a reduction of 53% over 10 years. From 2001 to 2008, the rate remained constant (Fig 1) and then declined from 54 per 100 000 live births in 2009 to 40 in 2013 (the latest year that data are available). In 2013, 1561 infants died of SIDS.[13] Although SIDS rates have declined by >50% since the early 1990s, SIDS remains the leading cause of postneonatal (28 days to 1 year of age) mortality.

The all-cause postneonatal death rate follows a trend similar to the SIDS and SUID rates, with a 26% decline from 1992 to 2001 (from 314 to 231 per 100 000 live births). From 2001 until 2009, postneonatal mortality

rates also remained fairly unchanged (from 231 to 222 per 100 000 live births), and then have declined yearly since 2009 to a rate of 193 per 100 000 live births in 2013.[14] Several studies have observed that some deaths previously classified as SIDS (ICD-10 R95) are now being classified as other causes of sleep-related infant death (eg, accidental suffocation and strangulation in bed [ASSB; ICD-10 W75] or other ill-defined or unspecified causes [ICD-10 R99]),[15,16] and that at least some of the decline in SIDS rates may be explained by increasing rates of these other assigned causes of SUID.[15,17] To account for variations in death certifier classification and to more consistently track SIDS and other sleep-related infant deaths, the National Center for Health Statistics has created the special cause-of-death category SUID. The SUID category captures deaths with an underlying cause coded as ICD-10 R95, R99, and W75.[13] In 2013, SIDS accounted for 46% of the 3422

SUIDs in the United States. Similar to the SIDS rate, the SUID rate also declined in the late 2000s, from 99 per 100 000 live births in 2009 to 87 in 2013.

Racial and Ethnic Disparities

SIDS and SUID mortality rates, like other causes of infant mortality, have notable and persistent racial and ethnic disparities.[14] Despite the decline in SIDS and SUIDs in all races and ethnicities, the rate of SUIDs among non-Hispanic black (172 per 100 000 live births) and American Indian/Alaska Native (191 per 100 000 live births) infants was more than double that of non-Hispanic white infants (84 per 100 000 live births) in 2010–2013 (Fig 2). SIDS rates for Asian/Pacific Islander and Hispanic infants were much lower than the rate for non-Hispanic white infants. Furthermore, similar racial and ethnic disparities are seen with deaths attributed to both ASSB and ill-defined or unspecified deaths (Fig 2). Differences in the prevalence of supine positioning and other sleep environment conditions between racial and ethnic populations may contribute to these disparities.[18] The prevalence of supine positioning in 2010 data from the National Infant Sleep Position Study in white infants was 75%, compared with 53%, 73%, and 80% among black, Hispanic, and Asian infants, respectively (Fig 3).[19] The Pregnancy Risk Assessment Monitoring System also monitors the prevalence of infant sleep position in several states (http://www.cdc.gov/prams/pramstat/index.html). In 2011, 78% of mothers reported that they most often lay their infants on their backs for sleep (26 states reporting and most recent year available), with 80.3% of white mothers and 54% of black mothers reporting supine placement. Parent-infant bed-sharing[20-22] and the use of soft bedding are also more common among black families

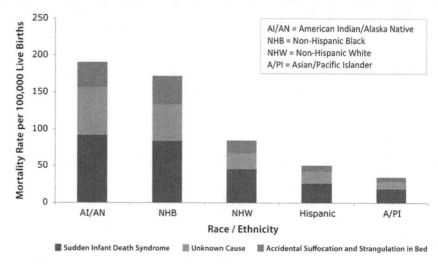

FIGURE 2

SUID by race/ethnicity, 2010–2013. Source: Centers for Disease Control and Prevention/National Center for Health Statistics, National Vital Statistics System, period-linked birth/infant death data. (Figure duplicated from http://www.cdc.gov/sids/data.htm.)

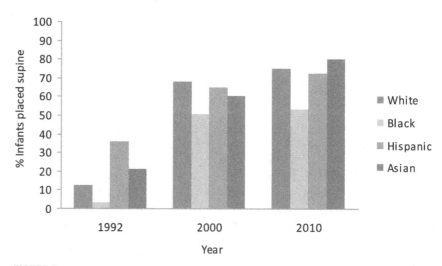

FIGURE 3

Prevalence of supine sleep positioning by maternal race and ethnic origin, 1992–2010. Source: National Infant Sleep Position Study. Note that data collection for the National Infant Sleep Position Study ended in 2010.

than among other racial/ethnic groups.[23-25]

Age at Death

Ninety percent of SIDS cases occur before an infant reaches the age of 6 months.[16] SIDS peaks between 1 and 4 months of age. Although SIDS was once considered a rare event during the first month after birth, in 2004–2006 nearly 10% of cases that were coded as SIDS occurred during this period. SIDS is uncommon after 8 months of age.[16] A similar age distribution is seen for ASSB.[16]

PATHOPHYSIOLOGY AND GENETICS OF SIDS

A working model of SIDS pathogenesis includes a convergence of exogenous triggers or "stressors" (eg, prone sleep position, overbundling, airway obstruction), a critical period of development, and dysfunctional

SIDS AND OTHER SLEEP-RELATED INFANT DEATHS:
EVIDENCE BASE FOR 2016 UPDATED RECOMMENDATIONS FOR A SAFE INFANT SLEEPING ENVIRONMENT

379

and/or immature cardiorespiratory and/or arousal systems (intrinsic vulnerability) that lead to a failure of protective responses (Fig 4).[26] The convergence of these factors may ultimately result in a combination of progressive asphyxia, bradycardia, hypotension, metabolic acidosis, and ineffectual gasping, leading to death.[27] Thus, death may occur as a result of the interaction between a vulnerable infant and a potentially asphyxiating and/or overheating sleep environment.[28]

The mechanisms responsible for intrinsic vulnerability (ie, dysfunctional cardiorespiratory and/or arousal protective responses) remain unclear but may be the result of in utero environmental conditions and/or genetically determined maldevelopment or delay in maturation. Infants who die of SIDS are more likely to have been born preterm and/or were growth restricted, which suggests a suboptimal intrauterine environment. Other adverse in utero environmental conditions include exposure to nicotine or other components of cigarette smoke and alcohol.[29]

Recent studies have explored how prenatal exposure to cigarette smoke may result in an increased risk of SIDS. In animal models, exposure to cigarette smoke or nicotine during fetal development alters the expression of the nicotinic acetylcholine receptors in areas of the brainstem important for autonomic function and alters the numbers of orexin receptors in piglets,[30,31] reduces the number of medullary serotonergic (5-hydroxytryptamine [5-HT]) neurons in the raphe obscurus in mice,[32] increases 5-HT and 5-HT turnover in Rhesus monkeys,[33] alters neuronal excitability of neurons in the nucleus tractus solitarius (a brainstem region important for sensory integration) in guinea pigs,[34] and alters fetal autonomic activity

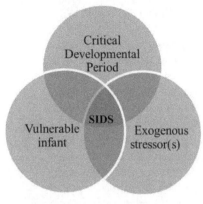

FIGURE 4
Triple risk model for SIDS. Adapted from Filiano and Kinney.[26]

and medullary neurotransmitter receptors, including nicotinic receptors, in baboons.[35-37] From a functional perspective, prenatal exposure to nicotine causes hypoventilation and increased apnea[38,39]; reduces hypercarbia and hypoxia-induced ventilator chemoreflexes in mice, rats,[38-40] and lambs[41]; and blunts arousal in response to hypoxia in rats[40] and lambs.[41]

In human infants, there are strong associations between nicotinic acetylcholine receptors and serotonergic (5-HT) receptors in the brainstem during development,[42] and there is important recent evidence of epigenetic changes in the placentas of infants with prenatal tobacco smoke exposure.[43] Prenatal exposure to tobacco smoke attenuates recovery from hypoxia in preterm infants,[44] decreases heart rate variability in preterm[45] and term[46] infants, and abolishes the normal relationship between heart rate and gestational age at birth.[45] Moreover, infants of smoking mothers exhibit impaired arousal patterns to trigeminal stimulation in proportion to urinary cotinine concentrations.[47] It is important to also note that prenatal exposure to tobacco smoke alters the normal programming of cardiovascular reflexes, such that the increase in blood pressure and heart rate in response to breathing

4% carbon dioxide or a 60° head-up tilt is greater than expected.[48] These changes in autonomic function, arousal, and cardiovascular reflexes may all increase an infant's vulnerability to SIDS.

A recent large systematic review of the neuropathologic features of unexplained SUDI, including only studies that met strict criteria, concluded that "the most consistent findings, and most likely to be pathophysiologically significant, are abnormalities of serotonergic neurotransmission in the caudal brain stem."[49] Brainstem abnormalities that involve the 5-HT system in up to 70% of infants who die of SIDS have now been confirmed in several independent data sets and laboratories.[29,50-52] These include decreased 5-hydroxytryptamine 1A (5-HT1A) receptor binding, a relative decreased binding to the 5-HT transporter, increased numbers of immature 5-HT neurons, and decreased tissue levels of 5-HT and the rate-limiting enzyme for 5-HT synthesis, tryptophan hydroxylase.[53] Moreover, there is no evidence of excessive serotonin degradation as assessed by levels of 5-hydroxyindoleacetic acid (the main metabolite of serotonin) or ratios of 5-hydroxyindoleacetic acid to serotonin.[35] This area of the brainstem plays a key role in coordinating many respiratory, arousal, and autonomic functions, and when dysfunctional, might prevent normal protective responses to stressors that commonly occur during sleep. Importantly, these findings are not confined to nuclei containing 5-HT neurons but also include relevant projection sites. Other abnormalities in brainstem projection sites have been described as well. For example, abnormalities of Phox2B immune-reactive neurons have been reported in the homologous human retrotrapezoid nucleus, a region of the brainstem that receives important 5-HT projections and is critical to carbon dioxide chemoreception and implicated in human congenital central hypoventilation syndrome.[54]

The brainstem has important reciprocal connections to the limbic system comprising both cortical and subcortical components, including the limbic cortex, hypothalamus, amygdala, and hippocampus. These areas of the brain are important in the regulation of autonomic function, particularly in response to emotional stimuli. Thus, the brainstem and limbic system constitute a key network in controlling many aspects of autonomic function. Recently, abnormalities in the dentate gyrus (a component of the hippocampus) were observed in 41% of 153 infants who died unexpectedly with no apparent cause and 43% of the subset of deaths classified as SIDS. This finding suggests that dysfunction of other brain regions interconnected with the brainstem may participate in the pathogenesis of SIDS.[55] Dentate gyrus bilamination is also found in some cases of temporal lobe epilepsy. A future potential line of investigation is a possible link in brainstem-limbic–related homeostatic instability between SIDS and sudden unexpected death in epilepsy and febrile seizures noted in some cases of sudden unexpected death in childhood.[55]

There are significant associations between brainstem 5-HT1A receptor binding abnormalities and specific SIDS risk factors, including tobacco smoking.[52] These data confirm results from earlier studies in humans[29,53] and are also consistent with studies in piglets that reveal that postnatal exposure to nicotine decreases medullary 5-HT1A receptor immunoreactivity.[56] Serotonergic neurons located in the medullary raphe and adjacent paragigantocellularis lateralis play important roles in many autonomic functions, including the control of respiration, blood pressure,

heart rate, thermoregulation, sleep and arousal, and upper airway patency. Engineered mice with decreased numbers of 5-HT neurons and rats or piglets with decreased activity secondary to 5-HT1A autoreceptor stimulation show diminished ventilator responses to carbon dioxide, dysfunctional heat production and heat loss mechanisms, and altered sleep architecture.[57] The aberrant thermoregulation in these models provides evidence for a biological substrate for the risk of SIDS associated with potentially overheating environments. In addition, mice pups with a constitutive reduction in 5-HT–producing neurons (PET1 knockout) or rat pups in which a large fraction of medullary 5-HT neurons have been destroyed with locally applied neurotoxins have a decreased ability to auto-resuscitate in response to asphyxia.[58,59] Moreover, animals with 5-HT neuron deficiency caused by direct injection of a 5-HT–selective neurotoxin had impaired arousal in response to hypoxia.[60]

Some cases of SUID have a clear genetic cause, such as medium-chain acyl-coenzyme A dehydrogenase deficiency. A recent study in California showed that the frequency of mutations for undiagnosed inborn errors of metabolism was similar in SIDS and controls and that newborn screening was effectively detecting medium-chain and very-long-chain acyl-coenzyme A dehydrogenase deficiencies that could potentially lead to SUID.[61] There is no evidence of a strong heritable contribution for SIDS; however, genetic alterations that may increase the vulnerability to SIDS have been observed. Genetic variation can take the form of common base changes (polymorphisms) that alter gene function or rare base changes (mutations) that often have highly deleterious effects. (For a comprehensive review, see Opdal

and Rognum.[62]) Several categories of physiologic functions relevant to SIDS have been examined for altered genetic makeup. Genes related to the serotonin transporter, cardiac channelopathies, and the development of the autonomic nervous system are the subject of current investigation.[63] The serotonin transporter recovers serotonin from the extracellular space and largely serves to regulate overall serotonin neuronal activity. There are reports that polymorphisms in the promoter region that enhance the efficacy of the transporter (L) allele seem to be more prevalent in infants who die of SIDS compared with polymorphisms that reduce efficacy (S)[62]; however, at least 1 study did not confirm this association.[64] It has also been reported that a polymorphism (12-repeat intron 2) of the promoter region of the serotonin transporter, which also enhances serotonin transporter efficiency, was increased in black infants who died of SIDS[63] but not in a Norwegian population.[62]

It has been estimated that 5% to 10% of infants who die of SIDS have novel mutations in the cardiac sodium or potassium channel genes, resulting in long QT syndrome, as well as in other genes that regulate channel function.[63] Some of these mutations may represent an actual cause of death, but others may contribute to causing death when combined with environmental factors, such as acidosis.[65] There is molecular and functional evidence that implicates specific *SCN5A* (sodium channel gene) β subunits in SIDS pathogenesis.[66] In addition, 2 rare mutations in connexin 43, a major gap junction protein, have been found in SIDS cases and not in ethnically matched controls.[67] In vitro assays of 1 mutation showed a lack of gap junction function, which could lead to ventricular arrhythmogenesis. The other mutation did not appear to have functional consequences.

SIDS AND OTHER SLEEP-RELATED INFANT DEATHS:
EVIDENCE BASE FOR 2016 UPDATED RECOMMENDATIONS FOR A SAFE INFANT SLEEPING ENVIRONMENT

381

A recent study also adds weight to the need to perform functional assays and morphologic studies of the altered gene products. Several of the missense variants in genes encoding cardiac channels that have been found in SIDS cases had a high prevalence in the National Heart, Lung, and Blood Institute GO Exome Sequencing Project Database.[68] A large study in a nonreferred nationwide Danish cohort estimated that up to 7.5% of SIDS cases may be explained by genetic variants in the sodium channel complex.[69] These estimates are in the range of those previously reported. However, it is important that for each channelopathy variant discovered, the biological plausibility for pathogenicity is investigated to consider it as a cause of or contributor in SIDS.

The identification of polymorphisms in genes pertinent to the embryologic origin of the autonomic nervous system in SIDS cases also lends support to the hypothesis that a genetic predisposition contributes to the etiology of SIDS. The *PACAP* (pituitary adenylate cyclase-activation polypeptide) gene and the gene of 1 of its receptors (*PAC1*) have received recent attention because of the apparent racial differences in their expression. For example, there were no associations between *PACAP* and SIDS found in white infants, but in SIDS cases in black infants a specific allele was significantly associated.[70] Although in a recent study, a strong association between variants in the *PAC1* gene and SIDS was not found, a number of potential associations between race-specific variants and SIDS were identified; these warrant further study.[71] There have also been a number of reports of polymorphisms or mutations in genes regulating inflammation,[72,73] energy production,[74–76] and hypoglycemia[77] in infants who died of SIDS, but these associations require more study to determine their importance.

RECOMMENDATIONS TO REDUCE THE RISK OF SIDS AND OTHER SLEEP-RELATED INFANT DEATHS

The recommendations outlined herein were developed to reduce the risk of SIDS and sleep-related suffocation, asphyxia, and entrapment among infants in the general population. As defined by epidemiologists, risk refers to the probability that an outcome will occur given the presence of a particular factor or set of factors. Although all recommendations are intended for all who care for infants, some recommendations are also directed toward health policy makers, researchers, and professionals who care for or work on behalf of infants. In addition, because certain behaviors, such as smoking, can increase risk for the infant, some recommendations are directed toward women who are pregnant or may become pregnant in the near future.

The recommendations, along with the strength of the recommendation, are summarized in the accompanying policy statement.[78] It should be noted that there are no randomized controlled trials with regard to SIDS and other sleep-related deaths; instead, case-control studies are the standard.

The recommendations are based on epidemiologic studies that include infants up to 1 year of age. Therefore, recommendations for sleep position and the sleep environment, unless otherwise specified, are for the first year after birth. The evidence-based recommendations that follow are provided to guide health care practitioners in conversations with parents and others who care for infants. Health care practitioners are encouraged to have open and nonjudgmental conversations with families about their sleep practices. Individual medical conditions may warrant that a health care provider make different recommendations

after weighing the relative risks and benefits.

INFANT SLEEP POSITION

To reduce the risk of SIDS, infants should be placed for sleep in the supine position (wholly on the back) for every sleep period by every caregiver until 1 year of age. Side sleeping is not safe and is not advised.

The prone or side sleep position can increase the risk of rebreathing expired gases, resulting in hypercapnia and hypoxia.[79–82] The prone position also increases the risk of overheating by decreasing the rate of heat loss and increasing body temperature more than the supine position.[83,84] Evidence suggests that prone sleeping alters the autonomic control of the infant cardiovascular system during sleep, particularly at 2 to 3 months of age,[85] and may result in decreased cerebral oxygenation.[86] The prone position places infants at high risk of SIDS (odds ratio [OR]: 2.3–13.1).[87–91] In 1 US study, SIDS risk associated with the side position was similar in magnitude to that associated with the prone position (ORs: 2.0 and 2.6, respectively),[88] and a higher population-attributable risk has been reported for the side sleep position than for the prone position.[90,92] Furthermore, the risk of SIDS is exceptionally high for infants who are placed on the side and found on the stomach (OR: 8.7).[88] The side sleep position is inherently unstable, and the probability of an infant rolling to the prone position from the side sleep position is significantly greater than rolling prone from the back.[90,93] Infants who are unaccustomed to the prone position and who are placed prone for sleep are also at greater risk than those usually placed prone (adjusted OR: 8.7–45.4).[88,94,95] It is therefore critically important that every caregiver use the supine sleep position for every sleep period.

This is particularly relevant in situations in which a new caregiver is introduced: for example, when an infant is placed in foster care or an adoptive home or when an infant enters child care for the first time.

Despite these recommendations, the prevalence of supine positioning has remained stagnant for the past decade.[19] One reason often cited by parents for not using the supine sleep position is the perception that the infant is uncomfortable or does not sleep well.[96-104] However, an infant who wakes frequently is normal and should not be perceived as a poor sleeper. Physiologic studies show that infants are less likely to arouse when they are sleeping in the prone position.[105-113] The ability to arouse from sleep is an important protective physiologic response to stressors during sleep,[114-118] and the infant's ability to sleep for sustained periods may not be physiologically advantageous.

The supine sleep position does not increase the risk of choking and aspiration in infants, even in those with gastroesophageal reflux.

Parents and caregivers continue to be concerned that the infant will choke or aspirate while supine.[96-104] Parents often misconstrue coughing or gagging, which is evidence of a normal protective gag reflex, for choking or aspiration. Multiple studies in different countries have not shown an increased incidence of aspiration since the change to supine sleeping.[119-121] Parents and caregivers are often concerned about aspiration when the infant has been diagnosed with gastroesophageal reflux. The AAP concurs with the North American Society for Pediatric Gastroenterology and Nutrition that "the risk of SIDS outweighs the benefit of prone or lateral sleep position on GER [gastroesophageal reflux]; therefore, in most infants from birth to 12 months of age, supine positioning during sleep is recommended…. Therefore, prone

positioning is acceptable if the infant is observed and awake, particularly in the postprandial period, but prone positioning during sleep can only be considered in infants with certain upper airway disorders in which the risk of death from GERD [gastroesophageal reflux disease] may outweigh the risk of SIDS."[122] Examples of such upper airway disorders are those in which airway-protective mechanisms are impaired, including infants with anatomic abnormalities, such as type 3 or 4 laryngeal clefts, who have not undergone antireflux surgery. There is no evidence that infants receiving nasogastric or orogastric feedings are at increased risk of aspiration if placed in the supine position. Elevating the head of the infant's crib while the infant is supine is not effective in reducing gastroesophageal reflux[123,124]; in addition, elevating the head of the crib may result in the infant sliding to the foot of the crib into a position that may compromise respiration and therefore is not recommended.

Preterm infants should be placed supine as soon as possible.

Infants born preterm have an increased risk of SIDS,[125,126] and the association between the prone position and SIDS among low birth weight and preterm infants is equal to, or perhaps even stronger than, the association among those born at term.[94] Therefore, preterm infants should be placed supine for sleep as soon as clinical status has stabilized. The task force concurs with the AAP Committee on Fetus and Newborn that "preterm infants should be placed supine for sleeping, just as term infants should, and the parents of preterm infants should be counseled about the importance of supine sleeping in preventing SIDS. Hospitalized preterm infants should be kept predominantly in the supine position, at least from the postmenstrual age of 32 weeks onward, so that they become

acclimated to supine sleeping before discharge."[127] Furthermore, the task force believes that neonatologists, neonatal nurses, and other health care providers responsible for organizing the hospital discharge of infants from NICUs should be vigilant about endorsing the SIDS risk-reduction recommendations from birth. They should model the recommendations as soon as the infant is medically stable and significantly before the infant's anticipated discharge from the hospital. In addition, NICUs are encouraged to develop and implement policies to ensure that supine sleeping and other safe sleep practices are modeled for parents beforeo discharge from the hospital.[128,129]

As stated in the AAP clinical report, "skin-to-skin care is recommended for all mothers and newborns, regardless of feeding or delivery method, immediately following birth (as soon as the mother is medically stable, awake, and able to respond to her newborn), and to continue for at least an hour."[130] Thereafter, or when the mother needs to sleep or take care of other needs, infants should be placed supine in a bassinet.

Placing infants on the side after birth in newborn nurseries or in mother-infant rooms continues to be a concern. The practice likely occurs because of a belief among nursery staff that newborn infants need to clear their airways of amniotic fluid and may be less likely to aspirate while on the side. No evidence that such fluid will be cleared more readily while in the side position exists. Perhaps most importantly, if parents observe health care providers placing infants in the side or prone position, they are likely to infer that supine positioning is not important[131] and therefore may be more likely to copy this practice and use the side or prone position at home.[101,104,132] Infants who are

SIDS AND OTHER SLEEP-RELATED INFANT DEATHS:
EVIDENCE BASE FOR 2016 UPDATED RECOMMENDATIONS FOR A SAFE INFANT SLEEPING ENVIRONMENT

383

rooming in with their parents or cared for in a separate newborn nursery should be placed in the supine position as soon as they are ready to be placed in the bassinet. To promote breastfeeding, placing the infant skin-to-skin with mother after delivery, with appropriate observation and/or monitoring, is the best approach. When the mother needs to sleep or take care of other needs, the infant should be placed supine in a bassinet.

Once an infant can roll from supine to prone and from prone to supine, the infant may remain in the sleep position that he or she assumes.

Parents and caregivers are frequently concerned about the appropriate strategy for infants who have learned to roll over, which generally occurs at 4 to 6 months of age. As infants mature, it is more likely that they will roll. In 1 study, 6% and 12% of 16- to 23-week-old infants placed on their backs or sides, respectively, were found in the prone position; among infants ≥24 weeks of age, 14% of those placed on their backs and 18% of those placed on their sides were found in the prone position.[133] Repositioning the sleeping infant to the supine position can be disruptive and may discourage the use of the supine position altogether. Because data to make specific recommendations as to when it is safe for infants to sleep in the prone position are lacking, the AAP recommends that all infants continue to be placed supine until 1 year of age. If the infant can roll from supine to prone and from prone to supine, the infant can then be allowed to remain in the sleep position that he or she assumes. One study analyzing sleep-related deaths reported to state child death review teams found that the predominant risk factor for sleep-related deaths in infants 4 to 12 months of age was rolling into objects in the sleep area.[134] Thus, parents and caregivers should continue to keep the infant's sleep environment

clear of soft or loose bedding and other objects. Parents may be reassured in being advised that the incidence of SIDS begins to decline after 4 months of age.[16]

SLEEP SURFACES

Infants should be placed on a firm sleep surface (eg, a mattress in a safety-approved crib) covered by a fitted sheet with no other bedding or soft objects to reduce the risk of SIDS and suffocation.

To avoid suffocation, rebreathing, and SIDS risk, infants should sleep on a firm surface (eg, safety-approved crib and mattress). The surface should be covered by a fitted sheet without any soft or loose bedding. A firm surface maintains its shape and will not indent or conform to the shape of the infant's head when the infant is placed on the surface. Soft mattresses, including those made from memory foam, could create a pocket (or indentation) and increase the chance of rebreathing or suffocation if the infant is placed in or rolls over to the prone position.[81,135]

A crib, bassinet, portable crib, or play yard that conforms to the safety standards of the Consumer Product Safety Commission (CPSC) is recommended.

Cribs should meet safety standards of the CPSC,[136] including those for slat spacing, snugly fitting and firm mattresses, and no drop sides. The AAP recommends the use of new cribs, because older cribs may no longer meet current safety standards, may have missing parts, or may be incorrectly assembled. If an older crib is to be used, care must be taken to ensure that there have been no recalls on the crib model, that all of the hardware is intact, and that the assembly instructions are available.

For some families, the use of a crib may not be possible for financial or space considerations. In addition, parents may be reluctant to place the

infant in the crib because of concerns that the crib is too large for the infant or that "crib death" (ie, SIDS) only occurs in cribs. Alternate sleep surfaces, such as portable cribs, play yards, and bassinets that meet safety standards of the CPSC,[137,138] can be used and may be more acceptable for some families because they are smaller and more portable.

Bedside sleepers are attached to the side of the parental bed. The CPSC has published safety standards for bedside sleepers,[139] and they may be considered by some parents as an option. There are no CPSC safety standards for in-bed sleepers. The task force cannot make a recommendation for or against the use of either bedside sleepers or in-bed sleepers, because there have been no studies examining the association between these products and SIDS or unintentional injury and death, including suffocation. Studies of in-bed sleepers are currently underway, but results are not yet available. Parents and caregivers should adhere to the manufacturer's guidelines regarding maximum weight of infants who use these products.[140,141] In addition, with the use of any of these products, other AAP guidelines for safe sleep outlined in this document, including supine positioning and avoidance of soft objects and loose bedding, should be followed.

Mattresses should be firm and maintain their shape even when the fitted sheet designated for that model is used, such that there are no gaps between the mattress and the wall of the bassinet, playpen, portable crib, play yard, or bedside sleeper. Only mattresses designed for the specific product should be used. Pillows or cushions should not be used as substitutes for mattresses or in addition to a mattress. Soft materials or objects, such as pillows, quilts, comforters, or sheepskins, even if covered by a sheet, should not be placed under a sleeping infant.

Mattress toppers, designed to make the sleep surface softer, should not be used for infants younger than 1 year. Any fabric on the crib walls or a canopy should be taut and firmly attached to the frame so as not to create a suffocation risk for the infant.

Infants should not be placed for sleep on adult-sized beds because of the risk of entrapment and suffocation.[142] Portable bed rails (railings installed on the side of the bed that are intended to prevent a child from falling off of the bed) should not be used with infants because of the risk of entrapment and strangulation.[143] The infant should sleep in an area free of hazards, including dangling cords, electric wires, and window-covering cords, because these may present a strangulation risk.

Recently, special crib mattresses and sleep surfaces that claim to reduce the chance of rebreathing carbon dioxide when the infant is in the prone position have been introduced. Although there are no apparent disadvantages of using these mattresses if they meet the safety standards as described previously, there are no studies that show a decreased risk of SUID/SIDS. (See section entitled "Commercial Devices" for further discussion of special mattresses.)

Sitting devices, such as car seats, strollers, swings, infant carriers, and infant slings, are not recommended for routine sleep in the hospital or at home, particularly for young infants.

Some parents choose to allow their infants to sleep in a car seat or other sitting device. Sitting devices include, but are not restricted to, car seats, strollers, swings, infant carriers, and infant slings. Parents and caregivers often use these devices, even when not traveling, because they are convenient. One study found that the average young infant spends 5.7 hours/day in a

car seat or similar sitting device.[144] However, there are multiple concerns about the use of sitting devices as a usual infant sleep location. Placing an infant in such devices can potentiate gastroesophageal reflux[145] and positional plagiocephaly. Because they still have poor head control and often experience flexion of the head while in a sitting position, infants younger than 4 months in sitting devices may be at increased risk of upper airway obstruction and oxygen desaturation.[146-150] A recent retrospective study reviewed deaths involving sitting and carrying devices (car seats, bouncers, swings, strollers, and slings) reported to the CPSC between 2004 and 2008. Of the 47 deaths analyzed, 31 occurred in car seats, 5 occurred in slings, 4 each occurred in swings and bouncers, and 3 occurred in strollers. Fifty-two percent of deaths in car seats were attributed to strangulation from straps; the others were attributed to positional asphyxia.[151] In addition, analyses of CPSC data report injuries from falls when car seats are placed on elevated surfaces,[152-156] from strangulation on unbuckled or partially buckled car seat straps,[151] and from suffocation when car seats overturn after being placed on a bed, mattress, or couch.[155] There are also reports of suffocation in infants, particularly those who are younger than 4 months, who are carried in infant sling carriers.[151,157-159] When infant slings are used for carrying, it is important to ensure that the infant's head is up and above the fabric, the face is visible, and the nose and mouth are clear of obstructions. After nursing, the infant should be repositioned in the sling so that the head is up and is clear of fabric and the airway is not obstructed by the adult's body.[151] If an infant falls asleep in a sitting device, he or she should be removed from the product and moved to a crib or other appropriate flat surface as soon as is safe and practical. Car seats and similar products are not stable on

a crib mattress or other elevated surfaces.[152-156] Infants should not be left unattended in car seats and similar products, nor should they be placed or left in car seats and similar products with the straps unbuckled or partially buckled.[151]

BREASTFEEDING

Breastfeeding is associated with a reduced risk of SIDS. The protective effect of breastfeeding increases with exclusivity. Furthermore, any breastfeeding is more protective against SIDS than no breastfeeding.

The protective role of breastfeeding on SIDS is enhanced when breastfeeding is exclusive and without formula introduction.[160-162] Studies do not distinguish between direct breastfeeding and providing expressed milk. In the Agency for Healthcare Research and Quality's "Evidence Report on Breastfeeding in Developed Countries," 6 studies were included in the SIDS-breastfeeding meta-analysis, and ever having breastfed was associated with a lower risk of SIDS (adjusted summary OR: 0.64; 95% confidence interval [CI]: 0.51–0.81).[160] The German Study of Sudden Infant Death, the largest and most recent case-control study of SIDS, found that exclusive breastfeeding at 1 month of age halved the risk of SIDS (adjusted OR: 0.48; 95% CI: 0.28–0.82).[161] Another meta-analysis of 18 case-control studies found an unadjusted summary OR for any breastfeeding of 0.40 (95% CI: 0.35–0.44) and a pooled adjusted OR of 0.55 (95% CI: 0.44–0.69) (Fig 5).[162] The protective effect of breastfeeding increased with exclusivity, with a univariable summary OR of 0.27 (95% CI: 0.24–0.31) for exclusive breastfeeding of any duration.[162]

Physiologic sleep studies showed that breastfed infants are more easily aroused from sleep than their formula-fed counterparts.[163,164] In

SIDS AND OTHER SLEEP-RELATED INFANT DEATHS:
EVIDENCE BASE FOR 2016 UPDATED RECOMMENDATIONS FOR A SAFE INFANT SLEEPING ENVIRONMENT

385

addition, breastfeeding results in a decreased incidence of diarrhea, upper and lower respiratory infections, and other infectious diseases[165] that are associated with an increased vulnerability to SIDS and provides overall immune system benefits attributable to maternal antibodies and micronutrients in human milk.[166,167] Exclusive breastfeeding for 6 months has been found to be more protective against infectious diseases, compared with exclusive breastfeeding to 4 months of age and partial breastfeeding thereafter.[165] Furthermore, exclusive breastfeeding results in a gut microbiome that supports a normally functioning immune system and protection from infectious disease, and this commensal microbiome has been proposed as another possible mechanism or marker for protection against SIDS.[168]

INFANT SLEEP LOCATION

It is recommended that infants sleep in the parents' room, close to the parents' bed, but on a separate surface. The infant's crib, portable crib, play yard, or bassinet should be placed in the parents' bedroom, ideally for the first year of life, but at least for the first 6 months.

The terms bed-sharing and cosleeping are often used interchangeably, but they are not synonymous. Cosleeping is when parent and infant sleep in close proximity (on the same surface or different surfaces) so as to be able to see, hear, and/or touch each other.[169,170] Cosleeping arrangements can include bed-sharing or sleeping in the same room in close proximity.[170,171] Bed-sharing refers to a specific type of cosleeping when the infant is sleeping on the same surface with another person.[170] The shared surface can include a bed, sofa, or chair. Because the term cosleeping can be misconstrued and does not precisely describe sleep

Study or Subgroup	log[]	SE	Weight	IV, Fixed, 95% CI
Fleming 1996	0.058269	0.317657	12.6%	1.06 [0.57, 1.98]
Hauck 2003	-0.91629	0.319582	12.4%	0.40 [0.21, 0.75]
Klonoff-Cohen 1995	-0.89159812	0.3346305	11.4%	0.41 [0.21, 0.79]
Mitchell 1997	-0.07257	0.420337	7.2%	0.93 [0.41, 2.12]
Ponsonby 1995	-0.15082	0.401245	7.9%	0.86 [0.39, 1.89]
Vennemann 2009	-0.84397	0.239354	22.2%	0.43 [0.27, 0.69]
Wennergren 1997	-0.693147	0.21979	26.3%	0.50 [0.33, 0.77]
Total (95% CI)			100.0%	0.55 [0.44, 0.69]

Heterogeneity: Chi² = 10.08, df = 6 (P = .12); I² = 40%
Test for overall effect: Z = 5.28 (P < .00001)

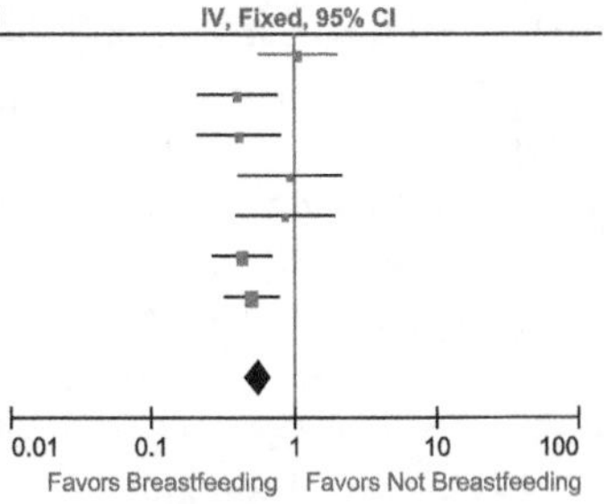

FIGURE 5

Multivariable analysis of any breastfeeding versus no breastfeeding. Adapted from Hauck et al.[162] log[ ], logarithm of the OR; Weight: weighting that the study contributed to the meta-analysis (by sample size); IV, Fixed, 95% CI, fixed-effect OR with 95% CI.

arrangements, the AAP recommends the use of the terms bed-sharing and room-sharing (when the infant sleeps in the parents' room but on a separate sleep surface [crib or similar surface] close to the parents' bed) (see Table 1).

The AAP recommends room-sharing, because this arrangement decreases the risk of SIDS by as much as 50%[89,91,172,173] and is safer than bed-sharing[89,91,172,173] or solitary sleeping (when the infant is in a separate room).[89,172] In addition, room-sharing is most likely to prevent suffocation, strangulation, and entrapment that may occur when the infant is sleeping in the adult bed. Furthermore, this arrangement allows close proximity to the infant, which will facilitate feeding, comforting, and monitoring of the infant. Most of the epidemiologic studies on which these recommendations are based include infants up to 1 year of age. Therefore, the AAP recommends that infants room-share, ideally for the first year after birth, but at least for the first 6 months. Although there is no specific evidence for moving an infant to his or her own room before 1 year of age, room-sharing during the first 6 months is especially critical because the rates of SIDS and other sleep-related deaths, particularly those occurring in bed-sharing situations, are highest during that period.

Parent-infant bed-sharing for all or part of sleep duration is common. In 1 national survey for the period

2001–2010, 46% of parents responded that they had shared a bed with their infant (8 months or younger) at some point in the preceding 2 weeks, and 13.5% reported that they usually bed-shared.[174] In another national survey, any bed-sharing was reported by 42% of mothers at 2 weeks of infant age and 27% of mothers at 12 months of infant age.[175] In a third study, almost 60% of mothers of infants from birth to 12 months of age reported bed-sharing at least once.[176] The rate of routine bed-sharing is higher among some racial/ethnic groups, including black, Hispanic, and American Indian/Alaska Native parents/infants.[20,22,174] There are often cultural and personal reasons why parents choose to bed-share, including convenience for feeding (breast or formula), comforting a fussy or sick infant, helping the infant and/or mother sleep better, bonding and attachment, and because it is a family tradition.[175,177] In addition, many parents may believe that their own vigilance is the only way that they can keep their infant safe and that the close proximity of bed-sharing allows them to maintain vigilance, even while sleeping.[178] Some parents will use bed-sharing specifically as a safety strategy if the infant sleeps in the prone position[23,178] or there is concern about environmental dangers, such as vermin or stray gunfire.[178]

Parent-infant bed-sharing continues to be highly controversial. Although electrophysiologic and behavioral studies offer a strong case for its effect in facilitating breastfeeding,[179-181] and although many parents believe that they can maintain vigilance of the infant while they are asleep and bed-sharing,[178] epidemiologic studies have shown that bed-sharing is associated with a number of conditions that are risk factors for SIDS, including soft bedding,[182-185] head covering,[186-189] and, for infants of smokers, increased exposure to tobacco smoke.[190] In addition, bed-sharing is associated with an increased risk of SIDS; a recent meta-analysis of 11 studies investigating the association of bed-sharing and SIDS showed a summary OR of 2.88 (95% CI: 1.99–4.18) with bed-sharing.[191] Furthermore, bed-sharing in an adult bed not designed for infant safety, especially when associated with other risk factors, exposes the infant to additional risks for unintentional injury and death, such as suffocation, asphyxia, entrapment, falls, and strangulation.[192,193] Infants younger than 4 months[194] and those born preterm and/or with low birth weight[195] are at the highest risk, possibly because immature motor skills and muscle strength make it difficult to escape potential threats.[191] In recent years, the concern among public health officials about bed-sharing has increased, because there have been increased reports of SUIDs occurring in high-risk sleep environments, particularly bed-sharing and/or sleeping on a couch or armchair.[196-198]

On the other hand, some breastfeeding advocacy groups encourage safer bed-sharing to promote breastfeeding,[199] and debate continues as to the safety of this sleep arrangement for low-risk, breastfed infants. In an analysis from 2 case-control studies in England (1993–1996 and 2003–2006), Blair et al[200] reported an adjusted OR of bed-sharing (excluding bed-sharing on a sofa) for infants in the absence of parental alcohol or tobacco use of 1.1 (95% CI: 0.6–2.9). For infants younger than 98 days, the OR was 1.6 (95% CI: 0.96–2.7).[200] These findings were independent of feeding method. The study lacked power to examine this association in older infants, because there was only 1 SIDS case in which bed-sharing was a factor in the absence of other risk factors. Breastfeeding was more common among bed-sharing infants, and the protective effect of breastfeeding was found only for infants who slept alone. The controls in these analyses were infants who were not bed-sharing/sofa-sharing regardless of room location; thus, they included infants who were room-sharing or sleeping in a separate room. In addition, the control infants included those whose parent(s) smoked or used alcohol. It is possible that this choice of controls overestimated their risk, leading to smaller ORs for risk among the cases (ie, biasing the results toward the null).

Carpenter et al[201] analyzed data from 19 studies across the United Kingdom, Europe, and Australasia to determine the risk of SIDS from bed-sharing when an infant is breastfed, the parents do not smoke, and the mother has not taken alcohol or drugs. When neither parent smoked, in the absence of other risk factors, the adjusted OR for bed-sharing versus room-sharing for all breastfed infants was 2.7 (95% CI: 1.4–5.3).[201] For breastfed infants younger than 3 months, in the absence of other risk factors, the adjusted OR for bed-sharing versus room-sharing was 5.1 (95% CI: 2.3–11.4). The study lacked power to examine this association in breastfed infants 3 months and older. Moreover, the large proportion of missing data for maternal alcohol and drug use is a limitation, although the authors used appropriate multiple imputation techniques for addressing these missing data.

The task force, recognizing the controversial nature of the recommendations about bed-sharing and the different methods and interpretations of these 2 sets of analyses outlined previously, requested an independent review of both articles by Dr Robert Platt, a biostatistician with expertise in perinatal epidemiology from McGill University in Canada. Dr Platt has no connection to the task force, nor does he have a vested interest in the recommendations. Dr Platt provided the following conclusion:

The fundamental difference in conclusions is that Blair et al conclude that bed-sharing in the absence of other risk factors (smoking, alcohol) does not convey an increased risk of SIDS, while Carpenter et al conclude the opposite. In both studies, the no-other-risk-factors group is limited in size, and the number of exposed cases is very small. In Blair et al, there are only 24 cases who bed-shared in the absence of these hazards. In Carpenter et al, although the total number of SIDS cases (1472) is more than 3 times the number of cases in the Blair study (400), the number of cases who bed-shared in the absence of these hazards was only 12 (personal communication, Professor Robert Carpenter, January 25, 2016). Therefore, the Carpenter results should be interpreted with some caution as well. In conclusion, both studies have strengths and weaknesses, and while on the surface the studies appear to contradict each other, I do not believe that their data support definitive differences between the 2 studies. There is some evidence of an increased risk in the no-other-risk-factor setting, in particular in the youngest age groups. However, based on concerns about sample size limitations, we are not able to say how large that increased risk is. Clearly, these data do not support a definitive conclusion that bed-sharing in the youngest

SIDS AND OTHER SLEEP-RELATED INFANT DEATHS:
EVIDENCE BASE FOR 2016 UPDATED RECOMMENDATIONS FOR A SAFE INFANT SLEEPING ENVIRONMENT

387

age group is safe, even under less hazardous circumstances.

There is insufficient evidence to recommend for or against the use of devices promoted to make bed-sharing "safe."

There is no evidence that devices marketed to make bed-sharing "safe" reduce the risk of SIDS or suffocation or are safe. Several products designed for in-bed use are currently under study, but results are not yet available. Bedside sleepers, which attach to the side of the parental bed and for which the CPSC published standards in 2013, may be considered by some parents as an option. The task force cannot make a recommendation for or against the use of either bedside sleepers or in-bed sleepers, because there have been no studies examining the association between these products and SIDS or unintentional injury and death, including suffocation. (See section entitled "Sleep Surfaces" for further discussion of sleepers.)

Infants who are brought into the bed for feeding or comforting should be returned to their own crib or bassinet when the parent is ready to return to sleep.

Studies have found an association between bed-sharing and longer duration of breastfeeding,[202] but most of these were cross-sectional studies, which do not enable the determination of a temporal relationship: that is, whether bed-sharing promotes breastfeeding or whether breastfeeding promotes bed-sharing, and whether women who prefer one practice are also likely to prefer the other.[203] However, a more recent longitudinal study provides strong evidence that bed-sharing promotes breastfeeding duration, with the greatest effect among frequent bed-sharers.[202] Another recent study has shown that, compared with mothers who room-shared without bed-sharing, mothers who bed-shared were more likely

to report exclusive breastfeeding (adjusted OR: 2.46; 95% CI: 1.76–3.45) or partial breastfeeding (adjusted OR: 1.75; 95% CI: 1.33–2.31).[204] Although bed-sharing may facilitate breastfeeding,[175] there are other factors, such as intent, that influence successful breastfeeding.[205] Furthermore, 1 case-control study found that the risk of SIDS while bed-sharing was similar among infants in the first 4 months of life, regardless of breastfeeding status, implying that the benefits of breastfeeding do not outweigh the increased risk associated with bed-sharing for younger infants.[194] The risk of bed-sharing is higher the longer the duration of bed-sharing during the night,[91] especially when associated with other risks.[89,90,206,207] Returning the infant to the crib after bringing the infant into the bed for a short period of time is not associated with increased risk.[90,207] Therefore, after the infant is brought into the bed for feeding, comforting, and bonding, the infant should be returned to the crib when the parent is ready for sleep.

Couches and armchairs are extremely dangerous places for infants.

Sleeping on couches and armchairs places infants at an extraordinarily high risk of infant death, including SIDS,[87,89,90,173,200,207] suffocation through entrapment or wedging between seat cushions, or overlay if another person is also sharing this surface.[197] Therefore, parents and other caregivers should be especially vigilant as to their wakefulness when feeding infants or lying with infants on these surfaces. It is important to emphasize this point to mothers, because 25% of mothers in 1 study reported falling asleep during the night when breastfeeding their infant on one of these surfaces.[176] Infants should never be placed on a couch or armchair for sleep.

Guidance for parents who fall asleep while feeding their infant.

The safest place for an infant to sleep is on a separate sleep surface designed for infants close to the parent's bed. However, the AAP acknowledges that parents frequently fall asleep while feeding the infant. Evidence suggests that it is less hazardous to fall asleep with the infant in the adult bed than on a sofa or armchair, should the parent fall asleep.[87,89,90,173,200,207] It is important to note that a large percentage of infants who die of SIDS are found with their head covered by bedding.[186] Therefore, there should be no pillows, sheets, blankets, or any other items in the bed that could obstruct infant breathing[87,182] or cause overheating.[208–211] Parents should follow safe sleep recommendations outlined elsewhere in this statement. Because there is evidence that the risk of bed-sharing is higher with longer duration, if the parent falls asleep while feeding the infant in bed the infant should be placed back on a separate sleep surface as soon as the parent awakens.[89,90,206,207]

There are specific circumstances that, in case-control studies and case series, have been shown to substantially increase the risk of SIDS or unintentional injury or death while bed-sharing, and these should be avoided at all times.

The task force emphasizes that certain circumstances greatly increase the risk of bed-sharing for both breastfed and formula-fed infants. Bed-sharing is especially dangerous in the following circumstances, and these should be avoided at all times:

- when one or both parents are smokers, even if they are not smoking in bed (OR: 2.3–21.6)[89,90,191,200,201,206,212];

- when the mother smoked during pregnancy[89,90,191,206,212];

- when the infant is younger than 4 months of age, regardless of parental smoking status (OR: 4.7–10.4)[89,91,173,191,201,207,213,214];

- when the infant is born preterm and/or with low birth weight[195];

- when the infant is bed-sharing on excessively soft or small surfaces, such as waterbeds, sofas, and armchairs (OR: 5.1–66.9)[87,89,90,173,200,207];

- when soft bedding accessories such as pillows or blankets are used (OR: 2.8–4.1)[87,215];

- when there are multiple bed-sharers (OR: 5.4)[87];

- when the parent has consumed alcohol (OR: 1.66–89.7)[91,196,200,201] and/or illicit or sedating drugs[201]; and

- when the infant is bed-sharing with someone who is not a parent (OR: 5.4).[87]

A retrospective series of SIDS cases reported that mean maternal body weight was higher for bed-sharing mothers than for non–bed-sharing mothers.[216] The only case-control study to investigate the relationship between maternal body weight and bed-sharing did not find an increased risk of bed-sharing with increased maternal weight.[217]

The safety and benefits of cobedding twins and higher-order multiples have not been established. It is prudent to provide separate sleep areas and avoid cobedding (sleeping on the same sleep surface) for twins and higher-order multiples in the hospital and at home.

Cobedding of twins and other infants of multiple gestation is a frequent practice, both in the hospital setting and at home.[218] However, the benefits of cobedding twins and higher-order multiples have not been established.[219–221] Twins and higher-order multiples are often born preterm and with low birth weights, so they are at increased risk of SIDS.[125,126] Furthermore, cobedding

increases the potential for overheating and rebreathing, and size discordance between multiples may increase the risk of unintentional suffocation.[220] Most cobedded twins are placed on the side rather than supine.[218] Finally, cobedding of twins and higher-order multiples in the hospital setting may encourage parents to continue this practice at home.[220] Because the evidence for the benefits of cobedding twins and higher-order multiples is not compelling and because of the increased risk of SIDS and suffocation, the AAP believes that it is prudent to provide separate sleep areas for these infants to decrease the risk of SIDS and unintentional suffocation.

USE OF BEDDING

Keep soft objects, such as pillows, pillow-like toys, quilts, comforters, sheepskins, and loose bedding, such as blankets and nonfitted sheets, away from the infant's sleep area to reduce the risk of SIDS, suffocation, entrapment, and strangulation.

Soft objects and loose bedding can obstruct an infant's airway and increase the risk of SIDS,[87,182] suffocation, and rebreathing.[79,81,82,135,222–224] In the United States, nearly 55% of infants are placed to sleep underneath or on top of bedding such as thick blankets, quilts, and pillows.[25] The prevalence of bedding use is highest among infants whose mothers are teenagers, from minority racial groups, and among those without a college education.

Pillows, quilts, comforters, sheepskins, and other soft bedding can be hazardous when placed under the infant[87,182,210,225–229] or left loose in the infant's sleep area.[90,182,215,224,228–234] Bedding in the sleeping environment increases SIDS risk fivefold, independent of sleep position,[87,182] and this risk increases to 21-fold when the infant is placed prone.[87,182] Many infants who die of SIDS are found in the supine position but with their heads

covered by loose bedding.[90,225,226,230] In addition, infants who bed-share (share a sleep surface) have a higher SIDS risk when sleeping on a soft as opposed to a firm surface.[215]

In addition to SIDS risk, soft objects and loose bedding in the sleeping environment may also lead to unintentional suffocation.[134,224,235] A review of 66 SUID case investigations in 2011 showed that soft bedding was the most frequently reported factor among deaths classified as possible and explained unintentional suffocation deaths.[224] In addition, a CPSC report of sleep-related infant deaths in 2009–2011 found that most deaths attributed to suffocation (regardless of whether infant was sleeping in a crib, on a mattress, or in a play yard) involved extra bedding, such as pillows or blankets.[235] Soft bedding (eg, blankets and stuffed animals) may also be a stronger risk factor for sleep-related deaths among infants older than 3 months than it is for their younger counterparts, especially when infants are placed in or roll to the prone position.[134]

Parents and caregivers are likely motivated by good intentions and perceived cultural norms when they opt to use bedding for infant sleep. Qualitative studies show that parents who use bedding want to provide a comfortable and safe environment for their infant.[236] For comfort, parents may use blankets to provide warmth or to soften the sleep surface. For safety, parents may use pillows as barriers to prevent falls from adult beds or sofas or as a prop to keep their infant on the side.[236] Images of infants sleeping with blankets, pillows, and other soft objects are widespread in popular magazines targeted to families with newborn infants.[237] Parents and caregivers who see these images may perceive the use of these items as the norm, both favorable and the ideal, for infant sleep.

To avoid suffocation, rebreathing, and SIDS risk, infants should sleep on a firm

SIDS AND OTHER SLEEP-RELATED INFANT DEATHS:
EVIDENCE BASE FOR 2016 UPDATED RECOMMENDATIONS FOR A SAFE INFANT SLEEPING ENVIRONMENT

389

surface (see section entitled "Sleep Surfaces" for a definition of a firm surface).[135] Because pillows, quilts, and comforters can obstruct the infant's airway (nose or mouth), they should never be used in the infant's sleeping environment. Infant sleep clothing, such as sleeping sacks, are designed to keep the infant warm and can be used in place of blankets to prevent the possibility of head covering or entrapment. However, care must be taken to select appropriately sized clothing and to avoid overheating. Nursing and hospital staff should model safe sleep arrangements to new parents after delivery.

Bumper pads are not recommended; they have been implicated in deaths attributable to suffocation, entrapment, and strangulation and, with new safety standards for crib slats, are not necessary for safety against head entrapment.

Bumper pads and similar products attaching to crib slats or sides are frequently used with the thought of protecting infants from injury. Initially, bumper pads were developed to prevent head entrapment between crib slats.[238] However, newer crib standards requiring crib slat spacing to be <2-3/8 inches have obviated the need for crib bumpers. In addition, infant deaths have occurred because of bumper pads. A case series by Thach et al,[239] which used 1985–2005 CPSC data, found that deaths attributed to bumper pads occurred as a result of 3 mechanisms: (1) suffocation against soft, pillow-like bumper pads; (2) entrapment between the mattress or crib and firm bumper pads; and (3) strangulation from bumper pad ties. However, a 2010 CPSC white paper that reviewed the same cases concluded that there were other confounding factors, such as the presence of pillows and/or blankets, that may have contributed to many of the deaths in this report.[240] The white paper pointed out that available

data from the scene investigations, autopsies, law enforcement records, and death certificates often lacked sufficiently detailed information to conclude how or whether bumper pads contributed to the deaths. Two more recent analyses of CPSC data also came to different conclusions. The CPSC review concluded again that there was insufficient evidence to support that bumper pads were primarily responsible for infant deaths when bumper pads were used per the manufacturer's instructions and in the absence of other unsafe sleep risk factors.[241] Scheers et al,[242] in their re-analysis, concluded that the rate of bumper pad–related deaths has increased, recognizing that changes in reporting may account for the increase, and that 67% of the deaths could have been prevented if the bumper pads had not been present. Limitations of CPSC data collection processes contribute to the difficulty in determining the risk of bumper pad use.

However, others[239,243] have concluded that the use of bumper pads only prevents minor injuries, and that the potential benefits of preventing minor injury with bumper pad use are far outweighed by the risk of serious injury, such as suffocation or strangulation. In addition, most bumper pads obscure infant and parent visibility, which may increase parental anxiety.[236,238] Other products exist that attach to crib sides or crib slats and claim to protect infants from injury; however, there are no published data that support these claims. Because of the potential for suffocation, entrapment, and strangulation and lack of evidence to support that bumper pads or similar products that attach to crib slats or sides prevent injury in young infants, the AAP does not recommend their use.

PACIFIER USE

Consider offering a pacifier at naptime and bedtime.

Multiple case-control studies[87,91,207,244–250] and 2 meta-analyses[251,252] have reported a protective effect of pacifiers on the incidence of SIDS, particularly when used at the time of the last sleep period, with decreased risk of SIDS ranging from 50% to 90%. Furthermore, 1 study found that pacifier use favorably modified the risk profile of infants who sleep in the prone/side position, bed-share, or use soft bedding.[253] The mechanism for this apparent strong protective effect is still unclear, but favorable modification of autonomic control during sleep[254] and maintaining airway patency during sleep[255] have been proposed. Physiologic studies of the effect of pacifier use on arousal are conflicting; 1 study found that pacifier use decreased arousal thresholds,[163] but others have found no effects on arousability with pacifier use.[256,257] It is common for the pacifier to fall from the mouth soon after the infant falls asleep; even so, the protective effect persists throughout that sleep period.[163,258] Two studies have shown that pacifier use is most protective when used for all sleep periods.[207,250] However, these studies also showed an increased risk of SIDS when the pacifier was usually used but not used the last time the infant was placed for sleep; the significance of these findings is yet unclear.

Although some SIDS experts and policy makers endorse pacifier use recommendations that are similar to those of the AAP,[259,260] concerns about possible deleterious effects of pacifier use have prevented others from making a recommendation for pacifier use as a risk-reduction strategy.[261] Although several observational studies[262–264] have shown a correlation between pacifiers and reduced breastfeeding duration, a recent Cochrane review comparing pacifier use and nonuse in healthy term infants who had initiated breastfeeding found that pacifier use had no effects on partial or exclusive breastfeeding rates at 3 and 4 months.[265] Furthermore, a systematic review found that the highest level of evidence (ie, from clinical trials) does not support an adverse relationship between pacifier use and breastfeeding duration or exclusivity.[266] The association between shortened duration of breastfeeding and pacifier use in observational studies likely reflects a number of complex factors, such as breastfeeding difficulties or intent to wean.[266,267] However, some have also raised the concern that studies that show no effect of pacifier introduction on breastfeeding duration or exclusivity may not account for early weaning or failure to establish breastfeeding.[268] The AAP policy statement "Breastfeeding and the Use of Human Milk" includes a recommendation that pacifiers can be used during breastfeeding but that implementation should be delayed until breastfeeding is well established.[269] Infants who are not being directly breastfed can begin pacifier use as soon as desired.

Some dental malocclusions have been found more commonly among pacifier users than nonusers, but the differences generally disappeared after pacifier cessation.[270] The American Academy of Pediatric Dentistry policy statement on oral habits states that nonnutritive sucking behaviors (ie, fingers or pacifiers) are considered normal in infants and young children and that, in general, sucking habits in children to the age of 3 years are unlikely to cause any long-term problems.[271] Pacifier use is associated with an approximate 1.2- to 2-fold increased risk of otitis media, particularly between 2 and 3 years of age.[272,273] The incidence of otitis media is generally lower in the first year after birth, especially the first 6 months, when the risk of SIDS is the highest.[274–279] However, pacifier use, once established, may persist beyond 6 months, thus increasing the risk of otitis media. Gastrointestinal tract

infections and oral colonization with *Candida* species were also found to be more common among pacifier users than nonusers.[275–277]

Because of the risk of strangulation, pacifiers should not be hung around the infant's neck. Pacifiers that attach to the infant's clothing should not be used with sleeping infants. Objects, such as stuffed toys, that may present a suffocation or choking risk, should not be attached to pacifiers.

There is insufficient evidence that finger sucking is protective against SIDS.

The literature on infant finger sucking and SIDS is extremely limited. Only 2 case-control studies have reported these results.[248,249] One study from the United States showed a protective effect of infant finger sucking (reported as "thumb sucking") against SIDS (adjusted OR: 0.43; 95% CI: 0.25–0.77), but it was less protective than pacifier use (adjusted OR: 0.07 [95% CI: 0.01–0.64] if the infant also sucked the thumb; adjusted OR: 0.08 [95% CI: 0.03–0.23] if the infant did not suck the thumb).[249] Another study from The Netherlands did not show an association between usual finger sucking (reported as "thumb sucking") and SIDS risk (OR: 1.38; 95% CI: 0.35–1.51), but the wide CI suggests that there was insufficient power to detect a significant association.[248]

PRENATAL AND POSTNATAL EXPOSURES (INCLUDING SMOKING AND ALCOHOL)

Pregnant women should obtain regular prenatal care.

There is substantial epidemiologic evidence linking a lower risk of SIDS for infants whose mothers obtain regular prenatal care.[280–283] Women should obtain prenatal care from early in the pregnancy, according to established guidelines for frequency of prenatal visits.[284]

Smoking during pregnancy, in the pregnant woman's environment, and in the infant's environment should be avoided.

Maternal smoking during pregnancy has been identified as a major risk factor in almost every epidemiologic study of SIDS.[285–288] Smoke in the infant's environment after birth has been identified as a separate major risk factor in a few studies,[286,289] although separating this variable from maternal smoking before birth is problematic. Third-hand smoke refers to residual contamination from tobacco smoke after the cigarette has been extinguished[290]; there is no research to date on the significance of third-hand smoke with regard to SIDS risk. Smoke exposure adversely affects infant arousal[291–297]; in addition, smoke exposure increases the risk of preterm birth and low birth weight, both risk factors for SIDS. The effect of tobacco smoke exposure on SIDS risk is dose-dependent. The risk of SIDS is particularly high when the infant bed-shares with an adult smoker (OR: 2.3–21.6), even when the adult does not smoke in bed.[89,90,191,200,201,206,212,298] It is estimated that one-third of SIDS deaths could be prevented if all maternal smoking during pregnancy was eliminated.[299,300] The AAP supports the elimination of all tobacco smoke exposure, both prenatally and environmentally.

Avoid alcohol and illicit drug use during pregnancy and after the infant's birth.

Several studies have specifically investigated the association of SIDS with prenatal and postnatal exposure to alcohol or illicit drug use, although substance abuse often involves more than one substance and it is often difficult to separate out these variables from each other and from smoking. However, 1 study in Northern Plains American Indian infants found that periconceptional

SIDS AND OTHER SLEEP-RELATED INFANT DEATHS:
EVIDENCE BASE FOR 2016 UPDATED RECOMMENDATIONS FOR A SAFE INFANT SLEEPING ENVIRONMENT

391

maternal alcohol use (adjusted OR: 6.2; 95% CI: 1.6–23.3) and maternal first-trimester binge drinking (adjusted OR: 8.2; 95% CI: 1.9–35.3)[211] were associated with increased SIDS risk, independent of prenatal cigarette smoking exposure. A retrospective study from Western Australia found that a maternal alcoholism diagnosis recorded during pregnancy (adjusted hazard ratio: 6.92; 95% CI: 4.02–11.90) or within 1 year postpregnancy (adjusted hazard ratio: 8.61; 95% CI: 5.04–14.69) was associated with increased SIDS risk, and the authors estimated that at least 16.41% of SIDS deaths were attributable to maternal alcohol use disorder.[301] Another study from Denmark, based on prospective data on maternal alcohol use, has also shown a significant relationship between maternal binge drinking and postneonatal infant mortality, including SIDS.[302] Parental alcohol and/or illicit drug use in combination with bed-sharing places the infant at particularly high risk of SIDS and unintentional suffocation.[91,196]

Rat models have shown increased arousal latency to hypoxia in rat pups exposed to prenatal alcohol.[303] Furthermore, postmortem studies in Northern Plains American Indian infants showed that prenatal cigarette smoking was significantly associated with decreased serotonin receptor binding in the brainstem. In this study, the association of maternal alcohol drinking in the 3 months before or during pregnancy was of borderline significance on univariate analysis but was not significant when prenatal smoking and case versus control status was in the model.[29] However, this study had limited power for multivariate analysis because of the small sample size. One study found an association of SIDS with heavy alcohol consumption in the 2 days before the death.[304] Several studies have found a particularly strong association when alcohol consumption or illicit drug use occurs in combination with bed-sharing.[89–91,305]

Studies investigating the relationship of illicit drug use and SIDS have focused on specific drugs or illicit drug use in general. One study found maternal cannabis use to be associated with an increased risk of SIDS (adjusted OR: 2.35; 95% CI: 1.36–4.05) at night but not during the day.[306] In utero exposure to opiates (primarily methadone and heroin) has been shown in retrospective studies to be associated with an increased risk of SIDS.[307,308] With the exception of 1 study that did not show an increased risk,[309] population-based studies have generally shown an increased risk with in utero cocaine exposure.[310–312] However, these studies did not control for confounding factors. A prospective cohort study found the SIDS rate to be significantly increased for infants exposed in utero to methadone (OR: 3.6; 95% CI: 2.5–5.1), heroin (OR: 2.3; 95% CI: 1.3–4.0), methadone and heroin (OR: 3.2; 95% CI: 1.2–8.6), and cocaine (OR: 1.6; 95% CI: 1.2–2.2), even after controlling for race/ethnicity, maternal age, parity, birth weight, year of birth, and maternal smoking.[313] In addition, a meta-analysis of studies investigating an association between in utero cocaine exposure and SIDS found an increased risk of SIDS to be associated with prenatal exposure to cocaine and illicit drugs in general.[314]

OVERHEATING, FANS, AND ROOM VENTILATION

Avoid overheating and head covering in infants.

The amount of clothing or blankets covering an infant and the room temperature are associated with an increased risk of SIDS.[208–211] Infants who sleep in the prone position have a higher risk of overheating than supine sleeping infants.[210] However,

the definition of overheating in the studies that found an increased risk of SIDS varies. It is therefore difficult to provide specific room temperature guidelines to avoid overheating.

It is unclear whether the relationship to overheating is an independent factor or merely a reflection of the increased risk of SIDS and suffocation with blankets and other potentially asphyxiating objects in the sleeping environment. Head covering during sleep is of particular concern. In 1 systematic review, the pooled mean prevalence of head covering among SIDS victims was 24.6%, compared with 3.2% among control infants.[186] It is not known whether the risk related to head covering is due to overheating, hypoxia, or rebreathing.

Some have suggested that room ventilation may be important. One study found that bedroom heating, compared with no bedroom heating, increases SIDS risk (OR: 4.5),[315] and another study showed a decreased risk of SIDS in a well-ventilated bedroom (windows and doors open; OR: 0.4).[316] In 1 study, the use of a fan appeared to reduce the risk of SIDS (adjusted OR: 0.28; 95% CI: 0.10–0.77).[317] However, because of the possibility of recall bias, the small sample size of controls who used fans ($n = 36$), a lack of detail about the location and types of fans used, and the weak link to a mechanism, this study should be interpreted with caution. On the basis of available data, the task force cannot make a recommendation on the use of a fan as a SIDS risk-reduction strategy.

IMMUNIZATIONS

Infants should be immunized in accordance with AAP and Centers for Disease Control and Prevention recommendations.

The incidence of SIDS peaks at a time when infants are receiving numerous immunizations. Case reports of a cluster of deaths shortly after immunization with diphtheria-tetanus toxoids-pertussis vaccine in the late 1970s created concern of a possible causal relationship between vaccinations and SIDS.[318–321] Case-control studies were performed to evaluate this temporal association. Four of the 6 studies showed no relationship between diphtheria-tetanus toxoids-pertussis vaccination and subsequent SIDS[322–325]; the other 2 suggested a temporal relationship, but only in specific subgroup analysis.[326,327] In 2003, the Institute of Medicine reviewed available data and concluded the following: "The evidence favors rejection of a causal relationship between exposure to multiple vaccinations and SIDS."[328] Several analyses of the US Vaccine Adverse Event Reporting System database have shown no relationship between vaccines and SIDS.[329–331] In addition, several large-population case-control trials consistently have found vaccines to be protective against SIDS[332–335]; however, confounding factors (social, maternal, birth, and infant medical history) may account for this protective effect.[336] It also has been theorized that the decreased SIDS rate immediately after vaccination was attributable to infants being healthier at the time of immunization, or "the healthy vaccinee effect."[337] Recent illness would both place infants at higher risk of SIDS and make them more likely to have immunizations deferred.[338]

Recent studies have attempted to control for confounding by social, maternal, birth, and infant medical history.[332,334,338] A meta-analysis of 4 studies found a multivariate summary OR for immunizations and SIDS to be 0.54 (95% CI: 0.39–0.76), indicating that the risk of SIDS is halved by immunization.[338] The evidence continues to show no causal relationship between immunizations and SIDS and suggests that vaccination may have a protective effect against SIDS.

COMMERCIAL DEVICES

Avoid the use of commercial devices that are inconsistent with safe sleep recommendations.

Risk-reduction strategies are based on the best-available evidence in large epidemiologic studies. These studies have been largely focused on the correlations between the sleep environment and SIDS. Our current understanding is that the cause of SIDS is multifactorial and that death results from the interaction between a vulnerable infant and a potentially asphyxiating sleep environment. Thus, claims that sleep devices, mattresses, or special sleep surfaces reduce the risk of SIDS must therefore be supported by epidemiologic evidence. At a minimum, any devices used should meet safety standards of the CPSC, the Juvenile Product Manufacturers Association, and ASTM International (known previously as the American Society for Testing and Materials). The AAP concurs with the US Food and Drug Administration and CPSC that manufacturers should not claim that a product or device protects against SIDS unless there is scientific evidence to that effect.

Wedges and positioning devices are often used by parents to maintain the infant in the side or supine position because of claims that these products reduce the risk of SIDS, suffocation, or gastroesophageal reflux. However, these products are frequently made with soft, compressible materials, which might increase the risk of suffocation. The CPSC has received reports of deaths attributable to suffocation and entrapment associated with wedges and positioning devices. Most of these deaths occurred when infants were placed in the prone or side position with these devices[339]; other incidents have occurred when infants have slipped out of the restraints or rolled into a prone position while using the device.[240,340] Because of

the lack of evidence that they are effective against SIDS, suffocation, or gastroesophageal reflux and because of the potential for suffocation and entrapment risk, the AAP concurs with the CPSC and the US Food and Drug Administration in warning against the use of these products. If positioning devices are used in the hospital as part of physical therapy, they should be removed from the infant sleep area well before discharge from the hospital.

Certain crib mattresses have been designed with air-permeable materials to reduce rebreathing of expired gases, in the event that an infant ends up in the prone position during sleep, and these may be preferable to those with air-impermeable materials. With the use of a head box model, Bar-Yishay et al[341] found that a permeable sleeping surface exhibited significantly better aeration properties in dispersing carbon dioxide and in preventing its accumulation. They also found the measured temperature within the head box to be substantially lower with the more permeable mattress, concluding that it was due to faster heat dissipation. This finding could be potentially protective against overheating, which has been identified as a risk factor for SIDS. Colditz et al[342] also performed studies both in vitro and in vivo, showing better diffusion and less accumulation of carbon dioxide with a mesh mattress. However, Carolan et al[343] found that even porous surfaces are associated with carbon dioxide accumulation and rebreathing thresholds unless there is an active carbon dioxide dispersal system. In addition, although rebreathing has been hypothesized to contribute to death in SIDS, particularly if the head is covered or when the infant is face down, there is no evidence that rebreathing, per se, causes SIDS and no epidemiologic evidence that these mattresses reduce the risk of SIDS. The use of "breathable" mattresses can be an

SIDS AND OTHER SLEEP-RELATED INFANT DEATHS:
EVIDENCE BASE FOR 2016 UPDATED RECOMMENDATIONS FOR A SAFE INFANT SLEEPING ENVIRONMENT

393

acceptable alternative as long as the other manufacturing requirements are met, including being designed for a particular crib, having a firm surface, and maintaining its shape even when the fitted sheet designated for that model is used, such that there are no gaps between the mattress and the side of the crib, bassinet, portable crib, or play yard.

HOME MONITORS, SIDS, AND BRIEF RESOLVED UNEXPLAINED EVENTS (FORMERLY APPARENT LIFE-THREATENING EVENTS)

There is no evidence that apparent life-threatening events are precursors to SIDS. Furthermore, infant home cardiorespiratory monitors should not be used as a strategy to reduce the risk of SIDS.

For many years, it was believed that brief resolved unexplained events (BRUEs; formerly known as apparent life-threatening events [ALTEs]) were the predecessors of SIDS, and home apnea monitors were used as a strategy for preventing SIDS.[344] However, the use of home cardiorespiratory monitors has not been documented to decrease the incidence of SIDS.[345-348] Home cardiorespiratory monitors are sometimes prescribed for use at home to detect apnea and bradycardia and, when pulse oximetry is used, decreases in oxyhemoglobin saturation for infants at risk of these conditions.[349] Routine in-hospital cardiorespiratory monitoring before discharge from the hospital has not been shown to detect infants at risk of SIDS. There are no data that other commercial devices that are designed to monitor infant vital signs reduce the risk of SIDS.

TUMMY TIME

Supervised, awake tummy time is recommended to facilitate development and to minimize development of positional plagiocephaly.

Positional plagiocephaly, or plagiocephaly without synostosis (PWS), can be associated with a supine sleeping position (OR: 2.5).[350] It is most likely to result if the infant's head position is not varied when placed for sleep; if the infant spends little or no time in awake, supervised tummy time; and if the infant is not held in the upright position when not sleeping.[350-352] Children with developmental delay and/or neurologic injury have increased rates of PWS, although a causal relationship has not been shown.[350,353-356] In healthy normal children, the incidence of PWS decreases spontaneously from 20% at 8 months to 3% at 24 months of age.[351] Although data to make specific recommendations as to how often and how long tummy time should be undertaken are lacking, the task force concurs with the AAP Section on Neurologic Surgery that "a certain amount of prone positioning, or 'tummy time,' while the infant is awake and being observed is recommended to help prevent the development of flattening of the occiput and to facilitate development of the upper shoulder girdle strength necessary for timely attainment of certain motor milestones."[357] The AAP clinical report "Prevention and Management of Positional Skull Deformities in Infants"[357] provides additional detail on the prevention, diagnosis, and management of positional plagiocephaly.

SWADDLING

There is no evidence to recommend swaddling as a strategy to reduce the risk of SIDS. Infants who are swaddled have an increased risk of death if they are placed in or roll to the prone position. If swaddling is used, infants should always be placed on the back. When an infant exhibits signs of attempting to roll, swaddling should no longer be used.

Many cultures and newborn nurseries have traditionally used swaddling, or wrapping the infant in a light blanket, as a strategy to soothe infants and, in some cases, to encourage sleep in the supine position. Swaddling, when done correctly, can be an effective technique to help calm infants and promote sleep.[358,359]

Some have argued that swaddling can alter certain risk factors for SIDS, thus reducing the risk of SIDS. For instance, it has been suggested that the physical restraint associated with swaddling may prevent infants placed supine from rolling to the prone position.[358] One study suggested a decrease in SIDS rate with swaddling if the infant was supine, but notably, there was an increased risk of SIDS if the infant was swaddled and placed in the prone position.[210] Although another study found a 31-fold increase in SIDS risk with swaddling, the analysis was not stratified by sleep position.[196] Although it may be more likely that parents will initially place a swaddled infant supine, this protective effect may be offset by the 12-fold increased risk of SIDS if the infant is either placed or rolls to the prone position when swaddled.[210,359] In addition, an analysis of CPSC data found that deaths associated with swaddling were most often attributed to positional asphyxia related to prone sleeping, and a large majority of sleep environments had soft bedding.[360] Thus, if swaddling is used, the infant should be placed wholly supine, and swaddling should be discontinued as soon as the infant begins to attempt to roll. Commercially available swaddle sacks are an acceptable alternative, particularly if the parent or caregiver does not know how to swaddle an infant with a conventional thin blanket. There is no evidence with regard to SIDS risk related to the arms swaddled in or out.

There is some evidence that swaddling may cause detrimental physiologic consequences. For example, it can cause an increase in respiratory rate,[361] and tight swaddling can reduce the infant's functional residual lung capacity.[358,362,363] Tight swaddling can also exacerbate hip dysplasia if the hips are kept in extension and adduction,[364–367] which is particularly important because some have advocated that the calming effects of swaddling are related to the "tightness" of the swaddling. In contrast, "loose" or incorrectly applied swaddling could result in head covering and, in some cases, strangulation if the blankets become loose in the bed. Swaddling may also possibly increase the risk of overheating in some situations, especially when the head is covered or there is infection.[368,369] However, 1 study found no increase in abdominal skin temperature when infants were swaddled in a light cotton blanket from the shoulders down.[362]

Impaired arousal has often been postulated as a mechanism contributing to SIDS, and several studies have investigated the relationship between swaddling and arousal and sleep patterns in infants. Physiologic studies have shown that, in general, swaddling decreases startling,[361] increases sleep duration, and decreases spontaneous awakenings.[370] Swaddling also decreases arousability (ie, increases cortical arousal thresholds) to a nasal pulsatile air-jet stimulus, especially in infants who are easily arousable when not swaddled.[361] One study found decreased arousability in infants at 3 months of age who were not usually swaddled and then were swaddled but no effect on arousability in routinely swaddled infants.[361] In contrast, another study has shown infants to be more easily arousable[370] and to have increased autonomic (subcortical) responses[371] to an auditory stimulus when swaddled.[371] Thus, although swaddling clearly promotes sleep and decreases the number of awakenings, the effects on arousability to an external stimulus remain unclear. Accumulating evidence suggests,

however, that routine swaddling has only minimal effects on arousal. In addition, there have been no studies investigating the effects of swaddling on arousal to more relevant stimuli such as hypoxia or hypercapnia. Finally, there is no evidence with regard to SIDS risk related to the arms swaddled in or out.

In summary, it is recognized that swaddling is one of many child care practices that can be used to calm infants, promote sleep, and encourage the use of the supine position. However, there is no evidence to recommend routine swaddling as a strategy to reduce the risk of SIDS. The risk of death is high if a swaddled infant is placed in or rolls to the prone position. If infants are swaddled, they should always be placed on the back. When an infant exhibits signs of attempting to roll, swaddling should no longer be used. Moreover, as many have advocated, swaddling must be correctly applied to avoid the possible hazards, such as hip dysplasia, head covering, and strangulation. Importantly, swaddling does not reduce the necessity to follow recommended safe sleep practices.

POTENTIAL TOXICANTS

There is no evidence substantiating a causal relationship between various toxicants to SIDS.

Many theories link various toxicants and SIDS.[372–374] Although 1 ecological study found a correlation of the maximal recorded nitrate levels of drinking water with local SIDS rates in Sweden,[375] no case-control study has shown a relationship between nitrates in drinking water and SIDS. Furthermore, an expert group in the United Kingdom analyzed data pertaining to a hypothesis that SIDS is related to toxic gases, such as antimony, phosphorus, or arsenic, being released from mattresses[376,377] and found the toxic gas hypothesis unsubstantiated.[378] Finally, 2

case-control studies found that wrapping mattresses in plastic to reduce toxic gas emission did not protect against SIDS.[230,379]

HEARING SCREENS

Current data do not support the use of newborn hearing screens as screening tests for SIDS.

One retrospective case-control study examined the use of newborn transient evoked otoacoustic emission hearing screening tests as a tool to identify infants at subsequent risk of SIDS.[380] Infants who subsequent died of SIDS did not fail their hearing tests but, compared with controls, showed a decreased signal-to-noise ratio score in the right ear only, at frequencies of 2000, 3000, and 4000 Hz. Methodologic concerns have been raised about the validity of the study methods used in this study,[381,382] and these results have not been substantiated by others. A larger, but non–peer-reviewed, report of hearing screening data in Michigan[383] and a peer-reviewed retrospective study in Hong Kong[383,384] showed no relationship between hearing screening test results and SIDS cases. Until additional data are available, hearing screening should not be considered as a valid screening tool to determine which infants may be at subsequent risk of SIDS. Furthermore, an increased risk of SIDS should not be inferred from an abnormal hearing screen result.

EDUCATIONAL INTERVENTIONS

Educational and intervention campaigns are often effective in altering practice.

Intervention campaigns for SIDS have been extremely effective, especially with regard to the avoidance of prone positioning.[385] Furthermore, primary care–based educational interventions, particularly those that address caregiver concerns and misconceptions about safe sleep recommendations,

SIDS AND OTHER SLEEP-RELATED INFANT DEATHS:
EVIDENCE BASE FOR 2016 UPDATED RECOMMENDATIONS FOR A SAFE INFANT SLEEPING ENVIRONMENT

395

can be effective in altering practice. For instance, addressing concerns about infant comfort, choking, and aspiration while the infant is sleeping supine is helpful.[19,96,97,386] However, many families report not receiving information consistent with AAP recommendations. When a nationally representative sample of mothers of young infants were asked about information received from their pediatricians, only 54.5% had received a recommendation to place their infant supine for sleep, 19.9% had received information about appropriate sleep location, and 11.0% had received information about pacifier use.[387] Primary care providers should be encouraged to develop quality-improvement initiatives to improve adherence to safe sleep recommendations among their patients.

In addition, modeling of unsafe sleep practices by health care and child care providers may increase the prevalence of these unsafe practices.[388–390] Modeling of unsafe practices may occur because professionals are not convinced of the utility of the safe sleep recommendations or have concerns about the supine sleep position, particularly with regard to infant comfort, choking, and aspiration.[391–395] Interventions that address provider concerns are effective in improving behavior.[391,396–398]

MEDIA MESSAGES

Media and manufacturers should follow safe sleep guidelines in their messaging and advertising.

A recent study found that, in magazines targeted toward childbearing women, more than one-third of pictures of sleeping infants and two-thirds of pictures of infant sleep environments portrayed unsafe sleep positions and sleep environments.[237] Media exposures (including movie, television, magazines, newspapers, and Web

sites), manufacturer advertisements, and store displays affect individual behavior by influencing beliefs and attitudes. Frequent exposure to health-related media messages can affect individual health decisions,[399,400] and media messages have been very influential in decisions regarding sleep position.[101,104] Media and advertising messages contrary to safe sleep recommendations may create misinformation about safe sleep practices.

Media and manufacturer messaging and advertising should follow safe sleep guidelines in text, photos, and illustrations. In addition, public health departments and organizations that provide safe sleep information should review, revise, and reissue this information at least every 5 years to ensure that each generation of new parents receives appropriate information.

RECOMMENDATIONS

The recommendations for a safe infant sleeping environment to reduce the risk of both SIDS and other sleep-related infant deaths are specified in the accompanying policy statement.[78]

ACKNOWLEDGMENTS

We acknowledge the contributions provided by others to the collection and interpretation of data examined in preparation of this report. We are particularly grateful for the independent biostatistical report submitted by Robert W. Platt, PhD.

LEAD AUTHOR

Rachel Y. Moon, MD, FAAP

TASK FORCE ON SUDDEN INFANT DEATH SYNDROME

Rachel Y. Moon, MD, FAAP, Chairperson
Robert A. Darnall, MD
Lori Feldman-Winter, MD, MPH, FAAP
Michael H. Goodstein, MD, FAAP
Fern R. Hauck, MD, MS

CONSULTANTS

Marian Willinger, PhD – Eunice Kennedy Shriver *National Institute for Child Health and Human Development*
Carrie K. Shapiro-Mendoza, PhD, MPH – *Centers for Disease Control and Prevention*

STAFF

James Couto, MA

ABBREVIATIONS

AAP: American Academy of Pediatrics
ASSB: accidental suffocation or strangulation in bed
CI: confidence interval
CPSC: Consumer Product Safety Commission
ICD: International Statistical Classification of Diseases and Related Health Problems
ICD-10: International Classification of Diseases, 10th Revision
OR: odds ratio
PWS: plagiocephaly without synostosis
SIDS: sudden infant death syndrome
SUDI: sudden unexpected death in infancy
SUID: sudden unexpected infant death
5-HT: 5-hydroxytryptamine (serotonin)
5-HT1A: 5-hydroxytryptamine 1A (serotonin 1A)

REFERENCES

1. Moon RY; Task Force on Sudden Infant Death Syndrome. SIDS and other sleep-related infant deaths: expansion of recommendations for a safe infant sleeping environment. *Pediatrics.* 2011;128(5). Available at: www.pediatrics. org/cgi/content/full/128/5/e1341

2. Moon RY; Task Force on Sudden Infant Death Syndrome. SIDS and other sleep-related infant deaths: expansion of recommendations for a safe infant sleeping environment. *Pediatrics.* 2011;128(5):1030–1039

3. Ebell MH, Siwek J, Weiss BD, et al. Strength of Recommendation

Taxonomy (SORT): a patient-centered approach to grading evidence in the medical literature. *Am Fam Physician*. 2004;69(3):548–556

4. Willinger M, James LS, Catz C. Defining the sudden infant death syndrome (SIDS): deliberations of an expert panel convened by the National Institute of Child Health and Human Development. *Pediatr Pathol*. 1991;11(5):677–684

5. Centers for Disease Control and Prevention. Sudden unexplained infant death investigation reporting form (SUIDIRF). Available at: www.cdc.gov/SIDS/SUIDRF.htm. Accessed January 10, 2016

6. Camperlengo LT, Shapiro-Mendoza CK, Kim SY. Sudden infant death syndrome: diagnostic practices and investigative policies, 2004. *Am J Forensic Med Pathol*. 2012;33(3):197–201

7. Krous HF, Chadwick AE, Haas EA, Stanley C. Pulmonary intra-alveolar hemorrhage in SIDS and suffocation. *J Forensic Leg Med*. 2007;14(8):461–470

8. Kim SY, Shapiro-Mendoza CK, Chu SY, Camperlengo LT, Anderson R. Differentiating cause-of-death terminology for deaths coded as SIDS, accidental suffocation, and unknown cause: an investigation using US death certificates, 2003-2004. *Am J Forensic Sci*. 2012;57(2):364–369

9. Shapiro-Mendoza CK, Kim SY, Chu SY, Kahn E, Anderson RN. Using death certificates to characterize sudden infant death syndrome (SIDS): opportunities and limitations. *J Pediatr*. 2010;156(1):38–43

10. Kattwinkel J, Brooks J, Myerberg D; American Academy of Pediatrics Task Force on Infant Positioning and SIDS. Positioning and SIDS [published correction appears in *Pediatrics*. 1992;90(2 pt 1):264]. *Pediatrics*. 1992;89(6 pt 1):1120–1126

11. National Institute of Child Health and Human Development/National Institutes of Health. Safe to Sleep campaign. Available at: www.nichd.nih.gov/sts. Accessed September 21, 2016

12. National Infant Sleep Position Study Web site. Available at: http://slone-web2.bu.edu/ChimeNisp/Main_Nisp.asp. Accessed January 10, 2016

13. Matthews TJ, MacDorman MF, Thoma ME. Infant mortality statistics from the 2013 period linked birth/infant death data set. *Natl Vital Stat Rep*. 2015;64(9):1–30

14. US Department of Health and Human Services. Linked birth/infant death records [CDC WONDER online database]. Available at: http://wonder.cdc.gov/lbd.html. Accessed June 1, 2016

15. Malloy MH, MacDorman M. Changes in the classification of sudden unexpected infant deaths: United States, 1992–2001. *Pediatrics*. 2005;115(5):1247–1253

16. Shapiro-Mendoza CK, Tomashek KM, Anderson RN, Wingo J. Recent national trends in sudden, unexpected infant deaths: more evidence supporting a change in classification or reporting. *Am J Epidemiol*. 2006;163(8):762–769

17. Shapiro-Mendoza CK, Kimball M, Tomashek KM, Anderson RN, Blanding S. US infant mortality trends attributable to accidental suffocation and strangulation in bed from 1984 through 2004: are rates increasing? *Pediatrics*. 2009;123(2):533–539

18. Hauck FR, Moore CM, Herman SM, et al. The contribution of prone sleeping position to the racial disparity in sudden infant death syndrome: the Chicago Infant Mortality Study. *Pediatrics*. 2002;110(4):772–780

19. Colson ER, Rybin D, Smith LA, Colton T, Lister G, Corwin MJ. Trends and factors associated with infant sleeping position: the National Infant Sleep Position Study, 1993-2007. *Arch Pediatr Adolesc Med*. 2009;163(12):1122–1128

20. Lahr MB, Rosenberg KD, Lapidus JA. Maternal-infant bedsharing: risk factors for bedsharing in a population-based survey of new mothers and implications for SIDS risk reduction. *Matern Child Health J*. 2007;11(3):277–286

21. Willinger M, Ko CW, Hoffman HJ, Kessler RC, Corwin MJ; National Infant Sleep Position Study. Trends in infant bed sharing in the United States, 1993-2000: the National Infant Sleep Position Study. *Arch Pediatr Adolesc Med*. 2003;157(1):43–49

22. Fu LY, Colson ER, Corwin MJ, Moon RY. Infant sleep location: associated maternal and infant characteristics with sudden infant death syndrome prevention recommendations. *J Pediatr*. 2008;153(4):503–508

23. Flick L, White DK, Vemulapalli C, Stulac BB, Kemp JS. Sleep position and the use of soft bedding during bed sharing among African American infants at increased risk for sudden infant death syndrome. *J Pediatr*. 2001;138(3):338–343

24. Rasinski KA, Kuby A, Bzdusek SA, Silvestri JM, Weese-Mayer DE. Effect of a sudden infant death syndrome risk reduction education program on risk factor compliance and information sources in primarily black urban communities. *Pediatrics*. 2003;111(4 pt 1). Available at: www.pediatrics.org/cgi/content/full/111/4/e347

25. Shapiro-Mendoza CK, Colson ER, Willinger M, Rybin DV, Camperlengo L, Corwin MJ. Trends in infant bedding use: National Infant Sleep Position Study, 1993–2010. *Pediatrics*. 2015;135(1):10–17

26. Filiano JJ, Kinney HC. A perspective on neuropathologic findings in victims of the sudden infant death syndrome: the triple-risk model. *Biol Neonate*. 1994;65(3-4):194–197

27. Kinney HC. Brainstem mechanisms underlying the sudden infant death syndrome: evidence from human pathologic studies. *Dev Psychobiol*. 2009;51(3):223–233

28. Goldstein RD, Trachtenberg FL, Sens MA, Harty BJ, Kinney HC. Overall postneonatal mortality and rates of SIDS. *Pediatrics*. 2016;137(1):1–10

29. Kinney HC, Randall LL, Sleeper LA, et al. Serotonergic brainstem abnormalities in Northern Plains Indians with the sudden infant death syndrome. *J Neuropathol Exp Neurol*. 2003;62(11):1178–1191

30. Browne CJ, Sharma N, Waters KA, Machaalani R. The effects of nicotine on the alpha-7 and beta-2 nicotinic acetycholine receptor subunits in the developing piglet brainstem. *Int J Dev Neurosci*. 2010;28(1):1–7

31. Hunt NJ, Waters KA, Machaalani R. Orexin receptors in the developing

SIDS AND OTHER SLEEP-RELATED INFANT DEATHS:
EVIDENCE BASE FOR 2016 UPDATED RECOMMENDATIONS FOR A SAFE INFANT SLEEPING ENVIRONMENT

397

piglet hypothalamus, and effects of nicotine and intermittent hypercapnic hypoxia exposures. *Brain Res.* 2013;1508:73–82

32. Cerpa VJ, Aylwin ML, Beltrán-Castillo S, et al. The alteration of neonatal raphe neurons by prenatal-perinatal nicotine: meaning for sudden infant death syndrome. *Am J Respir Cell Mol Biol.* 2015;53(4):489–499

33. Slotkin TA, Seidler FJ, Spindel ER. Prenatal nicotine exposure in rhesus monkeys compromises development of brainstem and cardiac monoamine pathways involved in perinatal adaptation and sudden infant death syndrome: amelioration by vitamin C. *Neurotoxicol Teratol.* 2011;33(3):431–434

34. Sekizawa S, Joad JP, Pinkerton KE, Bonham AC. Secondhand smoke exposure alters K+ channel function and intrinsic cell excitability in a subset of second-order airway neurons in the nucleus tractus solitarius of young guinea pigs. *Eur J Neurosci.* 2010;31(4):673–684

35. Duncan JR, Paterson DS, Hoffman JM, et al. Brainstem serotonergic deficiency in sudden infant death syndrome. *JAMA.* 2010;303(5):430–437

36. Duncan JR, Garland M, Myers MM, et al. Prenatal nicotine-exposure alters fetal autonomic activity and medullary neurotransmitter receptors: implications for sudden infant death syndrome. *J Appl Physiol (1985).* 2009;107(5):1579–1590

37. Duncan JR, Garland M, Stark RI, et al. Prenatal nicotine exposure selectively affects nicotinic receptor expression in primary and associative visual cortices of the fetal baboon. *Brain Pathol.* 2015;25(2):171–181

38. St-John WM, Leiter JC. Maternal nicotine depresses eupneic ventilation of neonatal rats. *Neurosci Lett.* 1999;267(3):206–208

39. Eugenín J, Otárola M, Bravo E, et al. Prenatal to early postnatal nicotine exposure impairs central chemoreception and modifies breathing pattern in mouse neonates: a probable link to sudden infant death syndrome. *J Neurosci.* 2008;28(51):13907–13917

40. Fewell JE, Smith FG, Ng VK. Prenatal exposure to nicotine impairs protective responses of rat pups to hypoxia in an age-dependent manner. *Respir Physiol.* 2001;127(1):61–73

41. Hafström O, Milerad J, Sundell HW. Prenatal nicotine exposure blunts the cardiorespiratory response to hypoxia in lambs. *Am J Respir Crit Care Med.* 2002;166(12 pt 1):1544–1549

42. Duncan JR, Paterson DS, Kinney HC. The development of nicotinic receptors in the human medulla oblongata: inter-relationship with the serotonergic system. *Auton Neurosci.* 2008;144(1–2):61–75

43. Wilhelm-Benartzi CS, Houseman EA, Maccani MA, et al. In utero exposures, infant growth, and DNA methylation of repetitive elements and developmentally related genes in human placenta. *Environ Health Perspect.* 2012;120(2):296–302

44. Schneider J, Mitchell I, Singhal N, Kirk V, Hasan SU. Prenatal cigarette smoke exposure attenuates recovery from hypoxemic challenge in preterm infants. *Am J Respir Crit Care Med.* 2008;178(5):520–526

45. Thiriez G, Bouhaddi M, Mourot L, et al. Heart rate variability in preterm infants and maternal smoking during pregnancy. *Clin Auton Res.* 2009;19(3):149–156

46. Fifer WP, Fingers ST, Youngman M, Gomez-Gribben E, Myers MM. Effects of alcohol and smoking during pregnancy on infant autonomic control. *Dev Psychobiol.* 2009;51(3):234–242

47. Richardson HL, Walker AM, Horne RS. Maternal smoking impairs arousal patterns in sleeping infants. *Sleep.* 2009;32(4):515–521

48. Cohen G, Vella S, Jeffery H, Lagercrantz H, Katz-Salamon M. Cardiovascular stress hyperreactivity in babies of smokers and in babies born preterm. *Circulation.* 2008;118(18):1848–1853

49. Paine SM, Jacques TS, Sebire NJ. Review: neuropathological features of unexplained sudden unexpected death in infancy: current evidence and controversies. *Neuropathol Appl Neurobiol.* 2014;40(4):364–384

50. Panigrahy A, Filiano J, Sleeper LA, et al. Decreased serotonergic receptor binding in rhombic lip-derived regions of the medulla oblongata in the sudden infant death syndrome. *J Neuropathol Exp Neurol.* 2000;59(5):377–384

51. Ozawa Y, Takashima S. Developmental neurotransmitter pathology in the brainstem of sudden infant death syndrome: a review and sleep position. *Forensic Sci Int.* 2002;130(suppl):S53–S59

52. Machaalani R, Say M, Waters KA. Serotoninergic receptor 1A in the sudden infant death syndrome brainstem medulla and associations with clinical risk factors. *Acta Neuropathol.* 2009;117(3):257–265

53. Paterson DS, Trachtenberg FL, Thompson EG, et al. Multiple serotonergic brainstem abnormalities in sudden infant death syndrome. *JAMA.* 2006;296(17):2124–2132

54. Lavezzi AM, Weese-Mayer DE, Yu MY, et al. Developmental alterations of the respiratory human retrotrapezoid nucleus in sudden unexplained fetal and infant death. *Auton Neurosci.* 2012;170(1–2):12–19

55. Kinney HC, Cryan JB, Haynes RL, et al. Dentate gyrus abnormalities in sudden unexplained death in infants: morphological marker of underlying brain vulnerability. *Acta Neuropathol.* 2015;129(1):65–80

56. Say M, Machaalani R, Waters KA. Changes in serotoninergic receptors 1A and 2A in the piglet brainstem after intermittent hypercapnic hypoxia (IHH) and nicotine. *Brain Res.* 2007;1152:17–26

57. Kinney HC, Richerson GB, Dymecki SM, Darnall RA, Nattie EE. The brainstem and serotonin in the sudden infant death syndrome. *Annu Rev Pathol.* 2009;4:517–550

58. Cummings KJ, Commons KG, Fan KC, Li A, Nattie EE. Severe spontaneous bradycardia associated with respiratory disruptions in rat pups with fewer brain stem 5-HT neurons. *Am J Physiol Regul Integr Comp Physiol.* 2009;296(6):R1783–R1796

59. Cummings KJ, Hewitt JC, Li A, Daubenspeck JA, Nattie EE. Postnatal loss of brainstem serotonin neurones compromises the ability of neonatal

rats to survive episodic severe hypoxia. *J Physiol.* 2011;589(pt 21):5247–5256

60. Darnall RA, Schneider RW, Tobia CM, Commons KG. Eliminating medullary 5-HT neurons delays arousal and decreases the respiratory response to repeated episodes of hypoxia in neonatal rat pups. *J Appl Physiol (1985).* 2016;120(5):514–525

61. Rosenthal NA, Currier RJ, Baer RJ, Feuchtbaum L, Jelliffe-Pawlowski LL. Undiagnosed metabolic dysfunction and sudden infant death syndrome—a case-control study. *Paediatr Perinat Epidemiol.* 2015;29(2):151–155

62. Opdal SH, Rognum TO. Gene variants predisposing to SIDS: current knowledge. *Forensic Sci Med Pathol.* 2011;7(1):26–36

63. Weese-Mayer DE, Ackerman MJ, Marazita ML, Berry-Kravis EM. Sudden infant death syndrome: review of implicated genetic factors. *Am J Med Genet A.* 2007;143A(8):771–788

64. Paterson DS, Rivera KD, Broadbelt KG, et al. Lack of association of the serotonin transporter polymorphism with the sudden infant death syndrome in the San Diego Dataset. *Pediatr Res.* 2010;68(5):409–413

65. Wang DW, Desai RR, Crotti L, et al. Cardiac sodium channel dysfunction in sudden infant death syndrome. *Circulation.* 2007;115(3):368–376

66. Tan BH, Pundi KN, Van Norstrand DW, et al. Sudden infant death syndrome-associated mutations in the sodium channel beta subunits. *Heart Rhythm.* 2010;7(6):771–778

67. Van Norstrand DW, Asimaki A, Rubinos C, et al. Connexin43 mutation causes heterogeneous gap junction loss and sudden infant death. *Circulation.* 2012;125(3):474–481

68. Andreasen C, Refsgaard L, Nielsen JB, et al. Mutations in genes encoding cardiac ion channels previously associated with sudden infant death syndrome (SIDS) are present with high frequency in new exome data. *Can J Cardiol.* 2013;29(9):1104–1109

69. Winkel BG, Yuan L, Olesen MS, et al. The role of the sodium current complex in a nonreferred nationwide cohort of

sudden infant death syndrome. *Heart Rhythm.* 2015;12(6):1241–1249

70. Cummings KJ, Klotz C, Liu WQ, et al. Sudden infant death syndrome (SIDS) in African Americans: polymorphisms in the gene encoding the stress peptide pituitary adenylate cyclase-activating polypeptide (PACAP). *Acta Paediatr.* 2009;98(3):482–489

71. Barrett KT, Rodikova E, Weese-Mayer DE, et al. Analysis of PAC1 receptor gene variants in Caucasian and African American infants dying of sudden infant death syndrome. *Acta Paediatr.* 2013;102(12). Available at: www.pediatrics.org/cgi/content/full/102/12/e546

72. Ferrante L, Opdal SH, Vege A, Rognum T. Cytokine gene polymorphisms and sudden infant death syndrome. *Acta Paediatr.* 2010;99(3):384–388

73. Ferrante L, Opdal SH, Vege A, Rognum TO. IL-1 gene cluster polymorphisms and sudden infant death syndrome. *Hum Immunol.* 2010;71(4):402–406

74. Opdal SH, Rognum TO, Vege A, Stave AK, Dupuy BM, Egeland T. Increased number of substitutions in the D-loop of mitochondrial DNA in the sudden infant death syndrome. *Acta Paediatr.* 1998;87(10):1039–1044

75. Opdal SH, Rognum TO, Torgersen H, Vege A. Mitochondrial DNA point mutations detected in four cases of sudden infant death syndrome. *Acta Paediatr.* 1999;88(9):957–960

76. Santorelli FM, Schlessel JS, Slonim AE, DiMauro S. Novel mutation in the mitochondrial DNA tRNA glycine gene associated with sudden unexpected death. *Pediatr Neurol.* 1996;15(2):145–149

77. Forsyth L, Hume R, Howatson A, Busuttil A, Burchell A. Identification of novel polymorphisms in the glucokinase and glucose-6-phosphatase genes in infants who died suddenly and unexpectedly. *J Mol Med (Berl).* 2005;83(8):610–618

78. American Academy of Pediatrics Task Force on Sudden Infant Death Syndrome. SIDS and other sleep-related infant deaths: updated 2016 recommendations for a safe infant

sleeping environment. *Pediatrics.* 2016;138(5):e20162938

79. Kanetake J, Aoki Y, Funayama M. Evaluation of rebreathing potential on bedding for infant use. *Pediatr Int.* 2003;45(3):284–289

80. Kemp JS, Thach BT. Quantifying the potential of infant bedding to limit CO2 dispersal and factors affecting rebreathing in bedding. *J Appl Physiol (1985).* 1995;78(2):740–745

81. Kemp JS, Livne M, White DK, Arfken CL. Softness and potential to cause rebreathing: differences in bedding used by infants at high and low risk for sudden infant death syndrome. *J Pediatr.* 1998;132(2):234–239

82. Patel AL, Harris K, Thach BT. Inspired CO(2) and O(2) in sleeping infants rebreathing from bedding: relevance for sudden infant death syndrome. *J Appl Physiol (1985).* 2001;91(6):2537–2545

83. Tuffnell CS, Petersen SA, Wailoo MP. Prone sleeping infants have a reduced ability to lose heat. *Early Hum Dev.* 1995;43(2):109–116

84. Ammari A, Schulze KF, Ohira-Kist K, et al. Effects of body position on thermal, cardiorespiratory and metabolic activity in low birth weight infants. *Early Hum Dev.* 2009;85(8):497–501

85. Yiallourou SR, Walker AM, Horne RS. Prone sleeping impairs circulatory control during sleep in healthy term infants: implications for SIDS. *Sleep.* 2008;31(8):1139–1146

86. Wong FY, Witcombe NB, Yiallourou SR, et al. Cerebral oxygenation is depressed during sleep in healthy term infants when they sleep prone. *Pediatrics.* 2011;127(3). Available at: www.pediatrics.org/cgi/content/full/127/3/e558

87. Hauck FR, Herman SM, Donovan M, et al. Sleep environment and the risk of sudden infant death syndrome in an urban population: the Chicago Infant Mortality Study. *Pediatrics.* 2003;111(5 pt 2):1207–1214

88. Li DK, Petitti DB, Willinger M, et al. Infant sleeping position and the risk of sudden infant death syndrome in California, 1997-2000. *Am J Epidemiol.* 2003;157(5):446–455

SIDS AND OTHER SLEEP-RELATED INFANT DEATHS:
EVIDENCE BASE FOR 2016 UPDATED RECOMMENDATIONS FOR A SAFE INFANT SLEEPING ENVIRONMENT

399

89. Blair PS, Fleming PJ, Smith IJ, et al; CESDI SUDI Research Group. Babies sleeping with parents: case-control study of factors influencing the risk of the sudden infant death syndrome. *BMJ.* 1999;319(7223):1457–1461

90. Fleming PJ, Blair PS, Bacon C, et al; Confidential Enquiry into Stillbirths and Deaths Regional Coordinators and Researchers. Environment of infants during sleep and risk of the sudden infant death syndrome: results of 1993-5 case-control study for confidential inquiry into stillbirths and deaths in infancy. *BMJ.* 1996;313(7051):191–195

91. Carpenter RG, Irgens LM, Blair PS, et al. Sudden unexplained infant death in 20 regions in Europe: case control study. *Lancet.* 2004;363(9404):185–191

92. Mitchell EA, Tuohy PG, Brunt JM, et al. Risk factors for sudden infant death syndrome following the prevention campaign in New Zealand: a prospective study. *Pediatrics.* 1997;100(5):835–840

93. Waters KA, Gonzalez A, Jean C, Morielli A, Brouillette RT. Face-straight-down and face-near-straight-down positions in healthy, prone-sleeping infants. *J Pediatr.* 1996;128(5 pt 1):616–625

94. Oyen N, Markestad T, Skaerven R, et al. Combined effects of sleeping position and prenatal risk factors in sudden infant death syndrome: the Nordic Epidemiological SIDS Study. *Pediatrics.* 1997;100(4):613–621

95. Mitchell EA, Thach BT, Thompson JMD, Williams S. Changing infants' sleep position increases risk of sudden infant death syndrome: New Zealand Cot Death Study. *Arch Pediatr Adolesc Med.* 1999;153(11):1136–1141

96. Oden RP, Joyner BL, Ajao TI, Moon RY. Factors influencing African American mothers' decisions about sleep position: a qualitative study. *J Natl Med Assoc.* 2010;102(10):870–872, 875–880

97. Colson ER, McCabe LK, Fox K, et al. Barriers to following the back-to-sleep recommendations: insights from focus groups with inner-city caregivers. *Ambul Pediatr.* 2005;5(6):349–354

98. Mosley JM, Daily Stokes S, Ulmer A. Infant sleep position: discerning knowledge from practice. *Am J Health Behav.* 2007;31(6):573–582

99. Moon RY, Omron R. Determinants of infant sleep position in an urban population. *Clin Pediatr (Phila).* 2002;41(8):569–573

100. Ottolini MC, Davis BE, Patel K, Sachs HC, Gershon NB, Moon RY. Prone infant sleeping despite the "Back to Sleep" campaign. *Arch Pediatr Adolesc Med.* 1999;153(5):512–517

101. Willinger M, Ko C-W, Hoffman HJ, Kessler RC, Corwin MJ. Factors associated with caregivers' choice of infant sleep position, 1994-1998: the National Infant Sleep Position Study. *JAMA.* 2000;283(16):2135–2142

102. Moon RY, Biliter WM. Infant sleep position policies in licensed child care centers after back to sleep campaign. *Pediatrics.* 2000;106(3):576–580

103. Moon RY, Weese-Mayer DE, Silvestri JM. Nighttime child care: inadequate sudden infant death syndrome risk factor knowledge, practice, and policies. *Pediatrics.* 2003;111(4 pt 1):795–799

104. Von Kohorn I, Corwin MJ, Rybin DV, Heeren TC, Lister G, Colson ER. Influence of prior advice and beliefs of mothers on infant sleep position. *Arch Pediatr Adolesc Med.* 2010;164(4):363–369

105. Kahn A, Groswasser J, Sottiaux M, Rebuffat E, Franco P, Dramaix M. Prone or supine body position and sleep characteristics in infants. *Pediatrics.* 1993;91(6):1112–1115

106. Bhat RY, Hannam S, Pressler R, Rafferty GF, Peacock JL, Greenough A. Effect of prone and supine position on sleep, apneas, and arousal in preterm infants. *Pediatrics.* 2006;118(1):101–107

107. Ariagno RL, van Liempt S, Mirmiran M. Fewer spontaneous arousals during prone sleep in preterm infants at 1 and 3 months corrected age. *J Perinatol.* 2006;26(5):306–312

108. Franco P, Groswasser J, Sottiaux M, Broadfield E, Kahn A. Decreased cardiac responses to auditory stimulation during prone sleep. *Pediatrics.* 1996;97(2):174–178

109. Galland BC, Reeves G, Taylor BJ, Bolton DP. Sleep position, autonomic function, and arousal. *Arch Dis Child Fetal Neonatal Ed.* 1998;78(3):F189–F194

110. Galland BC, Hayman RM, Taylor BJ, Bolton DP, Sayers RM, Williams SM. Factors affecting heart rate variability and heart rate responses to tilting in infants aged 1 and 3 months. *Pediatr Res.* 2000;48(3):360–368

111. Horne RS, Ferens D, Watts AM, et al. The prone sleeping position impairs arousability in term infants. *J Pediatr.* 2001;138(6):811–816

112. Horne RS, Bandopadhayay P, Vitkovic J, Cranage SM, Adamson TM. Effects of age and sleeping position on arousal from sleep in preterm infants. *Sleep.* 2002;25(7):746–750

113. Kato I, Scaillet S, Groswasser J, et al. Spontaneous arousability in prone and supine position in healthy infants. *Sleep.* 2006;29(6):785–790

114. Phillipson EA, Sullivan CE. Arousal: the forgotten response to respiratory stimuli. *Am Rev Respir Dis.* 1978;118(5):807–809

115. Kahn A, Groswasser J, Rebuffat E, et al. Sleep and cardiorespiratory characteristics of infant victims of sudden death: a prospective case-control study. *Sleep.* 1992;15(4):287–292

116. Schechtman VL, Harper RM, Wilson AJ, Southall DP. Sleep state organization in normal infants and victims of the sudden infant death syndrome. *Pediatrics.* 1992;89(5 pt 1):865–870

117. Harper RM. State-related physiological changes and risk for the sudden infant death syndrome. *Aust Paediatr J.* 1986;22(suppl 1):55–58

118. Kato I, Franco P, Groswasser J, et al. Incomplete arousal processes in infants who were victims of sudden death. *Am J Respir Crit Care Med.* 2003;168(11):1298–1303

119. Byard RW, Beal SM. Gastric aspiration and sleeping position in infancy and early childhood. *J Paediatr Child Health.* 2000;36(4):403–405

120. Malloy MH. Trends in postneonatal aspiration deaths and reclassification of sudden infant death syndrome:

impact of the "Back to Sleep" program. *Pediatrics*. 2002;109(4):661–665

121. Tablizo MA, Jacinto P, Parsley D, Chen ML, Ramanathan R, Keens TG. Supine sleeping position does not cause clinical aspiration in neonates in hospital newborn nurseries. *Arch Pediatr Adolesc Med*. 2007;161(5):507–510

122. Vandenplas Y, Rudolph CD, Di Lorenzo C, et al; North American Society for Pediatric Gastroenterology Hepatology and Nutrition; European Society for Pediatric Gastroenterology Hepatology and Nutrition. Pediatric gastroesophageal reflux clinical practice guidelines: joint recommendations of the North American Society for Pediatric Gastroenterology, Hepatology, and Nutrition (NASPGHAN) and the European Society for Pediatric Gastroenterology, Hepatology, and Nutrition (ESPGHAN). *J Pediatr Gastroenterol Nutr*. 2009;49(4):498–547

123. Meyers WF, Herbst JJ. Effectiveness of positioning therapy for gastroesophageal reflux. *Pediatrics*. 1982;69(6):768–772

124. Tobin JM, McCloud P, Cameron DJ. Posture and gastro-oesophageal reflux: a case for left lateral positioning. *Arch Dis Child*. 1997;76(3):254–258

125. Malloy MH, Hoffman HJ. Prematurity, sudden infant death syndrome, and age of death. *Pediatrics*. 1995;96(3 pt 1):464–471

126. Sowter B, Doyle LW, Morley CJ, Altmann A, Halliday J. Is sudden infant death syndrome still more common in very low birthweight infants in the 1990s? *Med J Aust*. 1999;171(8):411–413

127. American Academy of Pediatrics Committee on Fetus and Newborn. Hospital discharge of the high-risk neonate. *Pediatrics*. 2008;122(5):1119–1126

128. Gelfer P, Cameron R, Masters K, Kennedy KA. Integrating "Back to Sleep" recommendations into neonatal ICU practice. *Pediatrics*. 2013;131(4). Available at: www.pediatrics.org/cgi/content/full/131/4e1264

129. Hwang SS, O'Sullivan A, Fitzgerald E, Melvin P, Gorman T, Fiascone JM. Implementation of safe sleep practices

in the neonatal intensive care unit. *J Perinatol*. 2015;35(10):862–866

130. Feldman-Winter L, Goldsmith JP; AAP Committee on Fetus and Newborn; AAP Task Force on Sudden Infant Death Syndrome. Safe sleep and skin-to-skin care in the neonatal period for healthy term newborns. *Pediatrics*. 2016;138(3):e20161889

131. Moon RY, Oden RP, Joyner BL, Ajao TI. Qualitative analysis of beliefs and perceptions about sudden infant death syndrome (SIDS) among African-American mothers: implications for safe sleep recommendations. *J Pediatr*. 2010;157(1):92–97, e92

132. Brenner RA, Simons-Morton BG, Bhaskar B, et al. Prevalence and predictors of the prone sleep position among inner-city infants. *JAMA*. 1998;280(4):341–346

133. Willinger M, Hoffman HJ, Wu K-T, et al. Factors associated with the transition to nonprone sleep positions of infants in the United States: the National Infant Sleep Position Study. *JAMA*. 1998;280(4):329–335

134. Colvin JD, Collie-Akers V, Schunn C, Moon RY. Sleep environment risks for younger and older infants. *Pediatrics*. 2014;134(2). Available at: www.pediatrics.org/cgi/content/full/134/2/e406

135. Kemp JS, Nelson VE, Thach BT. Physical properties of bedding that may increase risk of sudden infant death syndrome in prone-sleeping infants. *Pediatr Res*. 1994;36(1 pt 1):7–11

136. US Consumer Product Safety Commission. *Crib Safety Tips: Use Your Crib Safely. CPSC Document 5030*. Washington, DC: US Consumer Product Safety Commission; 2011

137. Consumer Product Safety Commission. Safety standard for bassinets and cradles. *Fed Reg*. 2013;78(205):63019–63036

138. Consumer Product Safety Commission. Safety standard for play yards. *Fed Reg*. 2012;77(168):52220–52228

139. Consumer Product Safety Commission. Safety standards for bedside sleepers. *Fed Reg*. 2014;79(10):2581–2589

140. Jackson A, Moon RY. An analysis of deaths in portable cribs and playpens:

what can be learned? *Clin Pediatr (Phila)*. 2008;47(3):261–266

141. Pike J, Moon RY. Bassinet use and sudden unexpected death in infancy. *J Pediatr*. 2008;153(4):509–512

142. Nakamura S, Wind M, Danello MA. Review of hazards associated with children placed in adult beds. *Arch Pediatr Adolesc Med*. 1999;153(10):1019–1023

143. Consumer Product Safety Commission. Safety standard for portable bed rails: final rule. *Fed Reg*. 2012;77(40):12182–12197

144. Callahan CW, Sisler C. Use of seating devices in infants too young to sit. *Arch Pediatr Adolesc Med*. 1997;151(3):233–235

145. Orenstein SR, Whitington PF, Orenstein DM. The infant seat as treatment for gastroesophageal reflux. *N Engl J Med*. 1983;309(13):760–763

146. Bass JL, Bull M. Oxygen desaturation in term infants in car safety seats. *Pediatrics*. 2002;110(2 pt 1):401–402

147. Kornhauser Cerar L, Scirica CV, Stucin Gantar I, Osredkar D, Neubauer D, Kinane TB. A comparison of respiratory patterns in healthy term infants placed in car safety seats and beds. *Pediatrics*. 2009;124(3). Available at: www.pediatrics.org/cgi/content/full/124/3/e396

148. Côté A, Bairam A, Deschenes M, Hatzakis G. Sudden infant deaths in sitting devices. *Arch Dis Child*. 2008;93(5):384–389

149. Merchant JR, Worwa C, Porter S, Coleman JM, deRegnier RA. Respiratory instability of term and near-term healthy newborn infants in car safety seats. *Pediatrics*. 2001;108(3):647–652

150. Willett LD, Leuschen MP, Nelson LS, Nelson RM Jr. Risk of hypoventilation in premature infants in car seats. *J Pediatr*. 1986;109(2):245–248

151. Batra EK, Midgett JD, Moon RY. Hazards associated with sitting and carrying devices for children two years and younger. *J Pediatr*. 2015;167(1):183–187

152. Desapriya EB, Joshi P, Subzwari S, Nolan M. Infant injuries from child restraint safety seat misuse at British

SIDS AND OTHER SLEEP-RELATED INFANT DEATHS:
EVIDENCE BASE FOR 2016 UPDATED RECOMMENDATIONS FOR A SAFE INFANT SLEEPING ENVIRONMENT

401

Columbia Children's Hospital. *Pediatr Int.* 2008;50(5):674–678

153. Graham CJ, Kittredge D, Stuemky JH. Injuries associated with child safety seat misuse. *Pediatr Emerg Care.* 1992;8(6):351–353

154. Parikh SN, Wilson L. Hazardous use of car seats outside the car in the United States, 2003–2007. *Pediatrics.* 2010;126(2):352–357

155. Pollack-Nelson C. Fall and suffocation injuries associated with in-home use of car seats and baby carriers. *Pediatr Emerg Care.* 2000;16(2):77–79

156. Wickham T, Abrahamson E. Head injuries in infants: the risks of bouncy chairs and car seats. *Arch Dis Child.* 2002;86(3):168–169

157. Bergounioux J, Madre C, Crucis-Armengaud A, et al. Sudden deaths in adult-worn baby carriers: 19 cases. *Eur J Pediatr.* 2015;174(12):1665–1670

158. Madre C, Rambaud C, Avran D, Michot C, Sachs P, Dauger S. Infant deaths in slings. *Eur J Pediatr.* 2014;173(12):1659–1661

159. Consumer Product Safety Commission. Safety standard for sling carriers. *Fed Reg.* 2014;79(141):42724–42734

160. Ip S, Chung M, Raman G, Trikalinos TA, Lau J. A summary of the Agency for Healthcare Research and Quality's evidence report on breastfeeding in developed countries. *Breastfeed Med.* 2009;4(suppl 1):S17–S30

161. Vennemann MM, Bajanowski T, Brinkmann B, et al; GeSID Study Group. Does breastfeeding reduce the risk of sudden infant death syndrome? *Pediatrics.* 2009;123(3). Available at: www.pediatrics.org/cgi/content/full/123/3/e406

162. Hauck FR, Thompson JM, Tanabe KO, Moon RY, Vennemann MM. Breastfeeding and reduced risk of sudden infant death syndrome: a meta-analysis. *Pediatrics.* 2011;128(1):103–110

163. Franco P, Scaillet S, Wermenbol V, Valente F, Groswasser J, Kahn A. The influence of a pacifier on infants' arousals from sleep. *J Pediatr.* 2000;136(6):775–779

164. Horne RS, Parslow PM, Ferens D, Watts AM, Adamson TM. Comparison of evoked arousability in breast and formula fed infants. *Arch Dis Child.* 2004;89(1):22–25

165. Duijts L, Jaddoe VW, Hofman A, Moll HA. Prolonged and exclusive breastfeeding reduces the risk of infectious diseases in infancy. *Pediatrics.* 2010;126(1). Available at: www.pediatrics.org/cgi/content/full/126/1/e18

166. Heinig MJ. Host defense benefits of breastfeeding for the infant: effect of breastfeeding duration and exclusivity. *Pediatr Clin North Am.* 2001;48(1):105–123, ix

167. Kramer MS, Guo T, Platt RW, et al. Infant growth and health outcomes associated with 3 compared with 6 mo of exclusive breastfeeding. *Am J Clin Nutr.* 2003;78(2):291–295

168. Highet AR, Berry AM, Bettelheim KA, Goldwater PN. Gut microbiome in sudden infant death syndrome (SIDS) differs from that in healthy comparison babies and offers an explanation for the risk factor of prone position. *Int J Med Microbiol.* 2014;304(5–6):735–741

169. McKenna JJ, Thoman EB, Anders TF, Sadeh A, Schechtman VL, Glotzbach SF. Infant-parent co-sleeping in an evolutionary perspective: implications for understanding infant sleep development and the sudden infant death syndrome. *Sleep.* 1993;16(3):263–282

170. McKenna JJ, Ball HL, Gettler LT. Mother infant cosleeping, breastfeeding and sudden infant death syndrome: what biological anthropology has discovered about normal infant sleep and pediatric sleep medicine. *Yearb Phys Anthropol.* 2007;134(S4S):133–161

171. McKenna J. *Sleeping With Your Baby: A Parent's Guide to Cosleeping.* Washington, DC: Platypus Media, LLC; 2007

172. Mitchell EA, Thompson JMD. Co-sleeping increases the risk of SIDS, but sleeping in the parents' bedroom lowers it. In: Rognum TO, ed. *Sudden Infant Death Syndrome: New Trends in the Nineties.* Oslo, Norway: Scandinavian University Press; 1995:266–269

173. Tappin D, Ecob R, Brooke H. Bedsharing, roomsharing, and sudden infant death syndrome in Scotland: a case-control study. *J Pediatr.* 2005;147(1):32–37

174. Colson ER, Willinger M, Rybin D, et al. Trends and factors associated with infant bed sharing, 1993-2010: the National Infant Sleep Position Study. *JAMA Pediatr.* 2013;167(11):1032–1037

175. Hauck FR, Signore C, Fein SB, Raju TN. Infant sleeping arrangements and practices during the first year of life. *Pediatrics.* 2008;122(suppl 2): S113–S120

176. Kendall-Tackett K, Cong Z, Hale TW. Mother-infant sleep locations and nighttime feeding behavior: U.S. data from the Survey of Mothers' Sleep and Fatigue. *Clin Lactation.* 2010;1(1):27–31

177. Ward TC. Reasons for mother-infant bed-sharing: a systematic narrative synthesis of the literature and implications for future research. *Matern Child Health J.* 2015;19(3):675–690

178. Joyner BL, Oden RP, Ajao TI, Moon RY. Where should my baby sleep: a qualitative study of African American infant sleep location decisions. *J Natl Med Assoc.* 2010;102(10):881–889

179. Mosko S, Richard C, McKenna J. Infant arousals during mother-infant bed sharing: implications for infant sleep and sudden infant death syndrome research. *Pediatrics.* 1997;100(5):841–849

180. McKenna JJ, Mosko SS, Richard CA. Bedsharing promotes breastfeeding. *Pediatrics.* 1997;100(2 pt 1):214–219

181. Gettler LT, McKenna JJ. Evolutionary perspectives on mother-infant sleep proximity and breastfeeding in a laboratory setting. *Am J Phys Anthropol.* 2011;144(3):454–462

182. Scheers NJ, Dayton CM, Kemp JS. Sudden infant death with external airways covered: case-comparison study of 206 deaths in the United States. *Arch Pediatr Adolesc Med.* 1998;152(6):540–547

183. Unger B, Kemp JS, Wilkins D, et al. Racial disparity and modifiable risk factors among infants dying suddenly and unexpectedly. *Pediatrics.* 2003;111(2). Available at: www.pediatrics.org/cgi/content/full/111/2/e127

184. Kemp JS, Unger B, Wilkins D, et al. Unsafe sleep practices and an analysis of bedsharing among infants dying suddenly and unexpectedly: results of a four-year, population-based, death-scene investigation study of sudden infant death syndrome and related deaths. *Pediatrics.* 2000;106(3). Available at: www.pediatrics.org/cgi/content/full/106/3/e41

185. Drago DA, Dannenberg AL. Infant mechanical suffocation deaths in the United States, 1980-1997. *Pediatrics.* 1999;103(5). Available at: www.pediatrics.org/cgi/content/full/103/5/e59

186. Blair PS, Mitchell EA, Heckstall-Smith EM, Fleming PJ. Head covering—a major modifiable risk factor for sudden infant death syndrome: a systematic review. *Arch Dis Child.* 2008;93(9):778–783

187. Baddock SA, Galland BC, Bolton DP, Williams SM, Taylor BJ. Differences in infant and parent behaviors during routine bed sharing compared with cot sleeping in the home setting. *Pediatrics.* 2006;117(5):1599–1607

188. Baddock SA, Galland BC, Taylor BJ, Bolton DP. Sleep arrangements and behavior of bed-sharing families in the home setting. *Pediatrics.* 2007;119(1). Available at: www.pediatrics.org/cgi/content/full/119/1/e200

189. Ball H. Airway covering during bed-sharing. *Child Care Health Dev.* 2009;35(5):728–737

190. Kattwinkel J, Brooks J, Keenan ME, Malloy MH; American Academy of Pediatrics. Task Force on Infant Sleep Position and Sudden Infant Death Syndrome. Changing concepts of sudden infant death syndrome: implications for infant sleeping environment and sleep position. *Pediatrics.* 2000;105(3 pt 1):650–656

191. Vennemann MM, Hense HW, Bajanowski T, et al Bed sharing and the risk of sudden infant death syndrome: can we resolve the debate? *J Pediatr.* 2012;160(1):44–48, e42

192. Ostfeld BM, Perl H, Esposito L, et al. Sleep environment, positional, lifestyle, and demographic characteristics associated with bed sharing in sudden infant death syndrome cases: a population-based study. *Pediatrics.* 2006;118(5):2051–2059

193. Scheers NJ, Rutherford GW, Kemp JS. Where should infants sleep? A comparison of risk for suffocation of infants sleeping in cribs, adult beds, and other sleeping locations. *Pediatrics.* 2003;112(4):883–889

194. Ruys JH, de Jonge GA, Brand R, Engelberts AC, Semmekrot BA. Bed-sharing in the first four months of life: a risk factor for sudden infant death. *Acta Paediatr.* 2007;96(10):1399–1403

195. Blair PS, Platt MW, Smith IJ, Fleming PJ; CESDI SUDI Research Group. Sudden infant death syndrome and sleeping position in pre-term and low birth weight infants: an opportunity for targeted intervention. *Arch Dis Child.* 2006;91(2):101–106

196. Blair PS, Sidebotham P, Evason-Coombe C, Edmonds M, Heckstall-Smith EM, Fleming P. Hazardous cosleeping environments and risk factors amenable to change: case-control study of SIDS in south west England. *BMJ.* 2009;339:b3666

197. Rechtman LR, Colvin JD, Blair PS, Moon RY. Sofas and infant mortality. *Pediatrics.* 2014;134(5). Available at: www.pediatrics.org/cgi/content/full/134/5/e1293

198. Salm Ward TC, Ngui EM. Factors associated with bed-sharing for African American and white mothers in Wisconsin. *Matern Child Health J.* 2015;19(4):720–732

199. Bartick M, Smith LJ. Speaking out on safe sleep: evidence-based infant sleep recommendations. *Breastfeed Med.* 2014;9(9):417–422

200. Blair PS, Sidebotham P, Pease A, Fleming PJ. Bed-sharing in the absence of hazardous circumstances: is there a risk of sudden infant death syndrome? An analysis from two case-control studies conducted in the UK. *PLoS One.* 2014;9(9):e107799

201. Carpenter R, McGarvey C, Mitchell EA, et al. Bed sharing when parents do not smoke: is there a risk of SIDS? An individual level analysis of five major case-control studies. *BMJ Open.* 2013;3(5):e002299

202. Huang Y, Hauck FR, Signore C, et al. Influence of bedsharing activity on breastfeeding duration among US mothers. *JAMA Pediatr.* 2013;167(11):1038–1044

203. Horsley T, Clifford T, Barrowman N, et al. Benefits and harms associated with the practice of bed sharing: a systematic review. *Arch Pediatr Adolesc Med.* 2007;161(3):237–245

204. Smith LA, Geller NL, Kellams AL, et al. Infant sleep location and breastfeeding practices in the United States, 2011-2014. *Acad Pediatr.* 2016;16(6):540–549

205. Ball HL, Howel D, Bryant A, Best E, Russell C, Ward-Platt M. Bed-sharing by breastfeeding mothers: who bed-shares and what is the relationship with breastfeeding duration? *Acta Paediatr.* 2016;105(6):628–634

206. Scragg R, Mitchell EA, Taylor BJ, et al; New Zealand Cot Death Study Group. Bed sharing, smoking, and alcohol in the sudden infant death syndrome. *BMJ.* 1993;307(6915):1312–1318

207. McGarvey C, McDonnell M, Chong A, O'Regan M, Matthews T. Factors relating to the infant's last sleep environment in sudden infant death syndrome in the Republic of Ireland. *Arch Dis Child.* 2003;88(12):1058–1064

208. Fleming PJ, Gilbert R, Azaz Y, et al. Interaction between bedding and sleeping position in the sudden infant death syndrome: a population based case-control study. *BMJ.* 1990;301(6743):85–89

209. Ponsonby A-L, Dwyer T, Gibbons LE, Cochrane JA, Jones ME, McCall MJ. Thermal environment and sudden infant death syndrome: case-control study. *BMJ.* 1992;304(6822):277–282

210. Ponsonby A-L, Dwyer T, Gibbons LE, Cochrane JA, Wang Y-G. Factors potentiating the risk of sudden infant death syndrome associated with the prone position. *N Engl J Med.* 1993;329(6):377–382

211. Iyasu S, Randall LL, Welty TK, et al. Risk factors for sudden infant death syndrome among Northern Plains Indians. *JAMA.* 2002;288(21):2717–2723

212. Arnestad M, Andersen M, Vege A, Rognum TO. Changes in the epidemiological pattern of sudden infant death syndrome in southeast

SIDS AND OTHER SLEEP-RELATED INFANT DEATHS:
EVIDENCE BASE FOR 2016 UPDATED RECOMMENDATIONS FOR A SAFE INFANT SLEEPING ENVIRONMENT

403

Norway, 1984-1998: implications for future prevention and research. *Arch Dis Child*. 2001;85(2):108–115

213. McGarvey C, McDonnell M, Hamilton K, O'Regan M, Matthews T. An 8 year study of risk factors for SIDS: bed-sharing versus non-bed-sharing. *Arch Dis Child*. 2006;91(4):318–323

214. Academy of Breastfeeding Medicine Protocol Committee. ABM clinical protocol #6: guideline on co-sleeping and breastfeeding. Revision, March 2008. *Breastfeed Med*. 2008;3(1):38–43

215. Fu LY, Moon RY, Hauck FR. Bed sharing among black infants and sudden infant death syndrome: interactions with other known risk factors. *Acad Pediatr*. 2010;10(6):376–382

216. Carroll-Pankhurst C, Mortimer EAJ Jr. Sudden infant death syndrome, bedsharing, parental weight, and age at death. *Pediatrics*. 2001;107(3):530–536

217. Mitchell E, Thompson J. Who cosleeps? Does high maternal body weight and duvet use increase the risk of sudden infant death syndrome when bed sharing?. *Paediatr Child Health*. 2006;11(suppl 1):14A–15A

218. Hutchison BL, Stewart AW, Mitchell EA. The prevalence of cobedding and SIDS-related child care practices in twins. *Eur J Pediatr*. 2010;169(12):1477–1485

219. Hayward K. Cobedding of twins: a natural extension of the socialization process? *MCN Am J Matern Child Nurs*. 2003;28(4):260–263

220. Tomashek KM, Wallman C; American Academy of Pediatrics Committee on Fetus and Newborn. Cobedding twins and higher-order multiples in a hospital setting. *Pediatrics*. 2007;120(6):1359–1366

221. National Association of Neonatal Nurses Board of Directors. NANN Position Statement 3045: cobedding of twins or higher-order multiples. *Adv Neonatal Care*. 2008;9(6):307–313

222. Chiodini BA, Thach BT. Impaired ventilation in infants sleeping facedown: potential significance for sudden infant death syndrome. *J Pediatr*. 1993;123(5):686–692

223. Sakai J, Kanetake J, Takahashi S, Kanawaku Y, Funayama M. Gas dispersal potential of bedding as

a cause for sudden infant death. *Forensic Sci Int*. 2008;180(2-3):93–97

224. Shapiro-Mendoza CK, Camperlengo L, Ludvigsen R, et al. Classification system for the Sudden Unexpected Infant Death Case Registry and its application. *Pediatrics*. 2014;134(1):e210–e219

225. Ponsonby A-L, Dwyer T, Couper D, Cochrane J. Association between use of a quilt and sudden infant death syndrome: case-control study. *BMJ*. 1998;316(7126):195–196

226. Mitchell EA, Scragg L, Clements M. Soft cot mattresses and the sudden infant death syndrome. *N Z Med J*. 1996;109(1023):206–207

227. Mitchell EA, Thompson JMD, Ford RPK, Taylor BJ; New Zealand Cot Death Study Group. Sheepskin bedding and the sudden infant death syndrome. *J Pediatr*. 1998;133(5):701–704

228. Kemp JS, Kowalski RM, Burch PM, Graham MA, Thach BT. Unintentional suffocation by rebreathing: a death scene and physiologic investigation of a possible cause of sudden infant death. *J Pediatr*. 1993;122(6):874–880

229. Brooke H, Gibson A, Tappin D, Brown H. Case-control study of sudden infant death syndrome in Scotland, 1992-5. *BMJ*. 1997;314(7093):1516–1520

230. Wilson CA, Taylor BJ, Laing RM, Williams SM, Mitchell EA. Clothing and bedding and its relevance to sudden infant death syndrome: further results from the New Zealand Cot Death Study. *J Paediatr Child Health*. 1994;30(6):506–512

231. Markestad T, Skadberg B, Hordvik E, Morild I, Irgens LM. Sleeping position and sudden infant death syndrome (SIDS): effect of an intervention programme to avoid prone sleeping. *Acta Paediatr*. 1995;84(4):375–378

232. L'Hoir MP, Engelberts AC, van Well GTJ, et al. Risk and preventive factors for cot death in The Netherlands, a low-incidence country. *Eur J Pediatr*. 1998;157(8):681–688

233. Beal SM, Byard RW. Accidental death or sudden infant death syndrome? *J Paediatr Child Health*. 1995;31(4):269–271

234. Schlaud M, Dreier M, Debertin AS, et al. The German case-control scene investigation study on SIDS: epidemiological approach and main results. *Int J Legal Med*. 2010;124(1):19–26

235. Chowdhury RT. *Nursery Product-Related Injuries and Deaths Among Children Under Age Five*. Washington, DC: US Consumer Product Safety Commission; 2014

236. Ajao TI, Oden RP, Joyner BL, Moon RY. Decisions of black parents about infant bedding and sleep surfaces: a qualitative study. *Pediatrics*. 2011;128(3):494–502

237. Joyner BL, Gill-Bailey C, Moon RY. Infant sleep environments depicted in magazines targeted to women of childbearing age. *Pediatrics*. 2009;124(3). Available at: www.pediatrics.org/cgi/content/full/124/3/e416

238. Moon RY. "And things that go bump in the night": nothing to fear? *J Pediatr*. 2007;151(3):237–238

239. Thach BT, Rutherford GW Jr, Harris K. Deaths and injuries attributed to infant crib bumper pads. *J Pediatr*. 2007;151(3):271–274, 274.e1–274.e3

240. Wanna-Nakamura S. White paper—unsafe sleep settings: hazards associated with the infant sleep environment and unsafe practices used by caregivers: a CPSC staff perspective. Bethesda, MD: US Consumer Product Safety Commission; July 2010

241. US Consumer Product Safety Commission. *Staff Briefing Package, Crib Bumpers Petition*. Washington, DC: US Consumer Product Safety Commission; May 15, 2013

242. Scheers NJ, Woodard DW, Thach BT. Crib bumpers continue to cause infant deaths: a need for a new preventive approach. *J Pediatr*. 2016;169:93–97.e1

243. Yeh ES, Rochette LM, McKenzie LB, Smith GA. Injuries associated with cribs, playpens, and bassinets among young children in the US, 1990-2008. *Pediatrics*. 2011;127(3):479–486

244. Tappin D, Brooke H, Ecob R, Gibson A. Used infant mattresses and sudden infant death syndrome in

Scotland: case-control study. *BMJ.* 2002;325(7371):1007–1012

245. Arnestad M, Andersen M, Rognum TO. Is the use of dummy or carry-cot of importance for sudden infant death? *Eur J Pediatr.* 1997;156(12):968–970

246. Mitchell EA, Taylor BJ, Ford RPK, et al. Dummies and the sudden infant death syndrome. *Arch Dis Child.* 1993;68(4):501–504

247. Fleming PJ, Blair PS, Pollard K, et al; CESDI SUDI Research Team. Pacifier use and sudden infant death syndrome: results from the CESDI/SUDI case control study. *Arch Dis Child.* 1999;81(2):112–116

248. L'Hoir MP, Engelberts AC, van Well GTJ, et al. Dummy use, thumb sucking, mouth breathing and cot death. *Eur J Pediatr.* 1999;158(11):896–901

249. Li DK, Willinger M, Petitti DB, Odouli R, Liu L, Hoffman HJ. Use of a dummy (pacifier) during sleep and risk of sudden infant death syndrome (SIDS): population based case-control study. *BMJ.* 2006;332(7532):18–22

250. Vennemann MM, Bajanowski T, Brinkmann B, Jorch G, Sauerland C, Mitchell EA; GeSID Study Group. Sleep environment risk factors for sudden infant death syndrome: the German Sudden Infant Death Syndrome Study. *Pediatrics.* 2009;123(4):1162–1170

251. Hauck FR, Omojokun OO, Siadaty MS. Do pacifiers reduce the risk of sudden infant death syndrome? A meta-analysis. *Pediatrics.* 2005;116(5). Available at: www.pediatrics.org/cgi/content/full/116/5/e716

252. Mitchell EA, Blair PS, L'Hoir MP. Should pacifiers be recommended to prevent sudden infant death syndrome? *Pediatrics.* 2006;117(5):1755–1758

253. Moon RY, Tanabe KO, Yang DC, Young HA, Hauck FR. Pacifier use and SIDS: evidence for a consistently reduced risk. *Matern Child Health J.* 2012;16(3):609–614

254. Franco P, Chabanski S, Scaillet S, Groswasser J, Kahn A. Pacifier use modifies infant's cardiac autonomic controls during sleep. *Early Hum Dev.* 2004;77(1-2):99–108

255. Tonkin SL, Lui D, McIntosh CG, Rowley S, Knight DB, Gunn AJ. Effect of pacifier use on mandibular position in preterm infants. *Acta Paediatr.* 2007;96(10):1433–1436

256. Hanzer M, Zotter H, Sauseng W, Pfurtscheller K, Müller W, Kerbl R. Pacifier use does not alter the frequency or duration of spontaneous arousals in sleeping infants. *Sleep Med.* 2009;10(4):464–470

257. Odoi A, Andrew S, Wong FY, Yiallourou SR, Horne RS. Pacifier use does not alter sleep and spontaneous arousal patterns in healthy term-born infants. *Acta Paediatr.* 2014;103(12):1244–1250

258. Weiss PP, Kerbl R. The relatively short duration that a child retains a pacifier in the mouth during sleep: implications for sudden infant death syndrome. *Eur J Pediatr.* 2001;160(1):60–70

259. Nederlands Centrum Jeugdgezondheit. Safe sleeping for your baby. Available at: www.wiegedood.nl/files/download_vs_engels.pdf. Accessed January 10, 2016

260. Foundation for the Study of Infant Deaths. Factfile 2. Research background to the Reduce the Risk of Cot Death advice by the Foundation for the Study of Infant Deaths. Available at: www.cotmattress.net/SIDS-Guidelines.pdf. Accessed January 10, 2016

261. Canadian Paediatric Society Community Paediatrics Committee. Recommendations for the use of pacifiers. *Paediatr Child Health.* 2003;8(8):515–528

262. Aarts C, Hörnell A, Kylberg E, Hofvander Y, Gebre-Medhin M. Breastfeeding patterns in relation to thumb sucking and pacifier use. *Pediatrics.* 1999;104(4). Available at: www.pediatrics.org/cgi/content/full/104/4/e50

263. Benis MM. Are pacifiers associated with early weaning from breastfeeding? *Adv Neonatal Care.* 2002;2(5):259–266

264. Scott JA, Binns CW, Oddy WH, Graham KI. Predictors of breastfeeding duration: evidence from a cohort study. *Pediatrics.* 2006;117(4). Available at: www.pediatrics.org/cgi/content/full/117/4/e646

265. Jaafar SH, Jahanfar S, Angolkar M, Ho JJ. Pacifier use versus no pacifier use in breastfeeding term infants for increasing duration of breastfeeding. *Cochrane Database Syst Rev.* 2011;3:CD007202

266. O'Connor NR, Tanabe KO, Siadaty MS, Hauck FR. Pacifiers and breastfeeding: a systematic review. *Arch Pediatr Adolesc Med.* 2009;163(4):378–382

267. Alm B, Wennergren G, Möllborg P, Lagercrantz H. Breastfeeding and dummy use have a protective effect on sudden infant death syndrome. *Acta Paediatr.* 2016;105(1):31–38

268. Howard CR, Howard FM, Lanphear B, et al. Randomized clinical trial of pacifier use and bottle-feeding or cupfeeding and their effect on breastfeeding. *Pediatrics.* 2003;111(3):511–518

269. Eidelman AI, Schanler RJ; Section on Breastfeeding. Breastfeeding and the use of human milk. *Pediatrics.* 2012;129(3). Available at: www.pediatrics.org/cgi/content/full/129/3/e827

270. Larsson Erik. The effect of dummy-sucking on the occlusion: a review. *Eur J Orthodont.* 1986;8(2):127–130

271. American Academy of Pediatric Dentistry, Council on Clinical Affairs. Policy statement on oral habits. Chicago, IL: American Academy of Pediatric Dentistry; 2000. Available at: www.aapd.org/media/Policies_Guidelines/P_OralHabits.pdf. Accessed January 10, 2016

272. Niemelä M, Uhari M, Möttönen M. A pacifier increases the risk of recurrent acute otitis media in children in day care centers. *Pediatrics.* 1995;96(5 pt 1):884–888

273. Niemelä M, Pihakari O, Pokka T, Uhari M. Pacifier as a risk factor for acute otitis media: a randomized, controlled trial of parental counseling. *Pediatrics.* 2000;106(3):483–488

274. Jackson JM, Mourino AP. Pacifier use and otitis media in infants twelve months of age or younger. *Pediatr Dent.* 1999;21(4):255–260

275. Daly KA, Giebink GS. Clinical epidemiology of otitis media. *Pediatr Infect Dis J.* 2000;19(5 suppl):S31–S36

SIDS AND OTHER SLEEP-RELATED INFANT DEATHS:
EVIDENCE BASE FOR 2016 UPDATED RECOMMENDATIONS FOR A SAFE INFANT SLEEPING ENVIRONMENT

405

276. Darwazeh AM, al-Bashir A. Oral candidal flora in healthy infants. *J Oral Pathol Med.* 1995;24(8):361–364

277. North K, Fleming P, Golding J. Pacifier use and morbidity in the first six months of life. *Pediatrics.* 1999;103(3). Available at: www.pediatrics.org/cgi/content/full/103/3/E34

278. Niemelä M, Uhari M, Hannuksela A. Pacifiers and dental structure as risk factors for otitis media. *Int J Pediatr Otorhinolaryngol.* 1994;29(2):121–127

279. Uhari M, Mäntysaari K, Niemelä M. A meta-analytic review of the risk factors for acute otitis media. *Clin Infect Dis.* 1996;22(6):1079–1083

280. Getahun D, Amre D, Rhoads GG, Demissie K. Maternal and obstetric risk factors for sudden infant death syndrome in the United States. *Obstet Gynecol.* 2004;103(4):646–652

281. Kraus JF, Greenland S, Bulterys M. Risk factors for sudden infant death syndrome in the US Collaborative Perinatal Project. *Int J Epidemiol.* 1989;18(1):113–120

282. Paris CA, Remler R, Daling JR. Risk factors for sudden infant death syndrome: changes associated with sleep position recommendations. *J Pediatr.* 2001;139(6):771–777

283. Stewart AJ, Williams SM, Mitchell EA, Taylor BJ, Ford RP, Allen EM. Antenatal and intrapartum factors associated with sudden infant death syndrome in the New Zealand Cot Death Study. *J Paediatr Child Health.* 1995;31(5):473–478

284. American Academy of Pediatrics Committee on Fetus and Newborn; ACOG Committee on Obstetric Practice. *Guidelines for Perinatal Care.* 7th ed. Elk Grove Village, IL: American Academy of Pediatrics; 2012

285. MacDorman MF, Cnattingius S, Hoffman HJ, Kramer MS, Haglund B. Sudden infant death syndrome and smoking in the United States and Sweden. *Am J Epidemiol.* 1997;146(3):249–257

286. Schoendorf KC, Kiely JL. Relationship of sudden infant death syndrome to maternal smoking during and after pregnancy. *Pediatrics.* 1992;90(6):905–908

287. Malloy MH, Kleinman JC, Land GH, Schramm WF. The association of maternal smoking with age and cause of infant death. *Am J Epidemiol.* 1988;128(1):46–55

288. Haglund B, Cnattingius S. Cigarette smoking as a risk factor for sudden infant death syndrome: a population-based study. *Am J Public Health.* 1990;80(1):29–32

289. Mitchell EA, Ford RP, Stewart AW, et al. Smoking and the sudden infant death syndrome. *Pediatrics.* 1993;91(5):893–896

290. Winickoff JP, Friebely J, Tanski SE, et al. Beliefs about the health effects of "thirdhand" smoke and home smoking bans. *Pediatrics.* 2009;123(1). Available at: www.pediatrics.org/cgi/content/full/123/1/e74

291. Tirosh E, Libon D, Bader D. The effect of maternal smoking during pregnancy on sleep respiratory and arousal patterns in neonates. *J Perinatol.* 1996;16(6):435–438

292. Franco P, Groswasser J, Hassid S, Lanquart JP, Scaillet S, Kahn A. Prenatal exposure to cigarette smoking is associated with a decrease in arousal in infants. *J Pediatr.* 1999;135(1):34–38

293. Horne RS, Ferens D, Watts AM, et al. Effects of maternal tobacco smoking, sleeping position, and sleep state on arousal in healthy term infants. *Arch Dis Child Fetal Neonatal Ed.* 2002;87(2):F100–F105

294. Sawnani H, Jackson T, Murphy T, Beckerman R, Simakajornboon N. The effect of maternal smoking on respiratory and arousal patterns in preterm infants during sleep. *Am J Respir Crit Care Med.* 2004;169(6):733–738

295. Lewis KW, Bosque EM. Deficient hypoxia awakening response in infants of smoking mothers: possible relationship to sudden infant death syndrome. *J Pediatr.* 1995;127(5):691–699

296. Chang AB, Wilson SJ, Masters IB, et al. Altered arousal response in infants exposed to cigarette smoke. *Arch Dis Child.* 2003;88(1):30–33

297. Parslow PM, Cranage SM, Adamson TM, Harding R, Horne RS. Arousal and ventilatory responses to hypoxia in sleeping infants: effects of maternal smoking [published correction appears in *Respir Physiol Neurobiol.* 2004;143(1):99]. *Respir Physiol Neurobiol.* 2004;140(1):77–87

298. Zhang K, Wang X. Maternal smoking and increased risk of sudden infant death syndrome: a meta-analysis. *Leg Med (Tokyo).* 2013;15(3):115–121

299. Mitchell EA, Milerad J. Smoking and the sudden infant death syndrome. *Rev Environ Health.* 2006;21(2):81–103

300. Dietz PM, England LJ, Shapiro-Mendoza CK, Tong VT, Farr SL, Callaghan WM. Infant morbidity and mortality attributable to prenatal smoking in the U.S. *Am J Prev Med.* 2010;39(1):45–52

301. O'Leary CM, Jacoby PJ, Bartu A, D'Antoine H, Bower C. Maternal alcohol use and sudden infant death syndrome and infant mortality excluding SIDS. *Pediatrics.* 2013;131(3). Available at: www.pediatrics.org/cgi/content/full/131/3/e770

302. Strandberg-Larsen K, Grønboek M, Andersen AM, Andersen PK, Olsen J. Alcohol drinking pattern during pregnancy and risk of infant mortality. *Epidemiology.* 2009;20(6):884–891

303. Sirieix CM, Tobia CM, Schneider RW, Darnall RA. Impaired arousal in rat pups with prenatal alcohol exposure is modulated by GABAergic mechanisms. *Physiol Rep.* 2015;3(6):e12424

304. Alm B, Wennergren G, Norvenius G, et al. Caffeine and alcohol as risk factors for sudden infant death syndrome: Nordic Epidemiological SIDS Study. *Arch Dis Child.* 1999;81(2):107–111

305. James C, Klenka H, Manning D. Sudden infant death syndrome: bed sharing with mothers who smoke. *Arch Dis Child.* 2003;88(2):112–113

306. Williams SM, Mitchell EA, Taylor BJ. Are risk factors for sudden infant death syndrome different at night? *Arch Dis Child.* 2002;87(4):274–278

307. Rajegowda BK, Kandall SR, Falciglia H. Sudden unexpected death in infants of narcotic-dependent mothers. *Early Hum Dev.* 1978;2(3):219–225

308. Chavez CJ, Ostrea EM Jr, Stryker JC, Smialek Z. Sudden infant death syndrome among infants of drug-dependent mothers. *J Pediatr.* 1979;95(3):407–409

309. Bauchner H, Zuckerman B, McClain M, Frank D, Fried LE, Kayne H. Risk of sudden infant death syndrome among infants with in utero exposure to cocaine. *J Pediatr.* 1988;113(5):831–834

310. Durand DJ, Espinoza AM, Nickerson BG. Association between prenatal cocaine exposure and sudden infant death syndrome. *J Pediatr.* 1990;117(6):909–911

311. Ward SL, Bautista D, Chan L, et al. Sudden infant death syndrome in infants of substance-abusing mothers. *J Pediatr.* 1990;117(6):876–881

312. Rosen TS, Johnson HL. Drug-addicted mothers, their infants, and SIDS. *Ann N Y Acad Sci.* 1988;533:89–95

313. Kandall SR, Gaines J, Habel L, Davidson G, Jessop D. Relationship of maternal substance abuse to subsequent sudden infant death syndrome in offspring. *J Pediatr.* 1993;123(1):120–126

314. Fares I, McCulloch KM, Raju TN. Intrauterine cocaine exposure and the risk for sudden infant death syndrome: a meta-analysis. *J Perinatol.* 1997;17(3):179–182

315. Ponsonby AL, Dwyer T, Kasl SV, Cochrane JA. The Tasmanian SIDS Case-Control Study: univariable and multivariable risk factor analysis. *Paediatr Perinat Epidemiol.* 1995;9(3):256–272

316. McGlashan ND. Sudden infant deaths in Tasmania, 1980-1986: a seven year prospective study. *Soc Sci Med.* 1989;29(8):1015–1026

317. Coleman-Phox K, Odouli R, Li DK. Use of a fan during sleep and the risk of sudden infant death syndrome. *Arch Pediatr Adolesc Med.* 2008;162(10):963–968

318. Hutcheson R. DTP vaccination and sudden infant deaths—Tennessee. *MMWR Morb Mortal Wkly Rep.* 1979;28:131–132

319. Hutcheson R. Follow-up on DTP vaccination and sudden infant deaths—Tennessee. *MMWR.* 1979;28:134–135

320. Bernier RH, Frank JA Jr, Dondero TJ Jr, Turner P. Diphtheria-tetanus toxoids-pertussis vaccination and sudden infant deaths in Tennessee. *J Pediatr.* 1982;101(3):419–421

321. Baraff LJ, Ablon WJ, Weiss RC. Possible temporal association between diphtheria-tetanus toxoid-pertussis vaccination and sudden infant death syndrome. *Pediatr Infect Dis.* 1983;2(1):7–11

322. Griffin MR, Ray WA, Livengood JR, Schaffner W. Risk of sudden infant death syndrome after immunization with the diphtheria-tetanus-pertussis vaccine. *N Engl J Med.* 1988;319(10):618–623

323. Hoffman HJ, Hunter JC, Damus K, et al. Diphtheria-tetanus-pertussis immunization and sudden infant death: results of the National Institute of Child Health and Human Development Cooperative Epidemiological Study of Sudden Infant Death Syndrome risk factors. *Pediatrics.* 1987;79(4):598–611

324. Taylor EM, Emergy JL. Immunization and cot deaths. *Lancet.* 1982;2(8300):721

325. Flahault A, Messiah A, Jougla E, Bouvet E, Perin J, Hatton F. Sudden infant death syndrome and diphtheria/tetanus toxoid/pertussis/poliomyelitis immunisation. *Lancet.* 1988;1(8585):582–583

326. Walker AM, Jick H, Perera DR, Thompson RS, Knauss TA. Diphtheria-tetanus-pertussis immunization and sudden infant death syndrome. *Am J Public Health.* 1987;77(8):945–951

327. Jonville-Bera AP, Autret E, Laugier J. Sudden infant death syndrome and diphtheria-tetanus-pertussis-poliomyelitis vaccination status. *Fundam Clin Pharmacol.* 1995;9(3):263–270

328. Immunization Safety Review Committee. Stratton K, Almario DA, Wizemann TM, McCormick MC, eds. *Immunization Safety Review: Vaccinations and Sudden Unexpected Death in Infancy.* Washington, DC: National Academies Press; 2003

329. Miller ER, Moro PL, Cano M, Shimabukuro TT. Deaths following vaccination: what does the evidence show? *Vaccine.* 2015;33(29):3288–3292

330. Moro PL, Arana J, Cano M, Lewis P, Shimabukuro TT. Deaths reported to the Vaccine Adverse Event Reporting System, United States, 1997-2013. *Clin Infect Dis.* 2015;61(6):980–987

331. Moro PL, Jankosky C, Menschik D, et al. Adverse events following Haemophilus influenzae type b vaccines in the Vaccine Adverse Event Reporting System, 1990-2013. *J Pediatr.* 2015;166(4):992–997

332. Mitchell EA, Stewart AW, Clements M; New Zealand Cot Death Study Group. Immunisation and the sudden infant death syndrome. *Arch Dis Child.* 1995;73(6):498–501

333. Jonville-Béra AP, Autret-Leca E, Barbeillon F, Paris-Llado J; French Reference Centers for SIDS. Sudden unexpected death in infants under 3 months of age and vaccination status—a case-control study. *Br J Clin Pharmacol.* 2001;51(3):271–276

334. Fleming PJ, Blair PS, Platt MW, Tripp J, Smith IJ, Golding J. The UK accelerated immunisation programme and sudden unexpected death in infancy: case-control study. *BMJ.* 2001;322(7290):822

335. Müller-Nordhorn J, Hettler-Chen CM, Keil T, Muckelbauer R. Association between sudden infant death syndrome and diphtheria-tetanus-pertussis immunisation: an ecological study. *BMC Pediatr.* 2015;15:1

336. Fine PEM, Chen RT. Confounding in studies of adverse reactions to vaccines. *Am J Epidemiol.* 1992;136(2):121–135

337. Virtanen M, Peltola H, Paunio M, Heinonen OP. Day-to-day reactogenicity and the healthy vaccinee effect of measles-mumps-rubella vaccination. *Pediatrics.* 2000;106(5). Available at: www.pediatrics.org/cgi/content/full/106/5/e62

338. Vennemann MM, Höffgen M, Bajanowski T, Hense HW, Mitchell EA. Do immunisations reduce the risk for SIDS? A meta-analysis. *Vaccine.* 2007;25(26):4875–4879

339. Centers for Disease Control and Prevention. Suffocation deaths associated with use of infant sleep positioners—United States, 1997-2011. *MMWR Morb Mortal Wkly Rep.* 2012;61(46):933–937

340. US Consumer Product Safety Commission. Deaths prompt CPSC, FDA warning on infant sleep positioners. Available at: www.cpsc.gov/en/Newsroom/News-Releases/2010/

SIDS AND OTHER SLEEP-RELATED INFANT DEATHS:
EVIDENCE BASE FOR 2016 UPDATED RECOMMENDATIONS FOR A SAFE INFANT SLEEPING ENVIRONMENT

407

Deaths-prompt-CPSC-FDA-warning-on-infant-sleep-position. Accessed September 21, 2016

341. Bar-Yishay E, Gaides M, Goren A, Szeinberg A. Aeration properties of a new sleeping surface for infants. *Pediatr Pulmonol.* 2011;46(2):193–198

342. Colditz PB, Joy GJ, Dunster KR. Rebreathing potential of infant mattresses and bedcovers. *J Paediatr Child Health.* 2002;38(2):192–195

343. Carolan PL, Wheeler WB, Ross JD, Kemp RJ. Potential to prevent carbon dioxide rebreathing of commercial products marketed to reduce sudden infant death syndrome risk. *Pediatrics.* 2000;105(4 Pt 1):774–779

344. Steinschneider A. Prolonged apnea and the sudden infant death syndrome: clinical and laboratory observations. *Pediatrics.* 1972;50(4):646–654

345. Hodgman JE, Hoppenbrouwers T. Home monitoring for the sudden infant death syndrome: the case against. *Ann N Y Acad Sci.* 1988;533:164–175

346. Ward SL, Keens TG, Chan LS, et al. Sudden infant death syndrome in infants evaluated by apnea programs in California. *Pediatrics.* 1986;77(4):451–458

347. Monod N, Plouin P, Sternberg B, et al. Are polygraphic and cardiopneumographic respiratory patterns useful tools for predicting the risk for sudden infant death syndrome? A 10-year study. *Biol Neonate.* 1986;50(3):147–153

348. Ramanathan R, Corwin MJ, Hunt CE, et al; Collaborative Home Infant Monitoring Evaluation (CHIME) Study Group. Cardiorespiratory events recorded on home monitors: comparison of healthy infants with those at increased risk for SIDS. *JAMA.* 2001;285(17):2199–2207

349. American Academy of Pediatrics Committee on Fetus and Newborn. Apnea, sudden infant death syndrome, and home monitoring. *Pediatrics.* 2003;111(4 pt 1):914–917

350. Hutchison BL, Thompson JM, Mitchell EA. Determinants of nonsynostotic plagiocephaly: a case-control study. *Pediatrics.* 2003;112(4). Available at: www.pediatrics.org/cgi/content/full/112/4/e316

351. Hutchison BL, Hutchison LA, Thompson JM, Mitchell EA. Plagiocephaly and brachycephaly in the first two years of life: a prospective cohort study. *Pediatrics.* 2004;114(4):970–980

352. van Vlimmeren LA, van der Graaf Y, Boere-Boonekamp MM, L'Hoir MP, Helders PJ, Engelbert RH. Risk factors for deformational plagiocephaly at birth and at 7 weeks of age: a prospective cohort study. *Pediatrics.* 2007;119(2). Available at: www.pediatrics.org/cgi/content/full/119/2/e408

353. Miller RI, Clarren SK. Long-term developmental outcomes in patients with deformational plagiocephaly. *Pediatrics.* 2000;105(2). Available at: www.pediatrics.org/cgi/content/full/105/2/E26

354. Panchal J, Amirsheybani H, Gurwitch R, et al. Neurodevelopment in children with single-suture craniosynostosis and plagiocephaly without synostosis. *Plast Reconstr Surg.* 2001;108(6):1492–1498; discussion: 1499–1500

355. Balan P, Kushnerenko E, Sahlin P, Huotilainen M, Näätänen R, Hukki J. Auditory ERPs reveal brain dysfunction in infants with plagiocephaly. *J Craniofac Surg.* 2002;13(4):520–525; discussion: 526

356. Chadduck WM, Kast J, Donahue DJ. The enigma of lambdoid positional molding. *Pediatr Neurosurg.* 1997;26(6):304–311

357. Laughlin J, Luerssen TG, Dias MS; Committee on Practice and Ambulatory Medicine; Section on Neurological Surgery. Prevention and management of positional skull deformities in infants. *Pediatrics.* 2011;128(6):1236–1241

358. Gerard CM, Harris KA, Thach BT. Physiologic studies on swaddling: an ancient child care practice, which may promote the supine position for infant sleep. *J Pediatr.* 2002;141(3):398–403

359. van Sleuwen BE, Engelberts AC, Boere-Boonekamp MM, Kuis W, Schulpen TW, L'Hoir MP. Swaddling: a systematic review. *Pediatrics.* 2007;120(4). Available at: www.pediatrics.org/cgi/content/full/120/4/e1097

360. McDonnell E, Moon RY. Infant deaths and injuries associated with wearable blankets, swaddle wraps, and swaddling. *J Pediatr.* 2014;164(5):1152–1156

361. Richardson HL, Walker AM, Horne RS. Influence of swaddling experience on spontaneous arousal patterns and autonomic control in sleeping infants. *J Pediatr.* 2010;157(1):85–91

362. Richardson HL, Walker AM, Horne RS. Minimizing the risks of sudden infant death syndrome: to swaddle or not to swaddle? *J Pediatr.* 2009;155(4):475–481

363. Narangerel G, Pollock J, Manaseki-Holland S, Henderson J. The effects of swaddling on oxygen saturation and respiratory rate of healthy infants in Mongolia. *Acta Paediatr.* 2007;96(2):261–265

364. Kutlu A, Memik R, Mutlu M, Kutlu R, Arslan A. Congenital dislocation of the hip and its relation to swaddling used in Turkey. *J Pediatr Orthop.* 1992;12(5):598–602

365. Chaarani MW, Al Mahmeid MS, Salman AM. Developmental dysplasia of the hip before and after increasing community awareness of the harmful effects of swaddling. *Qatar Med J.* 2002;11(1):40–43

366. Yamamuro T, Ishida K. Recent advances in the prevention, early diagnosis, and treatment of congenital dislocation of the hip in Japan. *Clin Orthop Relat Res.* 1984;(184):34–40

367. Coleman SS. Congenital dysplasia of the hip in the Navajo infant. *Clin Orthop Relat Res.* 1968;56:179–193

368. Tronick EZ, Thomas RB, Daltabuit M. The Quechua manta pouch: a caretaking practice for buffering the Peruvian infant against the multiple stressors of high altitude. *Child Dev.* 1994;65(4):1005–1013

369. Manaseki S. Mongolia: a health system in transition. *BMJ.* 1993;307(6919):1609–1611

370. Franco P, Seret N, Van Hees JN, Scaillet S, Groswasser J, Kahn A. Influence of swaddling on sleep and arousal characteristics of healthy infants. *Pediatrics.* 2005;115(5):1307–1311

371. Franco P, Scaillet S, Groswasser J, Kahn A. Increased cardiac autonomic responses to auditory

challenges in swaddled infants. *Sleep.* 2004;27(8):1527–1532

372. Patriarca M, Lyon TD, Delves HT, Howatson AG, Fell GS. Determination of low concentrations of potentially toxic elements in human liver from newborns and infants. *Analyst (Lond).* 1999;124(9):1337–1343

373. Kleemann WJ, Weller JP, Wolf M, Tröger HD, Blüthgen A, Heeschen W. Heavy metals, chlorinated pesticides and polychlorinated biphenyls in sudden infant death syndrome (SIDS). *Int J Legal Med.* 1991;104(2):71–75

374. Erickson MM, Poklis A, Gantner GE, Dickinson AW, Hillman LS. Tissue mineral levels in victims of sudden infant death syndrome I. Toxic metals—lead and cadmium. *Pediatr Res.* 1983;17(10):779–784

375. George M, Wiklund L, Aastrup M, et al. Incidence and geographical distribution of sudden infant death syndrome in relation to content of nitrate in drinking water and groundwater levels. *Eur J Clin Invest.* 2001;31(12):1083–1094

376. Richardson BA. Sudden infant death syndrome: a possible primary cause. *J Forensic Sci Soc.* 1994;34(3):199–204

377. Sprott TJ. Cot death—cause and prevention: experiences in New Zealand 1995-2004. *J Nutr Environ Med.* 2004;14(3):221–232

378. Department of Health. *Expert Group To Investigate Cot Death Theories (Chair, Lady S. Limerick).* London, United Kingdom: HMSO; 1998

379. Blair P, Fleming P, Bensley D, Smith I, Bacon C, Taylor E. Plastic mattresses and sudden infant death syndrome. *Lancet.* 1995;345(8951):720

380. Rubens DD, Vohr BR, Tucker R, O'Neil CA, Chung W. Newborn oto-acoustic emission hearing screening tests: preliminary evidence for a marker of susceptibility to SIDS. *Early Hum Dev.* 2008;84(4):225–229

381. Hamill T, Lim G. Otoacoustic emissions does not currently have ability to detect SIDS. *Early Hum Dev.* 2008;84(6):373

382. Krous HF, Byard RW. Newborn hearing screens and SIDS. *Early Hum Dev.* 2008;84(6):371

383. Farquhar LJ, Jennings P. Newborn hearing screen results for infants that died of SIDS in Michigan 2004-2006. *Early Hum Dev.* 2008;84(10):699

384. Chan RS, McPherson B, Zhang VW. Neonatal otoacoustic emission screening and sudden infant death syndrome. *Int J Pediatr Otorhinolaryngol.* 2012;76(10):1485–1489

385. Hauck FR, Tanabe KO. Sids. *BMJ Clin Evid.* 2009;2009(315):1–13

386. Colson ER, Levenson S, Rybin D, et al. Barriers to following the supine sleep recommendation among mothers at four centers for the Women, Infants, and Children Program. *Pediatrics.* 2006;118(2). Available at: www.pediatrics.org/cgi/content/full/118/2/e243

387. Eisenberg SR, Bair-Merritt MH, Colson ER, Heeren TC, Geller NL, Corwin MJ. Maternal report of advice received for infant care. *Pediatrics.* 2015;136(2):e315–e322

388. Colson ER, Bergman DM, Shapiro E, Leventhal JH. Position for newborn sleep: associations with parents' perceptions of their nursery experience. *Birth.* 2001;28(4):249–253

389. Mason B, Ahlers-Schmidt CR, Schunn C. Improving safe sleep environments for well newborns in the hospital setting. *Clin Pediatr (Phila).* 2013;52(10):969–975

390. McKinney CM, Holt VL, Cunningham ML, Leroux BG, Starr JR. Maternal and infant characteristics associated with prone and lateral infant sleep positioning in Washington state, 1996-2002. *J Pediatr.* 2008;153(2):194–198, e191–e193

391. Moon RY, Calabrese T, Aird L. Reducing the risk of sudden infant death syndrome in child care and changing provider practices: lessons learned from a demonstration project. *Pediatrics.* 2008;122(4):788–798

392. Moon RY, Oden RP. Back to sleep: can we influence child care providers? *Pediatrics.* 2003;112(4):878–882

393. Lerner H, McClain M, Vance JC. SIDS education in nursing and medical schools in the United States. *J Nurs Educ.* 2002;41(8):353–356

394. Price SK, Gardner P, Hillman L, Schenk K, Warren C. Changing hospital newborn nursery practice: results from a statewide "Back to Sleep" nurses training program. *Matern Child Health J.* 2008;12(3):363–371

395. Cowan S, Pease A, Bennett S. Usage and impact of an online education tool for preventing sudden unexpected death in infancy. *J Paediatr Child Health.* 2013;49(3):228–232

396. Colson ER, Joslin SC. Changing nursery practice gets inner-city infants in the supine position for sleep. *Arch Pediatr Adolesc Med.* 2002;156(7):717–720

397. Voos KC, Terreros A, Larimore P, Leick-Rude MK, Park N. Implementing safe sleep practices in a neonatal intensive care unit. *J Matern Fetal Neonatal Med.* 2015;28(14):1637–1640

398. Goodstein MH, Bell T, Krugman SD. Improving infant sleep safety through a comprehensive hospital-based program. *Clin Pediatr (Phila).* 2015;54(3):212–221

399. Yanovitzky I, Blitz CL. Effect of media coverage and physician advice on utilization of breast cancer screening by women 40 years and older. *J Health Commun.* 2000;5(2):117–134

400. Magazine Publishers of America; Marketing Evolution. *Measuring Media Effectiveness: Comparing Media Contribution Throughout the Purchase Funnel.* New York, NY: Magazine Publishers of America; 2006

CLINICAL REPORT   Guidance for the Clinician in Rendering Pediatric Care

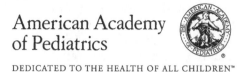

American Academy
of Pediatrics

DEDICATED TO THE HEALTH OF ALL CHILDREN™

Standard Terminology for Fetal, Infant, and Perinatal Deaths

Wanda D. Barfield, MD, MPH, COMMITTEE ON FETUS AND NEWBORN

abstract

Accurately defining and reporting perinatal deaths (ie, fetal and infant deaths) is a critical first step in understanding the magnitude and causes of these important events. In addition to obstetric health care providers, neonatologists and pediatricians should have easy access to current and updated resources that clearly provide US definitions and reporting requirements for live births, fetal deaths, and infant deaths. Correct identification of these vital events will improve local, state, and national data so that these deaths can be better addressed and prevented.

INTRODUCTION

Perinatal mortality is the combination of fetal deaths and neonatal deaths. In the United States in 2013, the fetal mortality rate for gestations of at least 20 weeks (5.96 fetal deaths per 1000 live births and fetal deaths)[1] was similar to the infant mortality rate (5.98 infant deaths per 1000 live births).[2] Depending on the definition used, fetal mortality contributes to approximately 40% to 60% of perinatal mortality. Understanding the etiologies of these events and predicting risk begins with accurately defining cases; the collection and analysis of reliable statistical data are an essential part of in-depth investigations on local, state, and national levels.

Fetal and infant deaths occur within the clinical practice of several types of health care providers. Although obstetric practitioners report fetal deaths, certain situations can occur during a delivery in which viability or possibility of survival is unclear; the pediatrician or neonatologist may attend the delivery to assess the medical condition of the fetus or infant, assess pre-viable gestational age, provide care as indicated, and report a subsequent infant death, if it occurs. Incorrectly defining and reporting fetal deaths and early infant deaths may contribute to misclassification of these important events and result in inaccurate fetal and infant mortality rates.[3] Within this context, the American Academy of Pediatrics provides definitions and reporting requirements of fetal death, live birth, and infant death to emphasize that neonatologists and pediatricians play an

This document is copyrighted and is property of the American Academy of Pediatrics and its Board of Directors. All authors have filed conflict of interest statements with the American Academy of Pediatrics. Any conflicts have been resolved through a process approved by the Board of Directors. The American Academy of Pediatrics has neither solicited nor accepted any commercial involvement in the development of the content of this publication.

The views expressed in this document are not necessarily those of the Centers for Disease Control and Prevention or the US Department of Health and Human Services.

Clinical reports from the American Academy of Pediatrics benefit from expertise and resources of liaisons and internal (AAP) and external reviewers. However, clinical reports from the American Academy of Pediatrics may not reflect the views of the liaisons or the organizations or government agencies that they represent.

The guidance in this report does not indicate an exclusive course of treatment or serve as a standard of medical care. Variations, taking into account individual circumstances, may be appropriate.

All clinical reports from the American Academy of Pediatrics automatically expire 5 years after publication unless reaffirmed, revised, or retired at or before that time.

DOI: 10.1542/peds.2016-0551

PEDIATRICS (ISSN Numbers: Print, 0031-4005; Online, 1098-4275).

To cite: Barfield WD and AAP COMMITTEE ON FETUS AND NEWBORN. Standard Terminology for Fetal, Infant, and Perinatal Deaths. *Pediatrics.* 2016;137(5):e20160551

important role in recording accurate and timely information surrounding these events. This role includes making the determination of the specific vital event during delivery, recording information surrounding the event on the appropriate certificate or report in compliance with state-specific requirements, and documenting information that is as complete and as accurate as possible, including the underlying cause of death, when known. Although guidance for these definitions is provided elsewhere,[4–6] it may not be readily available to pediatricians in the delivery room.

Both the collection and use of information about fetal, infant, and perinatal deaths have been hampered by lack of understanding of differences in definitions, statistical tabulations, and reporting requirements among providers and state, national, and international bodies. Distinctions can and should be made between the definition of an event and the reporting requirements for the event. The definition indicates the meaning of a term (eg, live birth, fetal death). A reporting requirement is that part of the defined event for which reporting is mandatory.

DEFINITIONS

Challenges in consistent definitions of fetal and infant death mostly stem from the perception of viability, which should not change the definition of the event. In other words, an extremely preterm infant born at 16 weeks' gestation may be defined as a live birth but is not currently viable outside of the womb. On the basis of international standards set by the World Health Organization,[7] the National Center for Health Statistics of the Centers for Disease Control and Prevention defines live birth, fetal death, infant death, and perinatal death as follows.[4]

Live Birth

A live birth is defined as the complete expulsion or extraction from the mother of a product of human conception, irrespective of the duration of pregnancy, which, after such expulsion or extraction, breathes or shows any other evidence of life, such as beating of the heart, pulsation of the umbilical cord, or definite movement of voluntary muscles, regardless of whether the umbilical cord has been cut or the placenta is attached. Heartbeats are to be distinguished from transient cardiac contractions; respirations are to be distinguished from fleeting respiratory efforts or gasps.

Fetal Death

A fetus is defined from 8 weeks after conception until term while in the uterus. Fetal death is defined as death before the complete expulsion or extraction from the mother of a product of human conception, irrespective of the duration of pregnancy that is not an induced termination of pregnancy. The death is indicated by the fact that, after such expulsion or extraction, the fetus does not breathe or show any other evidence of life such as beating of the heart, pulsation of the umbilical cord, or definite movement of voluntary muscles. Heartbeats are to be distinguished from transient cardiac contractions; respirations are to be distinguished from fleeting respiratory efforts or gasps.

For statistical purposes, fetal deaths are further subdivided as "early" (20–27 weeks' gestation) or "late" (≥28 weeks' gestation). The term "stillbirth" is also used to describe fetal deaths at 20 weeks' gestation or more. Stillbirth is not specifically divided into early and late gestations, but for international comparisons the World Health Organization defines stillbirth as at or after 28 weeks' gestation. Fetuses that die in utero before 20 weeks' gestation are categorized specifically as miscarriages.

Infant Death

A live birth that results in death within the first year (<365 days) is defined as an infant death. Infant deaths are characterized as neonatal (<28 days) and further subdivided into early neonatal (<7 days), late neonatal (7–27 days), or postneonatal (28–364 days).

Perinatal Death

Perinatal deaths refer to a combination of fetal deaths and live births with only brief survival (days or weeks) and are grouped on the assumption that similar factors are associated with these losses. Perinatal death is not a reportable vital event, per se, but is used for statistical purposes. Three definitions of perinatal deaths are in use:

- Definition I includes infant deaths that occur at less than 7 days of age and fetal deaths with a stated or presumed period of gestation of 28 weeks or more.

- Definition II includes infant deaths that occur at less than 28 days of age and fetal deaths with a stated or presumed period of gestation of 20 weeks or more.

- Definition III includes infant deaths that occur at less than 7 days of age and fetal deaths with a stated or presumed gestation of 20 weeks or more.

From national and international perspectives, perinatal deaths have important implications for both public health and clinical interventions. However, the interpretations of these definitions vary globally on the basis of cultural perspectives, clinical definitions of viability, and availability of information. The National Center for Health Statistics currently classifies perinatal deaths according to the first 2 definitions. Definition I is used by the National Center for Health

TABLE 1 Reporting Requirements for Fetal Death According to State or Reporting Area, 2014

Criteria	State/Reporting Area
Gestational age criteria only	
All periods	Arkansas, Colorado, Georgia, Hawaii, New York,[a] Rhode Island, Virginia, Virgin Islands
≥16 weeks	Pennsylvania
≥20 weeks	Alabama, Alaska, California, Connecticut, Florida, Illinois, Indiana, Iowa, Maine, Maryland,[b] Minnesota, Nebraska, Nevada, New Jersey, North Carolina, North Dakota, Ohio, Oklahoma, Oregon, Texas, Utah, Vermont,[c] Washington, West Virginia, Wyoming
≥5 months	Puerto Rico
Both gestational age and birth weight criteria	
≥20 weeks or ≥350 g	Arizona, Idaho, Kentucky, Louisiana, Massachusetts, Mississippi, Missouri, New Hampshire, New Mexico, South Carolina, Tennessee, Wisconsin, Guam
≥20 weeks or ≥400 g	Michigan
≥20 weeks or ≥500 g	District of Columbia
Birth weight criteria only	
≥350 g	Delaware,[d] Kansas, Montana[d]
≥500 g	South Dakota

Data source: National Center for Health Statistics, National Vital Statistics Reports.

[a] Includes New York city, which has separate reporting.

[b] If gestational age is unknown, weight of ≥500 g.

[c] If gestational age is unknown, weight of ≥400 g, ≥15 ounces.

[d] If weight is unknown, ≥20 weeks' completed gestation.

Statistics and the World Health Organization to make international comparisons to account for variability in registering births and deaths between 20 and 27 weeks' gestation.[8] However, definition II is more inclusive and hence is more appropriate for monitoring perinatal deaths throughout gestation, because the majority of fetal deaths occur before 28 weeks' gestation.

REPORTING REQUIREMENTS

In the United States, states and independent reporting areas (ie, New York City; Washington, DC; and the US territories) register the certificates of live birth, death, and fetal death. These certificates/reports include clinical information. Challenges in consistent reporting of fetal death, in particular, stem from the variation in reporting requirements among states.[9] Recommended definitions and reporting requirements are issued through the Model State Vital Statistics Act and Regulations (the Model Law).[10,11] The Model Law recommends fetal death reporting for deaths that occur at 350 g birth weight or more or, if the weight is

unknown, of 20 completed weeks' gestation or more. However, states have the authority to register these vital events and might not necessarily follow the Model Law, which results in differences in birth weight and gestational age criteria for reporting fetal deaths (Table 1). States also vary in the quality of the data reported, which include missing data.[9]

All live births, regardless of gestational age, are reported as vital record events. Infant deaths involve both the reporting of a live birth event and a death event using a certificate of live birth and a certificate of death, respectively. Information from the certificate of live birth, including demographic information, selected maternal risk factors, maternal labor and delivery information, and infant weight and gestational age, is linked to information on the infant death certificate to include cause-of-death information. The fetal death certificate or report, a single document, includes maternal demographic information, selected maternal risk factors, labor and delivery information, and information about the fetus to

include weight, gestational age, and cause of death. Accurate completion of these vital records is important for generating accurate data to determine the magnitude and causes of fetal, infant, and perinatal deaths.

PRACTICAL CONSIDERATIONS

A flow diagram for the determination of appropriate reporting of perinatal deaths was developed by the National Association for Public Health Statistics and Information Systems (Fig 1). The diagram delineates the sequence of reporting and can be used in delivery rooms to appropriately report perinatal events. Induced termination of pregnancy is included in the flow diagram but is beyond the scope of this report.

In the circumstance of delivery events in which the fetus is of uncertain viability, if the infant is determined to be a live birth, the event is reported regardless of birth weight, length of gestation, survival time, or other clinical information (eg, Apgar scores). If fetal death is determined, the event is reported by the obstetric health care provider on the basis of state criteria, including

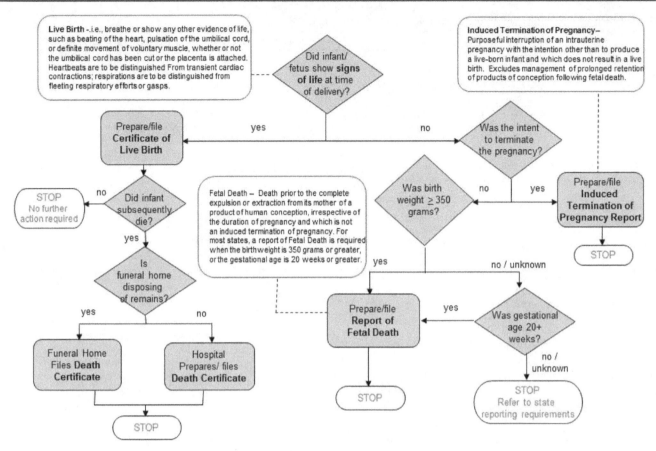

FIGURE 1

Hospital guidelines for reporting live births, infant deaths, fetal deaths, and induced terminations of pregnancy. (Adapted with permission from the National Association for Public Health Statistics and Information Systems; www.naphsis.org [available on request].)

both birth weight and gestational age. The careful use of accurate definitions is of utmost importance in medical record documentation of these events. Because there are no signs of life at delivery, fetal deaths are not assigned Apgar scores and are usually not admitted to the nursery or NICU. Postmortem examination of the fetus or infant and placenta may provide important information as to the cause of death; however, the actual evaluation and management of fetal and infant death are beyond the scope of this guidance and have been reported elsewhere.[12]

In summary, the accurate and timely reporting of live birth and fetal and infant death is the cornerstone of perinatal mortality data. Because reducing fetal and infant mortality is among the nation's health goals, accurate definitions of these events

are essential for understanding causes and researching potential solutions.

SUGGESTIONS

1. Vital events are best defined and reported as follows:

   o Live birth: The complete expulsion or extraction from the mother of a product of human conception, irrespective of the duration of pregnancy, which, after such expulsion or extraction, breathes or shows any other evidence of life such as beating of the heart, pulsation of the umbilical cord, or definite movement of voluntary muscles, regardless of whether the umbilical cord has been cut or the placenta is attached. Heartbeats are

to be distinguished from transient cardiac contractions; respirations are to be distinguished from fleeting respiratory efforts or gasps.

   o Fetal death: Death before the complete expulsion or extraction from the mother of a product of human conception, irrespective of the duration of pregnancy that is not an induced termination of pregnancy. The death is indicated by the fact that, after such expulsion or extraction, the fetus does not breathe or show any other evidence of life such as beating of the heart, pulsation of the umbilical cord, or definite movement of voluntary muscles. Heartbeats are to be distinguished from transient cardiac contractions; respirations are to be distinguished from fleeting respiratory efforts or gasps.

- o Infant death: A live birth that results in death within the first year (<365 days).

2. Obtain accurate information on state law to file the fetal death certificate/report according to state requirements.

3. Complete reporting of live births, infant deaths, and fetal deaths (in support of obstetrician reporters) with the most accurate information possible to include pertinent demographic information, maternal medical history, and fetal or infant diagnoses.

LEAD AUTHOR

Wanda Denise Barfield, MD, MPH, FAAP
wjb5@cdc.gov

COMMITTEE ON FETUS AND NEWBORN, 2014–2015

Kristi Watterberg, MD, FAAP, Chairperson
William Benitz, MD, FAAP
James Cummings, MD, FAAP
Eric Eichenwald, MD, FAAP
Brenda Poindexter, MD, FAAP
Dan L. Stewart, MD, FAAP
Susan W. Aucott, MD, FAAP
Karen M. Puopolo, MD, FAAP
Jay P. Goldsmith, MD, FAAP

LIAISONS

Kasper S. Wang, MD, FAAP – *AAP Section on Surgery*
Thierry Lacaze, MD – *Canadian Pediatric Society*
Maria Ann Mascola, MD – *American College of Obstetricians and Gynecologists*

Tonse N.K. Raju, MD, FAAP – *National Institutes of Health*
Wanda D. Barfield, MD, MPH, FAAP – *Centers for Disease Control and Prevention*
Erin Keels, MS, APRN, NNP-BC – *National Association of Neonatal Nurses*

STAFF

Jim Couto, MA

REFERENCES

1. MacDorman MF, Gregory ECW. Fetal and perinatal mortality: United States, 2013. *Natl Vital Stat Rep.* 2015;64(8):1–8

2. Centers for Disease Control and Prevention. Deaths: final data for 2013. Available at: www.cdc.gov/nchs/data/nvsr/nvsr64/nvsr64_02.pdf. Accessed July 2015

3. MacDorman MF, Martin JA, Mathews TJ, Hoyert DL, Ventura SJ. Explaining the 2001-02 infant mortality increase: data from the linked birth/infant death data set. *Natl Vital Stat Rep.* 2005;53(12):1–22

4. Centers for Disease Control and Prevention. State definitions and reporting requirements for live births, fetal deaths, and induced terminations of pregnancy. Hyattsville, MD: National Center for Health Statistics; 1997. Available at: www.cdc.gov/nchs/data/misc/itop97.pdf. Accessed July 7, 2015

5. American Academy of Pediatrics; American College of Obstetrics and Gynecology. Appendix F: standard terminology for reporting reproductive health statistics. In: *Guidelines for Perinatal Care.* 7th ed. Elk Grove Village, IL: American Academy of Pediatrics; 2012:497–512

6. Committee on Obstetric Practice. ACOG Committee opinion: perinatal and infant mortality statistics. Number 167, December 1995. *Int J Gynaecol Obstet.* 1996;53(1):86–88

7. World Health Organization. *International Statistical Classification of Diseases and Related Health Problems,* Tenth Revision. Vol 2. Geneva, Switzerland: World Health Organization; 2006

8. World Health Organization. *Neonatal and Perinatal Mortality: Country, Regional and Global Estimates.* Geneva, Switzerland: World Health Organization; 2006

9. Martin JA, Hoyert DL. The National Fetal Death File. *Semin Perinatol.* 2002;26(1):3–11

10. Centers for Disease Control and Prevention; National Center for Health Statistics. Model State Vital Statistics Act and Regulations: 1992 revision. Hyattsville, MD: National Center for Health Statistics; 1994. Available at: www.cdc.gov/nchs/data/misc/mvsact92b.pdf. Accessed July 7, 2015

11. Centers for Disease Control and Prevention; National Center for Health Statistics. 2003 Revisions of the U.S. Standard Certificates of Live Birth and Death and the Fetal Death Report. Hyattsville, MD: National Center for Health Statistics; 2014. Available at: www.cdc.gov/nchs/nvss/vital_certificate_revisions.htm. Accessed July 7, 2015

12. American College of Obstetricians and Gynecologists. ACOG Practice Bulletin No. 102: management of stillbirth. *Obstet Gynecol.* 2009;113(3):748–761

SECTION 9

Other Related Policies

American Academy
of Pediatrics

DEDICATED TO THE HEALTH OF ALL CHILDREN™

POLICY STATEMENT

Advanced Practice in Neonatal Nursing

Organizational Principles to Guide and
Define the Child Health Care System and/or
Improve the Health of All Children

Committee on Fetus and Newborn

ABSTRACT

The participation of advanced practice registered nurses in neonatal care continues to be accepted and supported by the American Academy of Pediatrics. Recognized categories of advanced practice neonatal nursing are the neonatal clinical nurse specialist and the neonatal nurse practitioner. *Pediatrics* 2009;123:1606–1607

INTRODUCTION

The American Academy of Pediatrics (AAP) endorses the role of the advanced practice registered nurse (APRN) and the current training and credentialing process developed by the National Association of Neonatal Nurses.[1,2] These guidelines were specifically designed to educate APRNs at the graduate level to manage critically ill and convalescing infants. These guidelines and standards include requirements for the completion of a graduate-level education program of study and supervised practice beyond the level of basic nursing. This preparation includes the attainment of a master's degree in the neonatal nursing specialty. The neonatal nurse practitioner (NNP) curriculum must have included a minimum of 200 neonatal-specific didactic hours plus a minimum of 600 directly supervised hours with critically ill neonates/infants in level II and III NICUs.[1-5] Currently credentialed NNPs who have graduated from non–master's degree programs or certificate programs should be allowed to maintain their practice and be encouraged to complete a formal graduate education.[6] The AAP supports the documented competency of the master's degree–prepared APRN for entry into practice as an NNP. Some APRNs may wish to pursue the highest level of educational preparation in nursing, either the doctor of philosophy (PhD) or the doctor of nurse practice (DNP). However, the AAP does not consider such a degree to be necessary for clinical practice.

Included in the category of neonatal APRNs are the following[1,2]:

www.pediatrics.org/cgi/doi/10.1542/peds.2009-0867

doi:10.1542/peds.2009-0867

All policy statements from the American Academy of Pediatrics automatically expire 5 years after publication unless reaffirmed, revised, or retired at or before that time.

This document is copyrighted and is property of the American Academy of Pediatrics and its Board of Directors. All authors have filed conflict of interest statements with the American Academy of Pediatrics. Any conflicts have been resolved through a process approved by the Board of Directors. The American Academy of Pediatrics has neither solicited nor accepted any commercial involvement in the development of the content of this publication.

Key Word
neonatal care

Abbreviations
AAP—American Academy of Pediatrics
APRN—advanced practice registered nurse
NNP—neonatal nurse practitioner
NCNS—neonatal clinical nurse specialist

PEDIATRICS (ISSN Numbers: Print, 0031-4005; Online, 1098-4275). Copyright © 2009 by the American Academy of Pediatrics

- Neonatal clinical nurse specialist (NCNS): a registered nurse with a master's degree who, through study and supervised practice at the graduate level, has become expert in the theory and practice of neonatal nursing. The NCNS is responsible for fostering continuous quality improvement in neonatal nursing care and developing and educating staff. The NCNS models expert nursing practice and applies and promotes evidence-based nursing practice.

- NNP: a registered nurse with clinical expertise in neonatal nursing who has obtained a master's degree with supervised clinical experience in the management of newborn infants and their families. The NNP manages patients in collaboration with a physician, usually a pediatrician or neonatologist. Using the acquired knowledge of pathophysiology, pharmacology, and physiology, the NNP may exercise independent judgment in the assessment, diagnosis, and management of infants and in the performance of certain procedures. The NNP may also be responsible for education of staff, research, and developing standards of nursing care.[6,7]

The spectrum of duties performed by the neonatal APRN will vary among institutions and may be governed by state regulations. Each of these roles currently requires advanced education and a master's degree. Nationally recognized certification examinations and requirements for maintenance education exist for each category.[8] Credentialing for practice is currently governed by individual states. Inpatient care privileges are granted by the individual institution. Each institution needs to develop a procedure for the initial granting and subsequent maintenance of privileges, ensuring that the proper professional credentials are in place. That procedure is best developed by the collaborative efforts of the nursing administration and the medical staff.

RECOMMENDATIONS

1. Medical care by the APRN for patients receiving level III newborn intensive care is provided in collaboration with, or under the supervision of, a physician, usually a neonatologist.

2. Medical care by the APRN for patients receiving level I and II care is provided in collaboration with, or under the supervision of, a physician with special interest and experience in neonatal medicine, usually a pediatrician or neonatologist.

3. Determination of whether the APRN practices in collaboration with, or under the supervision of, a physician should be determined in accordance with the board of nursing regulations in the state in which the APRN is practicing.[8]

4. The APRN should be certified by a nationally recognized organization and should maintain that certification.

5. The APRN should maintain clinical expertise and knowledge of current therapy by participating in continuing education and other scholarly activities as recommended by the National Certification Corporation.[9]

6. The APRN should comply with hospital policy regarding credentialing and recredentialing.[10]

COMMITTEE ON FETUS AND NEWBORN, 2008–2009

Ann R. Stark, MD, Chairperson
David H. Adamkin, MD
Jill E. Baley, MD
Vinod K. Bhutani, MD
Waldemar A. Carlo, MD
Praveen Kumar, MD
Richard A. Polin, MD
Rosemarie C. Tan, MD, PhD
Kristi L. Watterberg, MD

FORMER COMMITTEE MEMBERS

Daniel G. Batton, MD
Edward F. Bell, MD
Susan E. Denson, MD
Gilbert I. Martin, MD

LIAISONS

Ann L. Jefferies, MD
    Canadian Paediatric Society
Sarah J. Kilpatrick, MD, PhD
    American College of Obstetricians and Gynecologists
Tonse N. K. Raju, MD, DCH
    National Institutes of Health
Capt. Wanda D. Barfield, MD, MPH
    Centers for Disease Control and Prevention
*Carol Wallman, RN, MS, NNP-BC
    National Association of Neonatal Nurses and Association of Women's Health, Obstetric and Neonatal Nurses

FORMER LIAISONS

Keith J. Barrington, MB, ChB
    Canadian Paediatric Society
Gary D. V. Hankins, MD
    American College of Obstetricians and Gynecologists
Kay M. Tomashek, MD, MPH
    Centers for Disease Control and Prevention

CONSULTANT

Kasper S. Wang, MD

STAFF

Jim Couto, MA
    jcouto@aap.org

*Lead authors

REFERENCES

1. National Association of Neonatal Nurses. *Position Statement #3011: RN Practice Experience and Neonatal Advanced Nursing Practice*. Glenview, IL: National Association of Neonatal Nurses; 2004. Available at: www.nann.org/pdf/3011–04.doc. Accessed March 16, 2009

2. National Association of Neonatal Nurses. *Education Standards for Neonatal Nurse Practitioner Programs*. Glenview, IL: National Association of Neonatal Nurses; 2002. Available at: www.nann.org/pdf/NNP_Standards.pdf. Accessed March 8, 2007

3. National Association of Neonatal Nurses. *Position Paper: Requirement for Advanced Neonatal Nursing Practice in Newborn Intensive Care Units*. Glenview, IL: National Association of Neonatal Nurses; 2005. Available at: www.nann.org/pdf/2005final.pdf. Accessed March 16, 2009

4. Strodtbeck F, Trotter C, Lott JW. Coping with transition: neonatal nurse practitioner education for the 21st century. *J Pediatr Nurs*. 1998;13(5):272–278

5. American Academy of Pediatrics; American College of Obstetricians and Gynecologists. *Guidelines for Perinatal Care*. 6th ed. Washington, DC: American Academy of Pediatrics and American College of Obstetricians and Gynecologists; 2007

6. American Nurses Association, National Association of Neonatal Nurses. *Neonatal Nursing: Scope and Standards of Practice*. Washington, DC: nursesbooks.org; 2004

7. Pearson L. The Pearson report. *J Am Acad Nurse Pract*. 2007; 11(2):17–99

8. American Academy of Pediatrics, Committee on Pediatric Workforce. Scope of practice issues in the delivery of pediatric health care. *Pediatrics*. 2003;111(2):426–435

9. National Certification Corporation. Certificate maintenance requirements. Available at: www.nccnet.org/public/pages/index.cfm?pageid=442. Accessed March 16, 2009

10. O'Connor ME; American Academy of Pediatrics, Committee on Hospital Care. Medical staff appointment and delineation of pediatric privileges in hospitals. *Pediatrics*. 2002;110(2 pt 1): 414–418

AMERICAN ACADEMY OF PEDIATRICS

POLICY STATEMENT
Organizational Principles to Guide and Define the Child Health Care System and/or Improve the Health of All Children

Committee on Fetus and Newborn

Age Terminology During the Perinatal Period

ABSTRACT. Consistent definitions to describe the length of gestation and age in neonates are needed to compare neurodevelopmental, medical, and growth outcomes. The purposes of this policy statement are to review conventional definitions of age during the perinatal period and to recommend use of standard terminology including gestational age, postmenstrual age, chronological age, corrected age, adjusted age, and estimated date of delivery. *Pediatrics* 2004;114:1362–1364; *gestational age, postmenstrual age, chronological age, menstrual age, conceptional age, postconceptual age, corrected age, adjusted age, estimated date of delivery, estimated date of confinement.*

INTRODUCTION

Consistent definitions to describe the length of gestation and age in neonates are needed to compare neurodevelopmental, medical, and growth outcomes. The terms "gestational age," "postmenstrual age," "corrected age," and "postconceptional age" have frequently been defined unconventionally,[1,2] misapplied,[3–5] or left undefined.[6,7] Inconsistent use of terminology limits the accurate interpretation of data on health outcomes for newborn infants, especially for those born preterm or conceived using assisted reproductive technology. The purposes of this statement are to review conventional definitions of age during the perinatal period and to recommend standard terminology.

"Gestational age" (or "menstrual age") is the time elapsed between the first day of the last normal menstrual period and the day of delivery (Fig 1).[8–10] The first day of the last menstrual period occurs approximately 2 weeks before ovulation and approximately 3 weeks before implantation of the blastocyst. Because most women know when their last period began but not when ovulation occurred, this definition traditionally has been used when estimating the expected date of delivery. As long as menstrual dates are remembered accurately, this method of estimating the date of delivery is reliable.[11] Minor inaccuracy (4–6 days) in the expected date of delivery determined from menstrual dates is attributable to inherent biological variability in the relative timing of onset of the last menstrual period, fertilization of the egg, and implantation of the blastocyst.[12] Additional inaccuracy (weeks) may occur in women

who have menstrual cycles that are irregular or variable in duration or if breakthrough bleeding occurs around the time of conception. Gestational age is conventionally expressed as completed weeks. Therefore, a 25-week, 5-day fetus is considered a 25-week fetus. To round the gestational age of such a fetus to 26 weeks is inconsistent with national and international norms.[2] The term "gestational age" should be used instead of "menstrual age" to describe the age of the fetus or newborn infant.

"Chronological age" (or "postnatal" age) is the time elapsed after birth (Fig 1). It is usually described in days, weeks, months, and/or years. This is different from the term "postmenstrual age." Postmenstrual age is the time elapsed between the first day of the last menstrual period and birth (gestational age) plus the time elapsed after birth (chronological age). Postmenstrual age is usually described in number of weeks and is most frequently applied during the perinatal period beginning after the day of birth. Therefore, a preterm infant born at a gestational age of 33 weeks who is currently 10 weeks old (chronological age) would have a postmenstrual age of 43 weeks. When postmenstrual age is quantitated in weeks and days for postnatal management reasons, a 33-week, 1-day gestational age infant who is 10 weeks, 5 days chronological age would have a postmenstrual age of 43 weeks, 6 days.

"Corrected age" (or "adjusted age") is a term most appropriately used to describe children up to 3 years of age who were born preterm (Fig 1). This term is preferred to "corrected gestational age" or "gestational age" and represents the age of the child from the expected date of delivery.[13,14] Corrected age is calculated by subtracting the number of weeks born before 40 weeks of gestation from the chronological age. Therefore, a 24-month-old, former 28-week gestational age infant has a corrected age of 21 months according to the following equation:

$$24 \text{ months} - [(40 \text{ weeks} - 28 \text{ weeks}) \times 1 \text{ month}/4 \text{ weeks}]$$

Corrected age and chronological age are not synonymous in preterm infants. Additionally, the term "corrected age" should be used instead of "adjusted age."

"Conceptional age" is the time elapsed between the day of conception and the day of delivery. (The term "conceptual age" is incorrect and should not be

doi:10.1542/peds.2004-1915

PEDIATRICS (ISSN 0031 4005). Copyright © 2004 by the American Academy of Pediatrics.

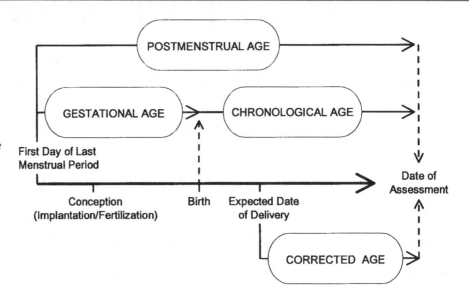

Fig 1. Age terminology during the perinatal period.

used.) Because assisted reproductive technologies accurately define the date of fertilization or implantation, a precise conceptional age can be determined in pregnancies resulting from such technologies. Much of the variability inherent in other methods of gestational age determination,[11–13] except for that attributed to timing of implantation, is eliminated when the date of conception is determined during assisted reproductive procedures. The convention for calculating gestational age when the date of conception is known is to add 2 weeks to the conceptional age.[10] Therefore, gestational age is 2 weeks longer than conceptional age; they are not synonymous terms. When describing the age of a fetus or neonate, "gestational age" is the term conventionally applied. This is particularly important for interpreting outcome studies of preterm infants. As an example, a preterm infant conceived using assisted reproductive technology who has a conceptional age of 25 weeks has a gestational age of 27 weeks. Outcomes for this infant should be compared with those of 27-week gestational age infants, not 25-week gestational age infants. To avoid confusion, the term "gestational age" should be used. The terms "conceptional age" and "postconceptional age," reflecting the time elapsed after conception, should not be used.

Gestational age is often determined by the "best obstetric estimate," which is based on a combination of the first day of last menstrual period, physical examination of the mother, prenatal ultrasonography, and history of assisted reproduction. The best obstetric estimate is necessary because of gaps in obstetric information and the inherent variability (as great as 2 weeks) in methods of gestational age estimation.[8,10,14–19] Postnatal physical examination of the infant is sometimes used as a method to determine gestational age if the best obstetric estimate seems inaccurate. Therefore, methods of determining gestational age should be clearly stated so that the variability inherent in these estimations can be considered when outcomes are interpreted.[8,10,14–19]

RECOMMENDATIONS

1. Standardized terminology should be used when defining ages and comparing outcomes of fetuses and newborns. The recommended terms (Table 1) are:

   - Gestational age (completed weeks): time elapsed between the first day of the last menstrual period and the day of delivery. If pregnancy was achieved using assisted reproductive technology, gestational age is calculated by adding 2 weeks to the conceptional age.
   - Chronological age (days, weeks, months, or years): time elapsed from birth.
   - Postmenstrual age (weeks): gestational age plus chronological age.
   - Corrected age (weeks or months): chronological age reduced by the number of weeks born before 40 weeks of gestation; the term should be used only for children up to 3 years of age who were born preterm.

2. During the perinatal period neonatal hospital stay, "postmenstrual age" is preferred to describe

TABLE 1.   Age Terminology During the Perinatal Period

Term	Definition	Units of Time
Gestational age	Time elapsed between the first day of the last menstrual period and the day of delivery	Completed weeks
Chronological age	Time elapsed since birth	Days, weeks, months, years
Postmenstrual age	Gestational age + chronological age	Weeks
Corrected age	Chronological age reduced by the number of weeks born before 40 weeks of gestation	Weeks, months

the age of preterm infants. After the perinatal period, "corrected age" is the preferred term.

3. "Conceptional age," "postconceptional age," "conceptual age," and "postconceptual age" should not be used in clinical pediatrics.

4. Publications reporting fetal and neonatal outcomes should clearly describe methods used to determine gestational age.

COMMITTEE ON FETUS AND NEWBORN, 2003–2004
Lillian R. Blackmon, MD, Chairperson
Daniel G. Batton, MD
Edward F. Bell, MD
Susan E. Denson, MD
*William A. Engle, MD
William P. Kanto, Jr, MD
Gilbert I. Martin, MD
Ann Stark, MD

LIAISONS
Keith J. Barrington, MD
    Canadian Paediatric Society
Tonse N. K. Raju, MD, DCH
    National Institutes of Health
Laura E. Riley, MD
    American College of Obstetricians and
    Gynecologists
Kay M. Tomashek, MD, MPH
    Centers for Disease Control and Prevention
Carol Wallman, MSN, RNC, NNP
    National Association of Neonatal Nurses

STAFF
Jim Couto, MA

*Lead author

REFERENCES

1. Malloy MH, Hoffman HJ. Prematurity, sudden infant death syndrome, and age of death. *Pediatrics.* 1995;96:464–471

2. Bernstein IM, Horbar JD, Badger GJ, Ohlsson A, Golan A. Morbidity and mortality among very-low-birth-weight neonates with intrauterine growth restriction. The Vermont Oxford Network. *Am J Obstet Gynecol.* 2000;182:198–206

3. Ellenhorn MJ, ed. Toxicokinetics. In: *Ellenhorn's Medical Toxicology: Diagnosis and Treatment of Human Poisoning.* 2nd ed. Philadelphia, PA: Williams and Wilkins; 1997:128–148

4. DeVivo DC, Koenigsberger MR. Intracranial hemorrhage. In: Rudolph AM, ed. *Rudolph's Pediatrics.* 20th ed. Stamford, CT: Appleton & Lange; 1996:1877

5. Moriette G, Paris-Llado S, Walti H, et al. Prospective randomized multicenter comparison of high-frequency oscillatory ventilation and conventional ventilation in preterm infants of less than 30 weeks with respiratory distress syndrome. *Pediatrics.* 2001;107:363–372

6. Ramanathan R, Corwin MJ, Hunt CE, et al. Cardiorespiratory events recorded on home monitors: comparison of healthy infants with those at increased risk for SIDS. *JAMA.* 2001;285:2199–2207

7. Pierrat V, Duquennoy C, van Haastert IC, Ernst M, Guilley N, deVries LS. Ultrasound diagnosis and neurodevelopmental outcome of localized and extensive cystic periventricular leucomalacia. *Arch Dis Child Fetal Neonatal Ed.* 2001;84:F151–F156

8. American Academy of Pediatrics, American College of Obstetricians and Gynecologists. *Guidelines for Perinatal Care.* 5th ed. Washington, DC: American College of Obstetricians and Gynecologists; 2002:378–379

9. Cunningham FG, Gant NF, Gilstrap LC III, Hauth JC, Wenstrom KD, Leveno KJ, eds. *Williams Obstetrics.* 21st ed. New York, NY: McGraw-Hill; 2001:129–165

10. Craven C, Ward K. Embryology, fetus and placenta: normal and abnormal. In: Scott JR, DiSaia PJ, Hammond CB, Spellacy WN, eds. *Danforth's Obstetrics and Gynecology.* 8th ed. Philadelphia, PA: Lippincott Williams & Wilkins; 1999:29–46

11. Rossavik IK, Fishburne JI. Conceptional age, menstrual age, and ultrasound age: a second-trimester comparison of pregnancies dated of known conception date with pregnancies dated from last menstrual period. *Obstet Gynecol.* 1989;73:243–249

12. Shepherd TH. Developmental pathology of the embryonic and previable fetal periods. In: Avery GB, Fletcher MA, MacDonald MG, eds. *Neonatology: Pathophysiology and Management of the Newborn.* 4th ed. Philadelphia, PA: JB Lippincott Co; 1994:109–125

13. Bennett FC. Developmental outcome. In: Avery GB, Fletcher MA, MacDonald MG, eds. *Neonatology: Pathophysiology and Management of the Newborn.* 4th ed. Philadelphia, PA: JB Lippincott Co; 1994:1367–1386

14. DiPietro JA, Allen MC. Estimation of gestational age: implications for developmental research. *Child Dev.* 1991;62:1184–1199

15. Sohaey R, Branch DW. Ultrasound in obstetrics. In: Scott JR, DiSaia PJ, Hammond CB, Spellacy WN, eds. *Danforth's Obstetrics and Gynecology.* 8th ed. Philadelphia, PA: Lippincott Williams & Wilkins; 1999:213–242

16. American Academy of Pediatrics, American College of Obstetrics and Gynecology. *Guidelines for Perinatal Care.* 5th ed. Washington, DC: American College of Obstetrics and Gynecology; 2002:199–202

17. Goldenberg RL, Davis RO, Cutter GR, Hoffman HJ, Brumfield CG, Foster JM. Prematurity, postdates, and growth retardation: the influence of use of ultrasonography on reported gestational age. *Am J Obstet Gynecol.* 1989;160:462–470

18. Berg AT. Menstrual cycle length and calculation of gestational age. *Am J Epidemiol.* 1991;133:585–589

19. Mustafa G, David RJ. Comparative accuracy of clinical estimate versus menstrual gestational age in computerized birth certificates. *Public Health Rep.* 2001;116:15–21

AMERICAN ACADEMY OF PEDIATRICS

POLICY STATEMENT

Organizational Principles to Guide and Define the Child Health Care System and/or Improve the Health of All Children

Committee on Fetus and Newborn

Controversies Concerning Vitamin K and the Newborn

ABSTRACT. Prevention of early vitamin K deficiency bleeding (VKDB) of the newborn, with onset at birth to 2 weeks of age (formerly known as classic hemorrhagic disease of the newborn), by oral or parenteral administration of vitamin K is accepted practice. In contrast, late VKDB, with onset from 2 to 12 weeks of age, is most effectively prevented by parenteral administration of vitamin K. Earlier concern regarding a possible causal association between parenteral vitamin K and childhood cancer has not been substantiated. This revised statement presents updated recommendations for the use of vitamin K in the prevention of early and late VKDB.

ABBREVIATION. VKDB, vitamin K deficiency bleeding.

BACKGROUND

Vitamin K deficiency may cause unexpected bleeding (0.25%–1.7% incidence) during the first week of life in previously healthy-appearing neonates (early vitamin K deficiency bleeding [VKDB] of the newborn [formerly known as classic hemorrhagic disease of the newborn]). The efficacy of neonatal vitamin K prophylaxis (oral or parenteral) in the prevention of early VKDB is firmly established. It has been the standard of care since the American Academy of Pediatrics recommended it in 1961.[1]

Late VKDB, a syndrome defined as unexpected bleeding attributable to severe vitamin K deficiency in infants 2 to 12 weeks of age, occurs primarily in exclusively breastfed infants who have received no or inadequate neonatal vitamin K prophylaxis. In addition, infants who have intestinal malabsorption defects (cholestatic jaundice, cystic fibrosis, etc) may also have late VKDB. The rate of late VKDB (often manifesting as sudden central nervous system hemorrhage) ranges from 4.4 to 7.2 per 100 000 births, according to reports from Europe and Asia.[2,3] When a single dose of oral vitamin K has been used for neonatal prophylaxis, the rate has decreased to 1.4 to 6.4 per 100 000 births. Parenteral neonatal vitamin K prophylaxis prevents the development of late VKDB in infants, with the rare exception of those with severe malabsorption syndromes.[2]

Oral administration of vitamin K has been shown to have efficacy similar to that of parenteral administration in the prevention of early VKDB.[4–6] However, several countries have reported a resurgence of late VKDB coincident with policies promoting the use of orally administered prophylaxis, even with multiple-dose regimens. In a 1997 review of these experiences by Cornelissen et al,[7] surveillance data from 4 countries revealed oral prophylaxis failures of 1.2 to 1.8 per 100 000 live births, compared with no reported cases after intramuscular administration. Newborns receiving incomplete oral prophylaxis tended to have a higher risk of developing VKDB, with rates of approximately 2 to 4 per 100 000. Small daily oral doses, as practiced in the Netherlands, may decrease the risk of late VKDB[8] and approach the efficacy of the parenteral route; however, this needs to be better studied.

Draper and Stiller,[9] using other data from Great Britain, have questioned the results of earlier studies of Golding et al[10,11] that attempted to show an association between intramuscular vitamin K administration in newborns and an increased incidence of childhood cancer. Using data from the National Registry of Childhood Tumors, they estimated the cumulative incidence of childhood leukemia. Three sources of data, including the estimates from Golding et al, provided rates of intramuscular vitamin K use over the same time frame. Their analyses failed to show a correlation between increased use of intramuscular vitamin K and the incidence of childhood leukemia.

The Vitamin K Ad Hoc Task Force of the American Academy of Pediatrics[12] reviewed the reports of Golding et al and other information regarding the US experience[13] and concluded that there was no association between the intramuscular administration of vitamin K and childhood leukemia or other cancers.

Additional studies that have since been conducted by other investigators have not supported a clinical relationship between newborn parenteral administration of vitamin K and childhood cancer. Ross and Davies[14] published a review of the evidence in 2000. They found no randomized or quasi-randomized evidence of an association between parenteral vitamin K prophylaxis and cancer in childhood. Ten case-control studies were identified, of which 7 found no relationship and 3 found only a weak relationship of neonatal administration of intramuscular or intravenous vitamin K with the risk of solid childhood tumors or leukemia.

PEDIATRICS (ISSN 0031 4005). Copyright © 2003 by the American Academy of Pediatrics.

Recent research on the pathogenesis of childhood leukemia additionally weakens the plausibility of a causal relationship between parenteral administration of vitamin K and cancer. Investigations by Wiemels et al[15] suggest a prenatal origin of childhood leukemia. They found an acute lymphocytic leukemia-associated gene in 12 children with newly diagnosed acute lymphocytic leukemia and postulated that an in utero chromosomal translocation event combined with a postnatal promotional event results in clinical leukemia. Although intramuscular administration of vitamin K could conceivably be a postnatal promotional event, a genetic etiologic explanation further lessens the likelihood of a clinically significant relationship between intramuscular administration of vitamin K and leukemia.

There is concern that adequate vitamin K prophylaxis be provided to the increasing numbers of newborns who are breastfed exclusively to avoid an increased risk of late VKDB with its associated intracranial hemorrhage.[7]

RECOMMENDATIONS

Because parenteral vitamin K has been shown to prevent VKDB of the newborn and young infant and the risks of cancer have been unproven, the American Academy of Pediatrics recommends the following:

1. Vitamin K_1 should be given to all newborns as a single, intramuscular dose of 0.5 to 1 mg.[16]
2. Additional research should be conducted on the efficacy, safety, and bioavailability of oral formulations and optimal dosing regimens of vitamin K to prevent late VKDB.
3. Health care professionals should promote awareness among families of the risks of late VKDB associated with inadequate vitamin K prophylaxis from current oral dosage regimens, particularly for newborns who are breastfed exclusively.

COMMITTEE ON FETUS AND NEWBORN, 2002–2003
Lillian Blackmon, MD, Chairperson
Daniel G. Batton, MD
Edward F. Bell, MD
William A. Engle, MD
William P. Kanto, Jr, MD
Gilbert I. Martin, MD
Warren Rosenfeld, MD
Ann R. Stark, MD

*Carol A. Miller, MD
   Past Committee Member

LIAISONS
Keith J. Barrington, MD
   Canadian Paediatric Society

Tonse Raju, MD, DCH
   National Institutes of Health
Laura E. Riley, MD
   American College of Obstetricians and Gynecologists
Kay M. Tomashek, MD
   Centers for Disease Control and Prevention
Carol Wallman, MSN, RNC, NNP
   National Association of Neonatal Nurses

STAFF
Jim Couto, MA

*Lead author

REFERENCES

1. American Academy of Pediatrics, Committee on Nutrition. Vitamin K compounds and the water-soluble analogues: use in therapy and prophylaxis in pediatrics. *Pediatrics*. 1961;28:501–507
2. von Kreis R, Hanawa Y. Neonatal vitamin K prophylaxis. Report of Scientific and Standardization Subcommittee on Perinatal Haemostasis. *Thromb Haemost*. 1993;69:293–295
3. Motohara K, Endo F, Matsuda I. Screening for late neonatal vitamin K deficiency by acarboxyprothrombin in dried blood spots. *Arch Dis Child*. 1987;62:370–375
4. O'Connor ME, Addiego JE Jr. Use of oral vitamin K_1 to prevent hemorrhagic disease of the newborn infant. *J Pediatr*. 1986;108:616–619
5. McNinch AW, Upton C, Samuels M, et al. Plasma concentrations after oral or intramuscular vitamin K_1 in neonates. *Arch Dis Child*. 1985;60:814–818
6. Schubiger G, Gruter J, Shearer MJ. Plasma vitamin K_1 and PIVKA-II after oral administration of mixed-micellar or cremophor EL-solubilized preparations of vitamin K_1 to normal breast-fed newborns. *J Pediatr Gastroenterol Nutr*. 1997;24:280–284
7. Cornelissen M, Von Kreis R, Loughnan P, Schubiger G. Prevention of vitamin K deficiency bleeding: efficacy of different multiple oral dose schedules of vitamin K. *Eur J Pediatr*. 1997;156:126–130
8. von Kreis R, Hachmeister A, Gobel U. Can 3 oral 2 mg doses of vitamin K effectively prevent late vitamin K deficiency bleeding? *Eur J Pediatr*. 1999;158(suppl 3):S183–S186
9. Draper GJ, Stiller CA. Intramuscular vitamin K and childhood cancer. *BMJ*. 1992;305:709
10. Golding J, Paterson M, Kinlen LJ. Factors associated with childhood cancer in a national cohort study. *Br J Cancer*. 1990;62:304–308
11. Golding J, Greenwood R, Birmingham K, Mott M. Childhood cancer, intramuscular vitamin K, and pethidine given during labour. *BMJ*. 1992;305:341–346
12. American Academy of Pediatrics, Vitamin K Ad Hoc Task Force. Controversies concerning vitamin K and the newborn. *Pediatrics*. 1993;91:1001–1003
13. Devesa SS, Silverman DT, Young JL Jr, et al. Cancer incidence and mortality trends among whites in the United States, 1947–84. *J Natl Cancer Inst*. 1987;79:701–770
14. Ross JA, Davies SM. Vitamin K prophylaxis and childhood cancer. *Med Pediatr Oncol*. 2000;34:434–437
15. Wiemels JL, Cazzaniga G, Daniotti M, et al. Prenatal origin of acute lymphoblastic leukaemia in children. *Lancet*. 1999;354:1499–1503
16. American Academy of Pediatrics, American College of Obstetricians and Gynecologists. *Guidelines for Perinatal Care*. 3rd ed. Washington, DC: American College of Obstetricians and Gynecologists; 1992

CLINICAL REPORT   Guidance for the Clinician in Rendering Pediatric Care

American Academy
of Pediatrics

DEDICATED TO THE HEALTH OF ALL CHILDREN™

Disaster Preparedness in Neonatal Intensive Care Units

Wanda D. Barfield, MD, MPH, FAAP, RADM USPHS,[a] Steven E. Krug, MD, FAAP,[b,c] COMMITTEE ON FETUS AND NEWBORN, DISASTER PREPAREDNESS ADVISORY COUNCIL

abstract

Disasters disproportionally affect vulnerable, technology-dependent people, including preterm and critically ill newborn infants. It is important for health care providers to be aware of and prepared for the potential consequences of disasters for the NICU. Neonatal intensive care personnel can provide specialized expertise for their hospital, community, and regional emergency preparedness plans and can help develop institutional surge capacity for mass critical care, including equipment, medications, personnel, and facility resources.

Disasters, whether natural or man-made, are especially threatening to the lives of people who are technology dependent. This is particularly true in the NICU. During a disaster, the provision of highly skilled and specialized care for preterm and critically ill newborn infants can be compromised by the loss of electrical power, physical facilities, specialized equipment, personnel, and other resources that can occur as a result of environmental disruption or large-scale illness, injury, or trauma. There is a paucity of data regarding the effect of disasters on the NICU population and practice implications for providers within the health care system.[1]

This clinical report first briefly reviews disasters that have affected NICUs in the United States and then examines how organizing concepts of mass critical care in pediatrics can be applied to the NICU, including the role of regionalized perinatal systems; disaster-based drills; and training, equipment, medication, and personnel needs. The objective of this report is to help neonatologists and other NICU providers and administrative leaders understand these organizing concepts and develop response plans within their units, hospital institutions, and geographic regions. This report builds on existing American Academy of Pediatrics policies concerning children in disasters, with a focus on the extremely vulnerable NICU population, and also discusses ethical issues related to surge capacity, altered standards, and atypical locations of care, evacuation, triage, and transport.

[a]Centers for Disease Control and Prevention, Atlanta, Georgia; [b]Northwestern University Feinberg School of Medicine, Evanston, Illinois; and [c]Department of Pediatric Emergency Medicine, Ann and Robert H. Lurie Children's Hospital, Chicago, Illinois

Drs Barfield and Krug were each responsible for all aspects of writing and editing the document and reviewing and responding to questions and comments from reviewers and the Board of Directors.

This document is copyrighted and is property of the American Academy of Pediatrics and its Board of Directors. All authors have filed conflict of interest statements with the American Academy of Pediatrics. Any conflicts have been resolved through a process approved by the Board of Directors. The American Academy of Pediatrics has neither solicited nor accepted any commercial involvement in the development of the content of this publication.

Clinical reports from the American Academy of Pediatrics benefit from expertise and resources of liaisons and internal (AAP) and external reviewers. However, clinical reports from the American Academy of Pediatrics may not reflect the views of the liaisons or the organizations or government agencies that they represent.

The guidance in this report does not indicate an exclusive course of treatment or serve as a standard of medical care. Variations, taking into account individual circumstances, may be appropriate.

All clinical reports from the American Academy of Pediatrics automatically expire 5 years after publication unless reaffirmed, revised, or retired at or before that time.

The findings and conclusions in this manuscript are those of the authors and do not necessarily represent the official position of the Centers for Disease Control and Prevention.

DOI: 10.1542/peds.2017-0507

Address correspondence to Wanda D. Barfield, MD, MPH, FAAP, RADM USPHS. E-mail: wjb5@cdc.gov

To cite: Barfield WD, Krug SE, AAP COMMITTEE ON FETUS AND NEWBORN, AAP DISASTER PREPAREDNESS ADVISORY COUNCIL. Disaster Preparedness in Neonatal Intensive Care Units. Pediatrics. 2017;139(5):e20170507

TABLE 1 Examples of Disaster Effects on NICU Populations

Disaster Type	General Examples	Potential Effects on NICU Patients
Natural disaster	Hurricane Katrina, Superstorm Sandy	Loss of electrical power and life-sustaining equipment
		Particulate matter or droplets from debris that can affect skin or airways[a,b]
		Increased risk of infection or injury during transfer or evacuation to another hospital
		Exposure to temperature extremes; inability to minimize effects of conduction, convection, evaporation, and radiation
		Constraints on adequate nutrition/caloric intake
		Limited medication doses available
		Increased risk of neonatal conditions related to maternal stress
		Loss of clean water
		Possible carbon monoxide poisoning from generators
Industrial disaster	Radiologic disasters, chemical spills	Disruption of fetus'/infant's growing organ systems
		Radiation/carcinogen exposure that may lead to long-term effects
		Contamination of water sources
Pandemic infectious diseases	H1N1 influenza, Ebola virus disease, Zika virus	Infection control and medical countermeasure challenges
		Need for patient isolation
		Increased maternal illness, preterm birth, or birth defects
		Risk to first responders, hospital staff, and caregivers
Bioterrorist event	2001 anthrax attacks, aerosol release of smallpox, 1995 sarin attack in Tokyo subway	Nonspecific syndromic symptoms
		Limited access to postexposure vaccination
		Selection criteria for administering vaccine
		Jeopardized safety of first-response team

[a] http://pediatrics.aappublications.org/content/early/2015/10/13/peds.2015-3112.long.
[b] www.fs.fed.us/rm/value/docs/health_economic_impact_wildfire.pdf.

BACKGROUND

A disaster is defined as a sudden, calamitous event, natural or man-made, that seriously disrupts the functioning of a community or society and causes human, material, and economic or environmental losses that exceed the community's or society's ability to cope using its own resources.[2] NICU patients are particularly vulnerable, not only because of their small size and physiologic immaturity, but also because of their baseline dependence on technology for warmth, nutritional supplementation, medication administration, cardiorespiratory monitoring, diagnostic information gathering, and life-sustaining physiologic support. Disasters not only can cause direct danger or injury to NICU patients, but may also affect their caregivers, parents, and families. Disasters may disrupt a NICU patient's protective surroundings, including light, warmth, electricity, oxygen, and air as well as diagnostic and therapeutic resources, such as medications, cardiorespiratory monitors, incubators, ventilators, blood gas machines, and imaging devices. Different types of disasters may affect NICU operations and capabilities in different ways (Table 1).

Natural Disasters (Hurricanes, Earthquakes, Superstorms, and Wildfires)

Hurricane Katrina was one of the largest threats to NICU patients in US history, because it disabled the health care system's ability to provide adequate care in a large, densely populated area because of the loss of supplies, personnel, communications, and infrastructure.[3] Hurricane Katrina caused extensive flood damage and electrical power loss to hospitals caring for critically ill newborn infants and resulted in mass evacuation efforts that were suboptimally coordinated.[4] Although all neonates in the affected hospitals survived, and many hospitals received evacuated neonates, there was a surge in NICU patients at the hospital receiving the most transports from the affected area, from 55 to 125 patients in 3 days.[4] This event illustrated the need for advance development of systemwide plans for maintenance of neonatal critical care under adverse conditions, local and regional neonatal care coordination and communication, interfacility patient transport, and NICU evacuation because of extensive flood damage and hospital closures.[5]

Hurricane Sandy also affected providers' ability to care for women with high-risk pregnancies and newborn infants in metropolitan New York.[6–8] However, in this instance, when Hurricane Sandy caused a power outage in a New York City medical center, 21 neonates were evacuated to other hospitals in the city in less than 5 hours. These transfers were accomplished with no known mortalities, which may be credited to that medical center's advance planning, with a clear command structure, overall regional coordination, and the availability of backups in the form of personnel, information, and equipment.[6]

Infectious Epidemics (H1N1 Pandemic Influenza, Ebola Virus Disease, and Other Emerging Infections)

Infectious disease outbreaks and pandemics may uniquely and disproportionately affect pregnant women and their fetuses as well as newborn and critically ill infants.[9,10] For example, the H1N1 influenza pandemic in 2009 was associated with significantly increased morbidity and mortality in otherwise healthy pregnant women and their infants. In addition, experts identified a potential risk of transmission from infected health care workers, family members, and mothers of high-risk newborn infants.[11] Most recently, Zika virus, a *Flavivirus* transmitted by *Aedes* mosquitoes, has been associated with significant congenital central nervous system abnormalities, including microcephaly, in some newborn infants of women infected during pregnancy.[12,13] Other emerging infections, such as Ebola, are rare, but can have severe effects; viral hemorrhagic fevers pose significant mortality risks to pregnant, laboring, and postpartum women, who may experience substantial bleeding and multiorgan system failure.[14] To date, the survival of newborn infants delivered to women with confirmed Ebola virus disease is poor; although the mechanism is not well understood, most infants are stillborn or die in the early neonatal period.[15–17] Strict adherence to infection control practices and the use of protective personnel equipment are critical for the safety of patients, family members, hospital staff, and the community.[18]

Bioterrorism (Anthrax, Smallpox, Other Biological Weapons, and Chemical Agents)

Certain biological or chemical agents dispersed by accident or intentionally would leave neonatal populations particularly vulnerable, because signs and symptoms in the newborn infant may be systemic and nonspecific. For example, anthrax (*Bacillus anthracis* infection) can present in several different ways because of multiple routes of infection (inhalational, cutaneous, and gastrointestinal). Infection can rapidly progress to systemic disease, which has a high mortality rate and requires rapid initiation of postexposure prophylaxis and/or antimicrobial treatment.[19] Data on anthrax in newborn populations are limited.[20–22] Many biologic (eg, plague and smallpox) or radiologic (eg, radioactive iodine) agents target dividing cells; therefore, the mass dispersion of such agents would particularly adversely affect growing children, especially infants.[23,24]

Defining Emergency Mass Critical Care for NICUs

Emergency mass critical care (EMCC) is defined as the immediate need for critical care resources, including staff, medical equipment, supplies, medications, and ICU space, to provide timely, effective care to a large population surge of critically ill victims during a disaster.[25] A mass casualty critical care event affecting the NICU may put many vulnerable patients at risk for limited life-sustaining interventions because of deficiencies in facilities, supplies, or staffing. If disaster events are prolonged, they can also affect the abilities of responders to provide sustained care for those affected. For optimal care of vulnerable NICU patients, specific advance plans for their acute care, stabilization, triage, transfer, and evacuation must be put in place. In 2010, a select pediatric task force developed a framework of pediatric EMCC capable of tripling critical care capabilities for a period of up to 10 days.[26] The unique challenges presented by pregnant women, newborn infants, and NICU patients were acknowledged, including concerns for surge capacity among these vulnerable populations.[1,27] Targeted surge capacity may be required in hospitals at varying distances from the affected hospital, depending on the nature of the disaster, so community and regional plans should be coordinated if possible.

During large and/or prolonged public health emergencies, crisis standards of care may be necessary. Crisis standards are defined as substantial changes in usual health care operations and the level of care delivered, made necessary by a pervasive or catastrophic disaster.[28] The institution of these standards is intended to optimize population outcomes rather than individual survival. In this scenario, available resources (eg, medications, ventilators, and staff) may become limited and could be substituted, adapted, or reallocated. Preparation for EMCC in NICUs must consider whether the initiation of life-saving interventions can be sustained in the context of a disaster scenario with limited resources as well as the effect on long-term survival. Changes in care and the ways in which such care is delivered may be made necessary by the nature of the disaster. In such circumstances, state and federal governmental entities may take steps to limit or eliminate some legal obligations and liabilities.[28–31] Therefore, coordinated planning with the hospital facility, community, state, and region is essential in preparing for disasters in NICUs.

THE ROLE OF NICU PROVIDERS IN EMCC PLANNING

Developing a Plan

Most NICUs are part of a larger department (eg, pediatrics or obstetrics) within an even larger facility (general or children's hospital). Nevertheless, a 2008 survey of US hospitals found that, although most facilities had memoranda of understanding between hospitals to transfer adult patients during an epidemic, fewer hospitals had memoranda of understanding for pediatric patients; in 2014, fewer than half of hospitals with an emergency department had a disaster plan for children.[32,33] Improving disaster preparedness for critically ill newborn infants will require neonatal care providers to participate in the larger plan of emergency preparedness within hospitals, communities, states, and regions. In certain disasters, the personnel and equipment necessary to care for critically ill patients may need to come from other facilities, including those across state lines, which may require plans for shared clinical credentialing within a region. When a governor declares a state of emergency and federal public health and medical resources are activated, licensed providers (physicians, nurses, pharmacists, and respiratory therapists) on emergency medical response teams from other regions can provide care to affected areas.[34] Therefore, regional plans may include a method to determine specific competencies within facilities so patients can be transferred to centers with appropriate capabilities.[35]

Several useful resources are available to help clinicians and hospitals prepare for disasters.

1. The Emergency Medical Services for Children Innovation and Improvement Center (https://emscimprovement.center/): This center is supported by the Health Resources and Services Administration of the US Department of Health and Human Services, and provides a comprehensive database of resources for pediatric disaster preparedness.

2. The California Hospital Association's Hospital Preparedness Program (www.calhospitalprepare.org/): This program is funded by the Office of the Assistant Secretary for Preparedness and Response (www.phe.gov/about/pages/default.aspx) to support California hospitals and other health systems in an all-hazards disaster planning approach. The Web site contains a large selection of resources for facility, regional, and state planning, including disaster drills, classes, and draft agreements. In addition to an annual conference, California Hospital Association's Hospital Preparedness Program provides classes and technical assistance and warehouses other regional, state, and federal resources.

3. The Pediatric Preparedness Resource Kit of the American Academy of Pediatrics (www.aap.org/en-us/advocacy-and-policy/aap-health-initiatives/Children-and-Disasters/Documents/PedPreparednessKit.pdf): This kit was developed to encourage partnerships and joint decision-making between pediatricians and state and/or local health department representatives, and includes information and strategies to promote strategic communications and effective messaging in disasters.

4. The New York City Pediatric Disaster Coalition's customizable Neonatal Critical Care Surge Capacity Plan (www.programinfosite.com/peds/files/2012/12/Pediatric-Disaster-Coalition-Template-NICU-Surge-Plan-docx.pdf): This plan provides a template for improving disaster-related surge capacity. The document outlines topics such as creating a rapid discharge team, enlisting additional staff, and ensuring availability of medications, code carts, and decontamination operations.

5. The Technical Resources, Assistance Center, and Information Exchange (TRACIE; https://asprtracie.hhs.gov/): This program is operated by the US Department of Health and Human Services, Office of the Assistant Secretary for Preparedness and Response, to address disaster medicine and emergency preparedness inquiries from health care providers and entities.

6. The National Library of Medicine Disaster Information Management Research Center (https://disaster.nlm.nih.gov): This site provides the most recent research regarding disaster impact and preparedness, emergency readiness tools, and research resources.

7. The Centers for Disease Control and Prevention (CDC) (www.cdc.gov): In addition to Web resources, the CDC provides technical assistance in response to public inquiries and clinician outreach calls as well as direct technical assistance for outbreak investigation and reporting and surveillance of disasters.

NICU Emergency Preparedness Plans

Developing and maintaining NICU emergency preparedness plans that include consideration of the total hospital patient populations, as well as community and regional resources, can improve the capacity to care for critically ill newborn infants during a disaster. Given the need of many NICU patients for intense technology support, planning for sufficient power during a disaster is critical, including backup generators. Backup power sources must be located in safe locations (protected by appropriate construction in earthquake-prone areas and high enough off the ground in flood-prone areas). Planning can also include discharge of relatively healthy newborn infants to the mother and family, with follow-up with a primary care provider, or transfer of convalescent patients to lower-level facilities.[35] In some circumstances, complete NICU evacuation may be indicated.

Certain epidemics (eg, H1N1) may disproportionately affect the population of pregnant women and may increase preterm deliveries and the need for NICU care.[36] Disasters may also increase demand for specialized equipment, such as ventilators, to care for all critically ill patients and may limit equipment and staffing available to newborn infants.[37] Because NICU bed capacity is not necessarily determined by a regional need–based formula, the strain of a major disaster could affect NICU resources in an unpredictable manner.[38]

Staffing Support for Safe and Effective Operations During a Disaster

Planning for a sustained disaster event involves calculating potential surge capacity, usually considered to be the ability to handle up to 3 times a facility's maximum capacity for a period of 10 days.[26,27] Because staff with highly specialized skills may be particularly limited during prolonged disaster situations, it is important to consider cross-training staff for the care of recovering preterm or critically ill infants. These care providers may include staff from other areas of the hospital who have either received training in advance or "just in time" to provide EMCC.[39] Cross-training of primary care pediatric, surgical, or ICU staff also may help to build surge capacity and institutional resilience. Clinical staff from other hospitals, including local volunteer groups or the Medical Reserve Corps, may be available.[34] Patient-provider ratios in disasters may need to be altered from the usual standards to address the needs of a larger number of patients. Depending on the type of disaster, alternative provider configurations (eg, non-NICU staff) may need to be considered.

Several hospitals have developed and tested disaster preparedness systems.[40] The Good Samaritan Hospital in Northern California developed a series of templates to assist in emergency operations, including staffing, bedside backpacks, mobile disaster boxes, and premade forms (eg, "go-kits") to document patient care (available at: www.calhospitalprepare.org/continuity-planning). These hospitals also provide resources for testing equipment, rotating inventory, and training staff in developing response protocols. The St Louis Children's Hospital has improved communication among physicians and families concerning bed availability and patient transport and has piloted a new computer-based bed management system to accelerate patient placement and service (BJC HealthCare, St. Louis Children's Hospital; available at: www.stlouischildrens.org/health-care-professionals/publications/doctors-digest/january-2012/surge-plan-readies-hospital-perio.)

Drills and exercises are important components of maintaining disaster readiness among NICU providers and staff, modifying scenarios and objectives for specific situations. The Federal Emergency Management Agency's Community Emergency Response Team drills and exercises (www.fema.gov/media-library/assets/documents/27997) are an excellent resource. These full-scale exercises include a sample scenario, the use of volunteers from outside agencies to fill various victim roles, altered site logistics, and postexercise feedback for participants. These exercises could be tailored to include NICU patients.

Family Care During Disasters

During major disasters, providers may need to identify and address additional psychosocial needs of family members beyond what may be anticipated in nondisaster settings.[41–46] Providers should consider and plan for the possibility that either the disaster itself or medical necessity will result in infants being separated from their mothers and/or other family members. Lessons learned from previous disasters include challenges because of forced relocation or evacuation, staffing shortages, and security concerns. Keeping mother and baby together is important to support bonding and breastfeeding. Opportunities to incorporate family-centered care principles should be considered because family members could assist in routine care and feeding of their infants during critical staff shortages.[41] When keeping the maternal-infant dyad together is not possible, a tracking system for patients who have been transferred should be in place. Safety and security should also be considered in disasters because standard modes of patient visitation may be compromised. In infectious outbreaks, if isolation is necessary, a postpartum mother and her newborn should be placed in isolation together if medically feasible. If separation is unavoidable, parents should receive written documentation of where their infant will be and how to contact their child's care providers.[42] Multiple family contact numbers should be obtained and kept with the infant's record, and efforts should be made to maintain contact with the parents and keep them as involved as possible in decision-making around the care of the infant.[43] Disaster planning should also include consideration of the psychosocial needs of families, who likely are already considerably stressed as a result of their critically ill child. Primary care providers should be considered as a potential resource for supporting affected families.[44–46]

Transfer/Evacuation

Because transfer of patients to unaffected locations or evacuation of both patients and personnel may be necessary in disasters, such plans should be arranged in advance whenever possible. NICU evacuation planning should ensure coordinated communication with transport teams and receiving hospitals. Planning may also include the use of specialized equipment (eg, moveable incubators or multiinfant carriers) for difficult terrain (eg, stairs). Planning should also prepare for possible separation of infants from their parents, families, or guardians. Evacuation plans should include a mechanism to identify and track NICU patients and caregivers during and after the disaster. Examples of evacuations plans specific to newborn infants include:

1. The New York City Pediatric Disaster Coalition NICU Evacuation Plan: This plan can be tailored to any institution (New York City Pediatric Disaster Coalition: A Plan Outline for NICU Evacuation [www. programinfosite.com/peds/files/ 2012/12/Pediatric-Disaster-Coalition-Template-NICU-Evacuation-Plan.pdf]). The plan outline includes maintaining emergency equipment, establishing a chain of command for urgent and nonurgent evacuations, assigning staff roles, and establishing designated evacuation areas.

2. A NICU/nursery evacuation tabletop exercise toolkit, created by Illinois Emergency Medical Services for Children, based on the Homeland Security Exercise and Evaluation Program (Illinois Emergency Medical Services for Children: NICU/Nursery Evacuation Tabletop Exercise Toolkit. 2013 [www.luhs.org/ depts/emsc/NICU_Nursery_ EvacuationTTX_Toolkit_FINAL. pdf]). These tabletop exercises are designed for training staff, gathering information to educate and improve emergency plans and responses, and identifying weaknesses in existing plans.

Sharing Resources With Hospital and Community

A mass critical care event may require a shift or reallocation of technology resources (Fig 1). Pooling resources from other departments and hospitals may also enable the provision of a more sustained response to an emergency. In the event of a major loss or depletion of medical countermeasures (MCMs), such as vaccines, antidotes, medications, and equipment, regional authorities can request support from the US Department of Health and Human Services, including support for the care of critically ill newborn infants. A national cache of medical supplies for use in disasters, the "Strategic National Stockpile," is maintained and can be dispersed as authorized by the CDC.[47]

Medical Countermeasures

In addition to maintaining surge capacity, there may be situations in which MCMs are warranted. MCMs are defined as medications, antitoxins, vaccines, immunoglobulins, medical devices, and age-appropriate life-saving medical equipment required to protect or treat children for possible chemical, biological, radiologic, nuclear, or explosive threats.[48] For example, during the H1N1 pandemic, the US Food and Drug Administration (FDA) provided emergency use authorization of oseltamivir for infants younger than 1 year of age.[49] In addition, in December 2012, the FDA approved raxibacumab to prevent and treat inhalational anthrax in adult and pediatric populations, using human safety and animal efficacy study results.[50] Although such emergency dosing may be warranted in disasters, additional research is needed to appropriately measure antimicrobial concentrations and assess the efficacy and safety of MCMs in newborn infants, including preterm infants. Agencies, such as the FDA,

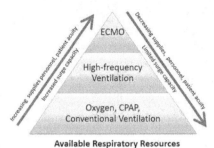

Available Respiratory Resources

FIGURE 1

Model of decision-making based on available supplies: example using respiratory support. The figure shows a model of decision-making based on available supplies, personnel, patient acuity, and surge capacity for pediatric EMCC. CPAP, continuous positive airway pressure; ECMO, extracorporeal membrane oxygenation. Reproduced with permission from Bohn D, Kanter RK, Burns J, Barfield WD, Kissoon N. Supplies and equipment for pediatric emergency mass critical care. *Pediatr Crit Care Med.* 2011;12(suppl 6):S120–S127. Copyright © 2011 Wolters Kluwer Health.

the CDC, and the National Institutes of Health, can collaborate to make specific medications available as needed during disasters, through state public health agencies. The Biomedical Advanced Research and Development Authority develops and procures needed MCMs against a broad array of public health threats, whether natural or intentional in origin. To meet the needs of neonates and children exposed to public health emergencies, sufficient amounts of MCMs appropriate for children of all ages should be present in caches, such as the Strategic National Stockpile.[37,47]

Nutrition and Human Milk

Nutritional supplies for NICU patients may become strained in disasters because of limited supplies of parenteral and enteral nutrition, including infant formula, supplemental vitamins, and trace elements. Agencies, such as the Supplemental Nutrition Program for Women, Infants, and Children, state health departments through the Maternal Child Health Bureau's Title V programs, milk banks, and private organizations, can assist with the provision of nutritional supplies.

Whenever feasible, a mother's own milk should be made available to infants, particularly those who are critically ill, because it is the safest form of nutrition in a disaster.

Ethical Considerations

Ethical dilemmas exist in the routine care of extremely preterm and medically complex infants,[51,52] but additional challenges occur during disasters. Ethics in medical practice include 4 key principles: (1) respect for autonomy; (2) nonmaleficence ("do no harm"); (3) beneficence; and (4) justice. During a disaster, the principle of justice becomes dominant, with 2 ethical theories mostly considered. The first theory, utilitarianism, states that actions are correct if they provide the greatest good for the greatest number of people. The second theory, egalitarianism, stresses equal distribution of resources for all individuals. These theories can be considered for a hospital's decision matrix to guide ethical questions and resolutions during a disaster.[53–55]

Providing a specific approach to ethical decision-making during disasters has been challenging. In 2010, the Pediatric Emergency Mass Critical Care Task Force met to discuss recommendations for US pediatric surge planning and allocation of resources.[56] The Task Force acknowledged the need for an objective tool to help predict the benefit of resource use. However, it noted that developing a reliable tool was challenging given the dependence of many tools on the use of technology for assessment (eg, response to ventilator support). The Task Force was reluctant to recommend expert opinion as a way to allocate limited resources and instead suggested either a system of queuing (eg, first come, first served) or lottery.

Nevertheless, NICU teams have a duty and opportunity to plan and anticipate ethical considerations before disasters. Because hospital ethics committees serve as advisory boards during dilemmas in neonatal care under standard operating conditions, these committees should become more familiar with potential disaster scenarios and assist with decisions in mass critical care, including altered standards of care and withholding or withdrawing life-sustaining treatment.[28,57] In disaster conditions, decisions for initiation or continuation of medical care may shift from the needs of the individual to the needs of the wider community, because decision-makers must determine how to allocate resources in a way that is substantial to all in need.[54,56] If decisions are made not to initiate or to withdraw support, families should be counseled and infants should be provided comfort care.[57]

Recovery From Prolonged Disaster Events

A disaster is a significant stressor, not only for patients and families, but also for NICU staff. In addition to the personal and family impact of a disaster, staff may be affected by their prolonged efforts and by the anguish of not being able to deliver usual intensive care and the resulting influence on patient outcomes. There are unique aspects that confront providers in an ICU setting in the context of a disaster. Altered standards of care include triage; decisions made because of limited resources may result in the death or disability of critically ill infants who might have otherwise survived under usual circumstances. Facing these difficult decisions may be extremely stressful to providers. It is important to consider the length of shifts, the length of response, incorporation of breaks, and psychosocial support of staff and their families. After a disaster event, the need for staff debriefing and counseling should be anticipated. Self-care, both during and after the event, is an important aspect of maintaining resilience in

disasters.[58,59] When possible in a prolonged disaster, relief teams can be brought in to allow respite for the on-site caretakers. Lastly, NICU providers will benefit from family preparedness planning before a disaster event because they will be better able to address the needs of patients and be aware of the well-being of loved ones.

CONCLUSIONS

Infants in the NICU are highly vulnerable in a disaster because of their need for specialized and highly technical support. As such, NICU preparedness is required for optimal disaster response.

1. Preparation before a disaster event is critical to optimizing outcomes of NICU patients during public health emergencies and disasters. Health care institutions and providers are strongly encouraged to know and prepare for the most likely disaster scenarios in their communities (eg, hurricane, earthquake, or flood) and also to consider unanticipated events (eg, bioterrorism) that could create a mass casualty event and similarly affect surge capacity and capabilities.

2. It is important for NICU teams to fully participate in the emergency- and disaster-planning activities of their facility, health care system, or regional, state, and local emergency management agency. Teams should be part of the periodic disaster simulation drills that are now required in every hospital. NICU teams should actively participate in the design of hospital drills to address the unique needs of NICU patients in situations involving "shelter-in-place," relocation, and/or evacuation. The use of an incident command structure within the NICU, facility, and community is

important to maintain structure and an organized response.

3. Neonatal care systems (providers, administration, information technology, and equipment) can develop appropriate staffing support for safe and effective operations during disasters. NICU care providers, in collaboration with their hospital facility, community practitioners, network, and region, need to identify the surge capacity to provide 3 times the baseline critical care resources and sustain this for 10 days during a major public health disaster. An effective response to specific disaster threats, including maintenance of adequate surge capacity, relies on sufficient supplies of age- and size-appropriate MCMs.

4. During a disaster, neonatal care providers can maintain situational awareness for decision-making, including patient volume and severity of illness, available equipment, medication, and staffing, transport, evacuation, recovery, and crisis standards of care. Maintaining flexibility is important in adjusting to new situations. Advance planning and coordination with local and state public health and emergency management agencies will additionally support situational awareness and timely decision-making. A process of ethical decision-making and altered standards of care needs to be included in disaster planning.

5. In addition to the needs of patients, NICU providers may need to consider the medical and psychosocial needs of postpartum mothers and families. To the extent it is feasible, parents and families should remain in contact with patients. Families may have unique needs and/or require assistance in unusual ways during a large-scale disaster. In addition, plans should be made to recognize and respond to the needs of NICU staff, including self-care and support.

6. Although some guidance in this report is based on systematic reviews (eg, H1N1 and mass critical care), much is based on lessons learned from previous disaster events. Preparedness is an ongoing process that changes on the basis of learned experience and evidence. NICU providers should continue to research best practices, neonatal medications and dosing, and the effects of altered standards of care in disasters.

AUTHORS

Wanda D. Barfield, MD, MPH, FAAP, RADM US Public Health Service
Steven E. Krug, MD, FAAP

COMMITTEE ON FETUS AND NEWBORN, 2016–2017

Kristi L. Watterberg, MD, FAAP, Chairperson
Susan W. Aucott, MD, FAAP
William E. Benitz MD, FAAP
Eric C. Eichenwald, MD, FAAP
Jay P. Goldsmith, MD, FAAP
Ivan L. Hand, MD, FAAP
Brenda B. Poindexter, MD, MS, FAAP
Karen M. Puopolo, MD, PhD, FAAP
Dan L. Stewart, MD, FAAP

LIAISONS

Wanda D. Barfield, MD, MPH, FAAP, RADM US Public Health Service – *Centers for Disease Control and Prevention*
Erin L. Keels, DNP, APRN, NNP-BC – *National Association of Neonatal Nurses*

Thierry Lacaze, MD – *Canadian Paediatric Society*
Maria A. Mascola, MD – *American College of Obstetricians and Gynecologists*
Tonse N.K. Raju, MD, DCH, FAAP – *National Institutes of Health*

STAFF

Jim Couto, MA

DISASTER PREPAREDNESS ADVISORY COUNCIL, 2016–2017

Steven E. Krug, MD, FAAP, Chairperson
Sarita A. Chung, MD, FAAP
Daniel B. Fagbuyi, MD, FAAP
Margaret C. Fisher, MD, FAAP
Scott M. Needle, MD, FAAP
David J. Schonfeld, MD, FAAP

LIAISONS

John James Alexander, MD, FAAP – *US Food and Drug Administration*
Daniel Dodgen, PhD – *Office of the Assistant Secretary for Preparedness and Response*
Eric J. Dziuban, MD, DTM, CPH, FAAP – *Centers for Disease Control and Prevention*
Andrew L. Garrett, MD, MPH, FAAP – *Office of the Assistant Secretary for Preparedness and Response*
Ingrid Hope, RN, MSN – *Department of Homeland Security Office of Health Affairs*
Georgina Peacock, MD, MPH, FAAP – *Centers for Disease Control and Prevention*
Erica Radden, MD – *US Food and Drug Administration*
David Alan Siegel, MD, FAAP – *National Institute of Child Health and Human Development*

STAFF

Laura Aird, MS
Tamar Magarik Haro

PEDIATRICS (ISSN Numbers: Print, 0031-4005; Online, 1098-4275).

FINANCIAL DISCLOSURE: The authors have indicated they have no financial relationships relevant to this article to disclose.

FUNDING: No external funding.

POTENTIAL CONFLICT OF INTEREST: The authors have indicated they have no potential conflicts of interest to disclose.

REFERENCES

1. Barfield WD, Krug SE, Kanter RK, et al. Emergency mass critical care in pediatrics: regionalized systems in neonatal and pediatric care. *Pediatr Crit Care Med.* 2011;12(suppl 6):S128–S134

2. International Federation of Red Cross and Red Crescent Societies. What is a disaster? Available at: www.ifrc.org/en/what-we-do/disaster-management/about-disasters/what-is-a-disaster/. Accessed September 24, 2016

3. Barkemeyer BM. Practicing neonatology in a blackout: the University Hospital NICU in the midst of Hurricane Katrina: caring for children without power or water. *Pediatrics.* 2006;117(5 pt 3):S369–S374

4. Ginsberg HG. Sweating it out in a level III regional NICU: disaster preparation and lessons learned at the Ochsner Foundation Hospital. *Pediatrics.* 2006;117(5 pt 3):S375–S380

5. Barkemeyer BM. NICU care in the aftermath of Hurricane Katrina: 5 years of changes. *Pediatrics.* 2011;128(suppl 1):S8–S11

6. Espiritu M, Patil U, Cruz H, et al. Evacuation of a neonatal intensive care unit in a disaster: lessons from Hurricane Sandy. *Pediatrics.* 2014;134(6). Available at: www.pediatrics.org/cgi/content/full/134/6/e1662

7. Powell T, Hanfling D, Gostin LO. Emergency preparedness and public health: the lessons of Hurricane Sandy. *JAMA.* 2012;308(24):2569–2570

8. Cohen E. N.Y. hospital staff carry sick babies down 9 flights of stairs during evacuation. CNN Health. October 30, 2012. Available at: www.cnn.com/2012/10/30/health/sandy-hospital. Accessed September 24, 2016

9. Jamieson DJ, Rasmussen SA, Uyeki TM, Weinbaum C. Pandemic influenza and pregnancy revisited: lessons learned from 2009 pandemic influenza A (H1N1). *Am J Obstet Gynecol.* 2011;204(6 suppl 1):S1–S3

10. Zapata L, Kendrick J, Jamieson D, MacFarlane K, Shealy K, Barfield WD. Review article: prevention of novel influenza infection in newborns: strategies based on the 2009 H1N1 pandemic. *Disaster Med Public Health Prep.* 2012;6(2):97–103

11. Callaghan WM, Creanga AA, Jamieson DJ. Pregnancy-related mortality resulting from influenza in the United States during the 2009-2010 pandemic. *Obstet Gynecol.* 2015;126(3):486–490

12. Schuler-Faccini L, Ribeiro EM, Feitosa IM, et al; Brazilian Medical Genetics Society–Zika Embryopathy Task Force. Possible association between Zika virus infection and microcephaly-Brazil, 2015. *MMWR Morb Mortal Wkly Rep.* 2016;65(3):59–62

13. Rasmussen SA, Jamieson DJ, Honein MA, Petersen LR. Zika virus and birth defects—reviewing the evidence for causality. *N Engl J Med.* 2016;374(20):1981–1987

14. Jamieson DJ, Uyeki TM, Callaghan WM, Meaney-Delman D, Rasmussen SA. What obstetrician-gynecologists should know about Ebola: a perspective from the Centers for Disease Control and Prevention. *Obstet Gynecol.* 2014;124(5):1005–1010

15. Mupapa K, Mukundu W, Bwaka MA, et al. Ebola hemorrhagic fever and pregnancy. *J Infect Dis.* 1999;179(suppl 1):S11–S12

16. Centers for Disease Control and Prevention. Guidance for screening and caring for pregnant women with Ebola virus disease for healthcare providers in U.S. hospitals. Available at: www.cdc.gov/vhf/ebola/healthcare-us/hospitals/pregnant-women.html. Accessed September 24, 2016

17. Nelson JM, Griese SE, Goodman AB, Peacock G. Live neonates born to mothers with Ebola virus disease: a review of the literature. *J Perinatol.* 2016;36(6):411–414

18. Centers for Disease Control and Prevention. Guidance on personal protective equipment (PPE) to be used by healthcare workers during management of patients with confirmed Ebola or persons under investigation (PUIs) for Ebola who are clinically unstable or have bleeding, vomiting, or diarrhea in U.S. Hospitals, including procedures for donning and doffing PPE. Available at: www.cdc.gov/vhf/ebola/healthcare-us/ppe/guidance.html. Accessed September 24, 2016

19. Centers for Disease Control and Prevention. Anthrax. Available at: www.cdc.gov/anthrax. Accessed September 24, 2016

20. Meaney-Delman D, Rasmussen SA, Beigi RH, et al. Prophylaxis and treatment of anthrax in pregnant women. *Obstet Gynecol.* 2013;122(4):885–900

21. Meaney-Delman D, Zotti ME, Creanga AA, et al; Workgroup on Anthrax in Pregnant and Postpartum Women. Special considerations for prophylaxis for and treatment of anthrax in pregnant and postpartum women. *Emerg Infect Dis.* 2014;20(2):e130611

22. Bradley JS, Peacock G, Krug SE, et al; AAP Committee on Infectious Diseases and Disaster Preparedness Advisory Council. Pediatric anthrax clinical management. *Pediatrics.* 2014;133(5). Available at: www.pediatrics.org/cgi/content/full/133/5/e1411

23. Inglesby TV, Dennis DT, Henderson DA, et al; Working Group on Civilian Biodefense. Plague as a biological weapon: medical and public health management. *JAMA.* 2000;283(17):2281–2290

24. Kurtoğlu S, Akin MA, Daar G, et al. Congenital hypothyroidism due to maternal radioactive iodine exposure during pregnancy. *J Clin Res Pediatr Endocrinol.* 2012;4(2):111–113

25. Devereaux AV, Dichter JR, Christian MD, et al; Task Force for Mass Critical Care. Definitive care for the critically ill during a disaster: a framework for allocation of scarce resources in mass critical care: from a Task Force for Mass Critical Care summit meeting, January 26-27, 2007, Chicago, IL. *Chest.* 2008;133(suppl 5):51S–66S

26. Kissoon N; Task Force for Pediatric Emergency Mass Critical Care. Deliberations and recommendations of the Pediatric Emergency Mass Critical Care Task Force: executive summary. *Pediatr Crit Care Med.* 2011;12(suppl 6):S103–S108

27. Kanter RK, Cooper A. Mass critical care: pediatric considerations in extending and rationing care in public

health emergencies. *Disaster Med Public Health Prep.* 2009;3(suppl 2):S166–S171

28. Institute of Medicine. *Guidelines for Establishing Crisis Standards of Care for Use in Disaster Situations: A Letter Report.* Washington, DC: The National Academies Press; 2009

29. Gardner AH, Krug SE. Pediatric emergency preparedness: are we ready? In: Graciano AL, Turner DA, eds. *Current Concepts in Pediatric Critical Care.* Mount Prospect, IL: Society of Critical Care Medicine; 2015:147–158

30. Courtney B, Hodge JG Jr; Task Force for Pediatric Emergency Mass Critical Care. Legal considerations during pediatric emergency mass critical care events. *Pediatr Crit Care Med.* 2011;12(suppl 6):S152–S156

31. McDonnell WM. EMTALA disaster rules and pandemic H1N1 influenza. *AAP News.* 2009;30(11):16–17

32. Niska RW, Shimizu IM. Hospital preparedness for emergency response: United States, 2008. *Natl Health Stat Rep.* 2011;37(37):1–14

33. Gausche-Hill M, Ely M, Schmuhl P, et al. A national assessment of pediatric readiness of emergency departments. *JAMA Pediatr.* 2015;169(6):527–534

34. US Department of Health and Human Services, Office of the Assistant Secretary for Preparedness and Response. Public health emergency: medical assistance. Available at: www.phe.gov/Preparedness/support/medicalassistance/Pages/default.aspx. Accessed September 21, 2016

35. Cohen R, Murphy B, Ahern T, Hackel A. Regional disaster planning for neonatology. *J Perinatol.* 2010;30(11):709–711

36. Daniels K, Oakeson AM, Hilton G. Steps toward a national disaster plan for obstetrics. *Obstet Gynecol.* 2014;124(1):154–158

37. Bohn D, Kanter RK, Burns J, Barfield WD, Kissoon N; Task Force for Pediatric Emergency Mass Critical Care. Supplies and equipment for pediatric emergency mass critical care. *Pediatr Crit Care Med.* 2011;12(suppl 6):S120–S127

38. Goodman DC, Fisher ES, Little GA, Stukel TA, Chang CH. Are neonatal intensive care resources located according to need? Regional variation in neonatologists, beds, and low birth weight newborns. *Pediatrics.* 2001;108(2):426–431

39. Tegtmeyer K, Conway EE Jr, Upperman JS, Kissoon N; Task Force for Pediatric Emergency Mass Critical Care. Education in a pediatric emergency mass critical care setting. *Pediatr Crit Care Med.* 2011;12(suppl 6):S135–S140

40. Phillips P, Niedergesaess Y, Powers R, Brandt R. Disaster preparedness: emergency planning in the NICU. *Neonatal Netw.* 2012;31(1):5–15

41. Mason KE, Urbansky H, Crocker L, Connor M, Anderson MR, Kissoon N; Task Force for Pediatric Emergency Mass Critical Care. Pediatric emergency mass critical care: focus on family-centered care. *Pediatr Crit Care Med.* 2011;12(suppl 6):S157–S162

42. Chung S, Shannon M. Reuniting children with their families during disasters: a proposed plan for greater success. *Am J Disaster Med.* 2007;2(3):113–117

43. American Academy of Pediatrics. Pediatric Preparedness Resource Kit. Elk Grove Village, IL: American Academy of Pediatrics; 2013. Available at: www.aap.org/en-us/advocacy-and-policy/aap-health-initiatives/Children-and-Disasters/Documents/PedPreparednessKit.pdf. Accessed October 4, 2016

44. Schonfeld DJ, Demaria T; Disaster Preparedness Advisory Council and Committee on Psychosocial Aspects of Child and Family Health. Providing psychosocial support to children and families in the aftermath of disasters and crises. *Pediatrics.* 2015;136(4). Available at: www.pediatrics.org/cgi/content/full/136/4/e1120

45. Disaster Preparedness Advisory Council; Committee on Pediatric Emergency Medicine. Ensuring the health of children in disasters. *Pediatrics.* 2015;136(5). Available at: www.pediatrics.org/cgi/content/full/136/5/e1407

46. Davies HD, Byington CL; Committee on Infectious Diseases. Parental

presence during treatment of Ebola or other highly consequential infection. *Pediatrics.* 2016;138(3):124–129

47. Centers for Disease Control and Prevention. Strategic national stockpile. Available at: www.cdc.gov/phpr/stockpile/stockpile.htm. Accessed April 22, 2016

48. Disaster Preparedness Advisory Council. Medical countermeasures for children in public health emergencies, disasters, or terrorism. *Pediatrics.* 2016;137(2):e20154273

49. US Food and Drug Administration. Emergency use authorization. Available at: www.fda.gov/EmergencyPreparedness/Counterterrorism/ucm182568.htm. Accessed September 20, 2016

50. Tsai CW, Morris S. Approval of raxibacumab for the treatment of inhalation anthrax under the US Food and Drug Administration "Animal Rule." *Front Microbiol.* 2015;6:1320

51. Nuffield Council on Bioethics. Critical care decisions in fetal and neonatal medicine: ethical issues. Available at: http://nuffieldbioethics.org/neonatal-medicine. Accessed September 20, 2016

52. Janvier A, Lantos J; POST Investigators. Ethics and etiquette in neonatal intensive care. *JAMA Pediatr.* 2014;168(9):857–858

53. Ytzhak A, Sagi R, Bader T, et al. Pediatric ventilation in a disaster: clinical and ethical decision making. *Crit Care Med.* 2012;40(2):603–607

54. Burkle FM Jr, Argent AC, Kissoon N; Task Force for Pediatric Emergency Mass Critical Care. The reality of pediatric emergency mass critical care in the developing world. *Pediatr Crit Care Med.* 2011;12(suppl 6):S169–S179

55. Jennings B, Arras JD. Ethical aspects of public health emergency preparedness and response. In: Jennings B, Arras JD, Barrett DH, Ellis BA, eds. *Emergency Ethics: Public Health Preparedness and Response.* New York, NY: Oxford University Press; 2016

56. Antommaria AHM, Powell T, Miller JE, Christian MD; Task Force for Pediatric

Emergency Mass Critical Care. Ethical issues in pediatric emergency mass critical care. *Pediatr Crit Care Med.* 2011;12(suppl 6):S163–S168

57. Bell EF; American Academy of Pediatrics Committee on Fetus and Newborn. Noninitiation or withdrawal of intensive care for high-risk newborns. *Pediatrics.* 2007;119(2):401–403

58. Madrid PA, Schacher SJ. A critical concern: pediatrician self-care after disasters. *Pediatrics.* 2006;117(5 pt 3):S454–S457

59. Markenson D, Reynolds S; American Academy of Pediatrics Committee on Pediatric Emergency Medicine; Task Force on Terrorism. The pediatrician and disaster preparedness. *Pediatrics.* 2006;117(2). Available at: www.pediatrics. org/cgi/content/full/117/2/e340

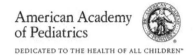

American Academy
of Pediatrics

DEDICATED TO THE HEALTH OF ALL CHILDREN™

Organizational Principles to Guide and Define the Child
Health Care System and/or Improve the Health of all Children

POLICY STATEMENT

Levels of Neonatal Care

COMMITTEE ON FETUS AND NEWBORN

KEY WORDS
neonatal intensive care, high-risk infant, regionalization, maternal and child health, health policy, very low birth weight infant, hospital newborn care services, nurseries

ABBREVIATIONS
AAP—American Academy of Pediatrics
aOR—adjusted odds ratio
CI—confidence interval
CON—certificate of need
ELBW—extremely low birth weight
TIOP—"Toward Improving the Outcome of Pregnancy"
VLBW—very low birth weight

www.pediatrics.org/cgi/doi/10.1542/peds.2012-1999

doi:10.1542/peds.2012-1999

PEDIATRICS (ISSN Numbers: Print, 0031-4005; Online, 1098-4275).

abstract

Provision of risk-appropriate care for newborn infants and mothers was first proposed in 1976. This updated policy statement provides a review of data supporting evidence for a tiered provision of care and reaffirms the need for uniform, nationally applicable definitions and consistent standards of service for public health to improve neonatal outcomes. Facilities that provide hospital care for newborn infants should be classified on the basis of functional capabilities, and these facilities should be organized within a regionalized system of perinatal care. *Pediatrics* 2012;130:1–11

OBJECTIVE

This revised policy statement reviews the current status of the designation of levels of newborn care definitions in the United States, which were delineated in a 2004 policy statement by the American Academy of Pediatrics (AAP).[1] Since publication of the 2004 policy statement, new data, both nationally and internationally, have reinforced the importance of well-defined regionalized systems of perinatal care, population-based assessment of outcomes, and appropriate epidemiologic methods to adjust for risk. This revised statement updates the designations to provide (1) a basis for comparison of health outcomes, resource use, and health care costs, (2) standardized nomenclature for public health, (3) uniform definitions for pediatricians and other health care professionals providing neonatal care, and (4) a foundation for consistent standards of service by institutions; state health departments; and state, regional, and national organizations focused on the improvement of perinatal care.

BACKGROUND

The availability of neonatal intensive care has improved the outcomes of high-risk infants born either preterm or with serious medical or surgical conditions.[2–4] Many of these improvements can be attributed to the concept and implementation of regionalized systems of perinatal care, broadly articulated in the 1976 March of Dimes report "Toward Improving the Outcome of Pregnancy" (TIOP I).[5] The TIOP I report included criteria that stratified maternal and neonatal care into 3 levels of complexity and recommended referral of high-risk patients to higher-level centers with the appropriate resources and personnel to address the required increased complexity of care. However, since the initial TIOP I report was published more than 3 decades ago, there have been signs of deregionalization, including (1) an increase in the number of NICUs and neonatologists, without a consistent relationship to the percentage of high-risk infants, (2) a proliferation of small NICUs in the same regions as large NICUs,[6–11] and (3) failure of states to reach the Healthy People 2010 goal that 90% of deliveries of very low birth weight (VLBW; <1500 g) infants occur at level III facilities.[12,13]

In the environment of deregionalization, preterm birth rates have increased 13% overall from 1990 to 2010 (10.6%–12.0%) as a result of a variety of factors, including increases in elective early cesarean deliveries, multiple births, advanced maternal age, and complications of pregnancy.[14–20] The majority of the increase in the preterm birth rate (>70%) is attributable to late preterm births.[21] Infants born late preterm can experience significant morbidity that may result in the need for specialized care and advanced neonatal services.[22,23] An increase in the supply of specialty staff[24,25] and availability of new neonatal therapies (eg, bubble continuous positive airway pressure), have expanded the scope of care in level II facilities.[26] Some have expressed concern that level II hospitals have expanded their scope of care without sufficient evidence of favorable outcome. Because most infant deaths in the United States occur among the most immature infants in the first few days after birth,[27,28] improvements in regionalized systems may reduce mortality among the most preterm newborn infants.

REVIEW OF THE LITERATURE ON NEONATAL LEVELS OF CARE SINCE THE 2004 AAP POLICY STATEMENT

In 2004, the AAP defined neonatal levels of care, including 3 distinct levels with subdivisions in 2 of the levels.[1] Level I centers provided basic care; level II

centers provided specialty care, with further subdivisions of IIA and IIB centers; and level III centers provided subspecialty care for critically ill newborn infants with subdivisions of level IIIA, IIIB, and IIIC facilities. Data published since the 2004 statement have informed the development of the levels of care in this new policy statement.

A meta-analysis of the published literature from 1978 to 2010 clearly demonstrates improved outcomes for VLBW infants and infants <32 weeks' gestational age born in level III centers. Lasswell et al reviewed 41 English-language US and international studies, which included >113 000 VLBW infants and found that VLBW infants born at non–level III hospitals had a 62% increase in odds of neonatal or predischarge mortality compared with those born at level III hospitals (adjusted odds ratio [aOR], 1.62; 95% confidence interval [CI], 1.44–1.83). Subset comparisons of studies identifying infants <32 weeks' gestation and extremely low birth weight (ELBW) infants (<1000 g) demonstrated similar effects (aOR, 1.55; 95% CI, 1.21–1.98; aOR, 1.64; 95% CI, 1.14–2.36, respectively). When only higher-quality studies were included, the findings were consistent (VLBW aOR, 1.60; 95% CI, 1.33–1.92; <32 weeks' gestation aOR, 1.42; 95% CI, 1.06–1.88; ELBW aOR, 1.80; 95% CI, 1.31–2.36). The effect of level of care on VLBW mortality did not vary by decade of publication[29]; hence, the risk of death for VLBW infants born in level I or II facilities remained higher than those born within a level III facility. Figures 1, 2, and 3 summarize the findings of these studies.

As Lasswell and colleagues found, part of the difficulty in collecting evidence to provide accurate assessments of VLBW outcomes has been in obtaining appropriate standardized measures. Heterogeneity among studies on

neonatal levels of care suggests the need for a quality standard for comparison which includes the following elements: (1) population-based studies within well-defined geographic regions, (2) clear definitions of the "intervention" or hospital level of care, and (3) appropriate adjustment for confounding factors to include maternal social and demographic risk factors, pregnancy and perinatal risks, and severity of illness at delivery.

Current Controversies in Levels of Care Designation

Although little debate exists on the need for advanced neonatal services for the most immature and surgically complex neonates, ongoing controversies exist regarding which facilities are qualified to provide these services and what is the most appropriate measure for such qualification. These issues are, in general, based on the need for comparison of facility experience (measured by patient volume or census), location (inborn/outborn deliveries, regional perinatal center, or children's hospital), or case mix (including stillbirths, delivery room deaths, and complex congenital anomalies).

Several studies have explored the topic of center experience as measured by volume or census of VLBW infants.[30–35] Phibbs et al conducted a population-based retrospective cohort study of 48 237 California VLBW infants to examine differences in neonatal mortality among NICUs with various levels of care and patient volumes. When compared with high-volume, high-level centers, the odds ratio of death was 1.19 (range, 1.04–1.37) for level IIIB, IIIC, or IIID centers with <100 annual admissions, 1.78 (range, 1.35–2.34) for level IIIA centers with 26 to 50 annual admissions, and 2.72 (range, 2.37–3.12) for level I centers with <10 annual admissions. The authors also found that the percentage of VLBW infants

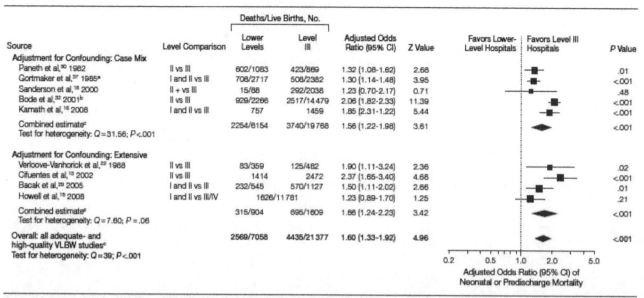

		Deaths/Live Births, No.							
Source	Level Comparison	Lower Levels	Level III	Adjusted Odds Ratio (95% CI)	Z Value	Favors Lower-Level Hospitals	Favors Level III Hospitals	P Value
Adjustment for Confounding: Case Mix								
Paneth et al,[30] 1982	II vs III	602/1083	423/869	1.32 (1.08-1.62)	2.68			.01
Gortmaker et al,[37] 1985[a]	I and II vs III	708/2717	508/2382	1.30 (1.14-1.48)	3.95			<.001
Sanderson et al,[16] 2000	II + vs III	15/88	292/2038	1.23 (0.70-2.17)	0.71			.48
Bode et al,[32] 2001[b]	II vs III	929/2266	2517/14 479	2.06 (1.82-2.33)	11.39			<.001
Kamath et al,[16] 2008	I and II vs III	757	1459	1.85 (2.31-1.22)	5.44			<.001
Combined estimate[c] Test for heterogeneity: Q=31.56; P<.001		2254/6154	3740/19 768	1.56 (1.22-1.98)	3.61			<.001
Adjustment for Confounding: Extensive								
Verloove-Vanhorick et al,[22] 1988	II vs III	83/359	125/482	1.90 (1.11-3.24)	2.36			.02
Cifuentes et al,[13] 2002	II vs III	1414	2472	2.37 (1.65-3.40)	4.68			<.001
Bacak et al,[29] 2005	I and II vs III	232/545	570/1127	1.50 (1.11-2.02)	2.66			.01
Howell et al,[15] 2008	I and II vs III/IV	1626/11 781		1.23 (0.89-1.70)	1.25			.21
Combined estimate[c] Test for heterogeneity: Q=7.60; P=.06		315/904	695/1609	1.66 (1.24-2.23)	3.42			<.001
Overall: all adequate- and high-quality VLBW studies[c] Test for heterogeneity: Q=39; P<.001		2569/7058	4435/21 377	1.60 (1.33-1.92)	4.96			<.001

Adjusted Odds Ratio (95% CI) of Neonatal or Predischarge Mortality
0.2   0.5   1.0   2.0   5.0

Case mix indicates adjustment for demographic and/or socioeconomic status variables; extensive indicates adjustment for case mix plus maternal/perinatal risk factors and infant illness severity. CI indicates confidence interval. Size of data markers indicates size of study population.
[a] Included data are for urban populations and combine reported black/white race strata and birth weight strata (750-1000 g and 1001-1500 g).
[b] Included data combine reported birth date interval strata (1980-1984, 1985-1989, and 1990-1994) and birth weight strata (500-1000 g and 1001-1500 g).
[c] Raw death counts are not reported in Cifuentes et al[13] and Kamath et al[16] and are not stratified by hospital level in Howell et al.[15] These studies are not included in combined death/birth counts.

FIGURE 1

Meta-analysis of adequate- and high-quality publications on VLBW infants, stratified by level of adjustment for confounding. (Reprinted with permission from Lasswell S, Barfield WD, Rochat R, Blackmon L. Perinatal regionalization for very low birth weight and very preterm infants: a meta-analysis. *JAMA.* 2010;304 [9]:992–1000.[29])

delivered in level IIIB, IIIC, or IIID centers decreased from 36% in 1991 to 22% in 2000 and estimated that shifting VLBW births in urban areas (92% of VLBW births) to level IIIC or IIID centers with >100 annual admissions would have prevented 21% of VLBW deaths in 2000.[30] In a secondary data analysis, Chung et al found that deregionalization of California perinatal services resulted in 20% of VLBW deliveries occurring in level I and level II hospitals, with lower-volume hospitals having the highest odds of mortality.[31]

A population-based study of 4379 VLBW infants who were born between 1991 and 1999 in Lower Saxony, Germany, evaluated neonatal mortality in relation to both the annual volume of births and NICU volume.[32] There was an increased odds ratio of mortality

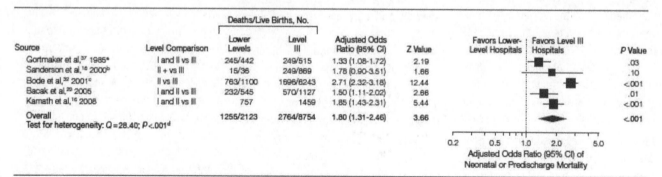

		Deaths/Live Births, No.							
Source	Level Comparison	Lower Levels	Level III	Adjusted Odds Ratio (95% CI)	Z Value	Favors Lower-Level Hospitals	Favors Level III Hospitals	P Value
Gortmaker et al,[37] 1985[a]	I and II vs III	245/442	249/515	1.33 (1.08-1.72)	2.19			.03
Sanderson et al,[16] 2000[b]	II + vs III	15/36	249/869	1.78 (0.90-3.51)	1.66			.10
Bode et al,[32] 2001[c]	II vs III	763/1100	1696/6243	2.71 (2.32-3.18)	12.44			<.001
Bacak et al,[29] 2005	I and II vs III	232/545	570/1127	1.50 (1.11-2.02)	2.66			.01
Kamath et al,[16] 2008	I and II vs III	757	1459	1.85 (1.43-2.31)	5.44			<.001
Overall Test for heterogeneity: Q=28.40; P<.001[d]		1255/2123	2764/8754	1.80 (1.31-2.46)	3.66			<.001

Adjusted Odds Ratio (95% CI) of Neonatal or Predischarge Mortality
0.2   0.5   1.0   2.0   5.0

CI indicates confidence interval. Size of data markers indicates size of study population.
[a] Included data are for urban populations and combine reported black/white race strata.
[b] Included data combine reported birth weight strata (500-749 g and 750-1000 g).
[c] Included data combine reported birth date interval strata (1980-1984, 1985-1989, and 1990-1994).
[d] The study by Kamath et al[16] does not report raw death count data and is not included in combined death/birth counts.

FIGURE 2

Meta-analysis of adequate- and high-quality publications on ELBW infants. (Reprinted with permission from Lasswell S, Barfield WD, Rochat R, Blackmon L. Perinatal regionalization for very low birth weight and very preterm infants: a meta-analysis. *JAMA.* 2010;304[9]:992–1000.[29])

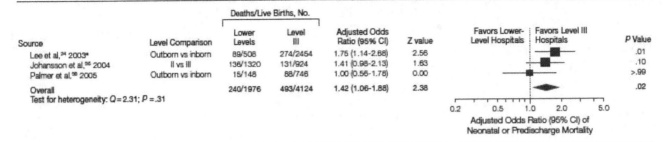

FIGURE 3

Meta-analysis of adequate- and high-quality publications on very preterm infants (<32 weeks' gestation). (Reprinted with permission from Lasswell S, Barfield WD, Rochat R, Blackmon L. Perinatal regionalization for very low birth weight and very preterm infants: a meta-analysis. *JAMA*. 2010;304[9]:992–1000.[29])

in centers with annual NICU admissions of fewer than 36 VLBW infants; the largest effect on mortality was for infants born at less than 29 weeks' gestation.

Other studies assessing NICU volume suggest caution in using this measure as an effective indicator of quality of care. Rogowski and colleagues assessed the potential usefulness of NICU volume as a quality indicator among 94 110 VLBW infants entered into the Vermont Oxford Network database between 1995 and 2000 and compared NICU volume with other indicators based on hospital characteristics and patient outcomes.[33] They found that although annual volume explained 9% of the variation in hospital mortality rates, other hospital characteristics explained another 7%. They suggested that direct measures based on patient outcomes are more useful quality indicators than volume for the purpose of selective referral.

Several studies assessed the effects of level of care, patient volume, and racial disparities on mortality of VLBW infants based on births in minority-serving hospitals. Morales[34] and Howell[35] evaluated mortality of VLBW infants born in minority-serving hospitals. In both studies, neonatal level of care and patient volume were

each independently associated with mortality, suggesting that delivery of all VLBW infants at high-volume hospitals would reduce black-white disparities in VLBW mortality rates. Rogowski and colleagues further suggest that the quality of care in poor-outcome hospitals could be improved through collaborative quality improvement, and evidence-based selective referral.[36]

Several studies have compared the short-term outcome of VLBW infants born in centers with level III units (inborn) compared with those born at lower level centers and soon transferred to a higher level (level III or children's hospital; outborn). Many of these studies are retrospective and may have selection bias because infants who were transferred most likely had the highest chance of survival and thus gave the impression of lower mortality.[24] In a secondary analysis of a randomized placebo-controlled study of preemptive morphine analgesia on neonatal outcomes, Palmer et al compared neonatal mortality as related to place of birth for 894 infants who were born at 23 to 32 weeks' gestation. Outborn babies were more likely to have severe intraventricular hemorrhage (P = .0005), and this increased risk persisted after controlling for severity

of illness. However, when adjusted for antenatal steroids, the effect of birth center was no longer significant.[37]

Evaluating and controlling for confounding variables and "case-mix" presents another set of challenges because these factors vary by population. For example, race and insurance status may have more of an effect on birth outcomes in the United States[34–36,38] than in countries with a more homogenous population and universal national health care.[39] There are also potential confounding factors for which measurement is frequently lacking, such as parental wishes regarding aggressive resuscitation of an infant. Arad et al noted that parental wishes varied by religious affiliation in their 2-hospital study. Because religious affiliation was unequally distributed between the 2 hospitals, fewer attempts at resuscitation may have been made at the level III hospital, with a result of improved survival at the level II facility.[40] More comprehensive studies controlling for confounding factors are needed.

Measured outcomes other than VLBW mortality (notably, fetal mortality, postdischarge mortality, and long-term physical and neurodevelopmental outcomes) may offer important information in assessing the evidence for newborn levels of care and perinatal regionalization. Studies measuring the effect of hospital level of birth on fetal and neonatal outcomes stratified by gestational age, as well as by birth weight, are also helpful, because gestational age is a better gauge of fetal maturity.[41–44] Although some studies include stillbirths and intrapartum fetal deaths, measurement and surveillance of fetal death varies widely.[3] Congenital anomalies are often excluded from studies of perinatal regionalization but should be considered in the provision of risk appropriate care.[45]

Additional studies are also needed to assess the effectiveness and potential cost savings of centralizing expensive technologies and provider expertise for relatively rare conditions at a few locations and to assess the effectiveness, including costs, of antenatal transport.

IMPORTANCE OF NEONATAL LEVELS OF CARE

Provision of Standardized Nomenclature for Public Health

Since 2004, efforts have been made to improve the comparison of health outcomes by hospital facility through the use of standardized nomenclature on the US birth certificate. The National Center for Health Statistics at the Centers for Disease Control and Prevention has worked with states to use the newly revised US Standard Certificate of Birth.[46] This 2003 revised certificate defines a NICU as a "hospital facility or unit staffed and equipped to provide continuous mechanical ventilatory support for a newborn infant." It also includes information on the use of antenatal therapies and postpartum surfactant, which may be useful in monitoring population-based utilization of technologies at birth.[47] In an analysis of 16 states using the revised certificate of birth, Barfield et al found that overall, 77.3% of VLBW infants were admitted to

NICUs; this estimate varied by state and ranged from 63.7% in California to 93.4% in North Dakota. Among VLBW infants of Hispanic mothers, 71.8% were admitted to NICUs, compared with 79.5% of VLBW infants of non-Hispanic black mothers and 80.5% of VLBW infants of non-Hispanic white mothers. In multivariable analysis, preterm delivery, multiple gestation, and cesarean delivery were associated with higher prevalence of NICU admission among VLBW infants.[13] State variations in the receipt of intensive care for VLBW infants may explain, in part, variation in VLBW outcomes across the country.

Use of Uniform Definitions of Levels of Care for Pediatricians and Other Health Care Professionals

Variation in definition, criteria, and state enforcement still occurs despite the TIOP I guidelines. Blackmon et al conducted an extensive review of all 50 states and the District of Columbia governmental Web sites to assess state definitions and levels terminology, functional and utilization criteria, regulatory compliance and funding measures, and citation of AAP documents on levels of neonatal care. The authors found that state definitions, criteria, compliance, and regulatory mechanisms for the specific type of care neonatal centers provide varied considerably, and they suggested a consistent national approach.[48] Lorch et al assessed all 50 states and the District of Columbia to identify state certificate of need (CON) legislation, a mechanism that regulates the expansion of NICU facilities and NICU beds. Thirty states regulated the construction of NICUs through CON programs, and non-CON program states were associated with more NICU facilities and more NICU beds (relative risk, 2.06; 95% CI, 1.74–2.45; and relative risk, 1.96; 95% CI, 1.89–2.03, respectively). In large metropolitan areas, non-CON states had higher infant mortality for all birth weight groups.[49]

The Maternal and Child Health Bureau has worked with state Title V agencies to document the percentage of VLBW infants delivered in high-risk facilities. In 2008, only 5 states met the goal of at least 90% of VLBW infants delivered at high-risk facilities, and some states reported less than 40% of VLBW infants being born at facilities with the highest level of care.[12] Recently, some states, in partnership with national organizations, have taken more definitive action in defining and regulating organization of perinatal care.[50]

Development of Consistent Standards of Service

Efforts by quality-improvement collaboratives, health services researchers, and public health officials will continue to improve the standards by which to measure quality of care.[51,52] Quality-improvement activities have begun to flourish at all levels to improve maternal and perinatal health and ideally prevent preterm births; this includes provider-level quality-improvement activities, hospital-level performance measures, and regional, state, and national performance measures.[53] Organizations such as the March of Dimes and others have promoted standard definitions of levels of care since the introduction of perinatal regionalization in the 1970s, reaffirmed its importance in 1993 (TIOP II),[54] and included the concept of quality care for the prevention of preterm birth with a new TIOP (TIOP III) in 2010.[53]

DEFINITIONS OF LEVELS OF NEONATAL CARE

The updated classification consists of basic care (level I), specialty care (level II), and subspecialty intensive care (level III, level IV; Table 1). These definitions reflect the overall evidence for risk-appropriate care through the availability of appropriate personnel, physical space, equipment, technology, and organization.[55] Each level reflects the minimal capabilities, functional criteria, and provider type required. Currently, there are 148 specialty care units and 809 subspecialty care units self-identified in the 2009 AAP perinatal section directory.

Level I

Level I units (well newborn nurseries) provide a basic level of care to neonates who are low risk. They have the capability to perform neonatal resuscitation at every delivery and to evaluate and provide routine postnatal care for healthy newborn infants. In addition, they can care for preterm infants at 35 to 37 weeks' gestation who are physiologically stable and can stabilize newborn infants who are less than 35 weeks of gestation or who are ill until they can be transferred to a facility at which specialty neonatal care is provided. Because late preterm infants (34–36 weeks' gestation) are at risk for increased neonatal morbidity and mortality, more evidence is needed to determine their outcomes by level of care.

Level II

Care in a specialty-level facility (level II) should be reserved for stable or moderately ill newborn infants who are born at ≥32 weeks' gestation or who weigh ≥1500 g at birth with problems that are expected to resolve rapidly and who would not be

TABLE 1 Definitions, Capabilities, and Provider Types: Neonatal Levels of Care

Level of Care	Capabilities	Provider Types[a]
Level I	• Provide neonatal resuscitation at every delivery	Pediatricians, family physicians, nurse practitioners, and other advanced practice registered nurses
Well newborn nursery	• Evaluate and provide postnatal care to stable term newborn infants • Stabilize and provide care for infants born 35–37 wk gestation who remain physiologically stable • Stabilize newborn infants who are ill and those born at <35 wk gestation until transfer to a higher level of care	
Level II Special care nursery	Level I capabilities plus: • Provide care for infants born ≥32 wk gestation and weighing ≥1500 g who have physiologic immaturity or who are moderately ill with problems that are expected to resolve rapidly and are not anticipated to need subspecialty services on an urgent basis • Provide care for infants convalescing after intensive care • Provide prompt and readily available access to a full range of pediatric medical subspecialists, pediatric surgical specialists, and pediatric anesthesiologists • Provide mechanical ventilation for brief duration (<24 h) or continuous positive airway pressure or both • Stabilize infants born before 32 wk gestation and weighing less than 1500 g until transfer to a neonatal intensive care facility	Pediatric hospitalists, neonatologist, and neonatal nurse practitioners.
Level III NICU	Level II capabilities plus: • Provide sustained life support • Provide comprehensive care for infants born <32 wk' gestation and weighing <1500 g and infants born at all gestational ages and birth weights with critical illness • Provide a full range of respiratory support that may include conventional and/or high-frequency ventilation and inhaled nitric oxide • Perform advanced imaging, with interpretation on an urgent basis, including computed tomography, MRI, and echocardiography	Pediatric medical subspecialists[b], pediatric anesthesiologists[b], and pediatric surgeons[b].
Level IV NICU	Level III capabilities plus: • Located within an institution with the capability to provide surgical repair of complex congenital or medical conditions • Maintain a full range of pediatric medical subspecialists, pediatric surgical subspecialists, and pediatric anesthesiologists on site • Facilitate transport and provide outreach education	Pediatric surgical subspecialists

[a] Includes all providers with relevant experience, training, and demonstrated competence.
[b] On site or at a closely related institution by prearranged consultative agreement.

anticipated to need subspecialty-level services on an urgent basis. These situations usually occur as a result of relatively uncomplicated preterm labor or preterm rupture of membranes. There is limited evidence to support the specific subdivision of level II care, in part because of the lack of studies with well-defined subdivisions. Level II facilities should take into consideration geographic constraints and population size when assessing the staffing resources needed to care appropriately for moderately ill newborn infants.

Level II nurseries may provide assisted ventilation on an interim basis until the infant's condition either soon improves or the infant can be transferred to a higher-level facility. Delivery of continuous positive airway pressure should be readily available by experienced personnel, and mechanical ventilation can be provided for a brief duration (less than 24 hours). Level II nurseries must have equipment (eg, portable chest radiograph, blood gas laboratory) and personnel (eg, physicians, specialized nurses, respiratory therapists, radiology technicians, laboratory technicians) continuously available to provide ongoing care as well as to address emergencies. Referral to a higher level of care should occur for all infants when needed for subspecialty surgical or medical intervention.

Level III

Evidence suggests that infants who are born at <32 weeks' gestation, weigh <1500 g at birth, or have complex medical or surgical conditions, regardless of gestational age, should be cared for at a level III facility. Designation of level III care should be based on clinical experience, as demonstrated by large patient volume, increasing complexity of care, and availability of pediatric medical subspecialists and

pediatric surgical specialists. Subspecialty care services should include expertise in neonatology and also ideally maternal-fetal medicine, if mothers are referred for the management of potential preterm birth. Level III NICUs are defined by having continuously available personnel (neonatologists, neonatal nurses, respiratory therapists) and equipment to provide life support for as long as necessary. Facilities should have advanced respiratory support and physiologic monitoring equipment, laboratory and imaging facilities, nutrition and pharmacy support with pediatric expertise, social services, and pastoral care.

Level III facilities should be able to provide ongoing assisted ventilation for periods longer than 24 hours, which may include conventional ventilation, high-frequency ventilation, and inhaled nitric oxide. Level III facility capabilities should also be based on a region's consideration of geographic constraints, population size, and personnel resources. If geographic constraints for land transportation exist, the level III facility should ensure availability of rotor and fixed-wing transport services to quickly and safely transfer infants requiring subspecialty intervention.[56] Potential transfer to higher-level facilities or children's hospitals, as well as back-transport of recovering infants to lower-level facilities, should be considered as clinically indicated.

A broad range of pediatric medical subspecialists and pediatric surgical specialists should be readily accessible on site or by prearranged consultative agreements. Prearranged consultative agreements can be performed by using telemedicine technology and/or telephone consultation, for example, from a distant location. Pediatric ophthalmology services and an organized program for the monitoring, treatment, and follow-up of retinopathy of prematurity

should be readily available in level III facilities.[57] Level III units should have the capability to perform major surgery (including anesthesiologists with pediatric expertise) on site or at a closely related institution, ideally in close geographic proximity. Because the outcomes of less complex surgical procedures in children, such as appendectomy or pyloromyotomy, are better when performed by pediatric surgeons compared with general surgeons, it is recommended that pediatric surgical specialists perform all procedures in newborn infants.[58]

Level III facilities should have the capability to perform advanced imaging with interpretation on an urgent basis, including CT, MRI, and echocardiography. Level III facilities should collect data to assess outcomes within their facility and to compare with other levels.

Level IV

Level IV units include the capabilities of level III with additional capabilities and considerable experience in the care of the most complex and critically ill newborn infants and should have pediatric medical and pediatric surgical specialty consultants continuously available 24 hours a day. Level IV facilities would also include the capability for surgical repair of complex conditions (eg, congenital cardiac malformations that require cardiopulmonary bypass with or without extracorporeal membrane oxygenation). More evidence is needed to assess the risk of morbidity and mortality by level of care for newborn infants with complex congenital cardiac malformations. A recent study by Burstein et al[59] was not able to note a difference in postoperative morbidity or mortality associated with dedicated pediatric cardiac ICUs versus NICUs and PICUs but did not separately assess the newborn and postneonatal periods. Although specific supporting data are not currently available, it is thought that concentrating the care of such infants at designated level IV centers will allow these centers to develop the expertise needed to achieve optimal outcomes.

Not all level IV hospitals need to act as regional centers; however, regional organization of perinatal health care services requires that there be coordination in the development of specialized services, professional continuing education to maintain competency, facilitation of opportunities for transport and back-transport,[60] and collection of data on long-term outcomes to evaluate both the effectiveness of delivery of perinatal health care services and the safety and efficacy of new therapies. These functions usually are best achieved when responsibility is concentrated in a single regional center with both perinatal and neonatal subspecialty services. In some cases, regional coordination may be provided adequately by the collaboration of a children's hospital with a subspecialty perinatal facility that is in close geographic proximity.[61]

STANDARDS OF SERVICE FOR HOSPITALS PROVIDING NEONATAL CARE

Current evidence indicates that family and cultural considerations are important for care of sick neonates.[62–65] These considerations include family- and patient-centered care, culturally effective care, family-based education, and opportunities for back-transport to level II facilities or transfer to the family's local community facility when medically and socially indicated.[64–67]

SUMMARY AND RECOMMENDATIONS

1. Regionalized systems of perinatal care are recommended to ensure that each newborn infant is delivered and cared for in a facility most appropriate for his or her health care needs, when possible, and to facilitate the achievement of optimal health outcomes.

   - Because VLBW and/or very preterm infants are at increased risk of predischarge mortality when born outside of a level III center, they should be delivered at a level III facility unless this is precluded by the mother's medical condition or there are geographic constraints.

2. The functional capabilities of facilities that provide inpatient care for newborn infants should be classified uniformly on the basis of geographic and population parameters in collaboration with state health departments, as follows:

   - Level I: a hospital nursery organized with the personnel and equipment to perform neonatal resuscitation, evaluate and provide postnatal care of healthy newborn infants, provide care for infants born at 35 to 37 weeks' gestation who remain physiologically stable, and stabilize ill newborn infants or infants born at less than 35 weeks' gestational age until transfer to a facility that can provide the appropriate level of neonatal care.
   - Level II: a hospital special care nursery organized with the personnel and equipment to provide care to infants born at 32 weeks' gestation or more and weighing 1500 g or more at birth who have physiologic immaturity, such as apnea of prematurity, inability to maintain body temperature, or inability to take oral feedings; who are moderately ill with problems that are expected to resolve rapidly and are not anticipated to need subspecialty services on an urgent basis; or who are convalescing from a higher level of intensive care. A level II center has the capability to provide continuous positive airway pressure and may provide mechanical ventilation for brief durations (less than 24 hours).

   - Level III: a hospital NICU organized with personnel and equipment to provide continuous life support and comprehensive care for extremely high-risk newborn infants and those with complex and critical illness. This includes infants born weighing <1500 g or at <32 weeks' gestation. Level III units have the capability to provide advanced medical and surgical care. Level III units routinely provide ongoing assisted ventilation; have ready access to a full range of pediatric medical subspecialists; have advanced imaging with interpretation on an urgent basis, including CT, MRI, and echocardiography; have access to pediatric ophthalmologic services with an organized program for the monitoring, treatment, and follow-up of retinopathy of prematurity; and have pediatric surgical specialists and pediatric anesthesiologists on site or at a closely related institution to perform major surgery. Level III units can facilitate transfer to higher-level facilities or children's hospitals, as well as back-transport recovering infants to lower-level facilities, as clinically indicated.
   - Level IV units have the capabilities of a level III NICU and are located within institutions that can provide on-site surgical repair of serious congenital malformations. Level IV units

can facilitate transport systems and provide outreach education within their catchment area.

3. The functional capabilities of facilities that provide inpatient care for newborn infants should be classified uniformly and with clear definitions that include requirements for equipment, personnel, facilities, ancillary services, training, and the organization of services (including transport) for the capabilities of each level of care.

4. Population-based data on patient outcomes, including mortality, morbidity, and long-term outcomes, should be obtained to provide level-specific standards for patients requiring various categories of specialized care, including surgery.

LEAD AUTHOR

CAPT Wanda Denise Barfield, MD, MPH

COMMITTEE ON FETUS AND NEWBORN, 2011–2012

Lu-Ann Papile, MD, Chairperson
Jill E. Baley, MD
William Benitz, MD
James Cummings, MD
Waldemar A. Carlo, MD
Praveen Kumar, MD
Richard A. Polin, MD

Rosemarie C. Tan, MD, PhD
Kristi L. Watterberg, MD

LIAISONS

CAPT Wanda Denise Barfield, MD, MPH – *Centers for Disease Control and Prevention*
George Macones, MD – *American College of Obstetricians and Gynecologists*
Ann L. Jefferies, MD – *Canadian Pediatric Society*
Rosalie O. Mainous, PhD, RNC, NNP – *National Association of Neonatal Nurses*
Tonse N. K. Raju, MD, DCH – *National Institutes of Health*
Kasper S. Wang, MD – *Section on Surgery*

STAFF

Jim Couto, MA

REFERENCES

1. Stark AR; American Academy of Pediatrics Committee on Fetus and Newborn. Levels of neonatal care. *Pediatrics*. 2004;114(5): 1341–1347

2. Bode MM, O'shea TM, Metzguer KR, Stiles AD. Perinatal regionalization and neonatal mortality in North Carolina, 1968–1994. *Am J Obstet Gynecol*. 2001;184(6):1302–1307

3. MacDorman MF, Kirmeyer S. Fetal and perinatal mortality, United States, 2005. *Natl Vital Stat Rep*. 2009;57(8):1–19

4. Clement MS. Perinatal care in Arizona 1950–2002: a study of the positive impact of technology, regionalization and the Arizona perinatal trust. *J Perinatol*. 2005;25 (8):503–508

5. March of Dimes, Committee on Perinatal Health. *Toward Improving the Outcome of Pregnancy: Recommendations for the Regional Development of Maternal and Perinatal Health Services*. White Plains, NY: March of Dimes National Foundation; 1976

6. Richardson DK, Reed K, Cutler JC, et al. Perinatal regionalization versus hospital competition: the Hartford example. *Pediatrics*. 1995;96(3 pt 1):417–423

7. Yeast JD, Poskin M, Stockbauer JW, Shaffer S. Changing patterns in regionalization of perinatal care and the impact on neonatal mortality. *Am J Obstet Gynecol*. 1998;178(1 pt 1):131–135

8. Goodman DC, Fisher ES, Little GA, Stukel TA, Chang CH. Are neonatal intensive care resources located according to need? Regional variation in neonatologists, beds, and low birth weight newborns. *Pediatrics*. 2001;108(2):426–431

9. Howell EM, Richardson D, Ginsburg P, Foot B. Deregionalization of neonatal intensive care in urban areas. *Am J Public Health*. 2002;92(1):119–124

10. Haberland CA, Phibbs CS, Baker LC. Effect of opening midlevel neonatal intensive care units on the location of low birth weight births in California. *Pediatrics*. 2006;118(6). Available at: www.pediatrics.org/cgi/content/full/118/6/e1667

11. Dobrez D, Gerber S, Budetti P. Trends in perinatal regionalization and the role of managed care. *Obstet Gynecol*. 2006;108(4): 839–845

12. US Department of Health and Human Services, Health Resources and Service Administration, Maternal and Child Health Bureau. National Performance Measure # 17. Available at: https://perfdata.hrsa.gov/mchb/TVISReports/. Accessed July 12, 2012

13. Centers for Disease Control and Prevention (CDC). Neonatal intensive-care unit admission of infants with very low birth weight—19 States, 2006. *MMWR Morb Mortal Wkly Rep*. 2010;59(44):1444–1447

14. Martin JA, Hamilton BE, Ventura SJ, et al. Births: final data for 2009. *Natl Vital Stat Rep*. 2011;60(1):1–70

15. Yoder BA, Gordon MC, Barth WH Jr. Late-preterm birth: does the changing obstetric paradigm alter the epidemiology of respiratory complications? *Obstet Gynecol*. 2008;111(4):814–822

16. Schieve LA, Ferre C, Peterson HB, Macaluso M, Reynolds MA, Wright VC. Perinatal outcome among singleton infants conceived through assisted reproductive technology in the United States. *Obstet Gynecol*. 2004; 103(6):1144–1153

17. Joseph KS, Marcoux S, Ohlsson A, et al; Fetal and Infant Heath Study Group of the Canadian Perinatal Surveillance System. Changes in stillbirth and infant mortality associated with increases in preterm birth among twins. *Pediatrics*. 2001;108(5):1055–1061

18. Kaaja RJ, Greer IA. Manifestations of chronic disease during pregnancy. *JAMA*. 2005;294(21):2751–2757

19. Shapiro-Mendoza CK, Tomashek KM, Kotelchuck M, et al. Effect of late-preterm birth and maternal medical conditions on newborn morbidity risk. *Pediatrics*. 2008;121 (2). Available at: www.pediatrics.org/cgi/content/full/121/2/e223

20. Yang Q, Greenland S, Flanders WD. Associations of maternal age- and parity-related factors with trends in low-birthweight rates: United States, 1980 through 2000. *Am J Public Health*. 2006;96(5):856–861

21. Davidoff MJ, Dias T, Damus K, et al. Changes in the gestational age distribution among U.S. singleton births: impact on rates of late preterm birth, 1992 to 2002. *Semin Perinatol*. 2006;30(1):8–15

22. Engle WA, Tomashek KM, Wallman C; Committee on Fetus and Newborn, American Academy of Pediatrics. "Late-preterm" infants: a population at risk. *Pediatrics*. 2007;120(6):1390–1401

23. Ramachandrappa A, Rosenberg ES, Wagoner S, Jain L. Morbidity and mortality in late preterm infants with severe hypoxic respiratory failure on extra-corporeal membrane oxygenation. *J Pediatr*. 2011;159(2):192–198, e3

24. Philip AG. The evolution of neonatology. *Pediatr Res.* 2005;58(4):799–815

25. Thompson LA, Goodman DC, Little GA. Is more neonatal intensive care always better? Insights from a cross-national comparison of reproductive care. *Pediatrics.* 2002;109(6):1036–1043

26. Gould JB, Marks AR, Chavez G. Expansion of community-based perinatal care in California. *J Perinatol.* 2002;22(8):630–640

27. Stoll BJ, Hansen NI, Bell EF, et al; Eunice Kennedy Shriver National Institute of Child Health and Human Development Neonatal Research Network. Neonatal outcomes of extremely preterm infants from the NICHD Neonatal Research Network. *Pediatrics.* 2010;126(3):443–456

28. Heron M, Sutton PD, Xu J, Ventura SJ, Strobino DM, Guyer B. Annual summary of vital statistics: 2007. *Pediatrics.* 2010;125(1):4–15

29. Lasswell SM, Barfield WD, Rochat RW, Blackmon L. Perinatal regionalization for very low-birth-weight and very preterm infants: a meta-analysis. *JAMA.* 2010;304(9):992–1000

30. Phibbs CS, Baker LC, Caughey AB, Danielsen B, Schmitt SK, Phibbs RH. Level and volume of neonatal intensive care and mortality in very-low-birth-weight infants. *N Engl J Med.* 2007;356(21):2165–2175

31. Chung JH, Phibbs CS, Boscardin WJ, Kominski GF, Ortega AN, Needleman J. The effect of neonatal intensive care level and hospital volume on mortality of very low birth weight infants. *Med Care.* 2010;48(7):635–644

32. Bartels DB, Wypij D, Wenzlaff P, Dammann O, Poets CF. Hospital volume and neonatal mortality among very low birth weight infants. *Pediatrics.* 2006;117(6):2206–2214

33. Rogowski JA, Horbar JD, Staiger DO, Kenny M, Carpenter J, Geppert J. Indirect vs direct hospital quality indicators for very low-birth-weight infants. *JAMA.* 2004;291(2):202–209

34. Morales LS, Staiger D, Horbar JD, et al. Mortality among very low-birthweight infants in hospitals serving minority populations. *Am J Public Health.* 2005;95(12):2206–2212

35. Howell EA, Hebert P, Chatterjee S, Kleinman LC, Chassin MR. Black/white differences in very low birth weight neonatal mortality rates among New York City hospitals. *Pediatrics.* 2008;121(3). Available at: www.pediatrics.org/cgi/content/full/121/3/e407

36. Rogowski JA, Staiger DO, Horbar JD. Variations in the quality of care for very-low-birthweight infants: implications for policy. *Health Aff (Millwood).* 2004;23(5):88–97

37. Palmer KG, Kronsberg SS, Barton BA, Hobbs CA, Hall RW, Anand KJ. Effect of inborn versus outborn delivery on clinical outcomes in ventilated preterm neonates: secondary results from the NEOPAIN trial. *J Perinatol.* 2005;25(4):270–275

38. Wall SN, Handler AS, Park CG. Hospital factors and nontransfer of small babies: a marker of deregionalized perinatal care? *J Perinatol.* 2004;24(6):351–359

39. Zeitlin J, Gwanfogbe CD, Delmas D, et al. Risk factors for not delivering in a level III unit before 32 weeks of gestation: results from a population-based study in Paris and surrounding districts in 2003. *Paediatr Perinat Epidemiol.* 2008;22(2):126–135

40. Arad I, Baras M, Bar-Oz B, Gofin R. Neonatal transport of very low birth weight infants in Jerusalem, revisited. *Isr Med Assoc J.* 2006;8(7):477–482

41. Institute of Medicine. *Preterm Birth: Causes, Consequences, and Prevention.* Washington, DC: National Academies Press; 2007

42. Rautava L, Lehtonen L, Peltola M, et al; PERFECT Preterm Infant Study Group. The effect of birth in secondary- or tertiary-level hospitals in Finland on mortality in very preterm infants: a birth-register study. *Pediatrics.* 2007;119(1). Available at: www.pediatrics.org/cgi/content/full/119/1/e257

43. Johansson S, Montgomery SM, Ekbom A, et al. Preterm delivery, level of care, and infant death in sweden: a population-based study. *Pediatrics.* 2004;113(5):1230–1235

44. Vieux R, Fresson J, Hascoet JM, et al; EPIPAGE Study Group. Improving perinatal regionalization by predicting neonatal intensive care requirements of preterm infants: an EPIPAGE-based cohort study. *Pediatrics.* 2006;118(1):84–90

45. Audibert F. Regionalization of perinatal care: did we forget congenital anomalies? *Ultrasound Obstet Gynecol.* 2007;29(3):247–248

46. Martin JA, Menacker F. Expanded health data from the new birth certificate, 2004. *Natl Vital Stat Rep.* 2007;55(12):1–22

47. Menacker F, Martin JA. Expanded health data from the new birth certificate, 2005. *Natl Vital Stat Rep.* 2008;56(13):1–24

48. Blackmon LR, Barfield WD, Stark AR. Hospital neonatal services in the United States: variation in definitions, criteria, and regulatory status, 2008. *J Perinatol.* 2009;29(12):788–794

49. Lorch SA, Maheshwari P, Even-Shoshan O. The impact of certificate of need programs on neonatal intensive care units. *J Perinatol.* 2012;32(1):39–44

50. Nowakowski L, Barfield WD, Kroelinger CD, et al. Assessment of state measures of risk-appropriate care for very low birth weight infants and recommendations for enhancing regionalized state systems. *Matern Child Health J.* 2012;16(1):217–227

51. Acolet D, Elbourne D, McIntosh N, et al; Confidential Enquiry Into Maternal and Child Health. Project 27/28: inquiry into quality of neonatal care and its effect on the survival of infants who were born at 27 and 28 weeks in England, Wales, and Northern Ireland. *Pediatrics.* 2005;116(6):1457–1465

52. Ohlinger J, Kantak A, Lavin JP Jr;et al. Evaluation and development of potentially better practices for perinatal and neonatal communication and collaboration. *Pediatrics.* 2006;118(suppl 2):S147–S152

53. March of Dimes. *Toward Improving the Outcome of Pregnancy III: Enhancing Perinatal Health Through Quality, Safety, and Performance Initiatives (TIOP3).* White Plains, NY: March of Dimes Foundation; 2010

54. Committee on Perinatal Health. *Toward Improving the Outcome of Pregnancy: The 90s and Beyond.* White Plains, NY: March of Dimes Foundation; 1993

55. American Academy of Pediatrics, American College of Obstetrics and Gynecology. *Guidelines for Perinatal Care.* 6th ed. Elk Grove Village, IL: American Academy of Pediatrics; 2007

56. American Academy of Pediatrics. *Section on Transport Medicine. Guidelines for Air and Ground Transport of Neonatal and Pediatric Patients.* 3rd ed. Elk Grove Village, IL: American Academy of Pediatrics; 2012

57. Fierson WM; Section on Ophthalmology American Academy of Pediatrics; American Academy of Ophthalmology; American Association for Pediatric Ophthalmology and Strabismus. Screening examination of premature infants for retinopathy of prematurity. *Pediatrics.* 2006;117(2):572–576

58. Kosloske A; American Academy of Pediatrics, Surgical Advisory Panel. Guidelines for referral to pediatric surgical specialists. *Pediatrics.* 2002;110(1 pt 1):187–191; *reaffirmed in* Pediatrics. 2007;119(5):1031

59. Burstein DS, Jacobs JP, Li JS, et al. Care models and associated outcomes in congenital heart surgery. *Pediatrics.* 2011;127(6). Available at: www.pediatrics.org/cgi/content/full/127/6/e1482

60. Attar MA, Lang SW, Gates MR, Iatrow AM, Bratton SL. Back transport of neonates:

effect on hospital length of stay. *J Perinatol.* 2005;25(11):731–736

61. Berry MA, Shah PS, Brouillette RT, Hellmann J. Predictors of mortality and length of stay for neonates admitted to children's hospital neonatal intensive care units. *J Perinatol.* 2008;28(4):297–302

62. American College of Obstetricians and Gynecologists. Cultural sensitivity and awareness in the delivery of health care. Committee Opinion No. 493. *Obstet Gynecol.* 2011;117(5):1258–1261

63. American College of Obstetricians and Gynecologists. Effective patient-physician communication. Committee Opinion No. 492. *Obstet Gynecol.* 2011;117(5):1254–1257

64. Tucker CM. *US Department of Health and Human Services Advisory Committee on Minority Health. Reducing Health Disparities by Promoting Patient-Centered Culturally and Linguistically Sensitive/Competent Health Care.* Rockville, MD: US Public Health Service; 2009

65. Britton CV; American Academy of Pediatrics Committee on Pediatric Workforce. Ensuring culturally effective pediatric care: implications for education and health policy. *Pediatrics.* 2004;114(6): 1677–1685

66. Eichner JM, Johnson BH; Committee on Hospital Care. American Academy of Pediatrics. Family-centered care and the pediatrician's role. *Pediatrics.* 2003;112(3 pt 1):691–697

67. Kattwinkel J, Cook LJ, Nowacek G, et al. Regionalized perinatal education. *Semin Neonatol.* 2004;9(2):155–165

INDEX

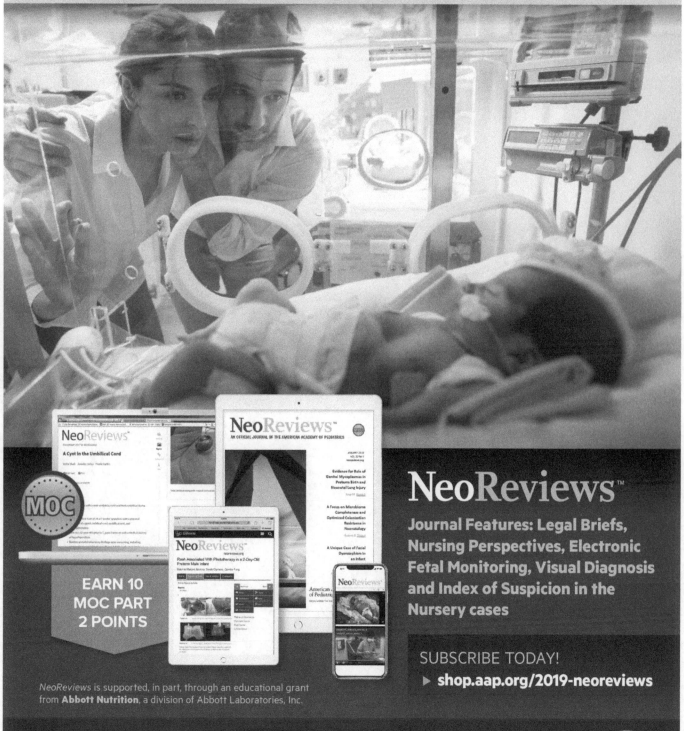
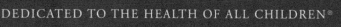